03/16/04

Laparoscopic Surgery of the Abdomen

Springer
New York
Berlin
Heidelberg
Hong Kong
London
Milan
Paris
Tokyo

Laparoscopic Surgery of the Abdomen

Bruce V. MacFadyen, Jr., MD

Professor, Department of Surgery, Chief, General Surgery, Director of Minimally Invasive Surgery, Medical College of Georgia, Augusta, Georgia

Maurice E. Arregui, MD

Director of Fellowship in Advanced Laparoscopy and Endoscopy and Ultrasound, St. Vincent's Hospital and Health Center, Indianapolis, Indiana

Steve Eubanks, MD

Associate Professor, Department of Surgery, Director of Surgical Endoscopy, Duke University Medical Center, Durham, North Carolina

Douglas O. Olsen, MD

Attending Surgeon, Centennial Medical Center, Nashville, Tennessee

Jeffrey H. Peters, MD

Professor, Department of Surgery, Chief, General Surgery, University of Southern California Keck School of Medicine, University of Southern California, Los Angeles, California

Nathaniel J. Soper, MD

Professor, Department of Surgery, Section of Hepatobiliary, Pancreatic, and Gastrointestinal Surgery, Washington University School of Medicine, St. Louis, Missouri

Lee L. Swanström, MD

Clinical Professor of Surgery, Oregon Health & Sciences University, Director, Department of Minimally Invasive Surgery, Legacy Health System, Portland, Oregon

Steven D. Wexner, MD

Chairman, Department of Colorectal Surgery, Chief of Staff, Cleveland Clinic Florida, Weston, Florida

Editors

With 252 Illustrations

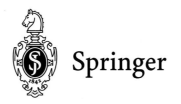

Springer

Bruce V. MacFadyen, Jr., MD
Professor
Department of Surgery
Chief, General Surgery
Director of Minimally Invasive Surgery
Medical College of Georgia
Augusta, GA 30912, USA

Maurice E. Arregui, MD
Director of Fellowship in Advanced
    Laparoscopy and Endoscopy and
    Ultrasound
St. Vincent's Hospital and Health Center
Indianapolis, IN 46260, USA

Steve Eubanks, MD
Associate Professor
Department of Surgery
Director of Surgical Endoscopy
Duke University Medical Center
Durham, NC 27710, USA

Douglas O. Olsen, MD
Attending Surgeon
Centennial Medical Center
Nashville, TN 37203, USA

Jeffrey H. Peters, MD
Professor, Department of Surgery
Chief, General Surgery
University of Southern California
Keck School of Medicine
University of Southern California
Los Angeles, CA 90033, USA

Nathaniel J. Soper, MD
Professor
Department of Surgery
Section of Hepatobiliary, Pancreatic, and
    Gastrointestinal Surgery
Washington University School of Medicine
St. Louis, MO 63110, USA

Lee L. Swanström, MD
Clinical Professor of Surgery,
Oregon Health & Sciences University
Director, Department of Minimally
Invasive Surgery
Legacy Health System
Portland, OR 97227, USA

Steven D. Wexner, MD
Chairman
Department of Colorectal Surgery
Chief of Staff
Cleveland Clinic Florida
Weston, FL 33331, USA

Library of Congress Cataloging-in-Publication Data

Laparoscopic surgery of the abdomen / editor, Bruce V. MacFadyen Jr. . . . [et al.].
        p. ; cm.
    Includes bibliographical references and index.
    ISBN 0-387-98468-2 (h/c : alk. paper)
        1. Digestive organs—Diseases.   2. Laparoscopy.   3. Gastrointestinal system—Diseases.
    I. MacFadyen, Bruce V., 1942–
        [DNLM: 1. Digestive System Diseases—surgery.   2. Laparoscopy—methods. WI 900
    L2998 2003]
    RC816.L37 2003
    617.4'3059—dc21
                                                                            2002029447

ISBN 0-387-98468-2   Printed on acid-free paper.

Printed in the United States of America.

9 8 7 6 5 4 3 2 1   SPIN 10664759

www.springer-ny.com

Springer-Verlag New York Berlin Heidelberg
A member of BertelsmannSpringer Science+Business Media GmbH

Preface

The use of laparoscopy to remove the gallbladder and appendix in the 1980s opened the door for the expanded application of this minimally invasive technique to be applied to abdominal operations that most surgeons have performed as an open procedure. Several textbooks have recorded the rapid development of these techniques in the 1990s. However, longer term data and experience has led to the development of new techniques, modifications of previous procedures, and changes in patient care. These changes resulted in the writing of this book, which addresses new patient management, as well as developments in abdominal and pelvic operations for the general surgeon. Positive and negative aspects of patient management, technique, and results are described. Because the field of laparoscopy continues to develop and expand, modification of this data will certainly be necessary. But, this book is the most up-to-date and comprehensive review in laparoscopic surgery of the abdomen now available.

Each section of the book is edited by an expert in the field who, along with the individual chapter authors, brings a wealth of experience to the book. All of the section editors and chapter authors are very busy clinical surgeons and integrate very well the theoretical and practical aspects of patient management, not only in the office but also in the operating room and in postoperative care. I want to particularly thank the section editors for their hard work and diligence in developing the large number and inclusiveness of each chapter. Without their help, this book would not have been possible.

This book is the "state of the art" in laparoscopic abdominal surgery, and I hope it will stimulate surgeons "to push the envelope" and advance the frontiers of this rapidly expanding field.

BRUCE V. MACFADYEN, JR., MD

Contents

SECTION I MINIMALLY INVASIVE SURGERY OF THE ESOPHAGUS AND STOMACH
Section Editor: Jeffrey H. Peters

Part I Esophageal Procedures

Part II Gastric Procedures

SECTION II   LAPAROSCOPIC CHOLECYSTECTOMY
Section Editor: Douglas O. Olsen

SECTION III   COMMON BILE DUCT
Section Editor: Lee L. Swanström

SECTION VII   DIAGNOSTIC LAPAROSCOPY AND ACUTE ABDOMEN
Section Editor: Steve Eubanks

Contributors

Peter I. Anderson, MD
Department of Emergency Medicine, Wilford Hall Medical Center, Lackland Air Force Base, TX 78236, USA.

Maurice E. Arregui, MD
St. Vincent's Hospital and Health Center, Indianapolis, IN 46260, USA.

Bruce Belin, MD
St. Joseph Office Park, Lexington, KY 40504, USA.

George Berci, MD
Department of Surgery, Cedars-Sinai Medical Center, Los Angeles, CA 90048, USA.

Sigurdur Blondal, MD
Department of Surgery, Landspitali-University Hospital, IS-101 Reykjavik, Iceland.

Luigi Bonavina, MD
Division of General Surgery, University of Milan, Istituto Policlinico San Donato, Milan, Italy.

L. Michael Brunt, MD
Department of Surgery, Washington University School of Medicine, St. Louis, MO 63110, USA.

Jo Buyske, MD
Department of Surgery, Presbyterian Medical Center, University of Pennsylvania Health System, Philadelphia, PA 19104, USA.

Margherita O. Cadeddu, MD
Department of Surgery, Hamilton General Hospital, Hamilton, Ontario, L8L 5G4, Canada.

W. Keat Cheah, MBBS
Department of Surgery, The National University Hospital, Singapore 119074.

Edward G. Chekan, MD
University of Virginia, Sewickley Valley Hospital, Sewickley, PA 15143. USA.

Roland N. Chen, MD
Carson City, NV 89703, USA.

Jonathan A. Cohen, MD
Nashville Surgical Associates, St. Thomas Medical Center, Nashville, TN 37205, USA.

Monty H. Cox, MD
Department of General Surgery, Medical University of South Carolina, Charleston, SC 29425, USA.

John R. Craig, MD
Department of Surgery, Deaconess Hospital, Billings MT, 59107, USA

David L. Crawford, MD
Department of Surgery, University of Illinois at Chicago, College of Medicine at Peoria, Peoria, IL 61603, USA.

Ara Darzi, MD
Department of Surgical Oncology and Technology, Imperial College School of Medicine, St. Mary's Hospital, Pattington, London W2 1NY, UK.

Jose Antonio Diaz-Elizondo, MD
Department of General Surgery, Instituto Tecnológico y de Estudios Superiores de Monterrey, Department Hospital San José—Tec de Monterrey, Monterrey, México, C.P. 64718.

Urs Diener, MD
Department of Gastrointestinal Surgery, University of California, San Francisco, San Francisco, CA 94143, USA.

Karen Draper-Stepanovich, MD
Department of Surgery, Lexington Clinical, Vanderbilt University Medical Center, Lexington, KY 40504, USA.

Jonathan E. Efron, MD
Department of Colorectal Surgery, Cleveland Clinic Florida, Naples, FL 34119, USA.

Steve Eubanks, MD
Department of Surgery, Duke University Medical Center, Durham, NC 27710, USA.

Edward L. Felix, MD
Department of Surgery, University of California, San Francisco, Fresno, CA 93710, USA.

Linda Fetko, MD
Department of Obstetrics and Gynecology, Duke University Medical Center, Durham, NC 27704, USA.

Charles J. Filipi, MD
Department of Surgery, Creighton University School of Medicine, Omaha, NE 68131, USA.

Aaron S. Fink, MD
Department of Surgery, Emory University School of Medicine, Atlanta Veterans Administration Medical Center, Decatur, GA 30033, USA.

Robert J. Fitzgibbons, MD
Department of Surgery, Division of General Surgery, Creighton University School of Medicine, Omaha, NE 68131, USA.

Morris E. Franklin, Jr., MD
Department of Surgery, University of Texas at San Antonio, San Antonio, TX 78222, USA.

James J. Gangemi, MD
Department of Surgery, University of Virginia Health System, Charlottesville, VA 22908, USA.

Luca Giordano, MD
Department of Minimally Invasive Surgery, Cedars-Sinai Medical Center, Los Angeles, CA 90048, USA.

Peter M.Y. Goh, MD
Universität zu Köln, II Lehrstuhl für Chirurgie, Klinikum Chirurgie—Köln-Merheim, Germany.

Mark K. Grove, MD
Department of General and Vascular Surgery, Cleveland Clinic Florida, Weston, FL 33331, USA.

Jeffrey A. Hagen, MD
Department of Surgery, Division of Thoracic and Foregut Surgery, University of Southern California Keck School of Medicine, Los Angeles, CA 90033-4612, USA.

Matthew F. Hansman, MD
Department of General Surgery, Virginia Mason Medical Center, Seattle, WA 98101, USA.

Kristín H. Haraldsdóttir, MD
Department of Surgery, Lunds University Hospital, Lund, Sweden.

John E. Hartley, MD
Department of Surgery, University of Hull, Academic Surgical Unit, Castle Hill Hospital, Cottingham, East Yorkshire, HU16 5JQ, UK.

Michael D. Hellinger, MD
Sylvester Comprehensive Cancer Center, Division of Colorectal Surgery, University of Miami, Miami, FL 33136, USA.

Daniel M. Herron, MD
Department of Surgery, Division of Laparoscopic Surgery, Mount Sinai School of Medicine, New York, NY 10029, USA.

Yik-Hong Ho, MBBS
Department of Surgery, James Cook University / The Townsville Hospital, Mater Misericordiae, Wesley Park Haven and Cairns Base Hospitals, Queensland 4810, Australia.

George W. Holcomb III, MD
Department of Surgery, Children's Mercy Hospital, Kansas City, MO 64108, USA.

Michael D. Holzman, MD, MPH
Department of Surgery, Vanderbilt University School of Medicine, St. Thomas Hospital, Nashville, TN 37232, USA.

Emina Huang, MD
Department of Surgery, Columbia Presbyterian Hospital, New York, NY 10032, USA.

Haruhiro Inoue, MD
First Department of Surgery, Tokyo Medical and Dental University, Tokyo, Japan.

Namir Katkhouda, MD
Department of Surgery, University of Southern California Keck School of Medicine, Los Angeles, CA 90033, USA.

Leena Khaitan, MD
Department of Surgery, Emory University School of Medicine, Atlanta, GA 30322, USA.

Sergio W. Larach, MD
Department of Surgery, University of Florida College of Medicine, Orlando, FL 32806, USA.

Demetrius Litwin, MD
Department of Surgery, University of Massachusetts School of Medicine, Worcester, MA 01655, USA.

Anthony Macaluso, Jr., MD
Texas Colon and Rectal Surgeons, Medical City Hospital, Dallas, TX 75230, USA.

Bruce V. MacFadyen, Jr., MD
Department of Surgery, Medical College of Georgia, Augusta, GA 30912, USA.

Joseph Mamazza, MD
Department of Surgery, University of Toronto, St. Michael's Hospital, Toronto, Ontario M5B 1W8, Canada.

Sharan Manhas, MD
Department of Surgery, University of Southern California Keck School of Medicine, Los Angeles, CA 90033, USA.

Peter W. Marcello, MD
Department of Surgery, Tufts University School of Medicine, Lahey Clinic, Burlington, MA 01805-0001, USA.

David W. McFadden, MD
Department of Surgery, West Virginia University, Morgantown, WV 26506-9238, USA.

Ross L. McMahon, MD
Department of Surgery, Duke University Medical Center, Durham, NC 27710, USA.

Brian J. Mehigan, MB
Department of Academic Surgery, Trinity College, Dublin 24, Ireland.

Juliane A. Miranda-Rassi, MD
Department of Gastroenterology, Division of Endoscopy, School of Medicine Universidade Federal de Goiás.; Department of Anorectal Physiology, CDI, Goiânia, Goiânia GO, 74140-020, Brazil.

J.R.T. Monson, MD
Department of Surgery, University of Hull, Academic Surgical Unit, Castle Hill Hospital, Cottingham, East Yorkshire, HU16 5JQ, UK.

Surendra Narne, MD
Division of ENT Endoscopic Surgery, Azienda Ospedaliera, Padova, 35100 Padova, Italy.

Juan J. Nogueras, MD
Department of Colorectal Surgery, Cleveland Clinic Florida, Weston, FL 33331, USA.

Lloyd M. Nyhus, MD
Department of Surgery, The Living Institute for Surgical Studies, College of Medicine, University of Illinois, Chicago, IL 60612-7322, USA.

Margret Oddsdottir, MD
Department of Surgery, Landspitali-University Hospital, IS-101 Reykjavik, Iceland.

Lucia Oliveira, MD
Department of Anorectal Physiology, Policlínica Geral do Rio de Janeiro, Titular Member Brazilian Society of Coloproctology, Titular Member Brazilian College of Surgeons, Lagoa, Rio de Janeiro, 22470-200, Brazil.

Douglas O. Olsen, MD
Centennial Medical Center, Nashville, TN 37203, USA.

Bruce A. Orkin, MD
Department of Surgery, George Washington University Medical Center, Washington, DC 20037, USA.

Marco G. Patti, MD
Department of Surgery, University of California, San Francisco, San Francisco, CA 94143, USA.

Carlos A. Pellegrini, MD
Department of Surgery, University of Washington School of Medicine, Seattle, WA 98195, USA.

Alberto Peracchia, MD
Department of Surgical Sciences, University of Milano, 20122 Milano, Italy.

Jeffrey H. Peters, MD
Department of Surgery, University of Southern California Keck School of Medicine, University of Southern California, Los Angeles, CA 90033, USA.

Johann Pfeifer, MD
Department of Surgery, Karl-Franzens University School of Medicine, A-8010 Graz, Austria.

Edward H. Phillips, MD
Department of Surgery, Center for Minimally Invasive Surgery, Cedars-Sinai Medical Center, Los Angeles, CA 90048, USA.

Alon J. Pikarsky, MD
Department of General Surgery, Hadassah Medical Center, Hadassah University Hospital, Jerusalem 91120, Israel.

Eric C. Poulin, MD
Department of Surgery, University of Toronto, St. Michael's Hospital, Toronto, Ontario M5B 1W8, Canada.

Aurora D. Pryor, MD
Department of Surgery, Duke University Medical Center, Durham, NC 27710, USA.

Thomas H. Quinn, PhD
Department of Biomedical Sciences, Creighton University School of Medicine, Omaha, NE 68178-0405, USA.

Petachia Reissman, MD
Department of Surgery, Shaare-Zedek University Medical Center, Jerusalem 91031, Israel.

William O. Richards, MD
Department of Surgery, Vanderbilt University School of Medicine, Nashville, TN 37232, USA.

Yoshihisa Saida, MD
The Third Department of Surgery, School of Medicine, Toho University, Tokyo 153-8515, Japan.

Mara R. Salum, MD
Anorectal Physiology Lab, Hospital Sírio-Libanês; Universidade Federal de São Paulo, Escola Paulista de Medicina; Hospital Sírio-Libanês, São Paulo 01433-010, Brazil.

Laurence R. Sands, MD
Department of Surgery, University of Miami School of Medicine, Miami, FL 33136, USA.

T. Cristina Sardinha, MD
Department of Surgery, Long Island Jewish Medical Center, New Hyde Park, NY 11042, USA.

Christopher M. Schlachta, MD
Department of Surgery, University of Toronto, St. Michael's Hospital, Toronto, Ontario M5B 1W8, Canada.

Mary E. Schultheis, MD
Department of Surgery, St. Agnes Hospital, Baltimore, MD 21229, USA.

Anthony J. Senagore, MD, MS
Department of Colorectal Surgery, Cleveland Clinic Foundation, Cleveland, OH 44195, USA.

Francis Seow-Choen, MBBS
Department of Colorectal Surgery, Singapore General Hospital, Nanyang Technological University, 169608, Singapore.

Pieter A. Seshadri, MD
Department of Surgery, University of Saskatchewan, Saskatoon, SK S7N 4R5, Canada.

Mark E. Sesto, MD
Department of General and Vascular Surgery, Cleveland Clinic Florida, Weston, FL 33331, USA.

Kenneth W. Sharp, MD
Department of Surgery, Vanderbilt University School of Medicine, Nashville, TN 37232, USA.

Marc E. Sher, MD
Department of Surgery, Long Island Jewish Medical Center, New Hyde Park, NY 11042, USA.

Jay J. Singh, MD
Piedmont Colorectal Associates, Atlanta, GA 30309, USA.

Nathaniel J. Soper, MD
Department of Surgery, Section of Hepatobiliary, Pancreatic, and Gastrointestinal Surgery, Washington University School of Medicine, St. Louis, MO 63110, USA.

Jonathan D. Spitz, MD
Department of Surgery, DuPage Medical Group, Glen Ellyn, IL 60137, USA.

Hubert J. Stein, MD, PhD
Chirurgische Klinik und Poliklinik, Klinikum rechts der Isar, Technische Universität München, D-81677 Munich, Germany.

Lee L. Swanström, MD
Department of Surgery, Oregon Health & Sciences University, Department of Minimally Invasive Surgery, Legacy Health System, Portland, OR 97227, USA.

Joerg Theisen, MD
Department of Surgery, Klinikum rechts der Isar, Munich, Germany.

Jared Torkington, MB, MS
Department of Colorectal Surgery, Cardiff and Vale NHS Trust, Cardiff, UK.

Shirin Towfigh, MD
Department of Surgery, University of Southern California Keck School of Medicine, Los Angeles, CA 90033, USA.

Frederick K. Toy, MD
Northeastern Surgical Consultants, P.C., Honesdale, PA 18431, USA.

L. William Traverso, MD
Section of General, Thoracic, and Vascular Surgery, Virginia Mason Medical Center, Seattle, WA 98101, USA.

Thadeus L. Trus, MD
Department of General Surgery, Dartmouth-Hitchcock Medical Center, Lebanon, NH 03756, USA.

Douglas S. Tyler, MD
Department of Surgery, Duke University School of Medicine, Durham, NC 27710, USA.

Selman Uranüs, MD
Department of General Surgery, Karl-Franzens University School of Medicine, A-8010 Graz, Austria.

Guy R. Voeller, MD
Department of Surgery, University of Tennessee, Memphis, TN 38120, USA.

Luca A. Vricella, MD
Department of Surgery, George Washington University Medical Center, Washington, DC 20037, USA.

Eric G. Weiss, MD
Department of Colorectal Surgery, Cleveland Clinic Florida, Weston, FL 33331, USA.

Carl Westcott, MD
Department of General Surgery, Wake Forest University School of Medicine, Winston-Salem, NC 27157, USA.

Steven D. Wexner, MD
Department of Colorectal Surgery, Cleveland Clinic Florida, Weston, FL 33331, USA.

R. Larry Whelan, MD
Division of Surgical Specialties, Columbia Presbyterian Hospital, New York, NY 10032, USA.

Rebekah R. White, MD
Department of Surgery, Duke University Medical Center, Durham, NC 27710, USA.

Eric D. Whitman, MD
Suburban Surgical Associates, St. Louis, MO 63131, USA.

Paul E. Wise, MD
Department of Surgery, Vanderbilt University Medical Center, Nashville, TN 37232, USA.

Renee S. Wolfe, MD
Department of Surgery, St. Elizabeth Medical Center, Boston, MA 02135, USA.

Steven M. Yood, MD, MPH
Department of Surgery, Yale University School of Medicine, New Haven, CT 06511, USA.

Karl A. Zucker, MD (deceased)
Formerly University of Arizona School of Medicine, Phoenix, AZ 85004, USA.

Section I
Minimally Invasive Surgery of the Esophagus and Stomach

Jeffrey H. Peters, MD
Section Editor

Part I
Esophageal Procedures

1
Endoscopic Mucosal Resection in the Esophagus

Haruhiro Inoue

Backgound and Historical Development

Endoscopic mucosal resection (EMR) is at present the only endoscopic treatment that provides a complete specimen for histopathological analysis. In general, a patient with mucosal cancer with no risk of lymph node metastasis is the best candidate for this procedure. The author developed the EMRC procedure (EMR using a transparent plastic cap) in 1992. Utilizing this technique, any part of the esophageal mucosa from the pharynx to the gastroesophageal junction, excluding the postlaryngeal mucosa, can be easily accessed and safely resected. This chapter describes the indications and technical details of the procedure, our clinical results, and the prevention of complications.

In clinical practice, most esophageal cancers are detected in an advanced stage with complaints of tumor-related symptoms such as chronic pain, gastrointestinal obstruction, and bleeding. The prognosis for advanced esophageal cancer is still poor, even when major surgery with wide-area lymph node dissection is carried out in combination with multidisciplinary treatments. To improve the prognosis for esophageal cancer, we must be able to detect the cancer as an early-stage, mucosal lesion before lymph node metastasis.[1]

Preoperative Investigations

Detection of Early-Stage Esophageal Cancer (Squamous Cell Carcinoma)

When observed by endoscopy, normal esophageal mucosa usually appears as a smooth, flat, and whitish lustrous surface. Early-stage esophageal cancer is characterized by changes of color and lusterless and rough surfaces with marginal stepup or stepdown in mucosal architecture. However, detection of a minute or early-stage lesion is extremely difficult because these characteristics are not visible. Actually, in IIb-type lesions, no changes can be seen even with meticulous observation using videoendoscopy. Fortunately, the iodine dye staining method is a very useful diagnostic technique for the esophagus. Normal esophageal epithelium, which contains glycogen-rich granules, stains dark brown when sprayed with 2% potassium iodide solution. In contrast, a cancerous lesion, which has lost glycogen granules in the epithelial cell layer, is clearly distinguished as an unstained area with a clear margin to the iodine-stained normal mucosa. This test is highly specific and sensitive for squamous cell carcinoma.[2] Endoscopic pinch biopsy is essential for histological confirmation of the disease.

Indications for Mucosal Resection

The infiltration depth should be no more than m1 or m2, and superficial spread should be less than half the circumference of the lesion. According to data from the Japanese national survey for histological evaluation of surgically resected esophageal cancer specimens,[3] only 4% of mucosal cancer cases that were limited to the mucosal layer had lymph node involvement. In contrast, 35% of cases of submucosally invading cancer had lymph node metastasis.

Mucosal cancer without lymph node involvement is considered to be an appropriate candidate for mucosal resection intending to achieve permanent cure of the disease. Among mucosal cancers, we have seen two lymph node-positive cases; these were massively invaded mucosal lesions in which the cancer contacted the muscularis mucosae over a wide area and superficial spread of the lesion was more than half its circumference. We restrict the indication to lesions no deeper than m2 that have spread less than half their circumference.

Even submucosal cancer, if it is lifted by submucosal saline injection, can be technically resected by this procedure. Submucosal cancer is then a candidate for mucosal resection if the patient has refused surgery or is a poor surgical risk.

Treatment of Barrett's Esophagus

EMR appears promising in the treatment of Barrett's mucosa. So far, few studies that discuss it directly have appeared in the literature. The first application of EMR for adenocarcinoma on short-segment Barrett's esophagus was reported in 1990 by the author.[4] Histopathological analysis of the endoscopically resected specimen showed that esophageal glands in the submucosa were totally resected. Therefore, this procedure is theoretically appropriate for eradication of Barrett's esophagus. In our experience of EMR for squamous cell carcinoma, however, totally circumferential mucosal resection often causes severe stenosis. Therefore, the division of the EMR session into a few sessions seems to be preferable. In the future, the author considers that major part resection of Barrett's mucosa by EMR will be preferred to obtain a histological specimen to analyze for cancer differentiation, infiltration depth, and vessel involvement. For residual parts, repeated EMR or other ablative therapy should be applied to completely eradicate Barrett's mucosa.

Endoscopic Mucosal Resection for Early-Stage Cancer in the Esophagus

Various local treatments such as laser ablation, argon plasma coagulator, and irradiation have been applied to treat mucosal cancer, but EMR is the only procedure that provides a complete resected specimen for histopathological analysis. We originally developed the EMRC procedure as a technique of mucosal resection. We believe it to be the simplest and safest technique to perform mucosectomy in any part of the gastrointestinal tract.

Principles

The gastrointestinal (GI) tract consists of two layers: the mucosal layer and the muscle layer. Embryologically, the mucosa is derived from the endodermal cell layer and the muscle layer from the middle germ layer of viviparity. The mucosal and the muscle layers are attached each other by loose connective tissue in the submucosa and can be separated by external force. For this reason, we can safely resect just mucosa from inside the cavity, leaving the muscle layer intact.

However, the gastrointestinal wall is less than 4 mm thick, so that special care to avoid perforation is extremely important during the procedure. Injection of saline solution into the submucosal layer is a simple and

effective technique to avoid muscle involvement. Lifting of the mucosa is always exhibited during submucosal saline injection in any part of the GI tract, without exception. After injection of a sufficient volume of saline, the mucosa, including the target lesion, can be safely captured in the cap, strangulated by a snare wire, and resected by electrocauterization.

History

In 1955, in the era of the rigid scope, Rosenberg[5] reported the importance of submucosal saline injection during polypectomy of rectal and sigmoidal polyps. Mucosal resection for superficial cancer using the fiberscope was first performed for early gastric cancer around 1983 in Japan. The original "strip-off biopsy" technique advocated by Tada et al.[6] was "injection and snaring" (Table 1.1). Submucosal saline injection was used to create a bleb; then, this bleb was cut by snare strangulation. This procedure had already been reported by Dehle et al. in 1973[7] as a technique for sessile colonic polyp resection. Another EMR technique recommended by Takekoshi et al.[8] was "grasping and snaring" (see Table 1.1), that is, retracting the mucosa by a grasper and then strangulating it by snare wire. Martin et al. in 1976[9] had also reported this technique. Now, these two procedures are combined and integrated as "strip biopsy," that is, submucosal saline injection to create a bleb, mucosal retraction by grasper, and capture of the mucosal lesion by a snare loop. Hirao et al.[10] reported an "injection, precutting, and snaring" technique, which means that after submucosal injection the target mucosa was cut by an electrocautery needle knife and the isolated mucosa was then captured by snare wire (see Table 1.1).

TABLE 1.1. Classification of endoscopic mucosal resection (EMR) techniques.

Without-suction techniques
1. Strip-off biopsy (injection and snaring)[6,7]
2. Lift and cut biopsy "double-snare polypectomy" (grasping and snaring)[8,9]
3. ERHSE (injection, precutting, and snaring)[10]
4. EMRT (grasping and snaring using overtube)[4a]

With-suction techniques
1. EEMR tube method (injection and snaring using overtube)[13a]
2. np-EEM (injection and snaring using overtube)[14a]
3. EMRC (injection and snaring using cap)[15–18]
4. EMRL (EVL and snaring)[20,21]
5. Simple-suction technique (snaring using stiff snare)[22a]

ERHSE, endoscopic resection with hypertonic saline-epinephrine solution; EMRT, EMR using a transparent overtube; EEMR, endoscopic esophageal mucosal resection; np-EEM, endoscopic esophageal mucosectomy under negative-pressure control; EMRC, endoscopic mucosal resection using a transparent plastic cap; EMRL, endoscopic mucosal resection using a ligating device.
[a] These techniques are only available for the esophagus.

Momma et al. and Makuuchi et al. reported the first application of EMR in the esophagus utilizing the strip-biopsy technique in 1989 (injection, lift, and snaring).[11,12] At the same time, the author reported the EMRT procedure, which uses a "lift and cut" method utilizing a specially designed EMRT tube[4] (Table 1.1). In the same paper,[4] the first application of EMR for adenocarcinoma on a short segment of Barrett's esophagus was reported. Makuuchi developed the endoscopic esophageal mucosal resection (EEMR) tube method[13] (Table 1.1). By this method, a larger specimen can be obtained than by other techniques. A modified Makuuchi tube is utilized in Kawano's technique.[14] This modified tube has a lateral window for mucosal trapping. We refined our EMRT procedure[4] to an EMR cap (EMRC) procedure[15–18] (see Table 1.1). EMRC made the surgical technique simpler and easier and made it possible to apply the procedure to any part of the GI tract from pharynx to anus, precluding the postlaryngeal mucosa and the small intestine. The principle of the EMRC procedure is based upon the endoscopic variceal ligating (EVL) technique developed by Stiegmann.[19]

EMR utilizing a variceal ligating device (EMRL) is a technically simple and safe procedure (see Table 1.1). Masuda et al. in Japan, Chaves et al.,[20] and Freischer et al.[21] reported experience utilizing the EVL device. This method is basically similar to the EMRC procedure but divides it into two steps. This method is appropriate to resect a relatively small lesion, less than 10 mm, because the size of the specimen is limited by the small capacity of the ligation cap.

Soehendra et al. introduced the extremely simple suction technique of mucosectomy.[22] In their method, no accessory device is necessary to perform the procedure except a specially designed snare, which is made of monofilament stainless steel wire with a diameter of 0.4 mm. A large-channel endoscope (Olympus GIF-1T) is utilized in combination with the special snare because that endoscope provides adequate suction alongside an inserted snare. The size of the resected specimen seems to be smaller than that with other techniques, but the simplicity of this procedure is potentially interesting.

EMRC Surgical Technique

In preparation for the EMRC procedure, a cap made from transparent plastic is attached to the tip of the forward-view endoscope and is fixed tightly with adhesive tape. A cap is commercially available from Olympus as the Distal attachment and is approved by the FDA in the United States.

For the initial session of EMR in the esophagus and stomach, an oblique-cut large-capacity cap with rim (MAJ297; Olympus, Tokyo, Japan) is fixed on the tip of the standard-size endoscope (Q240, Q140; Olympus) to obtain a larger sample. For trimming a residual lesion, a straight-cut medium-size cap with rim (MH595; Olympus) is appropriate.

Superficial extension of mucosal cancer is often difficult to recognize accurately in routine endoscopic observation but is clearly delineated by chromoendoscopy. For squamous cell carcinoma of the esophagus, iodine (2% iodine potassium solution) is the most promising dye, showing the lesion clearly as an unstained area. Spraying indigocarmine solution emphasizes surface relief in the stomach. The tip of the snare wire carefully marks the mucosal surface that surrounds the margin of the lesion. Markings are positioned 2 mm from the actual lesion margin. Visual enhancement during chromoendoscopy disappears within a couple of minutes, and therefore the markings by electrocoagulation become essential, especially to the flat lesion.

Epinephrine saline solution diluted 500,000 times (0.1% epinephrine solution 0.2 ml plus normal saline 100 ml) is injected into the submucosa with an injection needle (23 gauge, 4 mm tip length). Controlling the position of a needle tip in the submucosal layer is not technically difficult. The most important key to avoiding transmural penetration of the needle is to puncture the mucosa at a sharp angle. The total volume of injected saline depends on the size of the lesion, but it is necessary to inject enough saline to lift up the whole lesion. Usually more than 20 ml is injected. In principle, normal mucosa distal to the lesion is punctured first (Fig. 1.1). When saline is accurately injected into the submucosal layer in any part of the gastrointestinal tract, lifting of the mucosa or bulging of the mucosal surface is always observed. The injected area is also recognizable as a whitish swelling. With the injection of a sufficient volume of submucosal saline, any type of EMR procedure can be performed quite safely.

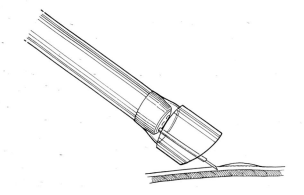

FIGURE 1.1. Submucosal saline injection. Puncture the distal part of the lesion first. Puncturing the mucosa at a sharp angle avoids transmural penetration.

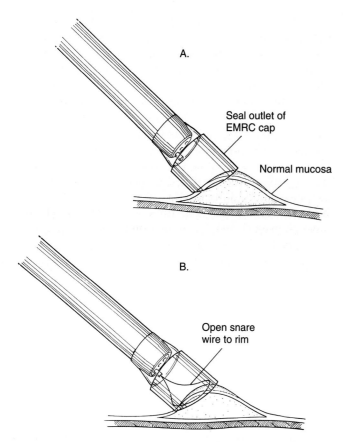

FIGURE 1.2. The endoscopic mucosal resection cap (EMRC) prelooping process. A. Suction the normal mucosa and seal the outlet of the EMRC cap. B. Open the snare wire; it then goes along the rim of the cap. The prelooping condition is created. The outer sheath of the snare wire is pushed up to the distal end of the cap, and the snare wire is fixed along the rim of the EMRC cap.

A specially designed small-diameter snare SD-7P (1.8 mm outer diameter; Olympus) is essential to the prelooping process. The snare wire is fixed along the rim of the EMRC cap. To start the prelooping process, moderate suction is applied to the normal mucosa to seal the outlet of the cap (Fig. 1.2A), and then the snare wire that passes through the instrumental channel of the endoscope is opened (Fig. 1.2B). The opened snare wire is fixed along the rim of the cap, and the outer sheath of the snare extends up to the rim of the cap (Fig. 1.2B). This step completes the prelooping process of the snare wire.

When the endoscope approaches, the target mucosa, including the lesion, is fully sucked inside the cap (Fig. 1.3) and is strangulated by simple closing of the prelooped snare wire. At this moment, the strangulated mucosa looks like a snared polypoid lesion. The pseudopolyp of the strangulated mucosa is cut by blend current electrocautery. The resected specimen can be

easily taken out by keeping it inside the cap without using any grasping forceps.

The smooth surface of the muscle layer is observed at the bottom of the artificial ulcer. In this case, a large vessel was observed at the center of the artificial ulcer; a hemostatic clip was applied to it to prevent bleeding.[23] Bleeding is usually nonexistent or minor and stops spontaneously with compression of the lateral wall of the transparent cap. To confirm complete resection of the lesion, iodine dye spraying is useful.

If additional resection is necessary to completely remove residual lesion, all procedures, including saline injection, should be repeated step by step. Injected saline usually infiltrates and disappears from the injection site within around 5 min, ending its role as a cushion between the mucosa and the muscle layer. Repeated saline injection, therefore, becomes necessary to reduce the risk of muscle involvement during the procedure. Our only experience of perforation of the esophagus hap-

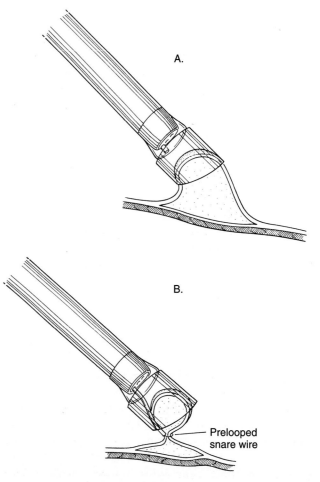

FIGURE 1.3. The EMRC procedure. A. After creating the prelooping condition, target mucosa is drawn inside the cap. B. The strangulated mucosa.

pened during the second strangulation, with no additional saline injection.

Histopathological Assessment

The resected specimen should be stretched and fixed on a rubber plate using fine needles and then bathed in 10% formalin solution. The fixated specimen is divided into 2-mm columns. Histopathological analysis of semiserial sections makes it possible to reconstruct the superficial extension of the cancer.

Postoperative Care

Three days after EMR, the artificial ulcer is covered by a white coating. Twelve days after EMR, the artificial ulcer is almost recovered with thin but normal squamous epithelium. Almost all patients complain of mild post-sternal pain and mild throat pain, which will disappear within a couple of days using medication.

Just after EMR, a mucosal protective agent (for example, Marlox) is prescribed four times a day. Antibiotics are also administered intravenously for the first 2 days, followed by 7 days of oral antibiotics. In our experience, one patient who received near-total circumferential resection in the esophagus, with only 2 days of antibiotics followed by no medication, suffered a severe stricture. That stricture was considered to have been caused by chronic, persistent inflammation.

A few hours after treatment, the patient can start to drink cold water. On the following day, the patient receives a soft meal. On the second day after treatment, the patient receives a normal diet.

In almost all cases of mucosal resection, quality of life can be maintained,[24] so we believe that early detection of cancerous lesions and treatment by endoscopic mucosal resection is an ideal means of cancer treatment.

Results

In our institute, more than 180 cases of early-stage esophageal cancer underwent mucosal resection, mainly by two techniques.[25] Of these cases, 72% were absolute indications for mucosal resection according to our criteria. The other cases were only relatively indicated because of poor risk for surgery or refusal of surgery. In absolutely indicated cases, no local or no distant metastasis occurred during the follow-up period. The 5-year survival rate was 95%, including other causes of death. All patients who died during the 5-year follow-up period suffered from other fatal diseases such as myocardial infarction, liver cirrhosis, and stroke.

As a major complication in the esophagus, one patient in our early series suffered perforation during the second cauterization. That patient recovered by conservative treatments such as intravenous hyperalimentation and antibiotic administration, resulting in no concomitant problems. Eight years later, she is healthy with no surgery-related complaints. Another patient who received near-total circumferential mucosal resection developed persistent stenosis that could not be controlled by repeated forceful balloon dilatation. He was finally treated by surgical esophagectomy. Five years after esophagectomy, he is in good health. In this case, antibiotics were administered for only 2 days, which may have allowed chronic inflammation to develop, resulting in stenosis.

Complications

Mechanism of Perforation

When the EMR procedure is performed without saline injection, the muscle layer beneath the surface mucosa is also drawn inside the cap, together with the covering mucosa, which risks muscle involvement at the moment of closure of the snare loop. A small-volume saline injection is not sufficient to avoid muscle involvement because this creates only a small bleb (Fig. 1.4A). Full suction for a small bleb causes muscle entrapment in the cap, resulting in muscle strangulation with the mucosa (Fig. 1.4B,C). An extra-large-volume saline injection creates a large bleb (Fig. 1.4D). This large cushion mechanically prevents muscle involvement during snare strangulation (Fig. 1.4D,E). In the other words, snaring of the mucosa should never be done at the base of the lifted mucosa (Fig. 1.4B) but rather should always be done at the middle part of the lifted mucosa (Fig. 1.4E,F).

To prevent perforation, a large-volume saline injection is important. In the esophagus, about 20 ml saline causes more than half-circumferential mucosal dissection, keeping the mucosal surface about 1 cm apart from the muscle layer. When saline is accurately injected into the submucosa in any part of the gastrointestinal tract, lifting or bulging of mucosa can be always observed.

The "with suction" techniques listed in Table 1.1 have a potentially greater risk of muscle involvement than the "without suction" techniques, and therefore injecting a larger volume of saline into the submucosa is highly recommended. The author usually injects at least 10 ml for each snaring. Large-volume saline injection is in itself a safe procedure. In our experience of removal of a creeping tumor in the rectum, a total of about 100 ml saline was injected, and the whole lesion was safely removed with inducing a half-circumferential ulceration. In this case, posttherapeutic treatment was uneventful, and therefore

Insufficient   Sufficient

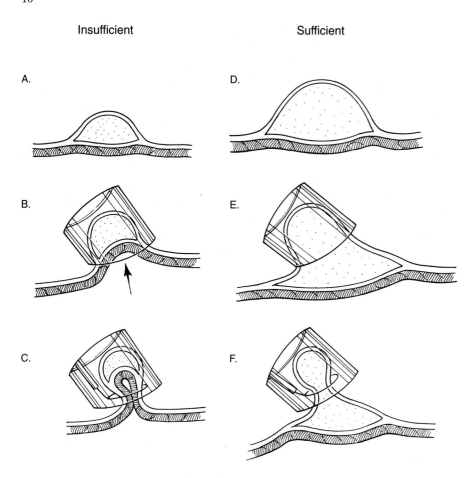

FIGURE 1.4. Submucosal saline injection. A. Small-volume injection of saline creates a small bleb. B. During suction of the target mucosa, the muscle layer is also sucked into the cap. C. Muscle layer entrapment at closure of the snare wire. D. Large-volume saline injection creates a large bleb. E. Even during full suction, only the top of the bleb is captured inside the cap. F. The mucosa is strangulated at the middle part of the bleb. This step makes the procedure safe.

large-volume saline injection is considered a safe procedure in itself.

Control of Bleeding from the Ulcer Bed

Low-concentration epinephrine saline solution (epinephrine saline solution diluted 500,000 fold) is definitely effective to control bleeding during EMR. In the esophagus, submucosal injection of this solution results in almost complete hemostasis, but in the stomach bleeding from an artificial ulcer sometimes cannot be controlled by the solution. At present, the hemostatic clip is the most reliable therapeutic modality to control spurting bleeding from the ulcer bed.[23] Consequently, bleeding from the ulcer bed can be relatively easily controlled.

Conclusion

Mucosal cancer in the esophagus generally has no risk of lymph node metastasis. It is cured by EMR, which provides a resected specimen for histopathological analysis.

References

1. Lambert R. Endoscopic detection and treatment of early esophageal cancer: a critical analysis. Endoscopy 1995;27: 12–18.
2. Endo M, Takeshita K, Yoshida M. How can we diagnose the early stage of esophageal cancer? Endoscopic diagnosis. Endoscopy 1986;18:11–18.
3. Endo M, Kawano T. Analysis of 1125 cases of early esophageal carcinoma in Japan. Dis Esoph 1991;4:71–76.
4. Inoue H, Endo M. Endoscopic esophageal mucosal resection using a transparent tube. Surg Endosc 1990;4:198–201.
5. Rosenberg N. Submucosal saline wheal as safety factor in fulguration of rectal and sigmoidal polypi. Arch Surg 1955; 70:120–122.
6. Tada M, Murakamai A, Karita M, et al. Endoscopic resection of early gastric cancer. Endoscopy 1993;25:445–450.
7. Dehle P, Largiader F, Jenny S, et al. A method for endoscopic electroresection of sessile colonic polyps. Endoscopy 1973;5:38–40.
8. Takekoshi T, Baba Y, Ota H, et al. Endoscopic resection of early gastric carcinomas: results of a retrospective analysis of 308 cases. Endoscopy 1994;26:352–358.

9. Martin TR, Onstad GR, Silvis SE, et al. Life and cut biopsy technique for submucosal samplings. Gastrointest Endosc 1976;23:29–30.

10. Hirao M, Masuda K, Asanuma T, et al. Endoscopic resection of early gastric cancer and other tumors with local injection of hypertonic saline-epinephrine. Gastrointest Endosc 1988;34:264–269.

11. Monma K, Sakaki N, Yoshida M. Endoscopic mucosectomy for precise evaluation and treatment of esophageal intra-epithelial cancer (in Japanese). Endosc Dig 1990;2:501–506.

12. Makuuchi H, Machimura T, Sugihara T, et al. Endoscopic diagnosis and treatment of mucosal cancer of the esophagus (in Japanese). Endosc Dig 1990;2:447–452.

13. Makuuchi H. Endoscopic mucosal resection for early esophageal cancer. Dig Endosc 1996;8:175–179.

14. Kawano T, Miyake S, Yasuno M, et al. A new technique for endoscopic esophageal mucosectomy using a transparent overtube with intraluminal negative pressure (np-EEM). Dig Endosc 1991;3:159–167.

15. Inoue H, Takeshita K, Hori H, et al. Endoscopic mucosal resection with a cap-fitted panendoscope for esophagus, stomach, and colon mucosal lesions. Gastrointest Endosc 1993:58–62.

16. Inoue H, Noguchi O, Saito N, et al. Endoscopic mucosectomy for early cancer using a pre-looped plastic cap. Gastrointest Endosc 1994;40:263–264.

17. Tada M, Inoue H, Endo M. Colonic mucosal resection using a transparent cap-fitted endoscope. Gastrointest Endosc 1996;44:63–65.

18. Izumi Y, Teramoto K, Ohshima M, et al. Endoscopic resection of duodenal ampulla with a transparent plastic cap. Surgery (St. Louis) 1998;123:109–110.

19. Stiegmann GV. Endoscopic ligation: now and the future. Gastrointest Endosc 1993;39:203–205.

20. Chaves DM, Sakai P, Mester M, et al. A new endoscopic technique for the resection of flat polypoid lesions. Gastrointest Endosc 1994;40:224–226.

21. Freischer DE, Dawsey S, Tio TL, et al. Tissue band ligation followed by snare resection (band and snare): a new technique for tissue acquisition in the esophagus. Gastrointest Endosc 1996;44:68–72.

22. Soehendra N, Binmoeller KF, Bohnacker S, et al. Endoscopic snare mucosectomy in the esophagus without any additional equipment: a simple technique for resection of flat early cancer. Endoscopy 1997;29:380–383.

23. Hachisu T, Yamada H, Satoh S, Kouzu T. Endoscopic clipping with a new rotatable clip device and a long clip. Dig Endosc 1996;8:172–173.

24. Takeshita K, Tani M, Inoue H, et al. Endoscopic treatment of early oesophageal or gastric cancer. Gut 1997;40:123–127.

25. Inoue H. Endoscopic mucosal resection for esophageal and gastric mucosal cancers. Can J Gastroenterol 1998;12:355–359.

2
Minimally Invasive Treatment of Zenker's Diverticulum

Luigi Bonavina, Surendra Narne, and Alberto Peracchia

Background and Historical Development of Endoscopic Treatment

Toward the end of the nineteenth century, Zenker and von Ziemssen formulated the hypothesis that a pharyngoesophageal diverticulum is caused by increased hypopharyngeal pressure producing herniation through an area of structural weakness, that is, the junction of the inferior pharyngeal constrictor and the cricopharyngeus muscle, also known as Killian's triangle. It is currently believed that inadequate opening of the upper esophageal sphincter, resulting from fibrosis of the cricopharyngeal muscle, considerably increases hypopharyngeal intrabolus pressure.[1,2] For this reason, when surgical resection or suspension of the diverticulum is performed without a concomitant myotomy, the procedure may fail to relieve dysphagia and to prevent complications or recurrence of the pouch.[3,4]

Unlike the traditional surgical approach, which varies depending on the preference of the individual surgeon, the endoscopic approach is by principle centered on the upper esophageal sphincter. First proposed early in the twentieth century by Mosher, it consists of division of the septum interposed between the pouch and the cervical esophagus, thus allowing the creation of a common cavity with simultaneous section of the upper esophageal sphincter. This procedure has been performed in some institutions using electrocoagulation or laser; although the results appear satisfactory, complications such as bleeding, perforation, and the need for repeated treatment have been reported. Moreover, postoperative pain is quite common, especially after electrocoagulation.[5,6]

During the last decade, interest in the transoral treatment of Zenker's diverticulum has been renewed by the introduction of endostaplers.[7–9] In fact, it has been shown that division of the septum can be safely and effectively performed through an endosurgical approach under general anesthesia.

Indications for Endoscopic Therapy

Treatment of Zenker's diverticulum is indicated to relieve symptoms such as dysphagia and pharyngo-oral regurgitation and to prevent the life-threatening complication of aspiration pneumonia. The tendency of the pouch to progressively enlarge and the possible, although rare, development of a squamous cell carcinoma represent additional arguments in favor of early treatment.

Myotomy is regarded today as an essential component of the operation. It has been shown that myotomy and virtual elimination of the pouch may be achieved via an endosurgical approach. The principle of this video-assisted operation is to establish a common cavity between the hypopharyngeal pouch and the adjacent esophageal lumen by means of a linear endostapler. Division of the common wall by stapling is a one-stage operation, requires a few minutes, and appears simpler and safer than using electrocoagulation or laser.

Compared to the conventional surgical operation, the advantages of endostapling include absence of skin incision, shorter operative time, minimal or no postoperative pain, quicker resumption of oral feeding, and shorter hospital stay. An additional advantage of this approach is expected in patients who present with recurrent diverticulum after conventional operation or in those who have undergone surgery in the left side of the neck. In such circumstances, the conventional operation may pose a major technical challenge to the surgeon and may be associated with a high risk of leakage or recurrent nerve palsy.

Diverticula smaller than 2 cm represent a formal contraindication to the endosurgical approach because the common wall is too short to accommodate one cartridge of staples and to allow complete division of the sphincter. The result would be an incomplete myotomy, causing persistent dysphagia.

Although the postoperative outcome of these patients, who often are elderly and compromised, suggests greater comfort and a quicker recovery compared to the con-

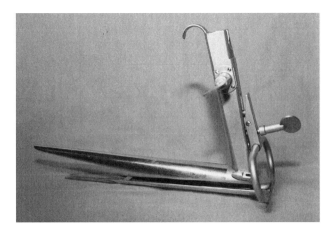

FIGURE 2.1. Weerda diverticuloscope.

ventional operation, it should be taken into account that the endosurgical approach requires general anesthesia. Therefore, in patients with excessive operative risk, a conventional operation carried out under simple local anesthesia still remains the procedure of choice.

Preoperative Assessment and Preparation

A barium swallow study and upper gastrointestinal endoscopy are routinely performed before operation. The diverticulum is carefully entered with the endoscope, and the mucosa is examined to rule out carcinoma. The length of the diverticulum is measured from the upper esophageal sphincter to the bottom of the pouch. The remaining esophagus is examined for the presence of hiatal hernia or esophagitis. A thin guidewire inserted at the end of the endoscopic examination may assist in positioning the manometric catheter within the esophageal lumen if a motility study is planned.

The patients are kept on a liquid diet the day before the operation. Intravenous antibiotics and intensive respiratory physiotherapy are recommended for a few days before surgery in patients admitted on an emergency basis for aspiration pneumonia. In some circumstances, especially in elderly individuals, preoperative nutritional support may be necessary. Short-term antibiotic prophylaxis is given before induction of anesthesia.

Surgical Technique

The operation is performed under general anesthesia with nasotracheal intubation. The patient is placed supine on the operating table, with a small pillow below the upper back and the head hyperextended. The surgeon is sitting behind the patient's head.

A modified Weerda endoscope (Karl Storz, Tuttlingen, Germany) is introduced into the hypopharynx under direct vision and gently pushed behind the endotracheal tube. The two self-retracting valves, which can be approximated and angulated to fit the patient's hypopharyngeal anatomy, are then allowed to enter the diverticulum and the esophageal lumen, respectively (Fig. 2.1). After visualization of the septum interposed between the diverticulum and the esophagus, the diverticuloscope is fixed and held in place by means of a chest support (Fig. 2.2).

A 5-mm wide-angle 0° telescope is inserted through the diverticuloscope and connected to a cold-light source and to a video camera to obtain a magnified vision of the operative field on a television screen. The depth of the diverticulum can be checked using a graduated rod. This maneuver also allows the surgeon to straighten the pouch and to elongate the common wall (Fig. 2.3).

The diverticulum esophagostomy is performed using a disposable linear endostapler (EndoGIA 30, Tyco, or ETS 35, Ethicon Endo-surgery) with a shorter anvil, thus allowing tissue stapling and sectioning down to the bottom of the septum. The anvil is placed in the lumen of the diverticulum and the cartridge of staples into the lumen of the cervical esophagus (Fig. 2.4). The instrument jaws are placed across the septum along the midline before firing. With a single application of the endostapler, the posterior esophageal wall is sutured to the wall of the diverticulum, and the tissue is transected between three rows of staples on each side. Multiple stapler applications may be necessary according to the size of the diverticu-

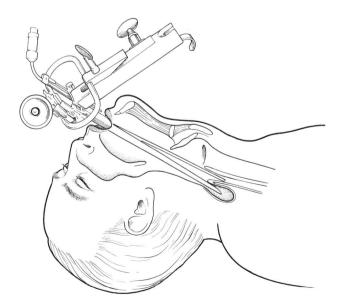

FIGURE 2.2. Position of the diverticuloscope. The lower valve is inserted into the Zenker diverticulum and the upper valve into the esophageal lumen.

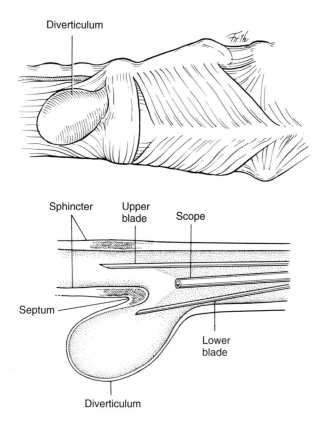

FIGURE 2.3. Visualization of the septum. The telescope is inserted through the instrument.

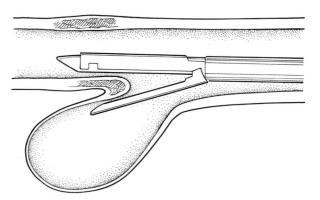

FIGURE 2.5. Suture section of the septum interposed between esophagus and diverticulum.

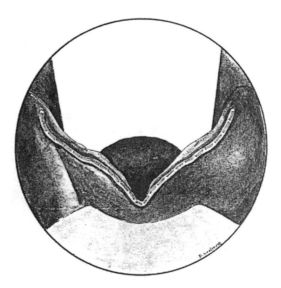

FIGURE 2.6. Frontal view of the stapled and divided septum. A common cavity has been created.

lum. Using the tip of the anvil, the bottom of the diverticulum can be pushed gently downward to lengthen the common wall and to minimize the size of the residual spur. Electrocoagulating endosurgical scissors may be used to complete the section at the distal end of the staple line (Fig. 2.5).

After removal of the stapler, the two wound edges retract laterally because of the division of the cricopharyngeal muscle (Fig. 2.6). Finally, the suture line is checked for hemostasis, and the hypopharynx is irrigated with saline solution.

Postoperative Care

A nasogastric tube is generally not required. A gastrographin swallow study is performed on the first postoperative day. The patient is then allowed to drink and eat and is discharged from the hospital. A soft diet is recom-

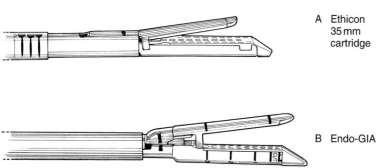

A Ethicon
   35 mm
   cartridge

B Endo-GIA

FIGURE 2.4. Endoscopic linear staplers. A. The Ethicon device has a shorter staple head and a 35-mm cartridge; this does not require any mechanical modification, making the instrument more suitable for the operation. B. The endo-GIA instrument required sawing off the anvil to avoid a residual spur. The shorter anvil allows tissue stapling and sectioning down to the bottom of the diverticulum.

mended during the first postoperative month. A barium swallow study is performed after 6 to 12 months.

Results

Conversion to open surgery was required in 3% of cases in a recent series[8]; the reason was a difficult exposure of the common wall in two cases and a mucosal tear in another. In these individuals, introduction of the endoscope and stapler manipulation were difficult due to limited mouth opening or reduced neck extension. No postoperative morbidity or mortality was recorded. In most patients, two applications of linear endostapler with a modified anvil were used. Before modication of the anvil of the endo-GIA stapler, five patient complained of persistent postoperative symptoms; three patients underwent repeat endosurgical operation, one underwent laser treatment by means of flexible endoscopy, and one eventually required open surgery.

Overall, this procedure has proven safe and effective. Radiologic, manometric, and scintigraphic studies over a follow-up period up to 5 years consistently show decreased outflow resistance at the pharyngoesophageal junction. The short hospital stay, lack of morbidity, minimal patient discomfort, and complete symptom relief associated with this operation have prompted us to change the approach to Zenker's diverticulum in our institution during the past decade.

References

1. Cook I, Dodds W, Dantas R. Opening mechanisms of the human upper esophageal sphincter. Am J Physiol 1989;257: G748–G759.
2. Mason R, Bremner C, DeMeester T, et al. Pharyngeal swallowing disorders. Selection for and outcome after myotomy. Ann Surg 1998;228:598–608.
3. Bonavina L, Khan N, DeMeester T. Pharyngoesophageal dysfunctions. Arch Surg 1985;120:541–549.
4. Shaw D, Jamieson G, Gabb M, Simula M, Dent J. Influence of surgery on deglutitive upper oesophageal sphincter mechanics in Zenker's diverticulum. Gut 1996;38:806–811.
5. Dohlman G, Mattson O. The endoscopic operation for hypopharyngeal diverticula. Arch Otolaryngol 1960;71: 744–752.
6. Van Overbeek J, Hoeksema P, Edens E. Microendoscopic surgery of the hypopharyngeal diverticulum using electrocoagulation of carbon dioxide laser. Ann Otol Rhinol Laryngol 1984;93:34–36.
7. Collard J, Otte J, Kestens P. Endoscopic stapling technique of esophagodiverticulostomy for Zenker's diverticulum. Ann Thorac Surg 1993;56:573–576.
8. Narne S, Bonavina L, Guido E, Peracchia A. Treatment of Zenker's diverticulum by endoscopic stapling. Endosurgery 1993;1:118–120.
9. Peracchia A, Bonavina L, Narne S, Segalin A, Antoniazzi L, Marotta G. Minimally invasive surgery for Zenker diverticulum. Analysis of results in 95 consecutive patients. Arch Surg 1998;133:695–700.

3
Laparoscopic Complete and Partial Fundoplication

Jeffrey A. Hagen and Jeffrey H. Peters

Background and Historical Development

Gastroesophageal reflux disease (GERD) is arguably one of the most common disorders in Western civilization. For reasons that are not clear, it appears to be increasing in prevalence. Historically, the treatment of GERD has included dietary modification, weight loss, and intermittent antacid therapy. These measures were often ineffective, however, and surgical therapy has been applied to those who failed. In the early days of surgical antireflux therapy, these were usually patients with refractory ulcers and severe fibrotic strictures. With the introduction of specific medical therapy with H_2 receptor antagonists and, more recently, proton pump inhibitors, the number of patients with these acid-pepsin-related complications of reflux disease has declined. In their place, patients with malignant complications of reflux disease have emerged as a larger problem, with the recognition of the relationship between GERD and Barrett's esophagus. Because cancer of the esophagus is frequently fatal, and because patients with Barrett's esophagus are often relatively asymptomatic, formal investigation of patients with a history of significant reflux symptoms and institution of effective therapy has become important.

Historically, two problems have prevented the widespread acceptance of antireflux surgery. The first was the observation that a fundoplication was frequently complicated by dysphagia and gas bloat, complications related to an overly competent lower esophageal high-pressure zone. Second was the perioperative morbidity and mortality associated with antireflux surgery. Hospital stays were routinely a week or more, with up to 6 or 8 weeks of additional disability from work. The development of more potent acid suppression medications further restricted the application of antireflux surgery, to the point where referral to surgery was limited to patients with complicated reflux disease who proved refractory to medical therapy.[1]

Two major developments over the past several decades have dramatically changed both the outcome and acceptance of antireflux surgery. The first was the appreciation that a shorter, loose, fundoplication markedly reduced the postoperative sequelae associated with antireflux surgery.[2-5] With these modifications in technique, most patients are able to belch normally and eat without long-term dysphagia, without sacrificing efficacy in controlling reflux of gastric contents into the esophagus. The second development that has revolutionized antireflux surgery was the introduction of the laparoscopic Nissen fundoplication.

Bernard Dallemagne first recreated the procedure that Nissen had serendipitously discovered in 1936.[6,7] Because of the diminished morbidity of these minimally invasive antireflux procedures, the threshold for referral to surgery for patients with GERD rapidly decreased. As a result, the laparoscopic Nissen fundoplication has become one of the most commonly performed laparoscopic procedures in everyday surgical practice. The explosion of laparoscopic antireflux surgery worldwide has stimulated a new interest in the study of surgical treatment of GERD. Through this experience, much has been learned, but significant controversies remain. Nonetheless, in the setting of relatively early GERD, laparoscopic antireflux procedures have been established as safe, highly effective, and long-lasting alternatives to lifelong medical therapy.

Clinical Features

GERD is a syndrome that includes a variety of clinical manifestations including symptoms and tissue injury patterns associated with abnormal esophageal exposure to gastric contents. The presenting symptoms can vary widely, but they can conveniently be grouped into three categories: typical symptoms, atypical symptoms, and complications. The indications for antireflux surgery and the results to be expected vary in these three groups, and as such they warrant separate consideration.

Heartburn and regurgitation are the most common typical symptoms of GERD. Heartburn is most often described as a substernal burning sensation that may radiate up into the throat. It may occur following meals, or with physical activity such as bending or stooping, and in some patients it occurs predominately at night. It has been estimated that 10% of the population experiences heartburn daily, with up to one-third experiencing heartburn at least once a month.[8] Patients with heartburn also frequently complain of regurgitation, which is described as the appearance of acid or bitter fluid, without warning, into the back of the throat. Regurgitation is particularly likely to occur after meals and when the patient lies down at night. The patient or their spouse may describe episodes of awakening from sleep coughing or choking. In addition to heartburn and regurgitation, the patient with typical symptoms of GERD may experience dysphagia. It is more common in patients with complicated reflux disease and stricture formation, but dysphagia may occur in the absence of segmental narrowing, as a result of either a large hiatal hernia[9] or the presence of reflux-induced esophageal peristaltic dysfunction. When present, the symptom of dysphagia warrants particular attention to exclude the possibility of cancer.

Atypical symptoms of reflux disease include chest pain, hoarseness, and pulmonary symptoms such as asthma, chronic cough, and aspiration pneumonia. Rarely, patients may present with protracted hiccups, night sweats, and erosions of their dental enamel. It has been shown, in patients with angina-like chest pain who have a negative cardiac evaluation, that abnormal gastroesophageal reflux will occur in up to 50%.[10] Thus, GERD is the most common abnormality in these patients. Chronic hoarseness or "reflux laryngitis" is associated with abnormal esophageal acid exposure in as many as 75% of patients studied by prolonged pH monitoring.[11] Ambulatory monitoring of pH in the cervical esophagus may be particularly helpful in these patients. Respiratory symptoms occasionally associated with GERD include repeated episodes of aspiration pneumonia, chronic cough, and, more commonly, nonallergic asthma. Recent studies have shown that as many as 20% of patients with chronic cough have abnormal reflux,[12] with reflux being documented in up to 80% of patients with chronic asthma.[13]

Complications of GERD include the development of esophageal ulcers or strictures, as well as the malignant complications of GERD, including the development of Barrett's esophagus and esophageal adenocarcinoma. It has been estimated that approximately 10% of unselected patients with reflux symptoms have evidence of Barrett's esophagus on endoscopy,[14] making endoscopic evaluation an important part of the evaluation of any patient presenting with chronic reflux symptoms.

Preoperative Investigations

To document that gastroesophageal reflux is responsible for symptoms, and to maximize the chances of success with antireflux surgery, patients suspected of having GERD should be carefully investigated before considering antireflux surgery. It has been shown that success in antireflux surgery is largely determined by two objectives: to achieve the long-term relief of reflux symptoms, and to do so without the development of complications or complaints induced by the operation. In practice, achieving these two deceptively simple goals is difficult. Both depend heavily upon establishing that the symptoms for which the operation is being performed are caused by excess esophageal exposure to gastric juice. In addition, it is critical that the appropriate antireflux procedure be performed in the proper fashion. Success can be expected in most patients if these two criteria are met.

To achieve these goals, the evaluation of patients suspected of having GERD who are being considered for antireflux surgery has four important components:

1. Establishing that GERD is the underlying cause of the patient's symptoms
2. Estimating the risk of progressive disease
3. Determining the presence or absence of esophageal shortening
4. Evaluating esophageal body function and, occasionally, gastric emptying function

Objective Documentation of GERD

In the past, patients referred for antireflux surgery had more advanced disease, usually associated with severe esophagitis, and often with stricture formation. Establishing reflux as the cause was generally not difficult. However, as the threshold for surgical referral has decreased, increasing numbers of patients without endoscopic esophagitis or other objective evidence of the presence of reflux are now considered for laparoscopic antireflux surgery.[15,16] In these patients, formal diagnostic testing is required to document the presence of abnormal esophageal exposure to gastric contents, the hallmark of GERD. The gold standard for diagnosing GERD is the use of ambulatory 24-h pH testing.[17]

Estimating the Risk of Progressive Disease

Identification of patients likely to develop progressive reflux disease in spite of medical therapy would allow us to prevent complications of GERD such as strictures or Barrett's esophagus by early application of antieflux surgery. Although absolute predictors do not as yet exist, a combination of 24-h pH testing, detection of abnormal esophageal exposure to duodenal contents (Bilitec monitoring), and the use of esophageal motility studies have provided us with some useful guidance. Patients with very high degrees of acid exposure, particularly at night, are at particular risk for the development of complicated reflux disease.[18] Thus, careful review of both the pattern and severity of acid reflux is important. Complications of reflux disease have also been shown to correlate with the presence of abnormal esophageal exposure to bilirubin.[19] As a result, before instituting long-term medical therapy in patients with GERD, consideration should be given to Bilitec monitoring. Finally, complicated reflux disease has also been shown to be more common in patients with a defective lower esophageal sphincter (LES),[20] and in those with impaired esophageal body function.[21] In patients with one or more of these risk factors for complications of reflux disease, early surgical therapy should be considered.

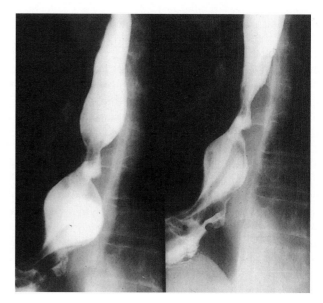

FIGURE 3.1. Radiograph showing esophageal shortening.

Detection of Esophageal Shortening

In a manner analogous to stricture formation, esophageal shortening can occur as a consequence of scarring and fibrosis associated with repetitive esophageal injury.[22,23] Recognition of anatomic shortening of the esophagus is important because it can compromise the ability to perform an adequate tension-free antireflux repair. In our experience,[24] and the experience of others,[25] unrecognized esophageal shortening is a major cause of recurrent herniation, a common cause of fundoplication failure. It is also the explanation for the "slipped" Nissen fundoplication. In many such instances, the initial repair is incorrectly constructed around the proximal tubularized stomach rather than the terminal esophagus. Although no ideal method exists to detect significant esophageal shortening, the combination of video roentgenographic contrast studies and endoscopic findings (Fig. 3.1) will alert the surgeon to a situation in which esophageal shortening is likely.[26] A large hiatal hernia on endoscopy or on video esophagram is likely to be associated with esophageal shortening, as is the presence of an esophageal stricture. Hernia size is measured endoscopically as the distance between the diaphragmatic crura (identified by having the patient sniff), and the gastroesophageal junction (identified as the loss of gastric rugal folds). We consider the possibility of a short esophagus in patients with strictures or those with large hiatal hernias (>5 cm), particularly when the latter fail to reduce in the upright position on a video barium esophagram. Because of the risk of failure due to excessive tension after transabdominal repair, these patients are best

treated by a thoracic approach that allows a more thorough mobilization of the esophagus. After complete mobilization, esophageal length can be appraised by assessing the ability to reduce the gastroesophageal (GE) junction beneath the diaphragm without excessive tension. When this is not possible, a Collis gastroplasty coupled with either a partial or complete fundoplication achieves excellent control of reflux in the majority of these patients.[27,28]

Evaluation of Esophageal Body Function

Selection of the appropriate antireflux operation in an individual patient requires a careful assessment of esophageal body function. Otherwise, the resistance to emptying imparted by a complete fundoplication will result in troublesome dysphagia in patients with poor peristaltic function. Assessment of esophageal body function is also important from a prognostic standpoint because esophageal body function has been shown to correlate with the likelihood of relief of regurgitation, dysphagia, and respiratory symptoms following surgery. When peristalsis is absent, or severely disordered (>50% simultaneous contractions), or the amplitude of the contractions in one or more of the lower esophageal segments in below 20mmHg, most surgeons would opt for a partial fundoplication. Persistent poor esophageal propulsive function and the continued regurgitation of esophageal contents may explain the less favorable response after fundoplication of atypical compared to typical reflux symptoms.[29-31]

Indications for Antireflux Surgery

Historically, antireflux surgery was reserved for patients with severe esophagitis or stricture or to those refractory to medical therapy, that is, to patients with relatively severe reflux disease, largely because of the relatively high morbidity and mortality associated with antireflux surgery in the era of open antireflux procedures. The demonstration of decreased morbidity and shorter hospital stays and periods of disability associated with minimally invasive antireflux surgery, coupled with the demonstration of the success of these procedures, have shifted the balance such that patients with less severe disease are now considered surgical candidates. In fact, it is likely that it is precisely these patients with less severe disease that are probably the best candidates for a laparoscopic Nissen (see following). Furthermore, the traditional concept, that a deficient lower esophageal sphincter is the primary cause of GERD and that a defective sphincter was a requirement before surgery, is no longer valid in the era of laparoscopic fundoplication.[29] It is now clear that reflux frequently occurs during temporary loss of the gastroesophageal barrier and that patients with normal resting sphicter parameters can have excellent outcomes following surgery.

The ideal candidate for a laparoscopic antireflux procedure is the patient with typical symptoms of heartburn or regurgitation (as opposed to atypical symptoms such as cough, asthma, or hoarseness), with a pH test-proven abnormal esophageal acid exposure, and who has responded to, but is dependent on, proton pump inhibitors for symptom relief. A multivariate analysis of the factors predicting a successful outcome after laparoscopic Nissen has identified these three parameters as the most important preoperative predictors of a successful outcome.[32] As mentioned, the most important aspect of patient selection is to be as certain as possible that gastroesophageal reflux is the underlying cause of their complaints. Taken in this context, it immediately becomes evident that each of the predictors of success just outlined helps do just that, to establish that gastroesophageal reflux disease is indeed the cause of the patient's symptoms.

There are several specific situations in which antireflux surgery should be considered. The first is the patient who has demonstrated the need for long-term medical therapy, particularly if escalating doses of proton pump inhibitors are needed to control symptoms; this is particularly true in patients who are less than 50 years of age, for whom the lifetime cost of medical therapy could easily exceed the cost of surgical therapy.[33] Patients who are noncompliant with medical therapy, those for whom the medications are a financial burden, or those who favor a single definitive intervention over long-term drug treatment, should also be offered the option of surgery.

Patients who are at high risk of progression to complications of GERD despite medical therapy (see earlier discussion) should also be considered for antireflux surgery. Minimally invasive antireflux surgery may be the treatment of choice in these patients.

Assuming the patient is physiologically fit, and that reflux has been carefully documented, there are no specific contraindications to laparoscopic antireflux surgery. Experience has shown, however, that difficulties may be encountered in patients who have a large left lateral segment of the liver, those who are morbidly obese, and those who have undergone prior upper gastrointestinal surgery. Patients with large paraesophageal hernias represent a specific technical challenge. Although the majority of these difficulties can be overcome with increasing experience, an open transabdominal or transthoracic approach may be the wisest choice in such patients. This decision, that is, when to abandon the laparoscopic approach in favor of the traditional open approach, is a difficult one that is currently under investigation.

Surgical Techniques

Laparoscopic Nissen Fundoplication

Port Positioning

The technique of laparoscopic Nissen fundoplication has been relatively well standardized. Access is via five upper abdominal ports (Fig. 3.2). We prefer an open technique

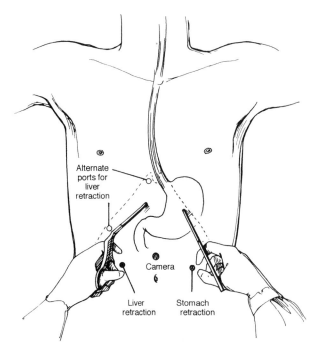

FIGURE 3.2. Port location.

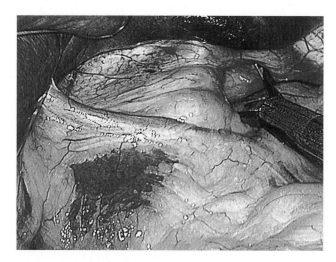

FIGURE 3.3. Intraoperative photograph of gastrohepatic ligament with replaced left hepatic artery. A hiatal hernia of moderate size can be seen in the *upper right corner.*

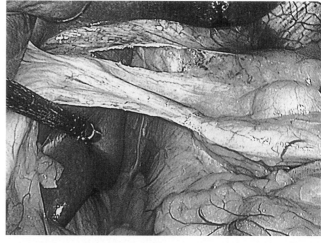

FIGURE 3.4. A window is created above and below the hepatic branch of the vagus nerve and any associated vascular structures. The right crus becomes evident.

for placement of the Hasson trochar used for camera access. Placement of this port through the left rectus abdominus muscle appears to result in more secure closure of the wound and fewer incisional hernias. Two lateral retracting ports are placed in the right and left anterior axillary lines, respectively. The right-sided liver retractor is best placed in the right midabdomen (midclavicular line), at or slightly below the camera port. This placement allows the proper angle toward the left lateral segment of the liver and thus the ability to push the instrument toward the operating table, lifting the liver. A second retraction port is placed at the level of the umbilicus, in the left anterior axillary line. The surgeon's right-handed trocar is placed in the left midclavicular line, 1 to 2 in. below the costal margin. The liver is then retracted, and the fifth and final port is placed just to the right of the falciform ligament in the subxyphoid area.

The esophageal hiatus is exposed by placement of a fan retractor in the right anterior axillary port. A table retractor can then be used to securely fix the liver in place, which minimizes trauma to the liver, and frees the hand of an assistant for other work. Mobilization of the left lateral segment by division of the triangular ligament is not necessary. A Babcock clamp is placed into the left anterior axillary port and the stomach retracted toward the patient's left foot. This maneuver exposes the esophageal hiatus. Commonly, a hiatal hernia will need to be reduced (Fig. 3.3). An atraumatic clamp should be used, and care should be taken not to grasp the stomach too vigorously, as gastric perforations can occur.

Hiatal Dissection

Identification of the right crus is the first and most important step in safe dissection of the hiatus. Metzenbaum-

type scissors and fine grasping forceps are preferred for dissection. In all except the most obese patients, a very thin portion of the gastrohepatic omentum overlies the caudate lobe of the liver. The right crus is exposed by incising the gastrohepatic omentum above and below the hepatic branch of the anterior vagal nerve, which we routinely spare. A large left hepatic artery arising from the left gastric artery will be present in about 25% of patients. It should be identified and avoided.

After incising the gastrohepatic omentum, the lateral surface of the right crus will become evident (Fig. 3.4). The peritoneum overlying the anterior aspect of the right crus is incised with scissors and electrocautery, and the right crus dissected as much as possible from anterior to posterior (Fig. 3.5). By blunt dissection along the medial surface of the right crus, the mediastinum is entered. The

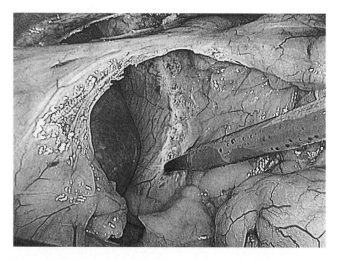

FIGURE 3.5. The peritoneum along the anterior border of the right crus is marked and incised.

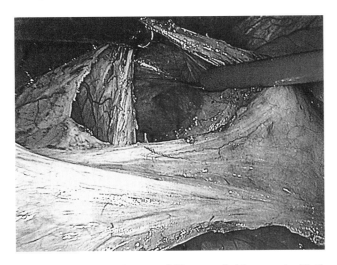

FIGURE 3.6. The anterior crural fibers are held upward with the left-handed grasper while the esophagus is swept downward and to the right.

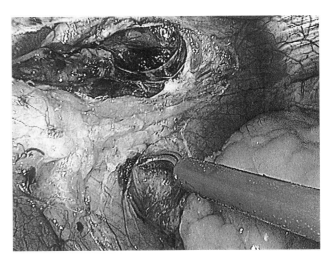

FIGURE 3.7. The left crural dissection and removal of the remaining portions of the gastroesophageal fat pad from the left crus as visualized from the left side.

esophagus will then become evident in the lower mediastinum. Lateral retraction of the right crus exposes the tissues behind the esophagus. No attempt is made at this point to dissect behind the gastroesophageal junction. Meticulous hemostasis is critical, as otherwise blood and fluid tend to pool in the hiatus, obscuring the view in this critical dissection. Irrigation should be kept to a minimum. Care must be taken not to injure the phrenic artery and vein as they course anterior to the hiatus. A large hiatal hernia makes this portion of the procedure easier, as it accentuates the diaphragmatic crura. On the other hand, dissection of a large mediastinal hernia sac can be difficult.

Once the right crus is fully mobilized, attention is turned toward the anterior crural confluence. The tissues anterior to the esophagus are held upward via the left-handed grasper and the esophagus is swept downward and to the patient's right, separating it from the left crus (Fig. 3.6). The anterior crural tissues are then divided and the left crus identified. The left crus is dissected as completely as possible from anterior to posterior. The attachments of the fundus to the left diaphragm should also be divided, to expose the left crus as far posteriorly as possible. A complete dissection of the lateral and inferior aspect of the left crus and fundus of the stomach is the key maneuver allowing circumferential mobilization of the esophagus (Fig. 3.7). Less than complete dissection will result in difficulty encircling the esophagus, particularly if it is approached from the right. Repositioning of the Babcock retractor toward the fundic side of the stomach facilitates retraction for this portion of the procedure.

The esophagus is now mobilized for several centimeters up into the mediastinum by careful dissection of the anterior and posterior soft tissues within the hiatus. If

the crura have been completely mobilized as described, a window posterior to the esophagus can be created without much difficulty (Fig. 3.8). With the esophagus retracted toward the patient's left, the hiatus is approached from the right. Anterior retraction on the esophagus with the surgeon's left-hand instrument allows posterior dissection with the right hand, creating an opening behind the gastroesophageal (GE) junction below the diaphragm. The posterior vagus nerve is left on the esophagus. The medical surface of the left crus is identified and the dissection kept caudal to it. There is a tendency to dissect into the mediastinum, and particular care must be taken to stay below the left crus in creating this posterior window. In the presence of severe esophagitis, transmural inflammation, esophageal shortening, a large

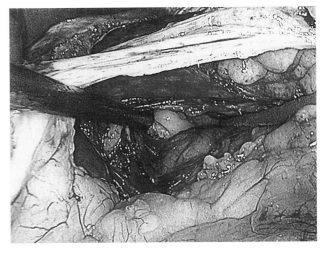

FIGURE 3.8. A window behind the gastroesophageal junction is made. The esophagus is anterior to the left-handed grasper, which points toward the spleen.

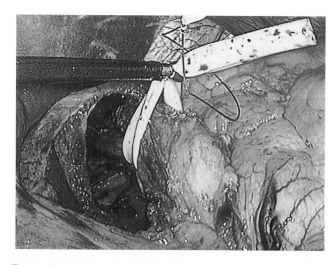

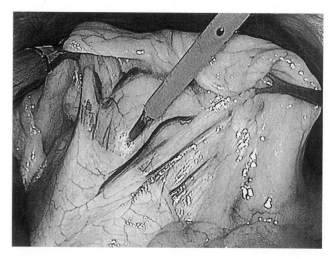

FIGURE 3.9. A Penrose drain is placed around the esophagus to aid in esophageal retraction and secured in place with a loop suture.

FIGURE 3.10. Initial retraction for short gastric division. A window is made between vessels with the electrocautery.

posterior fat pad, or some combination of these conditions, this dissection may be particularly difficult. If undue difficulty is encountered in this dissection, it should be abandoned and the hiatus approached from the left side after division of the short gastric vessels. Once this window has been created, a grasper is passed through the surgeon's left-handed port behind the esophagus and over the left crus. A Penrose drain is placed around the esophagus and used as an esophageal retractor for the remainder of the procedure (Fig. 3.9).

Fundic Mobilization

Once the hiatal dissection is completed, division of the short gastric vessels is performed to mobilize the fundus. Although the debate continues regarding the need to mobilize the short gastric vessels, at least one randomized trial has shown that failure to divide the short gastric vessels was associated with an increased risk of postoperative dysphagia.[34] Fundic mobilization is begun by replacing the liver retractor with a second Babcock forceps that is used to grasp the omentum along the greater curvature of the stomach just below the spleen. A second Babcock clamp placed through the left lower port is used to suspend the gastroplenic omentum in a clothesline fashion (Fig. 3.10). Short gastric vessels are sequentially divided with the aid of a Harmonic Scalpel (Ethicon Endo-Surgery, Cincinnati, OH, USA). As one approaches the last few short gastric vessels near the tip of the spleen, the Babcock placed in the liver retractor port is placed on the back wall of the stomach, while the other Babcock is moved sequentially further up the gastrosplenic ligament, suspending the short gastric vessels in a medial to lateral fashion (Fig. 3.11). Division of the pancreaticogastric branches that lie behind the upper

stomach completes mobilization of the fundus. The dissection is complete when the right crus and caudate lobe can be seen from the left side (Fig. 3.12). With caution and meticulous dissection, the fundus can be completely mobilized in virtually all patients.

Crural Closure

The crura are further dissected behind the esophagus, and the space behind the gastroesophageal junction is enlarged as much as possible. Recently, attention has been paid to mobilizing the esophagus into the mediastinum for several inches as well (Fig. 3.13). Care must be taken not to open the pleura, which can often be seen lateral to the esophagus. The esophagus is retracted ante-

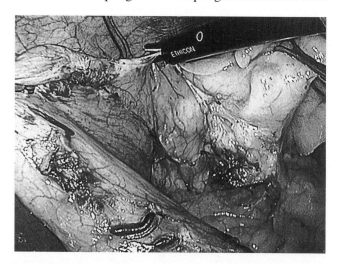

FIGURE 3.11. The proximal third of the fundus is mobilized from within the lesser sac. Sequential retraction of the stomach right laterally and the gastrosplenic omentum leftward provides excellent visualization.

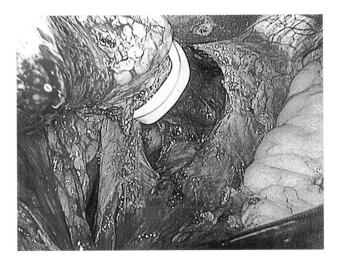

FIGURE 3.12. The fundic mobilization continues to include the panceaticogastric branches until the crura and caudate lobe can be seen from left posterior.

riorly and to the left, and the crura are approximated with three or four interrupted 0-silk sutures, starting just above the confluence of the right and left crura (Fig. 3.14). We prefer a large needle (CT1) passed down the left upper 10-mm port to facilitate a durable crural closure. Because the space behind the esophagus is limited, the surgeon must often use the left-handed instrument as a retractor. This maneuver facilitates placement of single bites through each crus with the surgeon's right hand. We prefer tying the knots extracorporeally, using a standard knot pusher, as this method appears to result in a more secure closure.

Although no randomized studies have evaluated the role of routine crural closure, compelling evidence indicates that closure should be standard. Failure to close the crura can result in paraesophageal herniation, which

Watson et al.[35] demonstrated in 17 of 253 (7%) patients undergoing laparoscopic Nissen. They found that 11% of those without crural closure suffered this complication, compared to only 3% in those who had undergone crural repair.

Creating the Fundoplication

The importance of proper geometry in constructing the fundoplication is not often emphasized. Failure to adhere to the techniques outlined will result in a Nissen that is more of a twisted wrap than a true fundoplication. This distortion of the GE junction can result in failure of relaxation of the lower esophageal high-pressure zone and the development of dysphagia. The key to maintaining the proper geometry is to use the posterior fundus for the posterior fundoplication, with the anterior surface of the fundus brought around anteriorly.

To ensure that the posterior fundus is used in the construction of the fundoplication, it is grasped and passed behind the esophagus from left to right rather than pulled from right to left. To accomplish this, a Babcock clamp is placed in the left lower port, grasping the midportion of the posterior fundus (Fig. 3.15). The Babcock is then passed up to the hiatal region, to the left of the esophagus, and the esophagus is then retracted to the patient's left. The posterior wall of the fundus can then be seen on the right side of the esophagus, coming through the window created posteriorly. The anterior wall of the fundus is brought over the anterior wall of the esophagus above the supporting Penrose drain. Both anterior and posterior fundic lips are manipulated so that the esophagus is enveloped without twisting the fundus (Fig. 3.16).

It is important to recognize that laparoscopic visualization has a tendency to exaggerate the size of the pos-

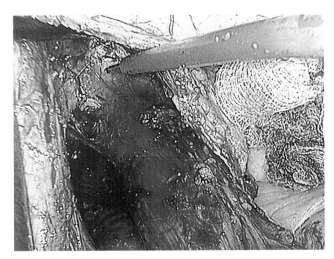

FIGURE 3.13. The esophagus is mobilized via mediastinal dissection for 3–4 in. to provide maximal intraabdominal length.

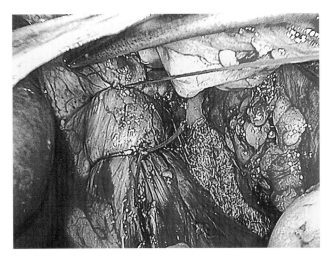

FIGURE 3.14. The crura are closed with three to five interrupted sutures.

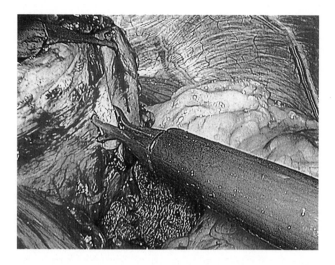

FIGURE 3.15. A suitable site on the midposterior fundus is chosen for passage behind the esophagus to the right side.

terior window, so that the space behind the esophagus may be smaller than thought. The result can be ischemia of the fundus when it is passed behind the esophagus. If the posterior lip of the fundoplication has a bluish discoloration, the stomach should be returned to its original position and the posterior window enlarged. A 60F bougie dilator is then carefully passed into the stomach. The anterior and posterior lips of the fundus are then brought together on the right anterolateral aspect of the esophagus, to properly size the fundoplication. There should be no tension when the fundoplication is brought together, but it should not be loose either. A double-armed 2-0 Prolene suture is then placed as a U-stitch, reinforced by a felt pledget. The suture is placed through the right-hand port, beginning in the anterior fundus, incorporating a bite of esophagus, before being placed in the posterior fundus. The second needle is then delivered through the same port, and it is secured in a similar fashion. Both needles are brought out through the right-handed working port, and they are passed through a second piece of felt. An extracorporeal knot is then tied down.

As mentioned, the most common error in constructing the fundoplication is grasping the anterior portion of the stomach and pulling it behind the esophagus, which results in twisting the gastric fundus around the esophagus. The esophagus should be enveloped by an *untwisted* fundus before suturing. Two anchoring sutures of 2-0 silk are placed about 0.5 cm above and below the U-stitch to complete the fixation of the fundoplication.

If the esophagus and fundus have been sufficiently wrapped, and if the wrap is not twisted, the stomach should remain in its original plane with the suture line of the fundoplication facing in the right anterior direction and the greater curvature, in the left posterior direction.

Before removing the ports, the abdomen is irrigated, hemostasis is assured, and the bougie is removed. A naso-gastric tube can then be inserted.

Laparoscopic Toupet Partial Fundoplication

A technique has been described for performing a partial fundoplication using laparoscopic techniques.[36] The port sites, the hiatal dissection, the fundic mobilization, and the crural closure are performed exactly as described in the technique of the Nissen fundoplication just outlined. The major difference is that the Toupet fundoplication involves a 270° fundoplication in contrast to the complete 360° wrap described in the Nissen.

Once the hiatus has been mobilized and the crura have been closed, and the fundus has been completely mobilized, the posterior fundus is passed behind the esophagus as described. The fundus is then secured to the right crural margin by a 3-0 silk suture, and three of four additional sutures are placed between the posterior lip of fundus and the right lateral wall of the esophagus. The anterior fundic lip is then sutured to the left crural margin, and three or four more interrupted sutures are placed between the fundus and the left anterolateral esophageal wall to complete a 270° fundoplication. A dilator is not necessary to calibrate this partial wrap, and when completed, a nasogastric tube can be inserted and the operation completed as described above.

Laparoscopic Collis Gastroplasty

The possibility of performing a Collis gastroplasty via laparoscopy has recently emerged as an alternative to open procedures in patients with esophageal shortening.[37] It has, however, been subjected to only occasional

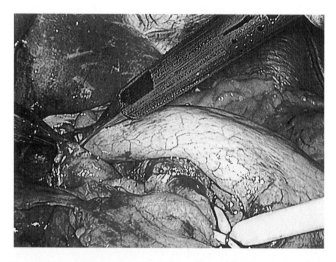

FIGURE 3.16. The geometry of the fundoplication is carefully oriented before passage of a 60F bougie. The fundoplication is then sutured in place.

clinical trials.[38,39] As a result, its appropriateness as a treatment option in GERD remains to be determined. Two techniques have been described, one pure laparoscopic and the other a combined thoracolaparoscopic approach. The pure laparoscopic procedure creates the gastroplasty segment by first making a circular gastrotomy 5 cm down from the angle of His with subsequent firing of a liner stapler toward the esophagus to create the neoesophageal segment. This maneuver is analogous to a vertical banded gastroplasty. It is a technically difficult procedure and requires placement of an 18-mm port and careful alignment of the EEA stapler onto the stomach.

The combined thoracolaparoscopic procedure creates the gastroplasty segment by passage of a linear endoscopic stapler blindly through a thoracic trochar through the fourth intercostal space. The right pleura is opened from below, and an articulating stapler is placed at the angle of His to create the neoesophageal segment. Whether one of these two approaches is superior remains to be seen. The complexity of the combined thoracolaparoscopic approach may mitigate against its use, as it appears to offer little advantage over an open transthoracic approach. Potential problems with the laparoscopic approach include the difficulty in placing the EEA stapler to create the neoesophagus and the risk of peritoneal contamination from the gastrotomy.

Until well-controlled trials demonstrate the safety and efficacy of these newly described techniques, the authors continue to consider an open transthoracic approach to be the best option in the setting of a suspected short esophagus. We have shown that the full esophageal mobilization afforded via thoracotomy often provides the extra 2 to 3 cm of esophageal length needed to avoid the need for a lengthening procedure. In patients suspected as having a short esophagus, we found that only about half of the patients needed a gastroplasty after complete transthoracic mobilization.[40] It has also been suggested that the gastroplasty segment continues to secrete acid, which may impact both symptomatic relief and healing of mucosal injury. Because preoperative indicators of esophageal shortening are present in only about 5% to 10% of patients with GERD, we continue to recommend an open approach in these patients. The laparoscopic gastroplasty procedure may occasionally be appropriate for patients in whom the short esophagus is unexpectedly encountered at the time of laparoscopic fundoplication.

Thoracoscopic Antireflux Procedures

Thoracoscopic creation of both the Belsey Mark IV and the Nissen fundoplication have been described.[41–43] However, neither has gained widespread acceptance. The rigidity of the thoracic cavity and the obliquity of the esophageal hiatus in relation to access via thoracoscopy leave much to be desired. Suturing, adequate fundic mobilization, and hiatal dissection are all considerably more difficult than they are by the laparoscopic approach. As a result, transthoracic access is best left for the minority of patients who require complete esophageal mobilization, in which case open thoracotomy should be performed.

Results

To be successful, antireflux surgery must provide long-term relief of reflux symptoms and not create complications or complaints secondary to the operation. Achieving these goals is more difficult than it seems. Careful attention to the principles of patient selection and to the technical details outlined will maximize the chances of success.

The decision as to whether to perform a complete or partial fundoplication is at times difficult. This issue continues to generate controversy. Proponents of the partial fundoplication argue that, when compared with a total fundoplication, partial wraps result in less postoperative bloating and dysphagia with equivalent reflux control. The former is possibly true, whereas the latter clearly is not. Recent reports have documented an unacceptably high prevalence of recurrent reflux following partial fundoplications.[44–46] In these studies, 24-h pH monitoring identified postoperative reflux in as many as 46% (22/48) of patients at an average of 2 to 3 years after surgery.[46] This finding is particularly true in patients with severe GERD. Risk factors for failure of the partial fundoplication were the presence of a defective lower esophageal sphincter, an aperistaltic distal esophagus, and the presence of erosive esophagitis (Savary–Miller grades 2–4).

Because they provide less effective reflux control, especially in advanced reflux disease, partial fundoplications should not be used routinely, and generally should be reserved for patients with mild reflux disease, such as those with a normal LES, small or absent hernia and no esophagitis, or those with abnormal esophageal motility. Even in the setting of poor motility, the use of partial fundoplication is being challenged, largely because the population of patients with GERD-induced motility abnormalities have the most severe reflux and thus are most likely to recur following a partial fundoplication. The clinician and the patient may be left with selecting the lesser of evils in such a circumstance, recurrent reflux versus postoperative dysphagia.

Postoperative complications occur in 8% to 10% (range, 2%–13%) of patients, and the rate of conversion to an open procedure is about 2% (range, 1%–10%). Mortality is uncommon. Symptomatic relief of typical reflux symptoms (heartburn, regurgitation, and dysphagia) can be expected in more than 90% of patients at follow-up intervals approaching 3 years (Table 3.1).

TABLE 3.1. Symptomatic outcome after laparoscopic fundoplication.

Author	Country	Relief of typical symptoms (%)	Relief of atypical symptoms (%)	Follow-up (months)
Watson (1995)[35]	Australia	98		16
Hunter (1996)[16]	USA	97	86	12
Gotley (1996)[72]	Australia	93		12
Cadiere (1997)[73]	Belgium	96		30
So (1998)[31]	USA	93	56	12
Allen (1998)[47]	Canada	93	83	6
Dallemagne (1998)[54]	Belgium	98		24
Peters (1998)[52]	USA	96		21
Ritter (1998)[29]	USA	97	50	18
Campos (1999)[32]	USA	92	67	15

These results compare favorably with those of the "modern" era of open fundoplication. Outcomes in patients with atypical reflux symptoms (cough, asthma, laryngitis) are less predictable, with relief expected in only about two-thirds of patients.[16,47,48]

Untoward side effects such as dysphagia (persisting >3 months) have been reported in 3% to 10% of patients. When dysphagia exists before surgery, it improves more often than not.[49] Temporary dysphagia is common after surgery (perhaps even desirable) and generally resolves within 3 months. In the authors' experience, occasional difficulty swallowing solids is present in 7% of patients at 3 months, 5% at 6 months, 2% at 12 months, and in a single patient at 24 months following surgery. Others have observed a similar improvement in postoperative dysphagia with time.

Objective studies have shown that more than 90% of patients will have negative pH studies 1 to 3 years following laparoscopic Nissen fundoplication.[50,51] We have recently shown that at follow-up approaching 2 years, 26 of 28 patients (93%) have negative pH studies.[52]

Mechanisms of Failure

Several authors have analyzed the most common reasons for failure following laparoscopic Nissen fundoplication.[53–56] Recurrent hernia of an intact or partially disrupted wrap has emerged as the most common anatomic reason for failure in the laparoscopic experience. Why this occurs is not clear, but it may be related to the selection of laparoscopic access in patients with a shortened esophagus, lack of or breakdown of the crural closure, less extensive esophageal mobilization, and, perhaps, a reduced tendency for adhesion formation after laparoscopic compared to open surgery. This finding is in contrast to the more common wrap disruption or "slippage" or the too long or too tight wraps that have plagued the open Nissen procedure. Dallemagne et al. suggested that technical quality of the operation was responsible for the majority of the failures (22/26, or 84.6%), most of which were secondary to the use of a Nissen–Rosetti fundopli-

cation (no short gastric division) and consequent dysphagia.[54] Horgan and Pellegrini have concluded that the most important technical factors preventing recurrence were effective crural closure, transhiatal esophageal mobilization, attention to the geometry of the fundoplication, and anchoring the wrap to the esophagus and surrounding tissues.[55]

One area that has received scant attention is the influence of body habitus on the outcome of laparoscopic fundoplication. A recent study identified obesity as a major factor in the failure of antireflux surgery. Perez et al. evaluated 224 patients after antireflux surgery, 187 after laparoscopic Nissen fundoplication, and 37 after open transthoracic Belsey repair.[56] At a mean follow-up time of 37 months, 12% of patients had objective evidence of recurrence. Patients with a body mass index (BMI) greater than 30 had a significantly higher recurrence rate (27%) than those with a BMI less than 25 (5%) or those with a BMI of 25 to 29 (8%).

Minimally Invasive Reoperative Antireflux Surgery

The results of remedial laparoscopic repair after failed open and laparoscopic primary procedures have been published.[53,57–60] Although it is clear that in many cases reoperative antireflux surgery can be accomplished, the wisdom of doing so remains to be established. It has been shown that the morbidity of laparoscopic redo fundoplication is considerably higher than after first-time procedures. However, on average 90% have been of reoperations completed laparoscopically when the initial procedure was laparoscopic, this figure dropping to 80% when the initial procedure was open. Only with additional experience can the wisdom of attempting reoperative antireflux surgery by laparoscopy be determined.

Cost

Laparoscopic antireflux surgery is also cost-effective. Three cost-utility analyses of long-term medical therapy versus laparoscopic fundoplication for GERD, one from the United States and two from Europe, have shown that the cost of open or laparoscopic surgery was less than that of lifelong daily therapy with proton pump inhibitors.[33,61,62] Even for men aged 65 to 69 years, the cost of lifelong omeprazole at either 20- or 40-mg dosage exceeded the costs of both open and laparoscopic surgery. Van Den Boom et al., reporting from the Netherlands, concluded that, when medical and surgical therapies were of similar cost, the break-even point was 4 years for open surgery and 17 months for laparoscopic surgery.[62] All three studies concluded that laparoscopic surgery was the most cost-effective form of treatment for patients likely to need lifelong therapy.

Future Prospects

Outpatient Laparoscopic Fundoplication

Compared to laparoscopic cholecystectomy, there has been more reticence to undertake laparoscopic fundoplication in an outpatient setting, which likely reflects the increased complexity of the surgery and the fact that laparoscopic fundoplication is a much less common procedure in most practice settings. Nonetheless, ambulatory laparoscopic fundoplication is being pursued with some success. In a consecutive series of 61 patients undergoing laparoscopic fundoplication, Milford and Paluch[63] found that all but 2 patients met the requirements for day-case surgery, and these 2 were excluded for reason of excessive driving distance from the hospital. Of the 59 patients considered suitable for day-case surgery, 54 (92%) were successfully treated and discharged on the same day. Two patients were admitted due to intraoperative complications (3%) (hemorrhage, esophageal perforation) and 3 (5%) were admitted because of excessive postoperative pain and nausea; all 5 admitted patients were discharged on the first postoperative day. The authors attributed their high success rate of day-case surgery to the use of preemptive anesthesia consisting of perioperative ketorolac and local anesthesia and careful attention to minimizing the use of parenteral narcotics. Several centers throughout the United States are exploring the feasibility of routine outpatient laparoscopic fundoplication.

Transoral Endoscopic Antireflux Procedures

Antireflux therapy delivered via flexible endoscopy is almost certainly on the horizon. Three approaches are currently under development: two are presently in phase III clinical trials and the third is about to begin phase II trials. These novel approaches include controlled scar formation at the GE junction, sphincter augmentation procedures, and creation of an endoscopic valvuloplasty.

Prevention of reflux by inducing scar formation was first described by Donahue and associates.[64] They attempted to increase the competence of the lower esophageal sphincter by injection of a sclerosant at the gastric cardia in dogs. Subsequent human studies failed to result in relief of reflux symptoms, however, and this approach has been abandoned. The concept has been revisited via the controlled delivery of multiple (50–200) small radiofrequency-induced lesions at the gastroesophageal junction.[65] This "controlled scar" is created after the introduction of a transoral delivery device fitted with a balloon for positioning at the gastroesophageal junction and eight radially oriented small needles for delivery of the energy. Phase II human trials have suggested considerable efficacy. A multicenter, placebo-controlled, phase III trial is currently underway.

In 1984, O'Connor and associates[66] investigated the use of both biodegradable and nonbiodegradable materials in the animal model as a means of preventing reflux by augmenting the lower esophageal sphincter pressure. Following the results of these experiments, collagen, the biodegradable substance, was injected into the lower esophagus in 10 patients with clinically documented severe gastroesophageal reflux disease.[67] The results were promising but short lived due to the absorption of the collagen. Shafik[68] later tried to bulk the esophagus at the level of the lower esophageal sphincter using a permanent Polytef material with marginal success. The major concern regarding the use of these permanent compounds is the demonstrated tendency for migration.

The final approach has been to create and endoluminal valvuloplasty using endoscopic or percutaneous transgastric sewing techniques. A mechanical aid, which allows passage of a needle and suturing via the biopsy port of an endoscope, has been developed and commercialized.[69] A neogastroesophageal valve is created by approximating the greater and lesser curve tissues around the body of the endoscope for 2 to 3 cm. Animal studies and phase II human trials have been completed with mixed success.[70] The main drawback of this technique is longevity. The stresses on the gastroesophageal junction created by belching, coughing, vomiting, and meals are significant, leading to suture failure in a substantial portion of patients. We have demonstrated both the efficacy and longevity of an endoluminal valvuloplasty performed via transgastric techniques in baboons.[71] Instrumentation necessary to perform this procedure percutaneously and/or endoscopically is currently in development.

Conclusion

Laparoscopic Nissen fundoplication has emerged as the procedure of choice for most surgical candidates with GERD. It is clear that laparoscopic fundoplication will abolish gastroesophageal reflux and relieve the typical symptoms of the disease in more than 90% of patients. Symptomatic relief has persisted for up to 4 years following surgery, and there is every reason to expect that the effect will persist for the life expectancy of most patients. Laparoscopic Nissen fundoplication is cost-effective, can be performed with little morbidity, and improves quality of life.

Given a high degree of confidence that a patient's symptoms are secondary to gastroesophageal reflux, selection of the appropriate procedure and operative approach, and careful operative technique on the part of their surgeons, most patients will wish they had undergone laparoscopic Nissen fundoplication years earlier.

References

1. DeVault KR, Castell DO. Guidelines for the diagnosis and treatment of gastroesophageal reflux disease. Practice Parameters Committee of the American College of Gastroenterology. Arch Intern Med 1995;155(20):2165–2173.

2. Rossetti M, Allgower M. Fundoplication for treatment of hiatal hernia. Prog Surg 1973;12:1–21.

3. Donahue PE, Samelson S, Nyhus LM, Bombeck CT. The floppy Nissen fundoplication. Effective long-term control of pathologic reflux. Arch Surg 1985;120(6):663–668.

4. DeMeester TR, Bonavina L, Albertucci M. Nissen fundoplication for gastroesophageal reflux disease. Evaluation of primary repair in 100 consecutive patients. Ann Surg 1986; 204(1):9–20.

5. Negre JB. Post-fundoplication symptoms. Do they restrict the success of Nissen fundoplication? Ann Surg 1983; 198(6):698–700.

6. Dallemagne B, Weerts JM, Jehaes C, Markiewicz S, Lombard R. Laparoscopic Nissen fundoplication: preliminary report. Surg Laparosc Endosc Percutan Tech 1991; 1(3):138–143.

7. Liebermann-Meffert DSH. Rudolf Nissen and the World Revolution of Fundoplication. St. Louis: Quality Medical, 1997.

8. Nebel OT, Fornes MF, Castell DO. Symptomatic gastroesophageal reflux: incidence and precipitating factors. Am J Dig Dis 1976;21(11):953–956.

9. Kaul BK, DeMeester TR, Oka M, et al. The cause of dysphagia in uncomplicated sliding hiatal and its relief by hiatal herniorrhaphy. A roentgenographic, manometric, and clinical study. Ann Surg 1990;211(4):406–410.

10. DeMeester TR, O'Sullivan GC, Bermudez G, Midell AI, Cimochowski GE, O'Drobinak J. Esophageal function in patients with angina-type chest pain and normal coronary angiograms. Ann Surg 1982;196(4):488–498.

11. Wiener GJ, Richter JE, Copper JB, Wu WC, Castell DO. The symptom index: a clinically important parameter of ambulatory 24-hour esophageal pH monitoring. Am J Gastroenterol 1988;83(4):358–361.

12. Irwin RS, Curley FJ, French CL. Chronic cough. The spectrum and frequency of causes, key components of the diagnostic evaluation, and outcome of specific therapy. Am Rev Respir Dis 1990;141(3):640–647.

13. Sontag SJ, O'Connell S, Khandelwal S, et al. Most asthmatics have gastroesophageal reflux with or without bronchodilator therapy [see comments]. Gastroenterology 1990;99(3):613–620.

14. Winters C Jr, Spurling TJ, Chobanian SJ, et al. Barrett's esophagus. A prevalent, occult complication of gastroesophageal reflux disease. Gastroenterology 1987;92(1): 118–124.

15. Jamieson GG, Watson DI, Britten-Jones R, Mitchell PC, Anvari M. Laparoscopic Nissen fundoplication. Ann Surg 1994;220(2):137–145.

16. Hunter JG, Trus TL, Branum GD, Waring JP, Wood WC. A physiologic approach to laparoscopic fundoplication for gastroesophageal reflux disease. Ann Surg 1996; 223(6):673–685; discussion 685–687.

17. Johnson LF, DeMeester TR. Development of the 24-hour intraesophageal pH monitoring composite scoring system. J Clin Gastroenterol 1986;8(suppl 1):52–58.

18. Campos GM, Peters JH, DeMeester TR, Oberg S, Crookes PF, Mason RJ. The pattern of esophageal acid exposure in gastroesophageal reflux disease influences the severity of the disease. Arch Surg 1999;134(8):882–887; discussion 887–888.

19. Nehra D, Howell P, Williams CP, Pye JK, Beynon J. Toxic bile acids in gastro-oesophageal reflux disease: influence of gastric acidity [see comments]. Gut 1999;44(5):598–602.

20. Costantini M, Zaninotto G, Anselmino M, Boccu C, Nicoletti L, Ancona E. The role of a defective lower esophageal sphincter in the clinical outcome of treatment for gastroesophageal reflux disease. Arch Surg 1996; 131(6):655–659.

21. Rakic S, Stein HJ, DeMeester TR, Hinder RN. Role of esophageal body function in gastroesophageal reflux disease: implications for surgical management. J Am Coll Surg 1997;185(4):380–387.

22. Kalloor GJ, Deshpande AH, Collis JL. Observations on oesophageal length. Thorax 1976;31(3):284–288.

23. Gozzetti G, Pilotti V, Spangaro M, et al. Pathophysiology and natural history of acquired short esophagus. Surgery (St. Louis) 1987;102(3):507–514.

24. Peters JH, DeMeester TR. The lessons of failed antireflux repairs. St. Louis: Quality Medical, 1994:188–196.

25. Stein HJ, Feussner H, Siewert JR. Failure of antireflux surgery: causes and management strategies. Am J Surg 1996;171(1):36–39; discussion 39–40.

26. Gastal OL, Hagen JA, Peters JH, et al. Short esophagus: analysis of predictors and clinical implications. Arch Surg 1999;134(6):633–636; discussion 637–638.

27. Swanstrom LL, Marcus DR, Galloway GQ. Laparoscopic Collis gastroplasty is the treatment of choice for the shortened esophagus [see comments]. Am J Surg 1996; 171(5):477–481.

28. Ritter MP, Peters JH, DeMeester TR, et al. Treatment of advanced gastroesophageal reflux disease with Collis gastroplasty and Belsey partial fundoplication. Arch Surg 1998;133(5):523–528; discussion 528–529.

29. Ritter MP, Peters JH, DeMeester TR, et al. Outcome after laparoscopic fundoplication is not dependent on a

structurally defective lower esophageal sphincter. J Gastrointest Surg 1998;2(6):567–572.

30. Johnson WE, Hagen JA, DeMeester TR, et al. Outcome of respiratory symptoms after antireflux surgery on patients with gastroesophageal reflux disease. Arch Surg 1996; 131(5):489–492.

31. So JB, Zeitels SM, Rattner DW. Outcomes of atypical symptoms attributed to gastroesophageal reflux treated by laparoscopic fundoplication. Surgery (St. Louis) 1998; 124(1):28–32.

32. Campos GM, Peters JH, DeMeester TR, Multivariate analysis of the factors predicting outcome after laparoscopic Nissen fundoplication. J Gastrointest Surg 1999;3: 292–300.

33. Viljakka M, Nevalainen J, Isolauri J. Lifetime costs of surgical versus medical treatment of severe gastro-oesophageal reflux disease in Finland. Scand J Gastroenterol 1997;32(8):766–772.

34. Dalenbak J, Lonroth H, Blomqvist A, Lundell L. Improved functional outcome after laparoscopic fundoplication by complete gastric fundus mobilization. Gastroenterology 1998;114:A1384 [abstract].

35. Watson DI, Jamieson GG, Devitt PG, Mitchell PC, Game PA. Paraoesophageal hiatus hernia: an important complication of laparoscopic Nissen fundoplication [see comments]. Br J Surg 1995;82(4):521–523.

36. Swanstrom LL. Laparoscopic partial fundoplications. Probl Gen Surg 1996;13:75–84.

37. Johnson AB, Oddsdottir M, Hunter JG. Laparoscopic Collis gastroplasty and Nissen fundoplication. A new technique for the management of esophageal foreshortening. Surg Endosc 1998;12(8):1055–1060.

38. Jobe BA, Horvath KD, Swanstrom LL. Postoperative function following laparoscopic collis gastroplasty for shortened esophagus. Arch Surg 1998;133(8):867–874.

39. Swanstrom LL, Marcus DR, Galloway GQ. Laparoscopic Collis gastroplasty is the treatment of choice for the shortened esophagus [see comments]. Am J Surg 1996; 171(5):477–481.

40. Gastal OL, Hagen JA, Peters JH, et al. Short esophagus: analysis of predictors and clinical implications. Arch Surg 1999;134(6):633–636; discussion 637–638.

41. Yang HK, Del Guercio LRM, Steichen FM. Thoracoscopic Belsey Mark IV fundoplication. Surg Rounds 1997: 277–291.

42. Demos NJ, Kulkarni VA, Arago A. A video assisted transthoracichiatal hernioplasty using stapled, uncut gastroplasty and fundoplication. Surg Rounds 1994: 427–436.

43. Salo JA, Kivulisko T, Heikkila L. Thoracoscopic fundoplication. Ann Chir Gynaecol 1993;82:199–201.

44. Bell RC, Hanna P, Mills MR, Bowrey D. Patterns of success and failure with laparoscopic Toupet fundoplication. Surg Endosc 1999;13(12):1189–1194.

45. Jobe BA, Wallace J, Hansen PD, Swanstrom LL. Evaluation of laparoscopic Toupet fundoplication as a primary repair for all patients with medically resistant gastroesophageal reflux. Surg Endosc 1999;11(11):1080–1083.

46. Horvath KD, Jobe BA, Herron DM, Swanstrom LL. Laparoscopic Toupet fundoplication is an inadequate pro-cedure for patients with severe reflux disease. J Gastrointest Surg 1999;3:583–591 [abstract].

47. Allen CJ, Anvari M. Gastro-oesophageal reflux related cough and its response to laparoscopic fundoplication. Thorax 1998;53(11):963–968.

48. Cornwell CJ, Trus T, Waring JP. Pattern of failure and results of redo fundoplication. Society of American Gastrointestinal Endoscopic Surgeon.

49. Patti MG, Feo CV, De Pinto M, et al. Results of laparoscopic antireflux surgery for dysphagia and gastroesophageal reflux disease. Am J Surg 1998;176(6):564–568.

50. Hinder RA, Filipi CJ, Wetscher G, Neary P, DeMeester TR, Perdikis G. Laparoscopic Nissen fundoplication is an effective treatment for gastroesophageal reflux disease. Ann Surg 1994;220(4):472–481; discussion 481–483.

51. Watson DI, Jamieson GG, Pike GK, Davies N, Richardson M, Devitt PG. Prospective randomized double-blind trial between laparoscopic Nissen fundoplication and anterior partial fundoplication [see comments]. Br J Surg 1999; 86(1):123–130.

52. Peters JH, DeMeester TR, Crookes P, et al. The treatment of gastroesophageal reflux disease with laparoscopic Nissen fundoplication: prospective evaluation of 100 patients with "typical" symptoms. Ann Surg 1998;228(1): 40–50.

53. Soper NJ, Dunnegan D. Anatomic fundoplication failure after laparoscopic antireflux surgery. Ann Surg 1999;229 (5):669–676; discussion 676–677.

54. Dallemagne B, Weerts JM, Jehaes C, Markiewicz S. Causes of failures of laparoscopic antireflux operations. Surg Endosc 1996;10(3):305–310.

55. Horgan S, Pohl D, Bogetti D, Eubanks T, Pellegrini C. Failed antireflux surgery: what have we learned from reoperations? Arch Surg 1999;134(8):809–815; discussion 815–817.

56. Perez AR, Moncure AC, Rattner DW. Obesity is a major cause of failure for both transabdominal and transthoracic antireflux operations. 100th Annual Meeting of the American Gastroenterological Association.

57. Curet MJ, Josloff RK, Schoeb O, Zucker KA. Laparoscopic reoperation for failed antireflux procedures. Arch Surg 1999;134(5):559–563.

58. DePaula AL, Hashiba K, Bafutto M, Machado CA. Laparoscopic reoperations after failed and complicated antireflux operations. Surg Endosc 1995;9(6):681–686.

59. Floch NR, Hinder RA, Klingler PJ, et al. Is laparoscopic reoperation for failed antireflux surgery feasible? Arch Surg 1999;134(7):733–737.

60. Watson DI, Jamieson GG, Game PA, Williams RS, Devitt PG. Laparoscopic reoperation following failed antireflux surgery. Br J Surg 1999;86(1):98–101.

61. Heudebert GR, Marks R, Wilcox CM, Centor RM. Choice of long-term strategy for the management of patents with severe esophagitis: a cost-utility analysis [see comments]. Gastroenterology 1997;112(4):1078–1086.

62. Van Den Boom G, Go PM, Hameeteman W, Dallemagne B, Ament AJ. Cost effectiveness of medical versus surgical treatment in patients with severe or refractory gastroesophageal reflux disease in the Netherlands. Scand J Gastroenterology 1996;31(1):1–9.

63. Milford MA, Paluch TA. Ambulatory laparoscopic fundo-plication. Surg Endosc 1997;11(12):1150–1152.

64. Donahue PE, Carvalho P, Yoshida J, et al. Endoscopic sclerosis of the cardia affects gastroesophageal reflux. Surg Endosc 1989;3(1):11–12.

65. Utley DS, Vierra MA, Kim MS, Triadafilopoulos G. Augmentation of the lower esophageal sphincter pressure and gastric yield pressure after radiofrequency energy delivery to the lower esophageal sphincter muscle; a porcine model. Gastrointest Endosc 1999;49:AB133.

66. O'Connor KW, Madison SA, Smith DJ, Ransburg RC, Lehman GA. An experimental endoscopic technique for reversing gastroesophageal reflux in dogs by injecting inert material in the distal esophagus. Gastrointest Endosc 1984; 30(5):275–280.

67. O'Conner KW, Lehman GA. Endoscopic placement of collagen at the lower esophageal sphincter to inhibit gastroe-sophageal reflux; a pilot study of 10 medically intractable patients. Gastrointest Endosc 1988;34(2):106–112.

68. Shafik A. Intraesophageal Polytef injection for the treatment of reflux esophagitis. Surg Endosc 1996;10(3):329–331.

69. Kadirkamanathan SS, Evans DF, Gong F, Yazaki E, Scott M, Swain CP. Antireflux operations at flexible endoscopy using endoluminal stitching techniques; an experimental study. Gastrointest Endosc 1996;44:133–143.

70. Kadirkamanathan SS, Yazaki E, Evans DF, Hepworth CC, Gong F, Swain CP. An ambulant porcine model of acid reflux used to evaluate endoscopic gastroplasty. Gut 1999; 44:782–788.

71. Mason RJ, Filipi CJ, DeMeester TR, et al. A new intraluminal antireflux procedure. Gastrointest Endosc 1997;45: 283–290.

4
Laparoscopic Esophageal Myotomy

Marco G. Patti, Urs Diener, and Carlos A. Pellegrini

Esophageal achalasia is a primary motility disorder of unknown etiology, characterized by the absence of esophageal peristalsis and increased resting pressure of the lower esophageal sphincter (LES), which fails to relax completely in response to swallowing. Treatment is palliative, and it is directed toward elimination of the outflow resistance at the level of the gastroesophageal junction caused by the abnormal LES function.

Clinical Features

Dysphagia is the most common symptom, experienced by virtually any patient.[1,2] It occurs mostly in response to solids, but it can also manifest for liquids. Some patients are able to adapt with changes in their diet, but others experience progressive increase of the dysphagia, which eventually leads to weight loss.

Regurgitation, the second most common symptom, is present in about 60% of patients.[1,2] It occurs more often in the supine position and exposes the patients to the risk of aspiration of undigested food.

Heartburn is experienced by about 40% of patients. It is quite common that patients are treated for a long time with acid-reducing medications, on the assumption that gastroesophageal reflux disease is the underlying problem. Interestingly, abnormal reflux is quite rare in untreated patients with achalasia,[3] and this symptom is usually caused by stasis and fermentation of food in the distal esophagus.[4,5]

Chest pain also occurs in about 40% of patients, and is usually experienced at the time of a meal.[1,2]

Preoperative Investigations

In addition to a careful symptomatic evaluation, the following tests should be routinely performed in the evaluation of a patient with suspected achalasia.[6]

Barium swallow should be the first test performed in the evaluation of dysphagia; it usually shows narrowing at the level of the gastroesophageal junction ("bird beak") and various degrees of dilatation of the esophageal body. Among 154 patients we treated between 1991 and 1998 by minimally invasive techniques,[1] we found that the esophageal diameter was less than 4 cm in 73 patients (48%), between 4 and 6 cm in 33 patients (21%), and more than 6 cm in 48 patients (31%). A barium swallow is also very important in the evaluation of a patient with persistent or recurrent dysphagia after a previous myotomy.

Endoscopy should follow the barium swallow. This test rules out the presence of a peptic or malignant stricture and gastroduodenal pathology.

Esophageal manometry is the key test for establishing the diagnosis. The classic manometric findings are (a) absence of esophageal peristalsis, and (b) hypertensive LES, which relaxes only partially in response to swallowing. When the esophagus is dilated and sigmoid in shape, it may be difficult to pass the catheter through the gastroesophageal junction into the stomach; in these case the catheter may be placed under fluoroscopic or endoscopic guidance.

Prolonged pH monitoring is very important for the evaluation of the following clinical situations.

1. Patients with heartburn. In patients with achalasia and heartburn, a positive score does not automatically imply the presence of abnormal gastroesophageal reflux. The tracings should always be carefully examined to distinguish between *false* reflux due to stasis and fermentation of food and *real* reflux caused by acid refluxing from the stomach into the esophagus.[4,5]

2. Patients with residual dysphagia after pneumatic dilatation, for whom a myotomy is planned. About 23% to 35% of patients develop abnormal reflux after pneumatic dilatation.[7,8] This information is of paramount importance for the surgeon planning an operation, as it indicates the need for a partial fundoplication in addition

to the myotomy. In our experience, a laparoscopic Heller myotomy and Dor fundoplication corrected abnormal reflux due to previous dilatations in 71% of patients.[1]

3. Any patient after Heller myotomy. About 60% of patients after thoracoscopic myotomy and 15% of patients after laparoscopic myotomy and partial fundoplication develop abnormal reflux.[1] Because the reflux is asymptomatic in the majority of patients, only pH monitoring, routinely performed postoperatively, can detect it. These patients should be treated with acid-reducing medications.

In patients with excessive weight loss, who are older than 60 years of age, and who have recent onset of dysphagia, *secondary achalasia* or *pseudoachalasia* should be ruled out.[9] Because a cancer of the gastroesophageal junction is the most common cause of pseudoachalasia, an endoscopic ultrasound and a CT scan of the gastroesophageal junction can help establish the diagnosis.[10]

Nonsurgical Therapeutic Techniques

Therapy is palliative and is directed toward relief of symptoms by decreasing the outflow resistance caused by the dysfunctional LES. Because peristalsis is absent, gravity becomes the key factor that allows progression of food from the esophagus into the stomach. The following treatment modalities are available to achieve this goal.

Pneumatic Dilatation

Pneumatic dilatation has been for many years the first line of treatment for esophageal achalasia. This technique was first popularized by Vantrappen, who reported good to excellent results in 77% of patients and a perforation rate of only 2.6%.[11] At that time, however, it became clear that these results were not easily reproducible in other centers. For instance, when we analyzed our own experience with pneumatic dilatation at the University of California San Francisco between 1977 and 1988, we found that the perforation rate was 12%.[12] In addition, at 4-year follow-up, only 50% of patients remained asymptomatic, but 20% had persistent dysphagia and 30% had symptoms of gastroesophageal reflux. More recent clinical series, using better and safer dilators, have shown that the success rate is between 70% and 85%, with a perforation rate of less than 5%.[13–15] The following issues must be taken into consideration before choosing pneumatic dilatation as the initial form of treatment for achalasia.

- Pneumatic dilatation is not as effective as surgery in relieving symptoms. In the past 20 years only a few studies have compared these two treatment modalities retrospectively[16,17] or prospectively[18] and have clearly shown the superiority of the surgical approach. Because of the fear of a long hospital stay, postoperative pain, and long recovery time, surgery previously had been relegated to a *remedial* form of treatment, mostly for patients who had suffered a perforation during dilatation or who had persistent dysphagia after multiple dilatations. Today, minimally invasive surgery has completely changed this treatment algorithm, as it is possible to achieve the same results obtained with open surgery, but with a short hospital stay, minimal postoperative discomfort, and fast recovery time.[1]

- Abnormal gastroesophageal reflux. When measured by pH monitoring, abnormal reflux after pneumatic dilatation has been found in 23% to 35% of patients.[7,8] It is important to stress the value of these studies, as the authors assessed objectively the incidence of post-dilatation reflux by pH monitoring, rather than relying on symptoms that are not a reliable indicator of the presence of reflux.[1,4,5]

- Esophageal perforation. About 5% of patients suffer a perforation at the time of the dilatation. These patients require open surgery to close the perforation and perform a myotomy, therefore losing the advantages of a minimally invasive operation.

Based on these considerations, we believe that today pneumatic dilatation should be used for patients who do not want surgery, or when adequate surgical expertise is not available, or to treat postmyotomy strictures.[19]

Intrasphincteric Injection of Botulinum Toxin

The pressure and relaxation of the LES are regulated by the interplay of excitatory (acetylcholine) and inhibitory neurotransmitters (nitric oxide and vasoactive intestinal peptide).[20] In achalasia, this balance is skewed by the loss of inhibitory nerves, resulting in a hypertensive and nonrelaxing LES.[21,22] The rationale for the intrasphincteric injection of botulinum toxin is to restore this balance by blocking acetylcholine release.[23] However, multiple clinical studies have shown that symptomatic relief is achieved in only 60% of patients after 6 months[23,24] and that only 30% of patients are still symptom free after 1 year.[25] In addition to the poor long-term efficacy, other concerns about this treatment modality are emerging.[26–28] Botulinum toxin injection may cause an inflammatory reaction at the level of the gastroesophageal junction, which can obliterate the anatomic planes. Consequently, a laparoscopic myotomy is more difficult, a mucosal perforation occurs more frequently, and the relief of dysphagia is less predictable. Because of these shortcomings, it is thought that botulinum toxin injections should be reserved for elderly and high-risk patients who are poor candidates for dilatation or surgery.[29]

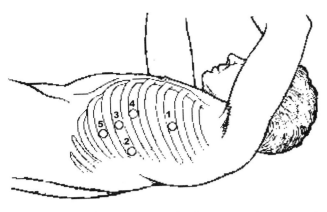

FIGURE 4.1. Position of trocars (1–5) for left thoracoscopic myotomy.

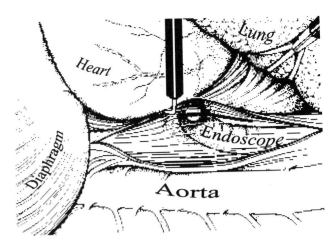

FIGURE 4.2. Intraoperative endoscopy.

Surgical Techniques

Open Surgery

A Heller myotomy involves the longitudinal division of the musculature of the distal 6 cm of the esophagus, extending onto the gastric wall for 0.5 to 2.0 cm. The procedure was traditionally performed through the left chest or the abdomen, alone or in combination with an antireflux procedure.[16–18,30–32] Excellent or good results were obtained in 90% to 94% of patients. Today, however, open surgery is mostly of historical interest, as it has been completely replaced by minimally invasive surgery.

Minimally Invasive Surgery

Cuschieri was the first to describe the technique of laparoscopic Heller myotomy for achalasia.[33] Subsequently, many centers in the world have shown that the results obtained with this new approach are as good as open surgery but with a shorter hospital stay, minimal postoperative discomfort, and faster return to work.[1,34–45] The success of minimally invasive surgery has resulted in a shift in practice, whereby today laparoscopic surgery is preferred by most gastroenterologists and surgeons as the primary treatment. The operation can be performed by either a thoracoscopic or laparoscopic approach.

Thoracoscopic Heller Myotomy

Technique

After induction of general endotracheal anesthesia with a double-lumen tube, the patient is positioned in a right lateral decubitus over an inflated beanbag, as for a left thoracotomy. A flexible endoscope is inserted into the esophagus. Four ports are used for the procedure (Fig. 4.1). Port 1, in the third intercostal space, about 2 cm ante-

rior to the posterior axillary line, is used for initial inspection of the thoracic cavity and to allow placement of the other ports under direct vision. Subsequently, port 1 is used for the insertion of the lung retractor. Port 2, in the seventh intercostal space 4 cm behind the posterior axillary line, is used for the scope. Port 3, in the sixth intercostal space in the anterior axillary line, is used for insertion of a grasper. Port 4, in the seventh intercostal space in the midaxillary line, is used for the insertion of the hook cautery (or bipolar scissors). An additional port (port 5) can be used to depress the diaphragm and improve the exposure of the gastroesophageal junction.

The procedure is started by dividing the inferior pulmonary ligament and retracting the left lung upward. By means of transillumination and tilting the tip of the endoscope, the esophagus is identified in the groove between the aorta and heart (Fig. 4.2). The mediastinal pleura is then incised. The myotomy is started in a point halfway between the diaphragm and the inferior pulmonary vein (Fig. 4.3). Once the submucosal plane is reached, the

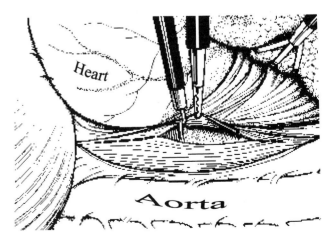

FIGURE 4.3. Starting the myotomy.

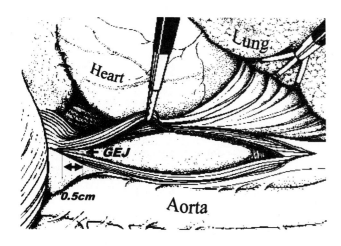

FIGURE 4.4. Completed myotomy. The myotomy extends for 0.5 cm onto the gastric wall. *GEJ*, gastroesophageal junction.

myotomy is extended downward and upward for about 7 cm. The distal extension of the myotomy is the most delicate part of the operation; if the myotomy is too short, the patient will have persistent dysphagia, but if it is too long abnormal reflux can occur postoperatively. Using the endoscopic view as a guide, we extend the myotomy for about 0.5 cm onto the gastric wall (Fig. 4.4). If there is any question about the integrity of the mucosa, the esophagus can be covered with water while air is insufflated through the endoscope. If a perforation is identified, it can be closed using fine absorbable sutures. The procedure is completed by inserting a 22 French chest tube through port 4. No nasogastric tube is left in place.

Hospital Course

We do not routinely obtain an esophagogram postoperatively. Patients are allowed to eat starting the morning of the first postoperative day. The chest tube is usually removed within 24 h. Pain control is achieved with narcotics initially and with oral pain medications after the chest tube is removed. Patients are discharged home between 48 and 72 h later.

Results

Between 1991 and 1994, we attempted 35 thoracoscopic myotomies. Thirty-three procedures were completed thoracoscopically, but a thoracotomy was performed in 2 patients to repair a mucosal perforation.[1] One patient, in whom a perforation developed postoperatively (probably caused by thermal damage by the hook cautery), underwent a transhiatal esophagectomy. Four patients had residual dysphagia due to a short myotomy. The myotomy was extended distally laparoscopically, with resolution of the dysphagia in all patients.

Postoperative function tests were performed in 10 patients. LES pressure decreased from 30 mmHg preop-

eratively to 9 mmHg postoperatively. Abnormal reflux was detected in 6 of 10 patients (60%), 5 of whom were asymptomatic.

Overall, 85% of patients considered their swallowing status as excellent or good at a median follow-up of 72 months.[1]

Laparoscopic Heller Myotomy and Partial Fundoplication

Technique

After induction of general endotracheal anesthesia with a single-lumen endotracheal tube, the patient is positioned supine on the operating table over an inflated beanbag. The legs are extended on stirrups. An orogastric tube is inserted after induction of anesthesia to keep the stomach decompressed, and it is removed at the end of the procedure. Pneumatic compression stockings are routinely used as prophylaxis against deep vein thrombosis. The procedure is performed with the patient in a steep reverse Trendelenburg position; the surgeon stands between the patient's legs. Five trocars are used for the procedure (Fig. 4.5). Trocar 1, about 15 cm below the xiphoid process in the midline, is used for the camera. Trocar 2, right midclavicular line, is used for the liver retractor. Trocar 3, left midclavicular line, is used for the Babcock clamp and for the laparosonic coagulating shears. Trocars 4 and 5, just below the costal margin, are used for the dissecting and suturing instruments.

The operation is started by dividing the gastrohepatic ligament. Subsequently, the right crus is separated by blunt dissection from the esophagus, the peritoneum overlying the esophagus is transected, and the left crus is dissected. Except in patients undergoing a posterior partial fundoplication, mobilization of the esophagus is

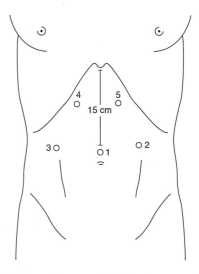

FIGURE 4.5. Position of trocars (*1–5*) for laparoscopic myotomy.

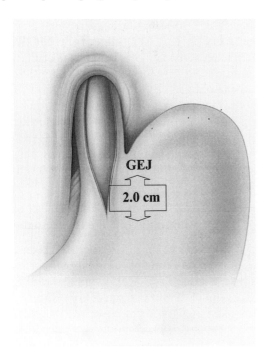

FIGURE 4.6. Completed myotomy. The myotomy extends for 2.0 cm onto the gastric wall.

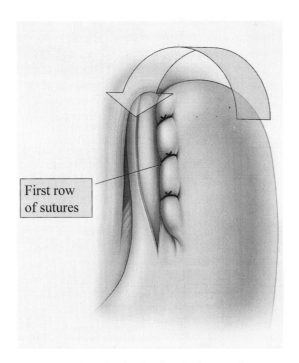

FIGURE 4.7. Dor fundoplication. Left row of sutures.

just proximal to the gastroesophageal junction and is extended proximally for about 6 cm and distally for about 2 cm onto the gastric wall (Fig. 4.6). The short gastric vessels are then divided, and a Dor fundoplication is constructed. The first row of sutures incorporates the gastric fundus and the left side of the esophageal wall (Fig. 4.7). The stomach is then folded over the myotomy, and a second row of sutures is placed between the fundus and the right side of the esophageal wall; the uppermost stitch also incorporates the right crus. Finally, two additional sutures are placed between the fundus and the anterior rim of the hiatus (Fig. 4.8).

Hospital Course

Patients are allowed to eat starting the morning of the first postoperative day. Pain control is usually achieved with narcotics for the first 12 h after the operation and with oral pain medications thereafter. Patients are discharged home between 24 and 48 h.

Results

Between 1993 and 1998, we attempted 133 laparoscopic myotomies.[1] A laparotomy was performed in 1 patient to evaluate a retroperitoneal hematoma caused by a Verress needle puncture of the inferior vena cava. A Dor fundoplication was performed in 125 patients (94%) and a posterior partial fundoplication in 8 patients (6%).

Mucosal perforations occurred in six patients (4.5%) and were all repaired laparoscopically. Three of the six patients had been treated with pneumatic dilatation, and

limited to the lateral and anterior aspects, leaving the posterior attachments intact. The myotomy can be performed in the 11 o'clock position (to the right of the anterior vagus nerve), or the 2 o'clock position (to the left of the anterior vagus nerver). The myotomy is started

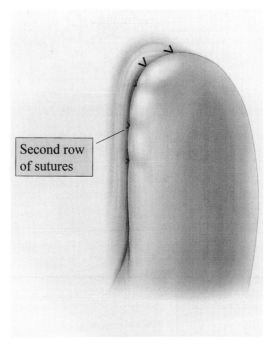

FIGURE 4.8. Completed Dor fundoplication.

a transmural stricture was found at the level of the gastroesophageal junction in two of them. The other three patients had been treated with intrasphincteric injections of botulinum toxin, and a severe inflammatory reaction had developed at the level of the gastroesophageal junction, which obliterated the normal anatomic planes.

Ten patients had *persistent* dysphagia after the first operation. The Dor fundoplication was considered the cause of the problem in 3 patients, which was taken down laparoscopically with resolution of symptoms. Pneumatic dilatation was effective in 1 patient only. Two patients had *recurrent* dysphagia after a symptom-free interval of 12 months, probably because of healing of the distal portion of the myotomy. Both patients are scheduled for a second operation, with the intent of extending the previous myotomy or performing a second myotomy on the opposite side of the esophagus.

Postoperative function tests were performed in 35 patients. LES pressure decreased from 28 mmHg preoperatively to 10 mmHg postoperatively. Abnormal reflux was detected in 6 patients (17%), 5 of whom were asymptomatic. Overall, 93% of patients considered their swallowing status as excellent or good at a median follow-up of 23 months.[1]

Comments

These results show that minimally invasive surgery allows the same excellent results traditionally obtained with open surgery but with a shorter hospital stay, minimal postoperative discomfort, and faster recovery. In addition, although the myotomy can be performed by either a thoracoscopic or laparoscopic approach, we believe that a laparoscopic Heller myotomy and Dor fundoplication is today the procedure of choice for the following reasons.

Exposure of the Gastroesophageal Junction

Exposure of the junction is clearly the most important and delicate part of the operation, because if the myotomy is too short the patient will have residual dysphagia but if it is too long gastroesophageal reflux will occur. When the myotomy is done through a left thoracoscopic approach, exposure of the gastroesophageal junction is difficult, even using an additional port to depress the diaphragm. Determination of the distal extent of the myotomy is often tricky, and even with the routine use of intraoperative endoscopy, problems with the distal endpoint of the myotomy occurred in 10 of the 35 patients (29%). Four patients, in fact, had a short myotomy that required laparoscopic extension; 6 patients had a too long myotomy with postoperative gastroesophageal reflux. In contrast, the laparoscopic approach

allows an excellent view of the distal esophagus, gastroesophageal junction, and stomach, even better than with open techniques. Dissection and removal of the fat pad increases the ability of the surgeon to identify clearly the transition between esophageal and gastric wall, and the longer extension onto the gastric wall ensures that the myotomy has been carried down through the entire high pressure zone. Intraoperative endoscopy is useful, particularly at the beginning of the laparoscopic experience or when scarring from previous treatment is encountered.[46,47]

Postoperative Gastroesophageal Reflux

In the past, the focus of surgery for achalasia was only on the *relief of dysphagia*; today, *prevention or correction of reflux* is also a recognized goal of the operation. In the past, the real incidence of postoperative reflux was probably underestimated as it was based on the presence of heartburn.[31] However, when objectively measured by pH monitoring, it became clear that the incidence of postoperative reflux was about 29% after transthoracic myotomy[32] but only 7% after transabdominal Heller and Dor fundoplication.[30] Our experience confirms that a fundoplication is an essential part of the operation, as postoperative reflux occurred in 60% of patients after a thoracoscopic myotomy but in only 17% of patients when a partial fundoplication was added to the myotomy.[1] Other groups have shown a low incidence of postoperative reflux after laparoscopic Heller myotomy and partial fundoplication.[37,38,40] For instance, Costantini and colleagues recently reported their experience with 100 laparoscopic Heller myotomies and Dor fundoplication for achalasia.[45] Excellent results were obtained in 93% of patients, with a incidence of postoperative reflux of only 6.3% (as measured by pH monitoring).

In addition, some patients have already abnormal reflux from previous dilatations. We encountered seven such patients, and five (71%) had normal reflux scores after laparoscopic Heller myotomy and Dor fundoplication.[1]

Operative and Postoperative Course

The positioning of the patient is much faster and anesthesia is simpler for a laparoscopic operation. After a laparoscopic operation patients are more comfortable (no chest tube), require fewer narcotics, and leave the hospital earlier.

Conclusions

The past 10 years have seen a tremendous evolution in the treatment of esophageal achalasia. We believe that the results obtained by minimally invasive surgery have convincingly put to rest the controversy between pneumatic dilatation and Heller myotomy. A laparoscopic Heller myotomy and partial fundoplication should be considered today the first line of treatment for patients with achalasia, relegating pneumatic dilatation to a secondary role for failures of surgery or when adequate surgical expertise is not available.

References

1. Patti MG, Pellegrini CA, Horgan, S, et al. Minimally invasive surgery for achalasia. An 8 year experience with 168 patients. Ann Surg 1999;230:587–594.
2. Wong RKH, Maydonovitch CL. Achalasia. In: Castell DO (ed) The Esophagus. Boston: Little, Brown, 1992:233–275.
3. Shoenut JP, Trenholm BG, Micflikier AB, et al. Reflux patterns in patients with achalasia without operation. Ann Thorac Surg 1988;45:303–305.
4. Crookes PF, Corkill S, DeMeester T. Gastroesophageal reflux in achalasia. When Is reflux really reflux? Dig Dis Sci 1997:1354–1361.
5. Patti MG, Arcerito M, Tong J, et al. Importance of preoperative and postoperative pH monitoring in patients with esophageal achalasia. J Gastrointest Surg 1997;1:505–510.
6. Patti MG, Way LW. Evaluation and treatment of primary esophageal motility disorders. West J Med 1997;166:263–269.
7. Benini L, Sembenini C, Castellani G, et al. Pathological esophageal acidification and pneumatic dilatation in achalasic patients. Too much or not enough? Dig Dis Sci 1996; 41:365–371.
8. Shoenut JP, Duerksen D, Yaffe CS. A prospective assessment of gastroesophageal reflux before and after treatment of achalasia patients: pneumatic dilation *versus* transthoracic limited myotomy. Am J Gastroenterol 1997;92: 1109–1112.
9. Kahrilas PJ, Kishk SM, Helm JF, et al. Comparison of pseudoachalasia and achalasia. Am J Med 1987;82:439–446.
10. Moonka R, Patti MG, Feo CV, et al. Clinical presentation and evaluation of malignant pseudoachalasia. J Gastrointest Surg 1999;3:456–461.
11. Vantrappen G, Hellemans J. Treatment of achalasia and related motor disorders. Gastroenterology 1980;79:144–154.
12. Sauer L, Pellegrini CA, Way LW. The treatment of achalasia. A current perspective. Arch Surg 1989;124:929–932.
13. Abid S, Champion G, Richter JE, et al. Treatment of achalasia: the best of both worlds. Am J Gastroenterol 1994; 89:979–985.
14. Spiess AE, Kahrilas PJ. Treating achalasia. From whalebone to laparoscope. JAMA 1998;280:638–642.
15. Katz PO, Gilber J, Castell DO. Pneumatic dilatation is effective long-term treatment for achalasia. Dig Dis Sci 1998; 43:1973–1977.
16. Okike N, Payne WS, Neufeld DM, et al. Esophagomyotomy versus forceful dilation for achalasia of the esophagus: results in 899 patients. Ann Thorac Surg 1979;28:119–125.
17. Ferguson MK. Achalasia: current evaluation and therapy. Ann Thorac Surg 1991;52:336–342.
18. Csendes A, Braghetto I, Henriquez A, et al. Late results of a prospective randomised study comparing forceful dilatation and oesophagomyotomy in patients with achalasia. Gut 1989;30:299–304.
19. Parkman HP, Ogorek CP, Harris AD, et al. Nonoperative management of esophageal strictures following esophagomyotomy for achalasia. Dig Dis Sci 1994;39:2102–2108.
20. Murthy KS, Makhlouf GM. Interplay of VIP and nitric oxide in the regulation of neuromuscular function in the gut. Regul Pept Lett 1995;VI:33–38.
21. Aggestrup S, Uddman R, Sundler F, et al. Lack of vasoactive intestinal polypeptide nerves in esophageal achalasia. Gastroenterology 1983;84:924–927.
22. Holloway RH, Dodds WJ, Helm JF, et al. Integrity of cholinergic innervation to the lower esophageal sphincter in achalasia. Gastroenterology 1986;90:924–929.
23. Pasricha PJ, Ravich WJ, Hendrix TR, et al. Intrasphincteric botulinum toxin for the treatment of achalasia. N Engl J Med 1995;322:774–778.
24. Cuilliere C, Ducrotte P, Metman EH, et al. Achalasia: outcome of patients treated with intrasphincteric injection of botulinum toxin. Gut 1997;41:87–92.
25. Vaezi MF, Richter JE, Wilcox CM, et al. Botulinum toxin versus pneumatic dilatation in the treatment of achalasia: a randomised trial. Gut 1999;44:231–239.
26. Eaker EY, Gordon JM, Vogel SB. Untoward effects of esophageal botulinum toxin injection in the treatment of achalasia. Dig Dis Sci 1997;42:724–727.
27. Horgan S, Hudda K, Eubanks T, et al. Does botulinum toxin injection make esophagomyotomy a more difficult operation? Surg Endosc 1999;13:576–579.
28. Patti MG, Feo CV, Arcerito M, et al. The effects of previous treatment on the results of myotomy for achalasia. Dig Dis Sci 1999;44:2270–2276.
29. Castell DO, Katzka DA. Botulinum toxin for achalasia: to be or not to be? Gastroenterology 1996;110:1650–1652.
30. Bonavina L, Nosadini A, Bardini R, et al. Primary treatment of esophageal achalasia. Long-term results of myotomy and Dor fundoplication. Arch Surg 1992;127:222–227.
31. Ellis FH Jr. Oesophagomyotomy for achalasia: a 22-year experience. Br J Surg 1993;80:882–885.
32. Streitz JM Jr, Ellis FH Jr, Williamson WA, et al. Objective assessment of gastroesophageal reflux after short esophagomyotomy for achalasia with the use of manometry and pH monitoring. J Thorac Surg 1996;111:107–113.
33. Shimi S, Nathanson LK, Cuschieri A. Laparoscopic cardiomyotomy for achalasia. J R Coll Surg Edinb 1991;36:152–154.
34. Pellegrini C, Wetter LA, Patti M, et al. Thoracoscopic esophagomyotomy. Initial experience with a new approach for the treatment of achalasia. Ann Surg 1992;216:291–299.
35. Ancona E, Anselmino M, Zaninotto G, et al. Esophageal achalasia: laparoscopic versus conventional open Heller–Dor operation. Am J Surg 1995;170:265–270.
36. Patti MG, Pellegrini CA, Arcerito M, et al. Comparison of medical and minimally invasive surgical therapy for primary esophageal motility disorders. Arch Surg 1995;130: 609–616.

37. Swanstrom LL, Pennings J. Laparoscopic esophagomyotomy for achalasia. Surg Endosc 1995;9:286–292.

38. Mitchell PC, Watson DI, Devitt PG, et al. Laparoscopic cardiomyotomy with a Dor patch for achalasia. CJS (Can J Surg) 1995;38:445–448.

39. Holzman MD, Sharp KW, Ladipo JK, et al. Laparoscopic surgical treatment of achalasia. Am J Surg 1997;173: 308–311.

40. Hunter JG, Trus TL, Branum GD, et al. Laparoscopic Heller myotomy and fundoplication for achalasia. Ann Surg 1997;225:655–665.

41. Vogt D, Curet M, Pitcher D, et al. Successful treatment of esophageal achalasia with laparoscopic Heller myotomy and Toupet fundoplication. Am J Surg 1997;174:709–714.

42. Patti MG, Arcerito M, De Pinto M, et al. Comparison of thoracoscopic and laparoscopic Heller myotomy for achalasia. J Gastrointest Surg 1998;2:561–566.

43. Rosati R, Fumagalli U, Bona S, et al. Evaluating results of laparoscopic surgery for esophageal achalasia. Surg Endosc 1998;12:270–273.

44. Stewart KC, Finley RJ, Clifton JC, et al. Thoracoscopic versus laparoscopic modified Heller myotomy for achalasia: efficacy and safety in 87 patients. J Am Coll Surg 1999;189:164–170.

45. Costantini M, Zaninotto G, Molena D, et al. One-hundred laparoscopic Heller–Dor operations: our experience in treating primary esophageal achalasia. Gastroenterology 1999;116:1305.

46. Alves A, Perniceni T, Godeberge P, et al. Laparoscopic Heller's cardiomyotomy in achalasia. Is intraoperative endoscopy useful, and why? Surg Endosc 1999;13:600–603.

47. Donahue PE, Teresi M, Patel S, et al. Laparoscopic myotomy in achalasia: intraoperative evidence for myotomy of the gastric cardia. Dis Esophag 1999;12:30–36.

5
Miscellaneous Esophageal Procedures

Hubert J. Stein and Joerg Theisen

Staging

Despite marked advances in the surgical therapy of esophageal and gastric carcinoma, the overall prognosis of these patients has not markedly improved during past decades, because, in most cases in the Western world, by the time esophageal or gastric cancer has been diagnosed, the tumor has already reached an advanced stage or has metastasized. Furthermore, systemic and local recurrences are common even after a complete tumor resection, extensive lymphadenectomy, or multidisciplinary approaches. Therefore, future improvements in the overall survival of patients with esophageal or gastric cancer can only be achieved by therapeutic strategies that are based on the individual histological tumor type, tumor location, and tumor stage at the time of presentation.[1–3] The need for precise pretherapeutic staging is evident. Only an accurate tumor staging allows selection of the right therapy for the right patient.

The goal of preoperative staging of esophageal and gastric cancer is to identify patients who will benefit from surgical resection or multimodal treatment protocols.[4] In patients with esophageal or gastric cancer, the presence of systemic or peritoneal tumor spread, incomplete tumor resection (i.e., R1 or R2 category according to the AJCC/UICC definition), and the presence of lymph node metastases are the major independent prognostic factors indicating poor survival after surgical resection.[3,5] Incomplete local tumor resection (R1 or R2 resection) and resection in patients with systemic or peritoneal tumor spread must be considered palliative and should be avoided because less invasive and safer methods for palliation are now available.[2,3] In contrast, long-term survival may still be possible in patients with a limited number of locoregional lymph node metastases, provided an extensive lymphadenectomy is performed.[6,7]

Although noninvasive imaging methods for detection of systemic tumor spread have markedly improved, diagnostic gaps remain in the detection of small liver metastases, peritoneal tumor spread, and lymph node involvement. It is not uncommon that a scheduled curative resection of an esophageal or gastric cancer must be abandoned because a tumor that is more advanced than appreciated on standard preoperative diagnostic tests is detected intraoperatively. Diagnostic laparoscopy and thoracoscopy have been assessed in recent years as tools to close these diagnostic gaps.

Laparoscopic Staging of Esophageal and Gastric Cancer

Several studies have shown, in patients with gastric cancer or adenocarcinoma of the esophagogastric junction, that diagnostic laparoscopy is superior to all other imaging modalities in the detection of liver metastases, intraabdominal lymph node metastases, and peritoneal tumor spread (Fig. 5.1).[8–13] Recent advances have made diagnostic laparoscopy an even more complete staging tool for gastrointestinal malignancies: laparoscopic ultrasonography with a flexible ultrasound probe and the use of diagnostic lavage to search for free tumor cells in the abdominal cavity. Some authors therefore recommend the use of diagnostic laparoscopy in every patient with esophageal or gastric cancer considered for surgical therapy.

More detailed studies show that the prevalence of intraabdominal tumor manifestations in patients with esophageal or gastric cancer is clearly related to the location of the primary tumor (esophagus, esophagogastric junction, stomach), the T category, and the histological tumor type (i.e., adenocarcinoma or squamous cell cancer).[13] Unrecognized peritoneal tumor dissemination and liver metastases can be found in up to 30% of patients with locally (i.e., uT3/T4 categories) advanced adenocarcinoma of the distal esophagus, esophagogastric junction, or stomach. In contrast to late-stage adenocarcinoma, the diagnostic yield of laparoscopy, in patients with squamous cell esophageal cancer (any T category)

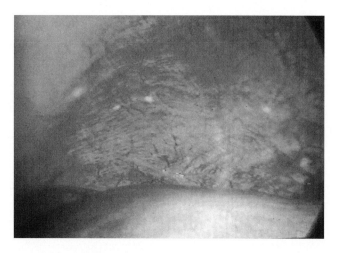

FIGURE 5.1. Laparoscopic diagnosis of peritoneal tumor spread in a patient with gastric cancer.

is low (below 5%) as it is in patients with early (i.e., uT1/T2 categories) adenocarcinoma of the distal esophagus, esophagogastric junction, or stomach.

Based on the available data, the proposed role of diagnostic laparoscopy for detecting and confirming intraabdominal nodal involvement is questionable at best. Biopsy of individual locoregional or celiac axis lymph nodes is potentially hazardous and has a low negative predictive value. Furthermore, the results of lymph node biopsies usually do not change the treatment plan.[14]

We therefore recommend performing laparoscopy only in patients in whom the potential diagnostic yield is high and truly relevant for the treatment plan, that is, patients with locally advanced adenocarcinoma of the esophagogastric junction or stomach who are considered for surgical resection or neoadjuvant treatment trials. The only goal of diagnostic laparoscopy in these patients is the exclusion of peritoneal tumor spread and liver metastases. These findings result in exclusion of the patient from potentially curative treatment strategies. A routine use of diagnostic laparoscopy in all other patients with esophageal or gastric cancer appears not justified in view of the potential complication rate of this invasive modality.[14] In our opinion, the still-unresolved issue of inadvertent tumor spread and the lack of therapeutic consequences argues against routine biopsy of regional lymph nodes during diagnostic laparoscopy.

Thoracoscopic Staging of Esophageal Cancer

None of the currently available conventional staging methods (including CT scan, endoscopic ultrasound, and MR scan) can reliably predict the presence of lymphatic spread of esophageal cancer.[4] Although positron emission tomography may indicate the presence of distant, that is, cervical and abdominal lymph node metastases, the spatial resolution of the current imaging technology does not allow differentiation of the primary tumor from local lymph node involvement.[15] For this reason, diagnostic thoracoscopy to identify lymphatic spread of esophageal cancer has been performed by a number of investigators.[10,11] Although these studies showed that thoracoscopic lymph node biopsy is feasible and increases the accuracy of pretherapeutic staging, the therapeutic consequences are still unclear. Consequently, diagnostic thoracoscopy for esophageal cancer remains investigational.

Thoracoscopic and Laparoscopic Enucleation of Esophageal Leiomyoma

Esophageal leiomyoma is the most common benign tumor of the esophagus, accounting for more than two-thirds of benign esophageal tumors. More than 95% of the leiomyomas originate from the muscularis propria of the esophagus. Because of the distribution of striated and smooth muscle in the esophagus, leiomyomas are usually located in the lower or middle portion of the esophagus.[16]

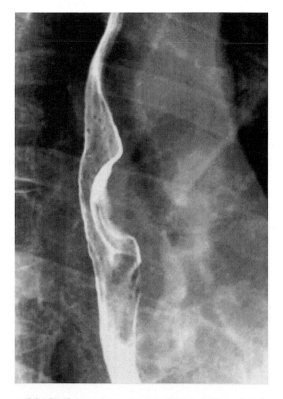

FIGURE 5.2. Barium contrast esophagography showing the typical image of a leiomyoma of the esophagus.

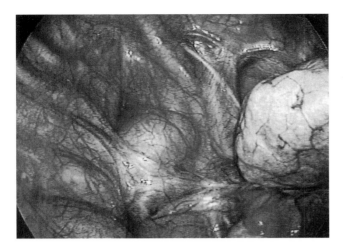

FIGURE 5.3. Thoracoscopic image of a leiomyoma in the proximal esophagus (*arrow*) above the level of the azygos vein (*double arrow*).

Some patients with leiomyoma present with dysphagia or chest pain, but the majority of patients are asymptomatic and the diagnosis is made incidentally on endoscopy performed for other reasons. The diagnosis is confirmed by barium swallow (Fig. 5.2), which shows a smooth indentation of the esophageal lumen, and endoscopic ultrasound, which shows a homogenous hypoechoic submucosal mass without signs of infiltration.[17] The overlying mucosa is usually intact. The major problem is the differentiation of the benign leiomyoma from the rare esophageal leiomyosarcoma. In contrast to stroma tumors elsewhere in the gastrointestinal tract, there is no clear correlation between the size of the lesion and the presence of malignancy.

Surgical enucleation of the leiomyoma is the treatment of choice in every symptomatic patient.[16] For asymptomatic tumors smaller than 3 cm, close follow-up can be justified with resection when the tumor increases in size. A transmucosal biopsy should not be performed because it is usually not representative of the tumor and may cause subsequent tumor enucleation without injury to the esophageal mucosa to be more difficult.

In the past, thoracotomy or laparotomy has been the access route of choice for leiomyoma enucleation. Recent studies have shown that minimally invasive enucleation by thoracoscopy or, for tumors located at the esophagogastric junction, laparoscopy is feasible (Fig. 5.3).[16,18] Intraoperative endoscopy may aid in locating small tumors. After limited incision of the outer longitudinal muscle layer, the tumor usually can be enucleated in toto. Particular attention must be paid to the integrity of the mucosa. If the mucosa is injured, it can be closed with one or two stitches. The muscle layers are approximated after removal of the tumor.

Minimally Invasive Esophagectomy and Reconstruction

Thoracoscopic esophagectomy has been performed successfully in several centers. However, questions remain regarding the safety, radicality, and benefits of this approach.[19] Due to a lack of comparative studies, minimally invasive esophagectomy currently remains an experimental procedure. In contrast, laparoscopic mobilization of the stomach and creation of a gastric tube for esophageal reconstruction constitute an attractive alternative to laparotomy that deserves further evaluation.[20]

References

1. Stein HJ, Sendler A, Fink U, Siewert JR. Multidisciplinary approach to esophageal and gastric cancer. Surg Clin N Am 2000;80:659–682.
2. Siewert JR, Stein HJ, Sendler A, Molls M, Fink U. Esophageal cancer: clinical management. In: Kelsen DA (ed) Principles and Practice of Gastrointestinal Oncology. Philadelphia: Lippincott Williams & Wilkins, 2001.
3. Siewert JR, Fink U, Sendler A, et al. Gastric cancer. Curr Probl Surg 1997;34:835–942.
4. Stein HJ, Brücher BLDM, Sendler A, Siewert JR. Esophageal cancer: patient evaluation and pretreatment staging. Surg Oncol 2001;10:103–111.
5. Stein HJ, Feith M. Cancer of the esophagus. In: Gospodarowicz M, et al. (eds) Prognostic Factors in Cancer. New York: Wiley-Liss, 2001:237–249.
6. Siewert JR, Stein HJ, Feith M, Brücher BLDM, Bartels H, Fink U. Tumor cell type is an independent prognostic in esophageal cancer: lessons learned from more than 1000 consecutive resections at a single institution in the Western world. Ann Surg 2001;234:360–369.
7. Siewert JR, Böttcher K, Stein HJ, Roder JD, and the German Gastric Carcinoma Study Group. Relevant prognostic factors in gastric cancer: 10-year results of the German Gastric Cancer Study. Ann Surg 1998;228:449–461.
8. Heath EI, Kaufmann HS, Talamini TT, et al. The role of laparoscopy in preoperative staging of esophageal cancer. Surg Endosc 2000;14:495–499.
9. Burke EC, Karpeh MS, Conlon KC, Brennan MF. Laparoscopy in the management of gastric adenocarcinoma. Ann Surg 1997;225:262–267.
10. Krasna MJ, Flowers JL, Attar S, McLaughlin J. Combined thoracoscopic/laparoscopic staging of esophageal cancer. J Thorac Cardiovasc Surg 1996;111:800–807.
11. Krasna MJ, Reed CE, Nedzwiecki D, et al. CALGB 9380: a prospective trial of the feasibility of thoracoscopy/laparoscopy in staging esophageal cancer. Ann Thorac Surg 2001;71:1073–1079.
12. Feussner H, Omote K, Fink U, Walker SJ, Siewert JR. Pretherapeutic laparoscopic staging in advanced gastric carcinoma. Endoscopy 1999;31:342–347.
13. Stein HJ, Kraemer SJM, Feussner H, Siewert JR. Clinical value of diagnostic laparoscopy with laparoscopic ultra-

sound in patients with cancer of the esophagus or cardia. J Gastrointest Surg 1997;1:167–173.

14. Stein HJ, Feussner H. Comment on The role of laparoscopy in preoperative staging of esophageal cancer. Surg Endosc 2001;15:528.

15. Lerut T, Flamen P, Ectors N, et al. Histopathologic validation of lymph node staging with FDG-PET scan in cancer of the esophagus and gastroesophageal junction: a prospective study based on primary surgery with extensive lymphadenectomy. Ann Surg 2000;232:743–752.

16. Bonavina I, Segalin A, Rosati R, Pavanello M, Peracchia A. Surgical therapy of esophageal leiomyoma. J Am Coll Surg 1995;181:257–262.

17. Massari M, De Simone M, Cioffi U, Gabrielli F, Boccasanta P, Bonavina. Endoscopic ultrasonography in the evaluation of leiomyoma and extramucosal cysts of the esophagus. Hepatogastroenterology 1998;45:938–943.

18. Tamura K, Takamori S, Tayama K, et al. Thoracoscopic resection of a giant leiomyoma of the esophagus with a mediastinal outgrowth. Ann Thorac Cardiovasc Surg 1998;4:351–353.

19. Peracchia A, Rosati R, Fumagalli U, Bona S, Chella B. Thoracoscopic esophagectomy: are there benefits? Semin Surg Oncol 1997;13:259–262.

20. Jagot P, Sauvanet A, Berthoux L, Belghiti J. Laparoscopic mobilization of the stomach for oesophageal replacement. Br J Surg 1996;83:540–542.

Part II
Gastric Procedures

6
Endoscopic Gastric Procedures: Endo-organ Surgery

Charles J. Filipi and Peter I. Anderson

Background and Historical Development

After the development of the percutaneous gastrostomy (PEG) by Ponsky and Gandevev,[1] but before the mini-invasive laparoscopic revolution, endoscopic foregut excision of early gastric cancer became commonplace in Japan.[2-4] The benefit of endoscopic mucosal resection (EMR) for mucosal malignancies has been significant, with the cure rate for T1 lesions being as high as 98%. However, lesions greater than 1 cm in diameter and lesions located in the posterior body of the stomach or the fundus became recognized limitations of EMR. As a result, mini-invasive gastric intraluminal surgery was developed by Ohashi in Japan.[5]

In the United States and Europe, after the advent of laparoscopic cholecystectomy, gastric access ports were developed in our laboratory with the intent to allow creation of an endo-organ antireflux nipple valve. It quickly became apparent that these access ports could provide access for a variety of intraluminal gastric procedures.[6] Concomitantly, Frimberger and Classen in Germany published a descriptive article on a metallic port that allowed intragastric procedures.[7]

Intraluminal rectal surgery was first introduced by Beuss et al.,[8] and subsequent publications have demonstrated the efficacy of this approach for benign and early malignant lesions.[9-11] Beuss uses a large sealing proctoscope with insufflation to gain visibility and introduces three or even four instruments through airtight ports. The equipment is expensive, and some debate its effectiveness compared to standard techniques of low anterior resection and transrectal open procedures. This same phenomenon has occurred with gastric intraluminal surgery, as some surgeons prefer laparoscopic, interventional radiologic, or open procedures for the treatment of disorders commonly treated by intraluminal gastric surgery. What then are the current appropriate indications for gastric intraluminal surgery and what will be the future direction of this new form of surgical intervention? That question can best be addressed by reviewing how gastric intraluminal surgery developed.

Endo-organ Access

Ohashi first developed laparoscopic intragastric surgery (LIGS) using an open technique through which minilaparotomy balloon trocars were introduced for access.[5] Way et al., with the assistance of Innerdyne Inc. (Sunnyvale, CA, USA), subsequently developed a radially expanding trocar that provided percutaneous laparoscopic-guided access to the gastric lumen for 5-mm instruments.[12] Other commercially available access devices now make intraluminal surgery possible in many countries. A sharp laparoscopic trocar can be introduced with the assistance of T fasteners that secure the stomach wall to the peritoneum. Gastric wall bleeding and inadvertent extraction are complications of this technique. Marlow (Cooper Surgical, Shellton, CT, USA) has developed a balloon port that is sharply introduced after T fasteners are placed. As industry provided access devices, surgeons have become more aware of the success of intraluminal surgery. Innovative ideas have produced additional intraluminal alternatives for various gastric procedures.

In our laboratory, we developed a traction large-diameter PEG for endo-organ surgery. This port provides access for larger instruments and allows extraction of tissue specimens. The port is secure in that an intraluminal balloon prevents inadvertent extraction. This access port can be placed pericutaneously; it has been used with success[13] but does have a 10% infection rate. With antibiotic ointment coating of the port, it is expected that the incidence of infection will be reduced by one-half. Intragastric stapling through a 12-mm-inner-diameter port in development may make possible the control of upper gastrointestinal (UGI) bleeding and gastroesophageal reflux disease by intraluminal means.

Gastric Tumors

Endo-organ gastric excision is minimally invasive while still providing surgical access. It is an alternative between transoral endoscopic loop cautery excision and laparotomy. This section addresses the current indications for endo-organ excision of the following lesions: gastric polyps, benign gastric wall tumors, Dieulafoy's lesion, and early gastric carcinoma.

Gastric polyps are divided into two main categories, hyperplastic and adenomatous polyps. Hyperplastic polyps, which constitute approximately 75% of all gastric epithelial polyps, are a product of regenerative glandular proliferation and have a low incidence of malignancy. Adenomatous polyps, for the most part, constitute the other 25% of gastric epithelial polyps and have a significantly higher risk of malignancy. Polyps, whether hyperplastic or adenomatous, are diagnosed by endoscopic biopsy. Current treatment includes endoscopic polypectomy, followed by open surgical resection if necessary. Endo-organ surgery provides the benefit of excision with wide accurate tissue margins, as opposed to loop cautery endoscopic excision, which obliterates histological margins. In addition, correct orientation of the endo-organ ports allows access to parts of the stomach that are inaccessible to the transoral endoscope, namely, the fundus, prepylorus, and posterior body. An endo-organ procedure can accomplish full-thickness resection up to 6cm in diameter if needed; this circumstance formerly required an open laparotomy.

Gastric wall tumors include gastric carcinoids, gastric lymphomas, and gastric leiomyogenic tumors. The incidence of these tumors is relatively unknown due to their often asymptomatic presentation. Bandoh and Isoyama[14] found that approximately 45% of these lesions are malignant and that surgery provided a significant survival advantage. Endo-organ procedures enable the surgeon to accomplish enucleation, mucosal resection, and full-thickness gastric excision (up to 6cm in diameter) for lesions in the prepyloric antrum, posterior body, or fundus.

Gastric carcinoids associated with hypergastrinemic states, because of their benign nature, are ideal for intraluminal surgery. Lesions up to 2cm can be safely excised. Naturally, larger lesions require wider margins if found to be malignant. Sporadic lesions or those associated with the multiple endocrine neoplasia (MEN) syndrome are more likely to be malignant; therefore, endo-organ surgery can only provide palliative resection of these often symptomatic lesions.[15]

Approximately 5% of gastric malignancies are lymphomas. Lymphomas are typically diagnosed by endoscopic biopsy; however, approximately 10% of endoscopically biopsied lymphomas are in fact pseudolymphomas. Endo-organ excision can provide adequate tissue for a complete and accurate histological diagnosis and will prevent the transformation of pseudolymphoma to lymphoma. Wide surgical resection is the treatment of choice for stage I and II gastric lymphomas, often coupled with radiation and chemotherapy. Intraluminal excisional gastric surgery can be of benefit for small lesions.

Gastric leiomyogenic tumors are typically asymptomatic and are diagnosed by endoscopy or laparotomy. Those that are excised have a high degree of malignancy, with rates ranging from 30% to 47%.[14,16] Endo-organ surgery is an important treatment option for these tumors because of the inability of endoscopic biopsy to obtain submucosal tissue. A definitive diagnosis and complete tumor excision up to 4cm in diameter are possible with intraluminal surgery.

Dieulafoy's lesion can cause severe upper gastrointestinal bleeding. As these lesions are small, they can be difficult to detect. Endoscopic electrocoagulation, angiographic embolization, and endoscopic sclerotherapy have all been used with limited success. Surgical intervention usually requires open gastrotomy to ligate the vessels or resect the tissue. Using the endo-organ approach, surgeons can ligate vessels or perform full-thickness excision under direct visualization. Very often, the lesion is difficult to find. If the intraluminal blood is fully evacuated and the gastric wall irrigated, the lesion is almost always identifiable: thus, the endo-organ approach is our preferred approach for occult gastric bleeding.

Early gastric cancer can be successfully resected using endoscopic mucosal resection (EMR). However, EMR is often not technically feasible for lesions larger than 2cm, or for those located in the fundus, posterior body, or on the lesser curvature of the antrum. Endo-organ surgery excels in these anatomic locations and for lesions larger than 2cm in diameter.[17] Ohashi has reported success with intraluminal excision in six patients with early gastric cancers ranging from 1.5 to 2.5cm.[5] In this series, he reported no complications and a mean hospital stay of 5 days. Intraluminal surgery of the stomach has also shown its utility in patients who have gastric myogenic tumors that are thought to be benign, although malignancy cannot be ruled out. Taniguchi et al. reported success enucleating an ulcerated 5-cm gastric leiomyoma.[18] Also, for medically unfit patients who would not be able to tolerate an open procedure, endo-organ surgery is an acceptable alternative for the excision of T2 and T3 lesions. Tomonaga et al. reported success with the excisions of a 1cm well-differentiated adenocarcinoma at the gastroesophageal junction in a patient with many comorbidities.[19] This report indicates the potential for the palliative intraluminal approach to gastric cancer.

Surgical Technique

Initial tissue diagnosis is important, especially for patients with early gastric cancer. Figure 6.1 shows ideal positions

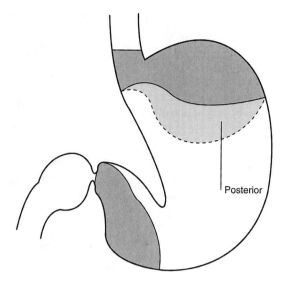

FIGURE 6.1. Ideal lesion locations for endo-organ surgery. The gray areas are optimal.

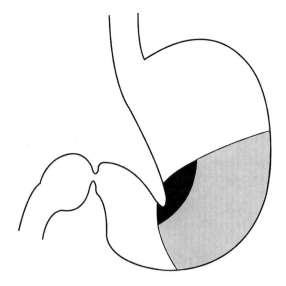

FIGURE 6.2. Suboptimal lesion locations for endo-organ surgery. The black area is the most difficult for endo-organ excision, and the gray area is suboptimal.

for lesions, and Figure 6.2 shows the suboptimal lesion locations for endo-organ surgery. The key feature of port placement is maximal displacement of the port from the lesion to be excised. This procedure provides a better panoramic view and instrument interaction, especially for intracorporeal suturing, and knot tying is improved.

Complete excision margins (both lateral and deep) are critical to the procedure's long-term success. If a low-grade early mucosal malignancy or a smooth muscle gastric wall tumor is to be excised, a 1-cm margin is usually adequate. Lesions requiring a bigger margin should, in general, be removed by open laparotomy. If the lesion is immediately adjacent to the gastroesophageal junction or the pyloric margin, clearance must be balanced against potential stenosis of the lumen. In patients requiring only mucosal resection, healing by secondary intention will suffice. For lesions requiring full-thickness excision, intraluminal patency must be assured; this is very possible with the intraluminal approach.

For full-thickness excision, the Harmonic Scalpel (Ethicon Endosurgery, Cincinnati, OH, USA) is ideal primarily for lesions near the lesser curvature where vasculature is increased. High-flow, high-pressure intragastric CO_2 insufflation makes this procedure possible even with a relatively large, full-thickness gastric wall defect. If there is a possibility that the intragastric secretions are

infected, a preliminary antibiotic irrigation is appropriate to prevent subsequent intraperitoneal infection because there is invariably some extragastric spillage with full-thickness excision. Gastric wall closure is best accomplished with interrupted monofilament sutures tied extracorporeally, especially if a large defect is present. Gastric wall tension makes intracorporeal knot security a problem because the first double throw (surgeon's knot) commonly slips. After gastric wall closure, insufflation testing of the suture line integrity is appropriate.

Results

A study to determine the efficacy of endoluminal surgery was initiated. After preliminary laboratory development of techniques and access devices, endoluminal gastric excision procedures were performed in 10 patients: 2 for gastric cancer, 3 for confluent polyps, 1 for a chronic benign ulcer, and 4 for leiomyoma (Table 6.1). Of the 10 patients, 2 were converted to an open procedure due to technical difficulties. In the first case there was inadequate exposure, and a heavier pair of disposable 10 mm scissors was needed but was not available. In the second case, gas insufflation of the stomach was lost due to scissors rupture of the modified PEG port balloon,

TABLE 6.1. Results of initial endo-organ gastric excision procedures.

Lesion	n	Conversion to laparotomy	Complications	Long-term results
Gastric cancer	2	0	1	One recurrence
Polyp	3	0	1	No recurrences
Ulcer	1	1	0	No recurrences
Leiomyoma	4	1	1	No recurrences

allowing gas to leak intraperitoneally and compromising exposure.

The average hospital stay was 12.2 days (range, 2–45 days). This figure is high because one patient underwent her procedure in Japan where patients typically are hospitalized for 14 to 21 days after gastrotomy. A second patient was hospitalized for 45 days because of an operative complication. This patient developed an intraperitoneal abscess secondary to premature pullout of a PEG. The average operative time was 3.1h and 30% of patients developed complications, which included the aforementioned abscess and two wound infections. No mortalities occurred, and with the exception of the abscess, the morbidities were minimal. These results confirm that endo-organ surgery is a feasible alternative to laparotomy. As more surgeons utilize this technique, hospital stay and morbidity should decrease, making this a viable alternative for open gastric excision.

Gastroesophageal Reflux Disease

Elderly patients unfit for general anesthesia could be well served with a procedure less invasive than laparoscopic Nissen fundoplication. Patients with respiratory problems, especially chronic obstructive pulmonary disease (COPD) patients on steroids, would benefit if the procedure results are long lasting and can be completed on an outpatient basis. Initial data show that the Swain valvuloplasty is effective in controlling regurgitation symptoms. Older patients unable to undergo open reoperative surgery for GERD may also be candidates.

Surgically adverse patients are probably going to comprise the majority receiving this procedure. Many patients are attracted by the possibility of receiving symptom relief without the need for expensive medication but are unwilling or unable psychologically to undergo a major operative procedure. An intraluminal valvuloplasty provides an attractive alternative for these patients.

Swain Valvuloplasty

Severe gastroesophageal reflux disease (GERD) is often associated with an incompetent lower esophageal sphincter (LES), which is characterized by one or more of the following conditions: an abnormally low resting LES pressure (LESP), an abnormally short length of the abdominal segment of the LES (AL), or an abnormally short total LES length (TL).[20,21] Many of the current procedures aimed at providing a surgical cure for GERD seek to improve one or all of these conditions. The laparoscopic Nissen fundoplication is currently considered the treatment of choice for severe GERD that is uncontrollable with medical therapy.[22] This procedure artificially lengthens both the AL and TL while increasing the LESP. A large portion of the success of laparoscopic Nissen fundoplication stems from its low morbidity and short convalescence.[23]

To reduce operative morbidity even further, many see the potential for a totally transoral endoluminal antireflux procedure that could be done without general anesthesia and in an outpatient setting. Swain and Mills[24] developed a device that makes just such a procedure possible. The Swain endoscopic sewing machine is a device that can pass suture through the muscularis propria. Methods of reinforcing the LES using this technique have yielded promising results in both animals[25,26] and humans.[27,28] Martinez-Serna et al.[29] undertook a study investigating the optimal placement and configuration of endoscopically placed sutures. Seventeen baboons underwent an endoscopic valvuloplasty, with 8 assigned to group I [three suture plications 1cm apart on the lesser curvature, with the most proximal suture just below the gastroesophageal junction (GEJ)], and the remaining 9 to group II (three suture plications 120° apart just distal to the GEJ). The procedure was performed in a manner similar to that described by Swain et al.[24,30,31]

Manometry (LESP, AL, and TL), fluoroscopic barium swallow, endoscopy, a pressure volume test, and gross and histological examination of the esophagus and stomach were employed to ascertain the competency of the LES both preoperatively and postoperatively. The results of postoperative manometry showed a statistically significant increase in the TL of group II, the LESP of group I, and the AL of both groups. Endoscopy revealed 62% and 37% retention of sutures for group I at 3 and 6 months, respectively; group II had a 67% (3 months) and 56% (6 months) retention of sutures. Fluoroscopic barium swallows were unremarkable. The pressure volume test showed no significant difference between groups I and II and a standardized control. Martinez-Serna et al.[29] reported no mortality or significant morbidity related to the operative procedure in this series. Total operative time was approximately 20min.

Kadirkamanathan et al.[25] performed a similar operation in animals that utilized a suture placement method similar to Martinez-Serna's group I. They noted very similar postoperative findings in which there was a statistically significant increase in TL and LESP, as well as a decrease in the time in which the patients' esophageal pH was less than 4. Currently, a 64-patient trial has been initiated and results are pending. The primary concerns are morbidities and plication durability.

Sphincter Augmentation

Many different intraluminal techniques have been used to augment the incompetent LES. Another endoscopic approach that has gained support is endoscopic sphincter augmentation, which encompasses different types of endoscopic bulking procedures such as the injection of collagen, Polytef, and sclerosing agent into the distal esophagus. These treatments all share a common mechanism; by inducing a submucosal fibrosis at the level of the LES, it was theorized that less acid reflux would occur. Endoscopic collagen placement has been shown to increase the LESP, improve symptom scores, and improve 24h pH monitoring test scores.[32] Shafik[33] had similar results using endoscopically placed Polytef injections and observed increased LESPs and symptom relief following treatment.

Other surgeons have chosen to induce native collagen formation through escharification, accomplished by the injection of sclerosing agents such as sodium morrhuate into the LES. This technique showed promising results with low morbidity in animal models.[34] An alternative method for excarification is laser energy. McGouran and Galloway induced fibrosis at the cardia with the Nd: YAG laser, which resulted in a higher yield pressure, supporting previous observations that a mechanical gastric wall barrier can diminish LES distraction with gastric distension.

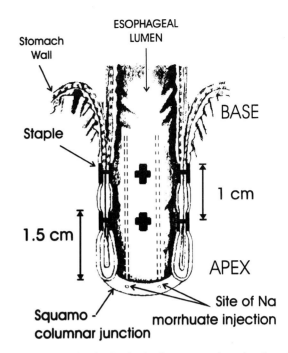

FIGURE 6.3. Intraluminal valvuloplasty procedure developed by Mason et al.[36] The esophagus is intussuscepted at the squamocolumnar junction to create a nipple-type valve.

Intussception Valvuloplasty

Building upon the success of the endoscopic bulking procedures, Mason et al. developed a new endoscopic intraluminal valvuloplasty procedure.[36] This procedure employs the assumption that a simple mechanical alteration can prevent the unfolding of the sphincter and improve its competency through the augmentation of the innate characteristics of the lower esophageal sphincter (LES) during periods of gastric distension. They noted that distension of the stomach is associated with a decrease in LES length and loss of competency. However, with the intraluminal valvuloplasty procedure, these factors were significantly improved.

Twenty adult chacma (*Papio ursinus*) baboons were used in their study. Thirteen of these baboons were placed in the valvuloplasty group and subsequently underwent an intraluminal antireflux procedure. One 12-mm operating percutaneous endoscopic gastrostomy (PEG) port and a 10-mm PEG port provide the surgeon with retrograde instrument access to the gastroesophageal (GE) junction. The 10-mm port accommodates a 45° laparoscope and the 12-mm port accommadates the stapling device. The esophagus is intussuscepted approximately 4cm into the stomach at the squamocolumnar junction to create a nipple-type valve. This valve was then transfixed using receivered staples and a sclerosing agent to induce fibrosis (Fig. 6.3).

The success of this procedure was measured by endoscopy, manometry, pathological analysis, and a pressure volume test. The later test consisted of a midline laparotomy followed by a ligature to completely occlude the duodenum. Then, a small gastrostomy was performed and a 24F Foley catheter was introduced into the stomach. A water-perfused manometry catheter was passed transnasally into the esophagus and stomach. As water was introduced into the stomach, producing distension, pressures were recorded in the stomach and esophagus and compared to each other. The volume of water that caused equalization of stomach and esophageal pressure was considered the yield pressure of the LES.

Endoscopic evaluation showed an intact nipple-type valve with complete integrity in 46% of the baboons at 6 months. The remaining six animals had a partial deterioration at the apex, which gave an overall assessment of valve circumference integrity of 86%. Manometry showed a longer total LES length, a longer intraabdominal length, and a higher LES vector volume pressure postoperatively. Pathological examination revealed a marked fibrotic "doughnut" at the cardia in the valvuloplasty group of animals. No fibrosis was evident in the control animals. The pressure volume test indicated a significantly higher median yield pressure of the valvuloplasty group over the controls, as well as a significantly higher median yield volume of the valvuloplasty group. The reason for these improvements is the protection against reduction in sphincter length following gastric distension provided by valvuloplasty.

It is well known that gastric distension causes failure of the LES, and so one hypothesis is that overeating and a high-fat diet can cause distension and over time significantly disrupt the LES, causing chronic gastric reflux. The intraluminal valvuloplasty procedure is one procedure aimed at providing a minimally invasive alternative to preventing or alleviating the symptoms of GERD. In the Mason study, the postoperative recovery time was short, and normal eating and behavior were noted just 12 h after the procedure. A short operative time and elimination of the need for dissection or mobilization around the stomach and cardia are major advantages of the endoluminal approach, which should ensure a low morbidity in patients.

Upper Gastrointestinal Bleeding

Patients with UGI bleeding requiring surgical intervention experience 20% mortality. A more definitive minimally invasive technique is needed. Currently, duodenal ulcer bleeding is the most common cause and often the most difficult to control endoscopically.[37] A variety of energy sources have been utilized with limited success, especially when there is visible vessel or active bleeding. Endoscopically placed hemoclips have been successful in some series,[38] but the clips can only penetrate 3 to 4 mm into the tissue. Open surgery has up to a 98% hemostasis success rate for posterior duodenal ulcer bleeding; it utilizes four or five deep sutures to surround the ulcer, followed by a pyloroplasty and truncal vagotomy. In our operating room, we have demonstrated by ultrasonography that these sutures commonly do not ligate the gastroduodenal artery but merely compress tissue. Nevertheless, they prove successful.

A deep staple or a specially designed suturing device that can place similar sutures in the confined space of the duodenal bulb is needed. Up to 12-mm gastric ports are available for such a device. The limitations are good visualization of the duodenum, if a 10- or 12-mm instrument is introduced through the stomach and pylorus, and sufficiently deep tissue compression. Until such a suturing device is available, open surgery or direct laparoscopic suturing through a duodenotomy are the only surgical options. The primary benefit of the endo-organ approach would be a decrease in infection rate and, if effective, an earlier definitive method that would limit blood loss and the morbidities associated with hemodynamic instability, namely, myocardial infarction and renal insufficiency.

Himpens (personal communication, 2000) has demonstrated that intraluminal endo-organ suturing can control bleeding in the human stomach. Lesions near the gastroesophageal junction and the pylorus are particularly accessible. A variety of bleeding causes can be treated, including Mallory–Weiss tears, channel ulcers, gastric and duodenal ulcers, and Dieulafoy's lesions. Theoretically gastritis and gastric varicies could also be treated successfully, but there are no reports of treatment for these entitites.

The technique includes port placement as far from the lesion in question as possible, being careful to place ports so that the needle holders are at right angles to each other. In hemodynamically unstable patients with type I, II, or III bleeding gastric ulcers, a generous biopsy and frozen section followed by oversewing of the ulcer is appropriate. Dieulafoy's lesions can either be ligated or excised. These difficult-to-find lesions can also be successfully treated by hemoclips,[39] but, if not, the endo-organ approach is ideal because the gastric lumen can be completely cleaned using a large-bore suction device for aspiration of blood clots, followed by irrigation and careful magnified inspection of the gastric mucosal surface. Mallory–Weiss tears can be simply suture ligated and pyloric channel ulcers similarly treated, being careful not to compromise the pyloric channel.

Pancreaticocystogastrostomy

There are numerous methods by which a pancreatic pseudocyst can be treated effectively. The endo-organ approach is particularly suited for the patient with debris within the cyst. Particulate matter prevents effective CT-controlled percutaneous drainage and may prevent complete decompression if the endoscopic needle knife technique is used. The endo-organ approach provides a 3- to 4-cm cystgastrostomy and access to the cyst cavity for debridement. The success rate has been satisfactory with this technique. In the rare circumstance in which the cyst wall is not fused to the stomach, conversion to laparoscopy or open laparotomy is necessary.

Conclusion

Intraluminal foregut surgery is feasible and safe. Nevertheless, it has not been applied frequently because cases for which the technique is applicable and preferable are rare. It is anticipated, however, with the advancement of technologies that this form of access and surgery for gastroesophageal reflux disease and UGI bleeding will become commonplace.

References

1. Ponsky JL, Gandevev MWL. Percutaneous endoscopic gastrostomy: a nonoperative technique for feeding gastrostomy. Gastrointest Endosc 1981;27:9–11.
2. Tada M, Shimada M, Yanai H, et al. A new technique of gastric biopsy. Stomach Intestine 1984;19:1107–1116.

3. Haruma K, Sumii K, Inoue K, Teshima H, Kajiyama G. Endoscopic therapy in patients with inoperable early gastric cancer. Am J Gastroenterol 1990:85:522–526.

4. Sano T, Kobori O, Muto T. Lymph node metastasis from early gastric cancer: endoscopic resection of tumor. Br J Surg 1992;79:241–244.

5. Ohashi S. Laparoscopic intraluminal (intragastric) surgery for early gastric cancer: a new concept in laparoscopic surgery. Surg Endosc 1995;9:169.

6. Filipi C, Wetscher G, DeMeester T, Peters J, Hinder R, Fitzgibbons R. Development of endo-organ surgery and potential clinical applications. In Peter JH, DeMesster TR (eds) Minimally Invasive Surgery of the Foregut. St. Louis: Quality Medical; 1995;288–308.

7. Frimberger E, Classen M. A new pull-through trocar technique for percutaneous operative endoscopy. Endoscopy 1991;23:338–341.

8. Buess G, Theiss R, Hutterer F, et al. Transanal endoscopic surgery of the rectum—testing a new method in animal experiments. Leber Magen Darm 1983;13:73.

9. Mentges B, Buess G, Schafer D, Mannke K, Becker HD. Local therapy of rectal tumors. Dis Colon Rectum 1996;39:886.

10. Banerjee AK, Jehle EC, Shorthouse AJ, Buess G. Local excision of rectal tumors. Br J Surg 1995;82:1165.

11 Swanstrom LL, Smiley P, Zelko J, Cagle L. Video endoscopic transanal-rectal tumor excision. Am J Surg 1997;173:383.

12 Way LW, Legha P, Mori T. Laparoscopic pancreatic cyst-gastrostomy: the first operation in the new field of intraluminal laparoscopic surgery [abstract]. Surg Endosc 1994;8:235.

13 Tomonaga T, Houghton SG, Filipi CJ, et al. A new form of access for endo-organ surgery: the initial experiences with percutaneous endoscopic gastrostomy. Surg Endosc 1999;13:738–741.

14. Bandoh T, Isoyama T. Submucosal tumors of the stomach: a study of 100 operative cases. Surgery (St. Louis) 1992;113:498–506.

15. Ahlman H, Kolby L, Lundell A, et al. Clinical management of gastric carcinoid tumors. Digestion 1994;55(suppl 3): 77–85.

16. Yamagiwa H, Matsuzaki O, Ishihara A, Yoshimura H. Clinicopathological study of gastric leiomyogenic tumors. Gastroenterol Jpn 1978;13:272–280.

17. Ohgami M. Abstract. SAGES, 1998.

18. Taniguchi E, Kamiike W, Yamanishi H, et al. Laparoscopic intragastric surgery for gastric leiomyoma. Surg Endosc 1997;11:287–289.

19. Tomonaga T, Filipi CJ, Marsh RE, Awad ZT, Shiino Y. Endo-organ full-thickness excision for gastric cancer: report of a case. Surg Today 1999;29(12):1248–1252.

20. Zaninotto G, DeMeester TR, Schwizer W, Johansson K, Cheng S. The lower esophageal sphincter in health and disease. Am J Surg 1988;155:104–111.

21. Mason RJ, Oberg S, Bremner CG, et al. Postprandial gastroesophageal reflux in normal volunteers and symptomatic patients. J Gastrointest Surg 1998;2:342–349.

22. DeMeester TR, Bonavina L, Albertucci M. Nissen fundoplication for gastroesophageal reflux disease. Evaluation of primary repair in 100 consecutive patients. Ann Surg 1986;204(1):9–20.

23. Hinder RA, Filipi CJ, Westcher G, Neary P, DeMeester TR, Perdikis G. Laparoscopic Nissen fundoplication is an effective treatment for gastroesophageal reflux disease. Ann Surg 1994;220:472–483.

24. Swain CP, Mills TN. An endoscopic sewing machine. Gastrointest Endosc 1986;32(1):36–38.

25. Kadirkamanathan SS, Yazaki E, Evans DF, Hepworth CC, Gong F, Swain CP. An ambulant porcine model of acid reflux used to evaluate endoscopic gastroplasty. Gut 1999;44(6):782–788.

26. Kadirkamanathan SS, Evans DF, Gong F, Yazaki E, Scott M, Swain CP. Antireflux operations at flexible endoscopy using endoluminal stitching techniques: an experimental study. Gastrointest Endosc 1996;44(2):133–143.

27. Kadirkamanathan SS, Evans DF, Gong F, Hepworth CC, Swain CP. Reflux control using endoluminal suturing at gastroscopy—early results in man [abstract]. Gastrointest Endosc 1995;41(4):352.

28. Swain CP, Kadirkamanathan SS, Brown G, Gong F, Evans DF, Mills TN. Sewing at flexible endoscopy in human gastrointestinal tract [abstract]. Gastrointest Endosc 1994;40(2 part 2):35.

29. Martinez-Serna T, Davis RE, Mason R, et al. An endoscopic valvuloplasty for gastroesophageal reflux disease. Gastrointest Endosc (in press).

30. Swain CP, Kadirkamanathan SS, Gong F, et al. Knot tying at flexible endoscopy. Gastrointest Endosc 1994;40(6):722–729.

31. Gong F, Swain P, Kadirkamanathan S, et al. Cutting thread at flexible endoscopy. Gastrointest Endosc 1996;44(6):667–674.

32. O'Connor KW, Lehman GA. Endoscopic placement of collagen at the lower escophageal sphincter to inhibit gastroesophageal reflux: a pilot study of 10 medically intractable patients. Gastrointest Endosc 1988;34:106–112.

33. Shafik A. Intraesophageal Polytef injection for the treatment of reflux esophagitis. Surg Endosc 1996;10:329–331.

34. Carvalho PJ, Donahue PE, Davis PE, et al. Endoscopic sclerosis prevents experimental reflux for longer than 12 months: reinforcement of the gastric component of the reflux barriers? Curr Surg 1990;47:20–22.

35. McGouran RCM, Galloway JM. A laser-induced scar at the cardia increases the yield pressure of the lower esophageal sphincter. Gastrointest Endosc 1990;36:439–443.

36. Mason RJ, Filipi CJ, DeMeester TR, et al. A new intraluminal antigastroesophageal reflux procedure in baboons. Gastrointest Endosc 1997;45:283–290.

37. Gostout CJ, Wang KK, Ahlquist DA, et al. Acute gastrointestinal bleeding. Experience of a specialized management team. J Clin Gastroenterol 1992;14:260–267.

38. Ohta S, Yukioka T, Ohta S, Miyagatani Y, Matsuda H, Shimazaki S. Hemostasis with endoscopic hemoclipping for severe gastrointestinal bleeding in critically ill patients. Am J Gastroenterol 1996;91:701–704.

39. Norton ID, Petersen BT, Sorbi D, Balm RK, Alexander GL, Gostout CJ. Management and long-term prognosis of Dieulafoy lesion. Gastrointest Endosc 1999;50:762–767.

7
Laparoscopic Approaches to Ulcer Therapy

Namir Katkhouda, Luca Giordano, and Sharon Manhas

Background and Historical Development

The pathogenesis of duodenal ulcer is multifactorial and complex. Although no study has demonstrated an immediate cause-and-effect relationship, *Helicobacter pylori* is always found in association with antral gastritis and is commonly associated with duodenal ulcer.[1-4]

The treatment of ulcers remains to be standardized. Therapy with proton pump inhibitors is controversial and has not been approved for long-term use. Triple antibiotic therapy, to eradicate *Helicobacter pylori*, may contain bismuth, which has a cicatrizational effect on gastric mucosae. Even following effective treatment, recent studies show reinfection rates of between 6% and 10% 1 year after the initial treatment.[3-5] The side effects of long-term medical treatment need to be considered. Carcinoid tumors have been demonstrated in the rat after long-term administration of proton pump inhibitors, and pseudomembranous colitis may complicate triple antibiotic therapy.

The mortality rate associated with peptic ulcer disease has been stable or increasing slightly over the course of the past few years despite improvements in medical therapy, as shown by Taylor et al.,[6] with an incidence of 4500 cases per year.

Several surgical options to treat peptic ulcer disease have been proposed: bilateral truncal vagotomy and antrectomy, highly selective vagotomy, posterior truncal vagotomy, and anterior seromyotomy. Today, with the advent of new advanced laparoscopic techniques and the development of new and more sophisticated laparoscopic tools, all these procedures can be performed safely, effectively, and reproducibly by an experienced surgeon.

In 1970 David Johnson popularized the highly selective vagotomy, which considered the treatment of choice for elective ulcer surgery.[7] The success of this operation is directly related to the skill of the surgeon. Johnson warned that recurrence rates would be unacceptably high if this operation were performed by the "occasional ulcer surgeon." Taylor et al.[8] in 1982 described the posterior truncal vagotomy and anterior seromyotomy. This procedure was performed laparoscopically for the first time in Nice, France in 1989, making it among the first advanced laparoscopic procedures.[9-12] In 1994, Katkhouda et al.[13] published a series of 90 patients treated electively for chronic duodenal ulcer with laparoscopic posterior vagotomy and anterior seromyotomy. This study reported minimal morbidity, no mortality, and a recurrence rate of 4.2% after a follow up of 2 to 41 months.

In 1997, Katkhouda et al.[14] introduced an improved technique for laparoscopic highly selective vagotomy (HSV) using harmonic shears. The authors demonstrated that this operation could be done expeditiously and taught safely. This procedure yields excellent results should become, in our opinion, the operation of choice for the treatment of chronic duodenal ulcer. The goal of the operation is to divide all vagal nerve fibers innervating the acid-producing cells of the stomach, while preserving the terminal branches of the main vagal trunks and the nerves of Latarjet, (thereby maintaining adequate antral motility). Success of HSV depends on meticulous technique because leaving a single fundic nerve branch intact will allow continued acid secretion in the corresponding gastric secretory zone, leading to early recurrence.[15,16]

The ideal laparoscopic technique is one that is safely taught, easily reproduced, and yields equivalent or better results than open surgery. The recent development of ultrasonically activated coagulating shears presents a new alternative to the tedious individual ligation of vagus nerve branches and associated vasculature.[17,18]

Indications and Patient Selection

In general, preoperative evaluation of patients with chronic duodenal ulcer disease is similar to that for laparoscopic cholecystectomy. In the elective setting, surgical intervention for duodenal ulcer disease is indicated in these patients:

1. Patients with the disease that is resistant to medical treatment despite pharmacologic therapy for at least 2 years and/or two or more documented recurrences after thorough medical treatment
2. Patients who cannot be followed regularly because of geographic or socioeconomic reasons or who cannot afford medications
3. Patients with complications such as perforation or hemorrhage

Laparoscopic Highly Selective Vagotomy

Preoperative Evaluation

As in elective open surgery, preoperative evaluation and preparation of the patient who is a candidate for a laparoscopic highly selective vagotomy (HSV) is of paramount importance. The general condition and operative risk factors of the patient are carefully investigated. Endoscopic and secretory studies are performed. Endoscopy documents the ulcer and rules out associated stenosis or hemorrhages. Secretory tests include measurement of basal acid output and peak acid output after stimulation with pentagastrin. These tests are necessary to evaluate the degree of acid hypersecretion in patients who are intractable to medical treatment. They are also useful as a baseline to compare a postoperative reduction of acid output. The serum gastrin level should always be assessed to rule out gastrinoma (Zollinger-Ellison Syndrome).

Surgical Technique

The patient is placed in the inverted Y position with the operating surgeon standing between the legs. The video monitor is positioned at the patient's shoulder. Pneumoperitoneum is established by the Veress needle technique at the umbilicus. Five trocars are placed. The video camera port is placed 2 cm above the umbilicus just to the left of the midline to avoid the falciform ligament. Two operative ports are placed in the right and left upper quadrant, respectively; a fan retractor is positioned in the subxifoid area; the last trocar is placed toward the left lower quadrant and is used to retract the stomach (Fig. 7.1). The procedure begins by elevation of the left lobe of the liver using the fan retractor. Laparoscopic

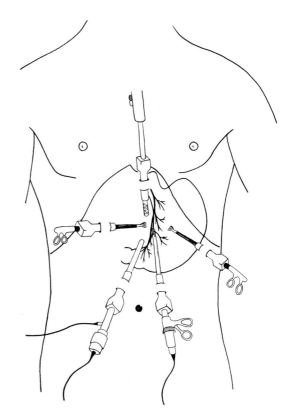

FIGURE 7.1. Trocar position for laparoscopic highly selective vagotomy (HSV).

Babcock clamps provide lateral traction of the greater curvature of the stomach. The lesser omentum is carefully inspected to identify several anatomic landmarks: the avascular aspect of the lesser omentum crossed by the hepatic branch of the anterior vagal nerve, the nerve of Latarjet (which runs parallel to the lesser curvature), and the terminal "crow's foot."

The anterior leaf of the omentum is incised between the nerve and the stomach proximal to the crow's foot, and the harmonic shears are introduced into this opening and positioned parallel to the nerve trunk (Fig. 7.2). The lesser omentum is retracted using an atraumatic grasper in order to ensure that the harmonic shears divide only the branches of the vagus nerve and not the nerve of latarjet. There is no need to identify and ligate individual neurovascular bundles. The important technical aspect is to ensure that the blunt jaws of the shears are applied and coapted beyond the vessel to avoid a partial welding that may lead to hemorrage. The tissues tend to separate automatically when the welding process is complete, so no traction needs to be applied on these fragile structures.

Four or five applications of the shears should suffice to clear the lesser curvature. This dissection then proceeds proximally to include the esophageal branches of the anterior vagus nerve. The fat pad of the cardioesophageal

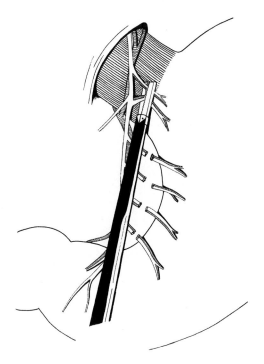

FIGURE 7.2. Laparoscopic HSV using harmonic shears (current technique).

junction containing the anterior nerve trunk is then raised upward and to the right, with care taken to divide the *criminal nerve of Grassi* near the angle of His. The division of those aberrant branches of the main vagal nerve is imperative to ensure complete vagotomy of the posterior fundus.

The dissection then return to the distal stomach. At this time retracting the opened anterior leaf of the lesser omentum exposes the posterior vagal branches. The posterior leaf is incised, as before, between the stomach and the posterior nerve of Latarjet, opening the lesser sac. Again, the harmonic shears are positioned parallel to, but not away from, the vagal trunk, dividing all the branches of the posterior vagus nerve proximal to the crow's foot. At the gastroesophageal junction, the main vagal trunk should be identified and retracted to avoid its injury. The esophagus is exposed circumferentially, and an electrocoagulation hook is used to denervate smaller branches easily recognized by the magnification provided by the laparoscope. At the end of the procedure, the distal esophagus should be clear of all nerve fibers for a length of 6 to 8 cm whereas the two trunks and their terminal gastric branches are preserved. To adhere to the concept of "extended highly selective vagotomy," use the magnification of the laparoscope to divide the proximal right anterior gastroepiploic nerve along the greater curvature of the stomach. Port sites are closed at the end of the operation, including fascial closure for the 10- and 11-mm trocars.

Postoperative Care

The nasogastric tube may be removed at the end of the procedure. The patient is encouraged to ambulate and resume a soft diet on the evening of surgery. Discharge is allowed the next day.

Laparoscopic Highly Selective Vagotomy Using Clips

The procedure described above can also be performed using the clip applier rather then the harmonic shears (Fig. 7.3). This technique is tedious, time consuming, and does not yield the same optimal results unless performed by a highly skilled surgeon.

Posterior Truncal Vagotomy and Anterior Seromyotomy

Taylor's Operative Procedure

With posterior truncal vagotomy and anterior seromyotomy, preoperative preparation, patient positioning, port placement, and initial abdominal cavity exploration are equivalent to the laparoscopic HSV.[19–25] Once the peritoneal cavity has been explored, the left lobe of the liver is retracted with the fan retractor placed through

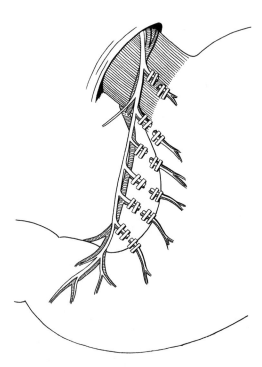

FIGURE 7.3. Laparoscopic HSV using clips.

the subxiphoid trocar. The lesser sac is entered opening the lesser omentum in the pars flaccida, the avascular area located anteriorly to the caudate lobe of the liver. Areolar tissue is divided using the hook dissector or harmonic shears with two angulated graspers. The dissection is continued until the muscular portion of the right crus is reached. The left gastric veins may be divided if encountered. Injury of the hepatic branch of the vagus nerve should be avoided if possible, although it has not been demonstrated that division causes clinically significant postoperative complication.

The two major landmarks for the posterior truncal vagotomy are the *caudate lobe* and the *right crus*. They should be grasped with the right-angle forceps and held to the right while the dissection is carried to open the phrenoesophageal membrane. The abdominal esophagus is retracted to the left, allowing visualization of the areolar tissue. The posterior vagus nerve is now identified, as it is easily recognized by its white color. With gentle traction on the nerve, adhesions are coagulated and divided and the nerve transected between two clips if the electrodissector is used; otherwise, the nerve can be simply divided if harmonic shears are available. A segment of the nerve is retrieved and sent for histological verification.

The anterior seromyotomy is started by spreading the anterior aspect of the stomach between two grasping forceps. Starting at the esophagogastric junction, the line of incision is outlined by light electrocoagulation parallel to and 1.5 cm from the lesser curvature. The line stops 5 to 7 cm from the pylorus, at the level of the crow's foot. The two most distal branches of the nerve are left intact to be sure that antropyloric innervation is preserved. Seromyotomy is then performed with the hook coagulator, successively incising the serosal layer, the oblique muscle layer, and the circular muscle layer. The two borders of the incision are then grasped and gently pulled apart, dividing the remaining deep circular fibers. Once the last muscular fibers have been divided, the mucosa will appear bluish with a tendency to bulge out of the incision. The submucosal layer should not be incised, as the mucosa is strongly adherent to it. With the help of the magnification offered by the laparoscope, inspection of the mucosa is carried out for the possibility that, inadvertently, holes have been made. Air or methylene blue can also be injected through the nasogastric tube to confirm that there are no leaks. Two or three short vessels may be encountered during the dissection. They should be divided. It is of utmost importance that the incision is anatomically accurate and hemostasis ensured. The seromyotomy is closed with an overlapping running suture, which prevents postoperative adhesion, allows perfect hemostasis, and prevents nerve regeneration. The abdomen is closed without drainage. Postoperative care is the same as for the laparoscopic HSV.

Treatment of Complications of Peptic Ulcer Disease

Gastric Outlet Obstruction by Intractable Chronic Duodenal Ulcer

Gastric outlet obstruction by intractable chronic duodenal ulcer, a frequent complication of chronic duodenal ulcer disease, has been successfully treated with bilateral truncal vagotomy and stapled gastrojejunostomy.

The posterior truncal vagotomy is performed as described in the previous section. The anterior (left) truncal vagotomy is performed using five trocars. The phrenoesophageal membrane is freed on the anterior aspect of the lower esophagus. It is of great importance to identify, together with the trunk of the left vagus nerve, all its numerous branches because they usually divide in a plexiform manner in the abdomen. The esophagus should be cleared of any nerve fibers on both the anterior and posterior aspects to ensure that any aberrant criminal nerve of Grassi is not missed. At completion of the dissection, several centimeters of the lower esophagus should appear skeletonized. A specimen of the nerve should always be sent for histological confirmation.

The gastrojejunostomy must be performed on the greater curvature of the lowest part of the antrum as close to the pylorus as possible. The second loop of jejunum is identified and approximated to the body of the stomach. To approximate the ends of the stomach and jejunum, a hernia stapler, a Babcock clamp, or a simple stich can be used. Two small incisions are made in both the stomach and the jejunum to allow the endolinear cutter 65 to be introduced. Before firing, the instrument is closed and rolled to confirm that the anastomosis is in a good position. The inner aspect of the anastomosis is checked for bleeding or inappropriate stapling. The same stapler is fired again to complete the anastamosis. If there is a risk of stenosis at this anastomotic site, the incisions should be closed with a running suture technique.

Laparoscopic Bilateral Truncal Vagotomy and Antrectomy for Treatment of Complications of Benign Gastric Ulcers

Gastric ulcers may be complicated by perforation and bleeding. Before definitive treatment is instituted, malignancy should be excluded. Gastric ulcers do not respond well to medical treatment, and surgical intervention is frequently indicated. Historically, bilateral truncal vagotomy and antrectomy have been used to treat intractable duodenal ulcers after multiple recurrences. This operation can also be used to resect distal gastric ulcers by extending the antrectomy to a hemigastrectomy using a laparoscopic approach. Because we have already described the bilateral truncal vagotomy, we focus now on description of the distal gastrectomy.

The procedure begins by opening the gastrocolic ligament under the right gastroepiploic vessel using electric scissors or harmonic shears. If electric scissors have been used, clips are needed to secure all vessels and prevent hemorrhage. With harmonic shears we secure only vessels greater than 4 to 5mm in diameter. The dissection is carried toward the duodenum, and the stomach is retracted with a Babcock clamp, permitting dissection of the posterior aspect of the duodenum and placement of a tape to be held by one grasper. The tape assists in the transection of the duodenum using an endolinear cutter 60 with 3.8-mm staples. Division of the duodenum permits the retraction of the specimen via two Babcock clamps and the ligation of the right gastric artery and the distal branches of the left gastric artery. The right gastroepiploic artery is then ligated and the posterior aspect of the stomach freed from the pancreas. Two enterotomies are performed on the posterior aspect of the stomach and on the second jejunal loop to allow the introduction of the endolinear cutter 60 to perform a stapled gastrojejunostomy. The enterotomies are then closed using continuous 3-0 prolene sutures and curved needles. We do not recommend closing the enterotomies with staples in this case as it may narrow the anastomosis. The gastrectomy is completed by resection of the specimen using a sequence of endolinear cutters with reload. The specimen is removed from the abdomen, the area is irrigated generously, the trocars removed, and the incision closed.

Thoracoscopic Bilateral Truncal Vagotomy for Treatment of Recurrent Peptic Ulcers

Thoracoscopic bilateral truncal vagotomy may be indicated for recurrent ulceration following a Billroth II gastrectomy. Adhesion from the first operation may preclude reoperation via an abdominal approach. If the recurrent peptic ulcer is benign, a thoracoscopic bilateral truncal vagotomy may be a valid alternative for this surgical problem.

A left-side approach with the surgeon standing behind the patient is preferred. After general endotracheal anesthesia has been induced using a double-lumen endotracheal tube, the patient is positioned in a right lateral decubitus position, the anesthesiologist is asked to collapse the left lung of the patient. Four trocars are inserted in a triangular fashion with the thoracoscope between the two main operating ports. The fourth trocar is used for the irrigation and suction device and may also serve as a palpation probe. Adhesions are divided and the preaortic pleura is incised to allow dissection of the esophagus. The nasogastric tube can be used to localized the esophagus in the event of severe adhesion, as can an illuminated bougie or an endoscope. An atraumatic isolated hook can then be used. All the vagal nerves are dissected and divided. The white fibers are nerves and must not be confused with normal esophageal muscular fibers. When the operation is completed, the esophagus is peeled and freed from the nerve fibers. Hemostasis can be achieved by inserting a 4×4 or 2×2 in. gauze pad through one of the trocars.

Use of electrocautery in the vicinity of the esophagus should be limited to avoid the considerable danger of postoperative necrosis. The operation is completed by inserting a thoracic drain through one of the ports and by closing the other ports.

Conclusion

Laparoscopic vagotomy is as effective and safe as open vagotomy for the treatment of duodenal ulcer disease refractory to medical therapy and yields uniformly good results. Despite improvements in medical therapy, the recurrence rate for ulcer disease is approximately 90% per year without long-term medical treatment. Antiulcer drugs have not decreased the mortality rate or complications associated with ulcer disease, especially in the elderly. We believe that elective surgical treatment is a useful alternative to long-term maintenance therapy. Therefore, laparoscopic highly selective vagotomy or posterior truncal vagotomy with anterior seromyotomy is the procedure of choice if the patients are selected as carefully as they are for open surgery. A prospective multicenter study is warranted to evaluate clinical outcome and cost effectiveness.

References

1. Graham DY. *Helicobacter pylori:* its epidemiology and its role in duodenal ulcer disease. J Gastroenterol Hepatol 1991;6:105–113.
2. George LL, Borody TJ, Andrews PO, et al. Cure of duodenal ulcer after eradication of *Helicobacter pylori.* Med J Aust 1990;153:145–149.
3. Graham DY, Lew GM, Klein PD, et al. Effect of treatment of *Helicobacter pylori* infection on the long-term recurrence of gastric or duodenal ulcer: a randomized controlled study. Ann Intern Med 1992;116:705–708.
4. Hentschel E, Brandstater G, Dragosics B, et al. Effect of ranitidine and amoxicillin plus metronidazole on the

eradication of *Helicobacter pylori* and the recurrence of duodenal ulcer. N Engl J Med 1993;328:308–312.

5. Rauws EAJ, Tytgat GNG. Cure of the duodenal ulcer associated with eradication of *Helicobacter pylori*. Lancet 1990; 335:1233–1235.

6. Taylor TV, Gunn AA, MacLeod DAD, et al. Morbidity and mortality after anterior lesser curve seromyotomy and posterior truncal vagotomy for duodenal ulcer. Br J Surg 1985; 72:950–951.

7. Blackett R, Johnson D. Recurrent ulceration after highly selective vagotomy for duodenal ulcer. Br J Surg 1981;68: 705–710.

8. Taylor TV, MacLeod DAD, Gunn AA, et al. Anterior lesser curve seromyotomy and posterior truncal vagotomy in the treatment of chronic duodenal ulcer. Lancet 1982;2:846–848.

9. Katkhouda N, Mouiel J. A new surgical technique of treatment of chronic duodenal ulcer without laparotomy by videocoelioscopy. Am J Surg 1991;161:361–364.

10. Katkhouda N, Mouiel J. Laparoscopic treatment of peptic ulcer disease. In: Hunter J, Sackier J (eds) Minimally Invasive Surgery. New York: McGraw-Hill, 1994:123–130.

11. Katkhouda N, Mouiel J. Laparoscopic treatment of peritonitis. In: Zucker KA (ed) Surgical Laparoscopy Update. St. Louis: Quality Medical, 1992;287–300.

12. Mouiel J, Katkhouda N. Laparoscopic truncal and selective vagotomy. In: Zunker KA (ed) Surgical Laparoscopy. St. Louis: Quality Medical, 1991:263–279.

13. Katkhouda N, Heimbucher J, Mouiel J. Laparoscopic posterior vagotomy and anterior seromyotomy. Endosc Surg 1994;2:95–99.

14. Katkhouda N, Mouiel J, Waldrep PJ, et al. An improved technique for laparoscopic highly selective vagotomy using harmonic shears. Surg Endosc 1998;12:1051–1054.

15. Blackett RL, Johnston D. Recurrent ulceration after highly selective vagotomy for duodenal ulcer. Br J Surg 1981;68: 705–710.

16. Donahue PE, Richter HM, Liu KJM, Anan K, Nyhus LM. Experimental basis and clinical application of extended highly selective vagotomy for duodenal ulcer. Surgery (St. Louis) 1993;176:39–48.

17. Laycock WS, Trus TL, Hunter JG. New technology for the division of the short gastric vessels during laparoscopic Nissen fundoplication. Surg Endosc 1996;10:71–73.

18. Swanstrom LL, Pennings JL. Laparoscopic control of short gastric vessels. J Am Coll Surg 1995;181:347–351.

19. Taylor TV. Lesser curve superficial seromyotomy. An operation for chronic doudenal ulcer. Br J Surg 1979;66:733–737.

20. Hill GL, Barker MCJ. Anterior highly selective vagotomy with posterior truncal vagotomy: a simple technique for denervating the parietal cell mass. Br J Surg 1978;65:702–705.

21. Burge HW, Hutchinson JSF, Longland CJ, et al. Selective nerve section in the prevention of post-vagotomy diarrhea. Lancet 1964;1:577.

22. Taylor TV. Experience with the Lunderquist Ownman dilator in the upper gastrointestinal tract. Br J Surg 1983;70: 445.

23. Daniel EE, Sarna SK. Distribution of excitatory vagal fibers in canine gastric wall to central motility. Gastroenterology 1976;71:608–612.

24. Kahwaji F, Grange D. Ulcere duodenal chronique. Traitement par seromyotomie fundique anterieure avec vagotomie tronculaire posterieure. Presse Med 1987;161: 28–30.

25. OostVogel HJM, Van Vroonhoven TJMV. Anterior seromyotomy and posterior truncal vagotomy: technic and early results of a randomized trial. Neth J Surg 1985;37:69–74.

8
Laparoscopic Gastrojejunostomy

David W. McFadden and Shirin Towfigh

Background and Historical Development

Laparoscopic gastrojejunostomy is a recently adopted procedure in the history of minimally invasive surgery. Early research showed that laparoscopic gastrojejunostomy was technically feasible in animal models.[1,2] Case presentations were first published in 1992, applying laparoscopic gastrojejunostomy to palliation of pancreatic cancer.[3] Initially, this proved to be a technically difficult procedure reserved for experienced surgeons. Now, as surgeons are becoming increasingly comfortable with laparoscopy and as laparoscopic technology improves, the frequency of laparoscopic gastrojejunostomy has increased. Its application to different disease states has similarly expanded.

Indications and Patient Selection

Laparoscopic gastrojejunostomy has been applied to a wide variety of malignant and benign disorders (Table 8.1). Palliative laparoscopic gastrojejunostomy is of special benefit to those with a short life expectancy. The most common indication is for malignant gastric outlet obstruction. Most are secondary to periampullary carcinoma, but application to gastric carcinoma, lymphoma, and metastatic lesions has proven equally successful.[4] Benign obstructing lesions such as Crohn's disease and chronic pancreatitis are also amenable to laparoscopic gastrojejunostomy.[5–7] Similarly, peptic ulcer disease can be managed laparoscopically.[8,9] More recently, bariatric surgery has benefited from advances in laparoscopy for their gastric bypass procedures. Morbid obesity introduces multiple technical challenges that are not addressed in this chapter.

Periampullary Carcinoma

Pancreatic carcinoma is the fourth leading cause of cancer death, with an incidence of 9 per 100,000 in the United States.[10] Less than 20% of patients have small tumors limited to the pancreatic capsule, and the 5-year survival rate of resectable patients following surgery approaches 20%. As most patients present at late stages, the overall 5-year survival rate is well under 5%.[11] Surgery is often palliative and reserved for patients with obstructive lesions of the bile duct or proximal gastrointestinal tract. Laparoscopic staging may be necessary to identify patients with unresectable disease.

If the tumor is unresectable, palliative laparoscopic gastrojejunostomy may be indicated for gastric outlet obstruction. In those cases of gastric outlet obstruction where biliary stents have been placed endoscopically, a laparoscopic gastrojejunostomy is a useful alternative to open procedures.

If assessment of the tumor is incomplete preoperatively, laparoscopic ultrasound is also helpful. Endoscopic biliary stenting is an additional tool used intraoperatively to relieve biliary duct obstruction. If this is technically impossible, laparoscopic cholecystojejunostomy is an alternative.[12]

Peptic Ulcer Disease

Both Bilroth I and II gastrectomies have been performed laparoscopically.[13,14] In the case of peptic ulcer disease, some have shown successful outcomes with laparoscopic gastrojejunostomy with or without truncal vagotomy.[15] This technique has been used for intractable ulcer disease, pyloric stenosis, and duodenal ulcer disease. Two- to 24-month follow-ups were promising. There is no evidence to suggest that these patients have different outcomes when compared to the open procedure.

TABLE 8.1. Applications of laparoscopic gastrojejunostomy for gastric outlet obstruction.

Malignant
Pancreatic carcinoma
Gastric carcinoma
Lymphoma
Doudenal carcinoma
Metastatic lesions

Benign
Peptic ulcer disease
Chronic pancreatitis
Crohn's disease
Pyloric stenosis
Duodenal tumor

Surgical Technique

As with all laparoscopic procedures, the patient must undergo general endotracheal anesthesia. In the case of obstructing lesions, our patients have large-bore nasogastric tubes placed at least 24h in advance for gastric decompression and irrigation of the obstructed stomach. Intravenous antibiotics are administered prophylactically. A urinary drainage catheter is placed at the time of operation.

An increased risk of venous thromboembolic events occurs in laparoscopic surgery, related to the pneumoperitoneum. We routinely use sequential compression devices. If there is a past history of deep venous thrombosis or pulmonary embolism in a patient, we initiate heparin therapy.

The patient is placed in low modified lithotomy with a slight reverse Trendelenburg. The primary surgeon is positioned between the patient's legs with the first assistant at the patient's left; an optional second assistant stands to the patient's right. The peritoneum is insufflated via a Veress needle from a left subcostal puncture. If previous abdominal surgery has been performed, an open technique is used. A 10-mm supraumbilical port is the site of entry of the 30° laparoscope. From here, planning of the subsequent ports is based on the patient's body habitus.

A fan liver retractor is placed through a right lateral port, exposing the gastroduodenal junction. At the left lateral and epigastric regions, 12-mm ports are placed for use of atraumatic graspers and a harmonic scalpel, respectively. A 10-mm port is placed at the left subcostal region where the first assistant will place a large grasper (Fig. 8.1).

To mobilize the stomach, we take down the gastrocolic ligament using a harmonic hook scalpel. After this is complete, a loop of jejunum is mobilized to perform the gastrojejunostomy. To do this, the midtransverse colon is elevated using atraumatic bowel graspers, identifying the

ligament of Treitz. An appropriate length of jejunum is brought to the anterior wall of the stomach in an antecolic fashion. The loop must be sufficiently long to rest comfortably against the distal greater curvature of the stomach. The site of anastamosis of the jejunum is usually 15 to 20cm distal to the ligament of Treitz.

Choice of anastamotic approaches varies among surgeons. We prefer the antecolic side-to-side anastamosis. From the epigastric port, separate stab incisions are made in the jejunum and stomach using the harmonic scalpel or coagulating scissors. The viscera are approximated with two silk traction sutures. A 45-mm linear stapler through the left lateral port is deployed two to three times through the enterotomy and gastrotomy to ensure adequate luminal length (approximately 6cm) (Fig. 8.2). The laparoscope is passed through the gastrotomy to inspect the staple line for hemostasis. To sew the enterotomy/gastrotomy closed, pass the linear stapler with the blade removed through the left lateral port (Fig. 8.3). Alternatively, you may choose a handsewn closure. The staple line may be reinforced with additional silk sutures.

Some surgeons are more comfortable exteriorizing the anastamosis for hand suturing.[16] Others use a sleeve that allows placement of a hand in the abdominal cavity without losing pneumoperitoneum.[17] This method has

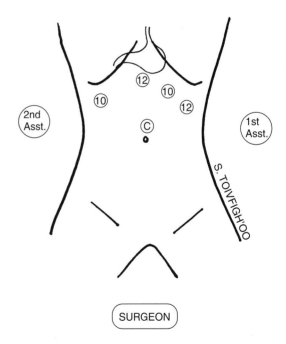

FIGURE 8.1. Laparoscopic gastrojejunostomy operative setup. With the patient in low lithotomy, the surgeon stands at the foot of the bed and the first assistant to the patient's left. Five trocars are placed as illustrated. The camera port (C) is placed supraumbilically. A liver retractor is placed laterally. Two 12-mm trocars are placed, one epigastrically and one left laterally, at least two fingerbreadths below the costal margin. Finally, a 10-mm trocar is placed between these two ports.

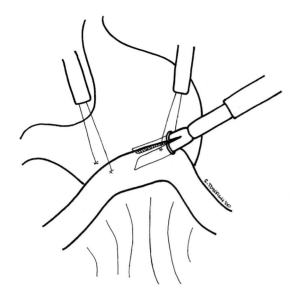

FIGURE 8.2. Gastrojejunal stapled anastamosis. Using stay sutures, a loop of jejunum is approximated with the greater curvature of the stomach. Gastrotomy and enterotomy are made using a harmonic hook scalpel. Two passes of the 45-mm linear stapler through the gastrotomy/enterotomy from the left lateral port ensure a 6-cm lumen.

been helpful with gastric tumors, where tactile sensation, finger dissection, and retraction improve the quality of the exploration of the abdominal cavity.

Additional utilities of the laparoscope, if clinically indicated, are laparoscopic placement of a feeding jejunostomy or a decompressive gastrostomy tube and laparoscopic cholecystojejunostomy.[18,19]

Problems and Controversies

Laparoscopic gastrojejunostomy is a relatively new technique and its applications to different disease states remain unfulfilled. Problems with this technique have been primarily a function of the surgeon's technical expertise and the patient's underlying pathology. Laparoscopic gastrojejunostomy is technically demanding and has not yet been widely adopted by the general surgical population. Most cases are performed by advanced laparoscopic surgeons in centers of excellence. With advanced surgical skills, improved instrumentation, and better operating room staff familiarity, this may become a readily performed laparoscopic procedure.

The introduction of any laparoscopic procedure must include formal analyses of safety, efficacy, operating time, hospital stay, and quality of life. Laparoscopic gastrojejunostomy is a recent phenomenon with few case reports and no large randomized trial.

The benefits of laparoscopic gastrojejunostomy lie in the presumed improvements in postoperative recovery.

As with any other laparoscopic procedure, there is less bowel manipulation, less postoperative pain, earlier mobilization of the patient, and earlier oral intake. Laparoscopic gastrojejunostomy offers fewer wound and respiratory complications, a quicker alimentation time, and earlier return to normal daily activities.[20] Operating time remains a function of the surgeon's expertise. Studies comparing laparoscopic with open Billroth II gastrectomies showed reduced morbidity, quicker recovery times, shorter hospital stays, and less postoperative pain.[21,22] Short-term quality of life after Billroth I and II were similar.[21] Because laparoscopic gastrojejunostomy remains a technically difficult procedure, we suggest that its use be reserved to surgeons with advanced technical skills and training in laparoscopic surgery.

With regard to patient selection, laparoscopic surgery in the morbidly obese patient adds new challenges to the surgeon. We believe that except for treatment of obesity when performed by a skilled bariatric surgeon, laparoscopic gastrojejunostomy should be contraindicated in the morbidly obese. Patients with portal hypertension and coagulation disorders are not suitable candidates. In addition, there is a relative contraindication to those who had undergone previous abdominal surgery or those who failed endoscopic biliary decompression.[23]

Laparoscopy in malignancy is controversial. Proceeding with palliative surgery is an option that must be discussed individually between the surgeon and the patient. Laparoscopic surgery with the intent to cure raises

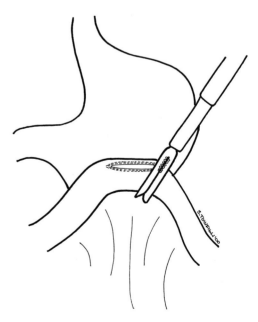

FIGURE 8.3. Stapled closure of gastrotomy/enterotomy is performed by approximating the two edges with a grasper. A linear stapler with the blade removed is placed through the left subcostal port to close this opening. An articulating linear stapler may be helpful to achieve awkward angles.

concern for tumor seeding at the port sites. In addition, laparoscopy for malignancy presents the following problems: lack of localization of the tumor, lack of tactile sensation, inadequate assessment of lymph node or liver metastases, and inadequate resection. With further experience, curative resection of malignancy may become an acceptable laparoscopic procedure with improved outcomes.

Postoperative Care

The patient remains with nasogastric tube decompression for at least 2 days postoperatively. Before beginning enteral nutrition, we perform an upper gastrointestinal study using water-soluble contrast to check for patency of the anastamosis and absence of leakage. Most patients are able to tolerate a diet as early as 3 to 5 days postoperatively,[24] compared to an average 6.5 days with the conventional open technique.[25] Hospital stay averages 7 to 10 days for malignancy, as compared to 13.3 days with conventional technique.[25]

Complications

Few data are available for laparoscopic gastrojejunostomy, as there are few case reports and no large randomized trials. Among reported cases, none had operative mortality; this compares to 8% to 17% average operative mortality for all cases using conventional techniques and a 22% operative mortality in malignancy.[25,26]

Morbidity for laparoscopic gastrojejunostomy varies depending on the underlying disease state and indications for operation. In malignancy, postoperative morbidities have included trocar site bleeding, delayed gastric emptying, congestive heart failure, pneumonia, and diarrhea.[20,23,27] With the conventional open technique in malignancy, there is 55% morbidity with 16% delayed gastric emptying.[26] Higher incidences of wound infections, chest infections, and prolonged ileus were found in the open approach when compared to the laparoscopic approach[4,25]; there seems to be no difference in delayed gastric emptying.[23]

In benign disease, the conventional open technique has 25% morbidity, with 16% delayed gastric emptying. Laparoscopic gastrojejunostomy in benign disease may be complicated by retrogastric fluid collection, incisional hernia, ulcer recurrences, and diarrhea. Complications related to pneumoperitoneum and positioning in reverse Trendelenburg include decreased venous return and cardiac output, increased chance of gastric reflux and aspiration, thromboembolic events, and decreased vital capacity. The small risk of carbon dioxide embolus on insufflation of the pneumoperitoneum results in cardiac arrhythmia, hypotension, pulmonary edema, hypoxemia, and right-sided heart failure.

Results

Few prospective data have been collated on laparoscopic gastrojejunostomy. This procedure is performed in few institutions by few surgeons, and the number of patients selected annually remains small.

The largest series of retrospective data for malignancy has been reported by Brune et al.[23] This studied 16 patients who were palliatively treated for malignant gastric outlet obstruction. Laparoscopic antecolic side-to-side gastrojejunostomy was performed in an average of 126 min with no intraoperative complications. One patient was converted to open procedure due to extensive adhesions. One postoperative complication, that of trocar site bleeding, required intervention. Median hospital stay was 7 days. Delayed gastric emptying was observed in 19%. Median survival was 87 days. Deaths were attributed to the underlying cancer, and patients were tolerating oral intake during their remaining survival time.

For benign disease, Wyman et al. retrospectively studied 12 patients with gastric outlet obstruction secondary to peptic ulcer disease and pyloric stenosis.[8] These patients underwent laparoscopic truncal vagotomy and gastrojejunostomy with a median operating time of 210 min. One patient required conversion to open technique. Median hospital stay was 6 days. Delayed gastric emptying was observed in 2 patients but resolved with conservative measures. All patients had a good symptomatic outcome at up to 12 months.

Conclusion

Laparoscopic gastrojejunostomy has been a successful minimally invasive procedure, although its applications have been limited. With increasing surgical experience, long-term studies can be performed to fully elucidate the indications and outcomes of such a procedure for the general surgical population.

References

1. Patel AG, McFadden DW, Hines OJ, Reber HA, Ashley SW. Palliation for pancreatic cancer: feasibility of laparoscopic cholecystojejunostomy and gastrojejunostomy in a porcine model. Surg Endosc 1996;10:639–643.
2. Soper NJ, Brunt LM, Brewer JD, Meininger TA. Laparoscopic Bilroth II gastrectomy in the canine model. Surg Endosc 1994;8(12):1395–1398.

3. Wilson RG, Varma JS. Laparoscopic gastroenterostomy for malignant duodenal obstruction. Br J Surg 1992;79: 1348.

4. Kum CK, Yap CHA, Goh PMY. Palliation of advanced gastric cancer by laparoscopic gastrojejunostomy. Singapore Med J 1995;36:228–229.

5. Reissman P, Salky BA, Edye M, Wexner SD. Laparoscopic surgery in Crohn's disease. Indications and results. Surg Endosc 1996;10(12):1201–1203.

6. Gagner M, Pomp A. Laparoscopic pylorus-preserving pancreatoduodenectomy. Surg Endosc 1994;8(5):408–410.

7. Reissman P, Salky BA, Pfeifer J, Edye M, Jagelman DG, Wexner SD. Laparoscopic surgery in the management of inflammatory bowel disease. Am J Surg 1996;171(1):47–50.

8. Wyman A, Stuart RC, Ng EK, Chung SC, Li AK. Laparoscopic truncal vagotomy and gastroenterostomy for pyloric stenosis. Am J Surg 1996;171(6):600–603.

9. McCloy R, Nair R. Minimal access surgery—the renaissance of gastric surgery? Yale J Biol Med 1994;67(3–4): 159–166.

10. Surveillance Research. Washington, DC: American Cancer Society, 1999.

11. Conlon KC, Klimstra DS, Brennan MF. Long-term survival after curative resection for pancreatic ductal adenocarcinoma: clinicopathologic analysis of 5-year survivors. Ann Surg 223(3):273–279.

12. Casaccia M, Diviacco P, Molinello P, Danovaro L, Casaccia M. Laparoscopic gastrojejunostomy in the palliation of pancreatic cancer: reflections on the preliminary results. Surg Laparosc Endosc 1998;8(5):331–334.

13. Ablaßmaier B, Gellert K, Tanzella U, Muller JM. Laparoscopic Bilroth-II gastrectomy. J Laparoendosc Surg 1996; 6(5):319–324.

14. Ballesta-Lopez C, Bastida-Vila X, Catarci M, Mato R, Ruggiero R. Laparoscopic Bilroth II distal subtotal gastrectomy with gastric stump suspension for gastric malignancies. Am J Surg 1996;171:289–292.

15. Lointier P, Leroux S, Ferrier C, Dapoigny M. A technique of laparoscopic gastrectomy and Bilroth II gastrojejunostomy. J Laparosc Endosc 1993;4:146–148.

16. Chung RS, Li P. Palliative gastrojejunostomy: a minimally invasive approach. Surg Endosc 1997;11:676–678.

17. Naitoh T, Gagner M. Laparoscopically assisted gastric surgery using the Dexterity Pneumo Sleeve. Surg Endosc 1997;11:830–833.

18. Shallmann R. Laparoscopic percutaneous gastrostomy. Gastrointest Endosc 1991;37:493–494.

19. Duh Q-Y, Senokozlieff-Engelhart AL, Choe YS, Siperstein AE, Rowland K, Way LW. Laparoscopic gastrostomy and jejunostomy. Arch Surg 1999;134:151–156.

20. Goh PMY, Alponat A, Mak K, Kum CK. Early international results of laparoscopic gastrectomies. Surg Endosc 1997;11: 650–652.

21. Adachi Y, Suematsu T, Shiraishi N, et al. Quality of life after laparoscolpy-assisted Bilroth I gastrectomy. Ann Surg 1999; 229(1):49–54.

22. Watson DI, Devitt PG, Game PA. Laparoscopic Bilroth II gastrectomy for early gastric cancer. Br J Surg 1995;82: 661–662.

23. Brune IB, Feussner H, Neuhaus H, Classen M, Siewert J-R. Laparoscopic gastrojejunostomy and endoscopic biliary stent placement for palliation of incurable gastric outlet obstruction with cholestasis. Surg Endosc 1997;11:834–837.

24. Rhodes M, Nathanson L, Fiedling G. Laparoscopic biliary and gastric bypass: a useful adjunct in the treatment of carcinoma of the pancreas. Gut 1995;36:778–780.

25. Lo NN, Kee SG, Nambiar R. Palliative gastrojejunostomy for advanced carcinoma of the stomach. Ann Acad Med Singapore 1991;20:356–358.

26. DeRooij DA, Rogatko A, Brennan MF. Evaluation of palliative surgical procedures in unresectable pancreatic cancer. Br J Surg 1991;78:1053–1058.

27. Nagy A, Brosseuk D, Hemming A, Scudamore C. Laparoscopic gastroenterostomy for duodenal obstruction. Am J Surg 1995;169:539–542.

9
Gastric Resection

Jo Buyske

Background and Historical Development of Laparoscopic Gastrectomy

Reports of laparoscopic wedge resections for small tumors of the stomach began to appear in the literature in 1991.[1] The majority of these were informal resections, primarily for benign or low-grade tumors. The more difficult formal gastrectomy was first reported in 1992 by Dr. Peter Goh from Singapore, who performed a laparoscopic hemigastrectomy for chronic ulcer disease.[2] The first laparoscopic gastrectomy for cancer was reported in 1993 by Azagra and Georgen.[3] Laparoscopic gastrectomy was then and continues to be a technically challenging operation, requiring advanced skills and instrumentation. Unlike laparoscopic cholecystectomy, laparoscopic gastectomy has not yet gained wide application. A 1997 worldwide survey of advanced laparoscopic surgeons uncovered a total of 118 such procedures, excluding wedge resections.[4] Several authors have now reported individual cases or small series of laparoscopic or lap-assisted total gastrectomy, hemigastrectomy, and Billroth I and Billroth II reconstructions.[5–12] Several other authors have reported laparoscopic wedge resections or limited gastrectomy procedures.[13–20] As technology continues to improve, and as future generations of surgical residents trained in laparoscopic skills alongside the traditional open skills of surgery go into practice, these procedures will likely increase in frequency.

Indications and Patient Selection

As these pioneers have demonstrated, laparoscopic gastric resection can be applied for all the same indications as can open gastric surgery, which include peptic ulcer disease complicated by gastric outlet obstruction, gastrectomy for gastric carcinoma, and gastric excision for definitive diagnosis of benign lesions or for management of signs or symptoms of obstruction or bleeding from the same.

In the era of H_2 antagonists and proton pump inhibitors, gastric resection for complications of peptic ulcer disease has become less common.[21] Surgical interventions such as highly selective vagotomy may have decreased the need for resective procedures even further. Those patients who do suffer from either untreated or medically resistant peptic ulcer disease, however, may still require surgical intervention.

More than 75% of patients with gastric outlet obstruction due to ulcer disease eventually require surgery.[21] Operative management requires both an antiulcer operation and a drainage procedure, commonly combined as a vagotomy and antrectomy with Billroth I or II reconstruction. Techniques of laparoscopic vagotomy have been described earlier, whereas those for formal laparoscopic gastric resection and reconstruction are described in this chapter.

Surgical resection for gastric cancer is primarily reserved for attempts at cure, although surgery for the palliation of bleeding or chronic obstruction is also indicated. T1 lesions may be good candidates for laparoscopic resection. More advanced tumors requiring wide lymph node dissection or extraction of a large or bulky tumor may be less well suited. As with other laparoscopic cases, patients with poor cardiac function, pulmonary disease with CO_2 retention, morbid obesity, or previous gastric surgery may pose a relative contraindication. Availability of surgical expertise in advanced laparoscopic procedures as well as adequate technical and staff support are essential to success.

Excision of benign gastric lesions can be technically quite straightforward. Lesions located on the greater curve of the stomach, away from either the cardia or the pylorus, are ideal for laparoscopic wedge resection. Lesions throughout the stomach, including those on the posterior wall or adjacent to the cardia or pylorus, can

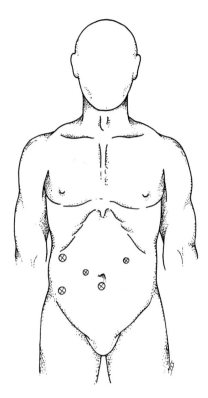

FIGURE 9.1. Location of port sites for laparoscopic gastric resections. (From Cuschieri A. Gastric resections. In: Scott-Conner C (ed) The SAGES Manual. New York: Springer-Verlag New York Inc., 1997:240.[22])

also be approached laparoscopically but may require an endoluminal or transgastric approach and are somewhat more difficult. Preoperative workup should include endoscopy with biopsy, endoscopic ultrasound if available, and MRI or CT imaging to demonstrate the benign nature of the lesion with as much certainty as possible before surgery. If there exists a high degree of suspicion for the presence of malignancy, even if it cannot be proven preoperatively, a plan should be made for formal resection rather than simple wedge.

Surgical Technique

Billroth I and II gastrectomy

The patient is placed in a modified lithotomy position, with the thighs as low as is feasible to allow for unrestricted movement of the instruments. The surgeon stands between the patient's legs, with the first assistant on the patient's right and the second assistant on the left. An umbilical trocar is used for the camera, which can be either a 30° or 0° laparoscope, according to the surgeon's preference. A second port is placed in the right upper quadrant in the anterior axillary line. This port is used for liver retraction. Operating ports are located in the

epigastrium and in the right and left upper quadrants in the midclavicular line. The left upper quadrant port should be 12 mm, to accommodate an endoscopic stapling device (Fig. 9.1).

The procedure is begun by examining the abdomen for evidence of unresectability, including viewing the surfaces of the liver as well as the peritoneal cavity at large. The stomach is evaluated for mobility, to ensure that the tumor is not fixed to adjacent organs. If available, laparoscopic ultrasound is used in the evaluation of the liver.

The greater curve of the stomach is taken down using ultrasonic shears, endoscopic clips, or vascular staples. After all short gastric vessels have been divided, the upper stomach and esophagus is encircled with one quarter inch. Penrose to facilitate control and retraction (Fig. 9.2). A generous Kocher maneuver is performed, elevating the second portion of the duodenum into the horizontal plane. This step is sometimes facilitated by moving the camera to the right upper quadrant port. The duodenum is divided using an endoscopic stapler through the left upper quadrant port. The proximal portion of the duodenum is then grasped and elevated, exposing the attachments of the stomach to the pancreas and retroperitoneum; these are divided using the electrocautery or ultrasonic shears. The previously placed Penrose is utilized at this point to retract the stomach anteriorly and superiorly. Any residual attachments are now cleared using the ultrasonic shears. The stomach is transected using the endoscopic stapler, from greater to lesser curvature. The specimen should be placed in a bag and placed in the right upper quadrant, to be extracted after completion of the anastomosis. Specimen extraction

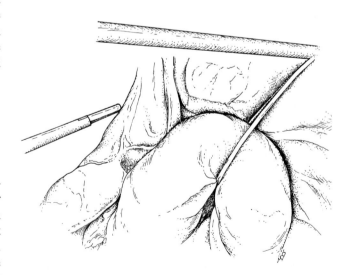

FIGURE 9.2. Sling retraction of stomach during laparoscopic gastrectomy. (From Cushieri A. Gastric resections. In: Scott-Conner C (ed) The SAGES Manual. New York: Springer-Verlag New York Inc., 1977:242.[22])

is facilitated by twisting the stomach up in a manner similar to wringing out a towel, to minimize bulkiness.

A Billroth II reconstruction is performed using the linear cutting stapler.[6] The ligament of Treitz is identified by placing the patient in Trendelenburg and reflecting the colon superiorly. A site for anastomosis on the jejunum is identified and marked with a suture; this is then drawn into the upper abdomen, and the patient is placed again in reverse Trendelenburg. Cautery is used to make an enterotomy in both the gastric remnant and the jejunum. One jaw of the stapler is insinuated into each defect and the stapler fired. The residual defect can be closed using a stapler or sutured closed. Alternatively, a midline epigastric extraction incision measuring 4 cm can be used to exteriorize the stomach remnant as well as the previously identified loop of jejunum, and the anastomosis can be performed in an extracorporeal manner.[22]

A Billroth I reconstruction can be facilitated by conversion of the left upper quadrant trocar to 33 mm to allow introduction of an endoscopic circular stapler.[8] The stapled duodenal stump is opened, and an endoscopic 25-mm circular anvil is placed and secured with an endoloop. An anterior gastrotomy is made, and the endoscopic circular stapler is introduced through the gastrotomy via the 33-mm port. It is advanced through the back wall of the stomach and docked to the anvil. The stapler is fired, and the device is checked to ensure complete donuts of tissue. The anterior gastrotomy can then be sutured or stapled closed.[8]

Wedge Resection

Techniques for resection of benign or low-grade tumors of the stomach vary slightly according to the location of the tumor. In general, the camera is placed at the umbilical port, and a 30° laparoscope is used. For lesions of the anterior wall in the body of the stomach, as few as two additional trocars may be used. Working ports are placed in the upper abdomen at a minimum distance of 8 cm from each other and from the camera. They are ideally placed such that the location of the camera, the working ports, and the location of the lesion as transposed to the abdominal wall form a diamond.[23] The stomach overlying the lesion is grasped and elevated with a Babcock, or alternatively it can be secured with a heavy suture that can in turn be used for elevation. A linear stapler is then fired across the tented-up stomach below the lesion, simultaneously amputating the lesion and sealing the stomach. The specimen is then placed in a bag and brought out through an enlarged trocar site.[15]

Lesions of the posterior wall can be removed in a similar manner where feasible, accomplished by dividing the greater omentum using either the ultrasonic shears or clips. The posterior wall can then be grasped and pulled away from the stomach as already described. Frequently,

however, this position is too awkward to be accomplished safely, in which case lesions of the posterior wall can be approached through an anterior gastrotomy. A small gastrotomy immediately overlying the lesion is made using electrocautery; this is then enlarged by firing an endoscopic stapler, thus making a hemostatic gastrotomy. The lesion is then grasped through the gastrotomy and everted, thus tenting up the posterior wall of the stomach (Fig. 9.3). A stapler is fired across the stomach below the lesion, and the lesion is placed in a bag and set in the right upper quadrant to be removed at the conclusion of the procedure. The gastrotomy is closed by apposing the edges with endoscopic Allis clamps, and firing the stapler across the defect; this commonly requires two firings. The specimen is then withdrawn through an enlarged port site and sent to pathology to confirm negative margins.

Lesions near either the pylorus or the gastroesophageal junction pose special problems, specifically that simple wedge resection may result in unacceptable narrowing of either the inlet or the outlet of the stomach. Under these circumstances, an endo-organ approach may help guide the extent and approach of the resection.[17] This technique is described elsewhere in this volume.

Problems and Controversies

Controversy about laparoscopic gastric resection revolves mainly around two issues: one, is it appropriate to perform laparoscopic resection for gastric malignancy, or indeed any malignancy, and two, is there any benefit to the patient of laparoscopic compared to open gastric surgery.

Laparoscopic surgery for early gastric cancer, specifically those tumors limited to the mucosa, appears to be as effective as open surgery. A 1999 study of 61 patients in Japan who underwent either laparoscopic wedge resection or laparoscopic intragastric mucosal resection reported no deaths and only 2 recurrences in 4 to 65-month follow-up.[18]

A retrospective study of 13 gastric carcinoma patients who underwent laparoscopic resection at one institution reported 84% of the patients to be alive at a mean follow-up of 27 months, with 69% being disease free.[5] The original tumor stage ranged from stage Ia (T1N0M0) to stage IV (Table 9.1). The results of this small series are not dissimilar to what might be expected from open surgery (Table 9.2). To date, there have been no reports of port site recurrences or unusual cases of intraperitoneal dissemination of tumor.

In terms of benefit, one study specifically addressed quality of life in patients undergoing laparoscopic versus open gastrectomy. Forty-one patients in the laparoscopic group and 35 in the open group were evaluated comparing

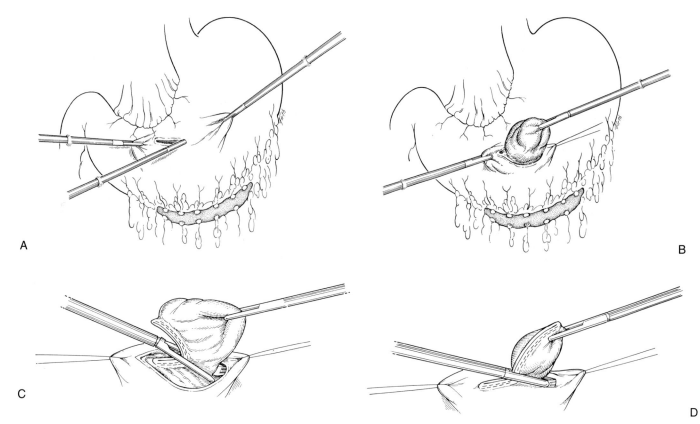

FIGURE 9.3. A. An anterior gastrotomy is made using electo-cautery and a linear stapler. B. A posterior mass is elevated through the gastrotomy. C. A stapler is fired across the posterior gastric wall. D. The gastrotomy is closed using a stapler.

(From Buyske J, McDonald M, Fernandez C, et al. Minimally invasive management of low-grade and benign gastric tumors. Surg Endosc 1997;11:1084–1087.[15])

TABLE 9.1. Laparoscopic gastric resections by patient stage.

Surgical procedure	No. (%)	Stage
Totally laparoscopic D_1 total gastrectomy (D_1 LTG)	2 (15.4)	1 Ia 1 Ib
Laparoscopy-assisted D_1 total gastrectomy (D_1 LATG)	7 (53.8)	1 Ib[a] 3 II 1 IIIa 2 IV
Laparoscopy-assisted D_2 total gastrectomy (D_2 LATG)	2 (15.4)	2 IIIa
Laparoscopy-assisted D_2 total gastrectomy + en bloc distal pancreatectomy (D_2 LATG + DP)	1 (7.7)	1 IIIb
Laparoscopy-assisted distal gastrectomy (LADG)	1 (7.7)	1 II[b]

[a] Major obesity.
[b] Pickwick syndrome.
Source: Azagra JS, Goergen M, DeSimone P, et al. Minimally invasive surgery for gastric cancer. Surg Endosc 1999;13:351–357, with permission.[5]

TABLE 9.2. Results of laparoscopic gastric resection for cancer.

Results	No. (%)
Mean duration of surgery	240 min
Conversions	0
Totally laparoscopic approach	2 (15.4%)
Mean blood losses	300 ml
Intraoperative complications	1 (7.7%)[a]
Surgery-related mortality	1 (7.7%)[b]
Mean postoperative stay	10 days (7–14)
Early postoperative complications	1 (7.7%)[b]
Late postoperative complications	1 (7.7%)[c]
Mean resumption of ambulation	1st day
Mean resumption of oral feeding	5th day
Mean follow-up	27.5 months (3–54)

[a] Inadvertent injury to proper hepatic artery.
[b] Acute hepatic failure and exitus on postoperative day 6 in HCV-related cirrhotic patient.
[c] Multiple splenic abscess treated by means of laparoscopic splenectomy 3 months after prior surgery.
Source: Azagra JS, Goergen M, DeSimone P, et al. Minimally invasive surgery for gastric cancer. Surg Endosc 1999;13:351–357, with permission.[5]

weight loss, dysphagia, dyspepsia, and performance status.[24] The laparoscopic group scored significantly better with regard to weight loss, dumping syndrome, dyspepsia, and overall quality of life. In a much less controlled study, an international survey of surgeons responding to a questionnaire about laparoscopic gastrectomy reported less pain, faster recovery, and better cosmesis. It was noted by the same group that the operation was very long and quite expensive.[4]

Postoperative Care

Early postoperative care for laparoscopic gastric resection is identical to that of open surgery and consists of pain control, intravenous fluids, and gastric decompression. A nasogastric tube is left in place according to the surgeon's preference. Several authors obtain a radiologic contrast study between days 3 and 7 to evaluate for leaks before feeding.[5,8,11] Ambulation, management of the bladder catheter, conversion to oral pain medication, advancement of diet, and discharge from the hospital are all individualized. Reported postoperative length of stay was quite variable, ranging from 3 to 31 days.[4,6,8,9] Return to full activity occurred as early as 1 week after surgery.[8] No formal records of postoperative pain measurements have been reported.

Complications

Morbidity

Complications of laparoscopic gastrectomy are similar to that of open gastrectomy. Reported complications include obstruction at the anastomosis, anastomotic leak, duodenal stump leak, pneumothorax, bleeding from the suture line, and gastric atony.[4,22] A 25% incidence of poor function of the anastomosis after intracorporeal reconstruction caused at least one author to change practice to routinely using extracorporeal anastomosis.[22] Injury to the hepatic artery requiring repair has been reported.[5] Postoperative pancreatitis may present as ileus, abdominal pain, fever, or hyperamylasemia and can be severe.[22]

Mortality

Reported mortality from laparoscopic gastric resection has been rare. Of 118 cases reported by 1997, there were only 3 mortalities[4]; these were due to duodenal stump leak with sepsis, subhepatic abscess, and pneumonia. There is 1 reported death from hepatic failure in a patient with cirrhosis and stage II gastric cancer.[5]

Results

Laparoscopic gastrectomy remains a challenging operation, with a steep learning curve. Operating times are reported between 90 and 360 min,[4,6,11] with cases early in a surgeon's experience taking longer.[6] Limited gastrectomy is a somewhat simpler procedure, and accordingly reported operating times range from 55 to 225 min.[15,17] Days in hospital appear to be similar to that expected for open gastrectomy, with some patients going home as early as postoperative day 3 but many staying a week or longer.[4] A few patients undergoing wedge resection were discharged on postoperative day 1 or 2.[17] Return to daily activities also varies widely, with reports of full activity as early as 7 days and as late as 90 days.

Conclusion

Laparoscopic gastric resection is a feasible alternative to open surgery, with low complication rates and excellent results. Wedge resections appear to offer a somewhat shorter hospital stay and recovery in some patients. Laparoscopic gastric surgery in general does not appear to offer the clear-cut advantages of other laparoscopic procedures such as laparoscopic cholecystectomy or antireflux surgery, in which hospitalization and recovery time have been dramatically reduced.[25] Nevertheless, it holds great promise as a minimally invasive alternative to open gastric surgery.

References

1. Fowler DL, White SA. Laparoscopic resection of a submucosal gastric lipoma: a case report. J Laparoendosc Surg 1991;1(5):303–306.
2. Goh P, Tekant Y, Kum CK, et al. Totally intra-abdominal laparoscopic Billroth II gastrectomy. Surg Endosc 1992;6:160.
3. Azagra JS, Georgen M. Laparoscopic total gastrectomy. In: Meinero M, Melotti G, Mouret PH (eds) Laparoscopic Surgery in the Nineties. Barcelona: Masson, 1994:289–296.
4. Goh P, Alponat A, Mak K, et al. Early international results of laparoscopic gastrectomies. Surg Endosc 1997;11:650–652.
5. Azagra JS, Goergen M, DeSimone P, et al. Minimally invasive surgery for gastric cancer. Surg Endosc 1999;13:351–357.
6. Fowler DL, White SA. Laparoscopic gastrectomy: five cases. Surg Laparosc Endosc 1996;2(6):98–101.
7. Kitano S, Yasunori I, Moriyama M, et al. Laparoscopy-assisted Billroth I gastrectomy. Surg Laparosc Endosc 1994;2(4):146–148.
8. Mayers M, Orebaugh M. Totally laparoscopic Billroth I gastrectomy. J Am Coll Surg 1998;1(186):100–103.
9. Naitoh T, Gagner M. Laparoscopically assisted gastric surgery using dexterity pneumo sleeve. Surg Endosc 1997;11:830–833.

10. Shimizu S, Uchiyama A, Mizumoto K, et al. Laparoscopically assisted distal gastrectomy for early gastric cancer. Surg Endosc 2000;14:27–31.

11. Taniguchi S, Koga K, Ibusuki K, et al. Laparoscopic pylorus-preserving gastrectomy with intracorporeal hand-sewn anastomosis. Surg Laparosc Endosc 1997;7(4):354–356.

12. Uyama I, Sugioka A, Fujita J, et al. Purely laparoscopic pylorus-preserving gastrectomy with extraperigastric lymphadenectomy for early gastric cancer: a case and technical report. Surg Laparosc Endosc Percutan Tech 1999;9(6):418–422.

13. Basso N, Sillecchia G, Pizzuto G, et al. Laparoscopic excision of posterior gastric wall leiomyoma. Surg Laparosc Endosc 1996;6(1):65–67.

14. Benitez LD, Edelman DS. Gastroscopic-assisted laparoscopic wedge resection of B-cell gastric mucosa-associated lymphoid tissue (MALT) lymphoma. Surg Endosc 1999;13:62–64.

15. Buyske J, McDonald M, Fernandez C, et al. Minimally invasive management of low-grade and benign gastric tumors. Surg Endosc 1997;11:1084–1087.

16. DiLorenzo N, Sica GS, Gaspari AL. Laparoscopic resection of gastric leiomyoblastoma. Surg Endosc 1996;10:662–665.

17. Geis WP, Baxt R, Kim HC. Benign gastric tumors minimally invasive approach. Surg Endosc 1996;10:407–410.

18. Ohgami M, Otani Y, Kumai K, et al. Curative laparoscopic surgery for early gastric cancer: five years experience. World J Surg 1999;23:187–193.

19. Otani Y, Ohgami M, Igarashi N, et al. Laparoscopic wedge resection of gastric submucosal tumors. Surg Laparosc Endosc Percutan Tech 2000;10(1):19–23.

20. Yoshida M, Otani Y, Ohgami M, et al. Surgical management of gastric leiomyosarcoma: evaluation of the propriety of laparoscopic wedge resection. World J Surg 1997;21:440–443.

21. Pappas TN. The stomach and duodenum. In: Sabiston DC (ed) Textbook of Surgery, 5th Ed. Philadelphia: Saunders, 1997:847–868.

22. Cuschieri A. Gastric resections. In: Scott-Conner C (ed) The SAGES Manual. Fundamentals of Laparoscopy and GI Endoscopy. New York: Springer, 1998:236–246.

23. Johnson AB, Oddsdottir M, Hunter JG. Laparoscopic Collis gastroplasty and Nissen fundoplication. Surg Endosc 1998;12:1055–1060.

24. Adachi Y, Suematsu T, Shiraishi N, et al. Quality of life after laparoscopy-assisted Billroth I gastrectomy. Am Surg 1999;229(1):49–54.

25. Trus TL, Hunter JG. Minimally invasive surgery of the esophagus and stomach. Am J Surg 1997;173:242–255.

Section II
Laparoscopic Cholecystectomy

Douglas O. Olsen, MD
Section Editor

10
Historical Overview and Indications for Cholecystectomy

Douglas O. Olsen

In 1882, Langenbuch performed one of the first cholecystectomies.[1] He was later quoted as saying "the gallbladder should be removed not because it contains stones, but because it forms stones."[2] Surgical removal of the gallbladder thus became the gold standard for management of biliary calculus disease. Although open cholecystectomy had been performed with minimal morbidity and mortality, physicians and patients alike continued to search for alternatives to what became known as a successful but often very painful means of treating gallbladder disease. A variety of approaches were attempted with little success.

With the widespread use and success of renal lithotripsy in the late 1970s, physicians began considering applying the same technology to gallstone disease. A large amount of money was spent, and many major institutions committed both resources and people to developing the technology of biliary lithotripsy. Before the technique ever became accepted, however, laparoscopic cholecystectomy was introduced and literally took the world by storm. Many have referred to the acceptance of laparoscopic cholecystectomy as a revolution because of the speed and energy with which the technique was accepted. With the introduction of laparoscopic cholecystectomy, patients were given the option of a treatment that managed their disease definitively without the morbidity of a surgical incision. This revolution has stimulated a growth in new technologies that has been unprecedented in surgical history.

Who discovered laparoscopic cholecystectomy is like asking who discovered America. Ultimately, it was a matter of time, technology, and climate in the medical community that brought about laparoscopic cholecystectomy. There had been great effort to search for alternatives to open cholecystectomy. Laparoscopy as a technique had been around for more than half a century and, as of the mid-1970s, was being utilized in gynecology with great success. Many surgeons were attempting to minimize the morbidity of open cholecystectomy by uti-

lizing a mini-lap approach.[3] It was only a matter of time before these efforts were brought together with the introduction of laparoscopic cholecystectomy.

Credit for performing the first procedure is now given to Dr. Erich Muhe of Germany.[4] In September 1985 he performed his first laparoscopic cholecystectomy, but his efforts were lost to the world. Because of local politics his efforts were rejected, and Muhe himself was persecuted for his efforts. In 1987, the French surgeon Philippe Mouret performed his first laparoscopic cholecystectomy while performing laparoscopy on one of his gynecology patients.[5] Once again, this effort went for the most part unrecognized until a French surgeon from Paris encountered this patient and inquired about her surgery. Dr. Francois DuBois had been extremely interested in finding minimal invasive techniques of performing cholecystectomy and was one of the early authors of papers about mini-lap cholecystectomies.[6] Thus, he was extremely interested in this patient and the surgery that she had undergone. Dr. DuBois sought out Dr. Mouret and continued to develop and perfect that technique. In May 1988, Dr. Dubois performed his first laparoscopic cholecystectomy,[5] and after presenting his work to his colleagues, awoke interest in France.

At approximately the same time, two American teams were also working on their own laparoscopic techniques. Drs. McKernan and Saye from Marietta, Georgia, and Drs. Olsen and Reddick from Nashville, Tennessee, were working on their own techniques of laparoscopic cholecystectomy. They performed their first laparoscopic procedures in June and August 1988, respectively.[7] Both the American teams and the French teams worked independently of each other without knowledge of each other's work. Once again, who "discovered" laparoscopic cholecystectomy?

The presentation of the technique at the American College of Surgeons Meeting in Atlanta, Georgia, in the fall of 1989 by Olsen and Reddick introduced the concept of laparoscopic cholecystectomy to the world. And, as contrasted to Dr. Muhe, who tried to convince his colleagues of the technique by lecture and slides, Olsen and Reddick were able to demonstrate their technique with video. Overnight, the technique was accepted and rapidly developed into a procedure that is now the standard for management of calculus biliary disease. In conclusion, one can say it was the video that discovered laparoscopic cholecystectomy.

Early reports of laparoscopic cholecystectomy were confined to a small series of selected groups of patients.[8,9] As a result, much of the early literature lists a variety of contraindications and relative contraindications to the procedure.[10–14] A number of articles report experience in these "difficult" patients to demonstrate that the laparoscopic procedure can be applied to virtually any patient who is a candidate for an open cholecystectomy.[15–18] The few contraindications that remain include the following:

1. A contraindication to open cholecystectomy
2. Inability to tolerate a pneumoperitoneum
3. Pregnancy
4. Inexperience of the surgeon

Contraindication to open cholecystectomy includes patients with recent myocardial infarction, inability to tolerate a general anesthesia, and coagulopathies. The inability to tolerate a pneumoperitoneum is difficult to evaluate preoperatively, but if a patient is found at the time of surgery to be in this category, it is possible to continue the procedure without a pneumoperitoneum by using an abdominal wall-lifting device. Pregnancy is a contraindication from a medicolegal standpoint and not from a technical concern. Although there are reports of laparoscopic cholecystectomy in the pregnant patient,[19,20] there are no studies that demonstrate the safety of a pneumoperitoneum with regard to long-term effects on the fetus.

Inexperience of the surgeon as a contraindication was more of an issue in the preceding years; now most surgeons have become familiar with the technique. The more important issue is that the surgeon realizes when he or she has reached the limits of their expertise and recognizes the proper time to convert the procedure to an open cholecystectomy. To summarize, virtually any patient who is a candidate for open cholecystectomy can be approached with a laparoscopic technique.

References

1. Langenbuch C. Ein Fall von Exterpation der Gallenblase wegen chronischer Cholelithiasis: Heilung. Klin Wochenschr 1882;19:725–727.
2. Halpert B. Fiftieth anniversary of the removal of the gallbladder. Arch Surg 1982;117:1526–30.
3. Olsen DO. Mini-lap cholecystectomy. Am J Surg 1993;165:440–443.
4. Litynski G. Erich Muhe—a surgeon ahead of his time. The first laparoscopic cholecystectomies. In: Highlights in the History of Laparoscopy. Frankfurt: Bernert, 1996.
5. Litynski G. Mouret, Dubois, and Perissat. The French connection. In: Highlights in the History of Laparoscopy Frankfurt: Bernert, 1996.
6. DuBois F, Berthelot B. Cholecystectomie par mini-laparotomie. Nouv Presse Med 1982;11:1139–1141.
7. Litynski G. The American spirit awakens. In: Highlights in the History of Laparoscopy. Frankfurt: Bernert, 1996.
8. Reddick EJ, Olsen DO. Laparoscopic laser cholecystectomy: a comparison with mini-lap cholecystectomy. Surg Endosc 1989;3:131.
9. Dubois F, Berthelot G, Levard H. Cholecystectomie par coelioscopie. Presse Med 1989;18:980–982.
10. Soper N. Effect of nonbiliary problems on laparoscopic cholecystectomy. Am J Surg 1993;165:522–526.
11. Cameron JC, Gadaez TR. Laparoscopic cholecystectomy. Ann Surg 1991;213:1–2.
12. Soper N. Laparoscopic cholecystectomy. In: Wells S (ed) Current Problems in Surgery. St. Louis: Mosby-Year Book 1991:583–655.
13. Baily R, Zucker K, et al. Laparoscopic cholecystectomy, experience with 375 consecutive patients. Ann Surg 1991;214:531–541.
14. Cushieri A, Berci G, McSherry C. Laparoscopic cholecystectomy. Am J Surg 1990;159:273.
15. Olsen D, Asbun H, Reddick E, Spaw A. Laparoscopic cholecystectomy for acute cholecystitis. Probl Gen Surg 1991;8:426–431.
16. Cooperman AM. Laparoscopic cholecystectomy for severe, acute, gangrenous cholecystitis. J Laparoendosc Surg 1990;1:37–40.
17. Unger S, Edelman D, Scott J, Hunger H. Laparoscopic treatment of acute cholecystitis. Surg Laparosc Endosc 1991;1:14–16.
18. Unger S, Unger H, Edelman D, et al. Obesity: an indication rather than contraindication to laparoscopic cholecystectomy. Obesity Surg 1992;2:29–31.
19. Arvidsson D, Gerdin E. Laparoscopic cholecystectomy during pregnancy. Surg Laparosc Endosc 1991;1:193–194.
20. Hunter JG. Laparoscopy in the pregnant patient. Surg Endosc 1992;6:52–53.

11
Surgical Anatomy of the Gallbladder, Liver, and Biliary Tree

Paul E. Wise and Michael D. Holzman

Discussion of laparoscopic cholecystectomy would not be complete without a thorough review of the anatomy of the liver, biliary tree, and gallbladder. Much of today's hepatobiliary anatomy was described by Couinaud in the mid-1900s and further delineated by corrosion casts, stereoscopic radiographs, and computerized three-dimensional imagery. The biliary system and hepatic vasculature are generally much more variable than any other part of the human anatomy.[1] The commonly described biliary system and potential anomalies from the cholangiocytes to the lower duodenal sphincter apparatus are the focus of this chapter. In addition, anatomic changes that result from pathophysiological processes requiring cholecystectomy are also addressed.

General Anatomy of the Liver

Grossly, the liver appears divided into two *lobes* (right and left) by the umbilical fissure and falciform ligament. This topographical lobar anatomy is misleading in comparison to the actual functional or segmental anatomy of the liver. Topographically, the inferior aspect of the right lobe is bound posteriorly by the transverse fissure, with the tissue lying anterior to this called the quadrate lobe. Also posteriorly, behind the portal vein, is another distinct region known as the caudate lobe. These four lobes (right, left, caudate, and quadrate) constitute the major topographical lobar anatomy of the liver. Use of the term lobes in the topographical sense has become routine in descriptions of the liver, but most hepatobiliary surgeons and endoscopists use either the French or American classification of hepatic anatomy (or both) to describe the liver's segmental anatomy.

French Segmental System

Couinaud most completely developed the functional anatomic description of the liver, which became known as the French segmental system for hepatic anatomy,[2] in the 1950s. This system shows more consideration for the hepatic venous drainage but also applies to the portal, biliary, and arterial anatomy.[3] Instead of four hepatic divisions, as in the topographical system, there are eight divisions or segments: four on the right, three on the left, and one corresponding to the topographical caudate lobe (segment I). Segments II through IV constitute the left lobe and segments V through VIII the right lobe (Fig. 11.1). The three main hepatic veins divide the liver into four sectors called *portal sectors*, each of which receives a portal vein pedicle (Fig. 11.2). The planes containing the right, middle, and left hepatic veins are called *portal scissurae* (right, main, and left), and the planes containing portal pedicles are called *hepatic scissurae.*[2]

American (Lobar) System

The American system of hepatic classification is based on the fact that the distribution of the major branches of the veins, arteries, or bile ducts of the liver does not conform precisely to the topographical anatomy. The relationships between the hepatic veins and portal vein branches therefore determine the lobar anatomy of the liver in this classification system.[4] The lobar anatomy of the liver is best demonstrated by direct injection of its blood supply with substances such as methylene blue or colored celloidin (Fig. 11.3). A plane called the portal fissure (Cantlie's line) passes from the left side of the gallbladder fossa to the left side of the inferior vena cava to divide the liver into its right and left lobes. The left lobe consists of a medial segment, which lies to the right of the falciform ligament and umbilical fissure, and a lateral segment, which lies to the left of the falciform ligament. The right lobe consists of an anterior and a posterior segment. No visible surface marking delineates the lobar segmental anatomy on the right. Conventionally, most of the topographical caudate lobe is in the medial segment of the left lobe, but it extends over the plane between the

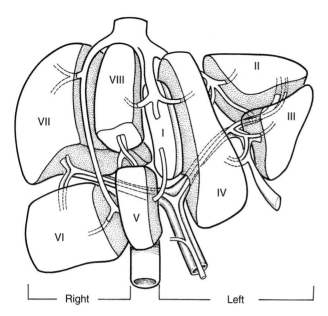

FIGURE 11.1. The French segmental system of hepatic anatomy described by Couinaud and determined by portal venous flow and hepatic venous drainage.

gallbladder and the inferior vena cava into the right lobe.[5] The conceptual division of the liver into lobes and segments forms the basis for the classic types of major hepatic resections (left or right lobectomy, left lateral segmentectomy, and right trisegmentectomy) (Fig. 11.4). The lobes may be further divided into subsegments that

correspond to the segments described in the French system.

Definitions

It is important to carefully define a number of terms utilized in this chapter and in surgical practice. The terms *proximal* and *distal* in the biliary system refer to the direction of biliary flow. Therefore, the proximal end would be within the parenchyma of the liver, the distal end being at the ampullary apparatus. As already described, the term *lobe* or *lobar* refers to the American system of anatomy, with the division of right and left lobes being the gallbladder fossa (Cantlie's line). Whenever the term lobe is used to describe topographical anatomy, it is used in conjunction with another term (e.g., caudate lobe). The term *segment* or *segmental* refers to the French segmental system. For clarity, the American meaning of segment is not used within this chapter unless specified.

The term *common bile duct* refers to the portion of the major biliary system only from the junction of the cystic duct to the duodenal communication. The portion of the biliary system above the junction of the cystic duct up to the hepatic duct confluence is the common hepatic duct. By definition, the term *common duct* includes the actual junctional area with the cystic duct but the *common hepatic duct* term does not. The *confluence* refers to the most predominant biliary junction of the right and left lobes of the liver; this may or may not be the last junction of the right and left lobe. For example, an accessory duct from segment VI may join the common hepatic duct or cystic duct considerably below the confluence. It is also

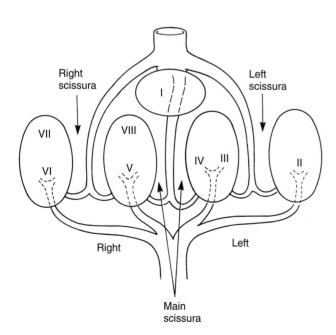

FIGURE 11.2. Another view of how the French segmental system divides the liver. Each *portal sector* receives one of four *portal pedicles*. The planes between these sectors are called the *portal scissurae* and contain the three hepatic veins.

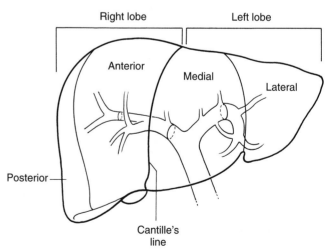

FIGURE 11.3. The American (lobar) system of hepatic anatomy is also determined by the relationships of the portal and hepatic veins, but this system does not routinely subsegment the liver as much as the French system.

FIGURE 11.4. Classic liver resections based on the American system of hepatic anatomy. A. Right lobectomy. B. Left lobectomy. C. Trisegmentectomy or right extended lobectomy. D. Left lateral segmentectomy.

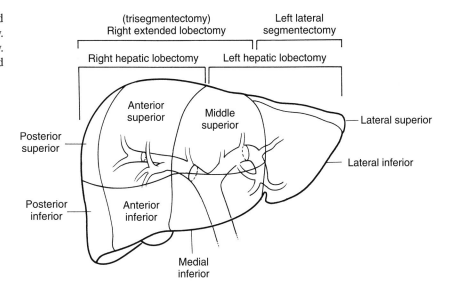

possible that there are more than two ducts which define the confluence. A segmental duct drains the parenchyma of a French segment, that is, segments I to VIII. Sectoral ducts have a similar meaning, except pertaining to the four parenchymal sectors of the French system.

The *cystic duct* refers to the entire ductal structure communicating between the gallbladder and the main extrahepatic biliary system. If an accessory or anomalous duct joins the cystic duct, the entire length of the duct until it joins the primary system is still the cystic duct. *Accessory* refers to an unusual location of an expected structure, such as a duct. The terms *anomalous* or *aberrant* are essentially synonymous and refer to additional unexpected variations of structures. For example, a segment VI duct joining the cystic duct before its junction with the common hepatic duct would be accessory, whereas a large duct of Luschka between the gallbladder and liver parenchyma is anomalous because it does not correspond to a specific segment or sector. Because the amount of duct necessary to drain a portion of liver has not been substantially determined on a physiological level, the term accessory should not connote simply an alternate route for bile. The gallbladder is determined by the presence of a cystic duct. For example, a septated gallbladder with only one cystic duct is one gallbladder, whereas multiple cystic ducts associated with blind sacs (e.g., fairly common in cows) refer to multiple gallbladders.

At the distal end of the biliary system, three terms are commonly used. *Ampulla* refers to dilatation of the biliary system just within the duodenal mucosa. The pancreatic duct may or may not join directly within the ampulla. The term *papilla* refers to the small, nipple-shaped tissue created by the ampulla and its associated muscle fibers that project into the duodenum. The *ampullary sphincter* refers to a ringlike band of muscle

fibers that constricts the biliary passage and may close the natural orifice.

Embryology

The first signs of the formation of the hepatobiliary system are noted at approximately the fifth week of intrauterine life when an outpouching forms from the ventral surface of the primitive gastrointestinal tract just beyond the junction of the foregut and midgut. This outpouching eventually forms both lobes of the liver, the entirety of the biliary tree, and a portion of the pancreatic head and uncinate process. As the outpouching progresses superiorly, it divides into a superior bud that leads to the formation of the liver and an inferior bud which forms the gallbladder and common duct. A separate third bud leads to formation of the ventral pancreas. If the inferior bud progresses too far superiorly, an intrahepatic gallbladder (usually in the right lobe) may form. The rotation of the ventral pancreas and the rest of the gastrointestinal tract brings the junction of the common bile duct and duodenum onto the posteromedial wall of the duodenum. By the seventh to eighth week of intrauterine life, a lumen has formed within the biliary tree and gallbladder. Bile starts to form in the liver and flow through the biliary system after 3 months of development.[1]

Intrahepatic Ducts

The biliary drainage system begins at the hepatocyte/cholangiocyte level where portions of the hepatocyte membrane form small channels called canaliculi. Bile drains from the canaliculi into intrahepatic

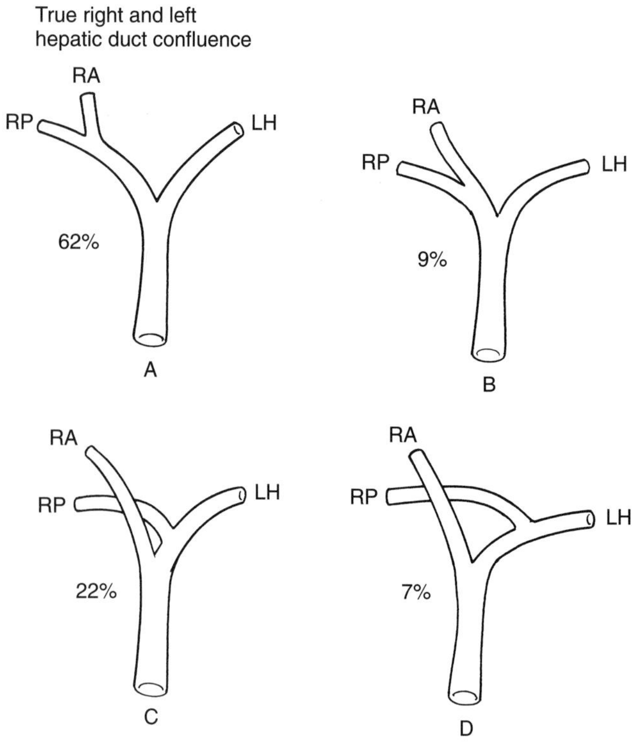

FIGURE 11.5. Primary variations of the hepatic duct confluence (percentages based on anatomic studies). A. "True" right and left hepatic duct confluence (62%). B. Triple branch confluence (9%). C. Right posterior sectoral duct draining into left or common hepatic duct (22%). D. Right anterior sectoral duct draining into left or common hepatic duct (7%).

ducts that follow the segmental anatomy determined primarily by the vascular supply.[6] The convergence of canaliculi and proximal ductal systems is called the canal of Hering. The smaller ducts unite to form a single channel called the segmental bile duct. The ductal patterns then become more variable as the biliary system travels distal from the canaliculi.

The right and left hepatic ducts are formed by the confluence of the segmental ducts within the substance of the liver. The left lobar duct forms in the umbilical fissure from the union of ducts from segments II, III, and IV and then passes to the right across the base of segment IV (medial portion of the left lobe, topographical quadrate lobe). Although there are numerous segmental variations in the left ductal system, the left side is less variable at the level of the confluence than the right ductal system[7] (Fig. 11.5). The right hepatic duct drains segments V to VIII and arises from the junction of the right anterior and posterior sectoral ducts. The early anatomic descriptions of the right anterior and posterior ducts as consistently failing to form a single right hepatic duct is probably inaccurate. These ducts of the right side join each other but are extremely variable with respect to the order and

site of the union. The most typical anatomy has the right posterior sectoral duct following an almost horizontal course before joining with the anterior duct, which descends more vertically. This junction is usually found above the right branch of the portal vein. In a minority of cases, the right ducts do not all incorporate into one right hepatic duct. Instead, a right segmental or sectoral duct joins the left hepatic duct and creates a third duct that seems to join the confluence. The biliary drainage of the caudate lobe (segment I) varies considerably, but enters both the right and left hepatic duct systems about 80% of the time. In about 15% of cases, the caudate lobe drains only into the left hepatic ductal system and in about 5% it drains only into the right hepatic duct.[8]

As the segmental ducts join to form right and left lobar (hepatic) ducts, it is not unusual for 1 to 3 cm of the lobar duct to lie within the hepatic tissue. In about 98% of cases, the right and left ducts unite in an extrahepatic position. The usual extrahepatic length of each hepatic duct varies from 0.5 to 1.5 cm. Most often, a shorter extrahepatic right duct joins a longer left duct at the level of the base of the right branch of the portal vein.[9] Because of this length discrepancy, the terminal intrahepatic segment of the left hepatic duct generally is easier to delineate than the similar segment of the right hepatic duct. This anatomic fact is of considerable importance in operative procedures in which an additional length of biliary duct is needed for an anastomosis to the intestinal tract.[10]

Depending partly upon their extrahepatic length, the right and left hepatic ducts join at a wide or acute angle, or even descend parallel to each other for a variable distance before their union. Most often they merge about 1 cm below the hepatic parenchyma to form the common hepatic duct. The angle at which the right and left ducts join is of clinical significance to both the endoscopist and hepatobiliary surgeon. When viewing the union of the lobar ducts from the level of the common hepatic duct, the right hepatic duct often is a "straight shot" relative to the more acute angle of the left hepatic duct. For this reason, the endoscopist at endoscopy and the surgeon during choledochoscopy frequently enter directly into the right lobe of the liver and have greater difficulty entering the left lobe.

Changes in the "typical" intrahepatic ductal anatomy caused by compensatory enlargement of liver tissue after damage or resection of a segment or lobe have been known for almost a century. The distorted configuration of the liver and the tendency of the lobe undergoing hypertrophy to rotate and extend across the midline causes diagnostic and operative difficulties. Vessels and ducts conform to this spatial lobar rearrangement with the following consequences: first, the portal vein lies more superficially and is therefore at risk for being injured; and second, the portal venous branches develop an anterior relationship to the bile ducts, making access to these ducts exceedingly difficult. In effect, the hilar vascular structures course obliquely anterior while the bile duct goes posteriorly.[11]

Common Hepatic Duct

The common hepatic duct is the length of biliary duct from the hepatic duct confluence to the cystic duct. The common hepatic duct makes up the left border of the triangle of Calot, which becomes important in any discussion of the laparoscopic cholecystectomy and is therefore described in greater detail in a separate section (following). The length of common hepatic duct varies from 1 to 10 cm depending on the location of the junction with the cystic duct, where it then becomes the common bile duct.[12] The common hepatic duct at the area of the confluence is separated anteriorly from the posterior aspect of the quadrate lobe by the "hilar plate." This structure is a fusion of Glisson's capsule and the connective tissue surrounding the biliary and vascular elements in this area, which, when opened, can allow excellent exposure to the confluence and common hepatic duct.[7]

The common hepatic duct can often be associated with accessory ducts. These accessory hepatic ducts are so common as to be found in up to 20% of people. They are readily injured at cholecystectomy if they traverse the triangle of Calot. In more than half of the cases in which an accessory duct is found, it joins the common hepatic duct somewhere along its course. Less frequently, the accessory duct joins the cystic duct. In the rarest of instances, it may join a duct in the opposite lobe. The majority of aberrant ducts are on the right side. True aberrant ducts (see definitions) are rare. One should have higher suspicion for aberrant hepatic ductal anatomy when there appears to be unusual arterial or distal biliary anatomy.[13]

Gallbladder

The gallbladder is a pear-shaped, distensible appendage of the extrahepatic biliary system, usually holding 30 to 50 ml of bile. It lies in a depression on the inferior, or visceral, surface of the right lobe of the liver. The position of the gallbladder marks the boundary of the right and left hepatic lobes in the American system. The gallbladder is attached to the liver by areolar connective tissue that contains multiple small lymphatics and veins. These lymphatic and veins connect the venous and lymphatic systems of the gallbladder with those of the liver. Rarely, one or more small accessory bile ducts pass through this tissue to enter the gallbladder directly (ducts of Luschka).[14] In extremely unusual cases, major hepatic ducts might even drain directly into the gallbladder.

Arbitrary definitions divide the gallbladder into a fundus, body, infundibulum, and neck. The fundus is the round, blind end of the gallbladder that usually projects about 1 cm beyond the free edge of the right lobe of the liver. The top of the fundus is often at the apex of an angle formed by the right lateral border of the rectus muscle and the ninth costal cartilage. In this position it comes into contact with the anterior peritoneum of the abdominal wall. The fundus becomes palpable in the right upper abdominal quadrant with gallbladder distension. Usually in association with stones or cholestasis, the fundus may become kinked upon itself, an anomaly referred to as a Phrygian cap. Grossly this may look like a fungating mass, but histologically the tissue only contains an abundance of fibrous tissue.

The fundus passes without a demonstrable transition into the body, which constitutes the largest segment of the organ. Unless a mesentery is present, the entire superior surface of the gallbladder body is closely attached to the visceral surface of the liver over the area of the gallbladder bed. This intimate relationship to the visceral surface of the liver easily permits direct spread of gallbladder inflammation, infection, or neoplasia into the parenchyma of the liver. This relationship also permits passage of a cholecystostomy catheter through the liver parenchyma into the gallbladder without spillage.

The infundibulum of the gallbladder is the tapering transitional area between the body and neck of the organ. It usually appears as a shallow diverticulum, lying close to the undersurface of the cystic duct, and occasionally obscuring the duct from view. It is attached to the right lateral surface of the second portion of the duodenum by an avascular peritoneal fold called the cholecystoduodenal ligament. The free surface of the body and the infundibulum of the gallbladder also lie in close approximation to the first portion of the duodenum as well as to the hepatic flexure and the right third of the transverse colon.

The infundibulum of the gallbladder rapidly tapers into the neck, which may be narrow and curve upon itself in the form of an "S." The neck is usually directed superiorly and to the left. It narrows into a sometimes poorly defined constriction at its junction with the cystic duct. The transition between the neck and the cystic duct can be gradual or abrupt. The neck is quite short, usually 5 to 7 mm.[15] An asymmetrical outpouching of the inferior surface of the infundibulum known as Hartmann's pouch lies close to the neck. It can often be used as a point of traction to provide exposure during cholecystectomy, but it is occasionally adherent to the cystic duct, making the operation difficult.[1] Hartmann's pouch may also trap large gallstones that are unable to enter the neck or cystic duct.[7]

Unusual morphologies of the gallbladder including septations or duplications or even agenesis may occa-

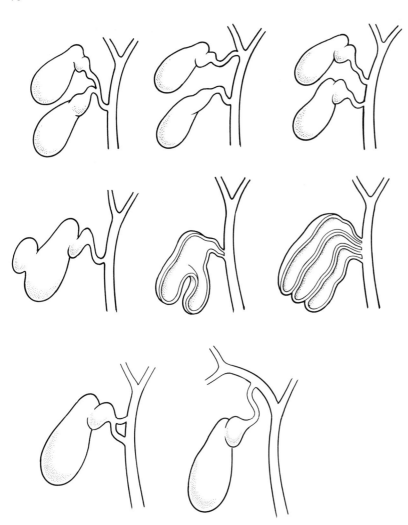

FIGURE 11.6. Unusual gallbladder morphologies occasionally encountered during laparoscopy or laparotomy.

sionally present during laparotomy or laparoscopy (Fig. 11.6). These are all rare anomalies with which the hepatobiliary specialist should be familiar. A septated gallbladder is by definition a bilobar gallbladder with a single cystic duct but two fundi. Duplication of the gallbladder means the presence of two cystic ducts. A double cystic duct draining a unilocular gallbladder has once been described. More frequently encountered anomalies of the cystic duct and gallbladder are intrahepatic gallbladders and a gallbladder within the left lobe of the liver.[16]

Cystic Duct

The cystic duct is the route by which the gallbladder fills and empties its bile. It connects the neck of the gallbladder to the common hepatic duct. In as many as 10% of cases, a portion of the right hepatic biliary system joins the cystic duct before its junction with the common hepatic duct. Past autopsy studies of this anatomy have been misleading, and most applicable information comes from recent clinical studies involving cholangiography.

Generally, the cystic duct is about 4 cm long. The length may vary from 0.5 to 8 cm depending on the site of the gallbladder and the junction with the common hepatic duct. The circumference of the duct varies from 3 to 12 mm.[17] The mucous membrane that lines the cystic duct usually has 4 to 10 folds, referred to as the spiral valves of Heister. The valves regulate bile flow, serving to prevent excess distension or collapse of the cystic duct, particularly as intraductal pressure changes. The valves may be extremely tortuous, complicating cannulation during intraoperative cholangiography.

The cystic duct usually runs dorsally, to the right, and inferiorly to the common hepatic duct. The course may be quite tortuous, mimicking other ducts until dissected. As a general rule, the cystic duct joins the right aspect of the common hepatic duct. The cystic duct may (1) join the common hepatic duct at various angles; (2) be parallel to the right side of the common hepatic duct before entering it; (3) be dorsal to the common duct and enter its dorsal surface; (4) be dorsal to the common duct and enter it from the left side; (5) enter the right or left hepatic duct directly; or (6) join the common duct just before it enters the posteromedial wall of the duodenum. The mode of entrance of the cystic duct into the common hepatic duct may be angular, parallel, or spiral. The angular type occurs in about 80% of people. The angle may vary from a right angle to an acute angle of 10°. With the parallel type of junction, the two ducts may run alongside each other for several centimeters. In such cases, the ducts may be closely adherent and impossible to separate without injuring the common bile duct. The complexity is compounded when a common sheath of dense connective tissue encircles the two ducts. In such cases it is considered safest to leave a long cystic duct stump attached to the common bile duct at the time of cholecystectomy. In the spiral type of junction, which occurs in about 2% of the population, the cystic duct may pass either ventral or dorsal to the common hepatic duct before joining it. Spiral cystic ducts may join on any surface of the common hepatic duct, including the left lateral side.[18]

The variable site of the union of the hepatic and cystic ducts determines the length of the common bile duct. If this union is low, that is, distal within the porta hepatis near the duodenum, the supraduodenal portion of the common bile duct is very short or even absent. If this is the case, the cystic and common hepatic ducts run parallel for a considerable length, causing difficulties during cholecystectomy. The cystic duct may also be very short or absent, in which case the gallbladder may appear to empty directly into the common hepatic duct.

Triangle of Calot and Rouviere's Sulcus

The region known as Calot's triangle differs today when compared to the area described by Calot in 1890 while he was a medical student. He described in his thesis a triangle bordered by the cystic artery, the cystic duct, and the common hepatic duct. The area described today as his triangle is the region bounded by the cystic duct, common (or right) hepatic duct, and inferior border of the liver. The change is thought to have occurred because of the practical use of the larger triangle that helps to frame and identify the cystic artery that lies within it.[19]

Recognition of critical structures and dissection within Calot's triangle is of great importance during cholecystectomy, especially at the apex of the triangle. The apex of the triangle contains the cystic artery, as discussed, as well as the right branch of the hepatic artery, 95% of accessory right hepatic arteries, and 90% of accessory bile ducts.[1] An anomalous hepatic artery arising from the superior mesenteric trunk (replaced right hepatic artery) usually courses superiorly in the groove posterolateral to the common bile duct. Therefore, it appears on the medial side of the apex of Calot's triangle, just behind the cystic duct where it is vulnerable to injury during cholecystectomy. Some degree of replacement is thought to occur in up to 10% of patients.[20]

Bile duct injuries during cholecystectomy most frequently occur because of poor exposure of Calot's triangle, leading to confusion between the common hepatic or common bile duct and the cystic duct. Similarly, vascular injuries or significant bleeding that can obscure the dissection can occur if the exposure of this anatomy is inadequate. Multiple styles and techniques are outlined in the literature to expand Calot's triangle to its greatest widths and thus improve exposure of the key structures while attempting to avoid tenting the common duct into the area of dissection. In the end, these various means are all dependent on repetition and the experience of the surgeon to avoid ductal or vascular injuries.[21]

Another landmark in this region that can be helpful in identifying the plane of the common bile duct and avoiding injuries during cholecystectomy is Rouviere's sulcus, identified by Rouviere in 1924 as a 2- to 5-cm sulcus lying anterior to the caudate lobe and running to the right of the liver hilum and usually containing the right portal triad. Based on anatomic studies by Couinaud and supported by subsequent laparoscopic cholecystectomy studies, this sulcus is identifiable in approximately 75% of patients and accurately identifies the plane of the common bile duct as substantiated by cholangiogram. Identification of the sulcus requires anterosuperior and leftward retraction of the neck of the gallbladder with exposure and dissection of the posterior hepatobiliary triangle bounded by the neck of the gallbladder, the liver surface, and the plane of the sulcus. Dissection maintained ventral to the plane of the common bile duct, with care taken to identify a possible posterior cystic artery branch or tortuous hepatic artery, is safe even with tenting of the common bile duct.[22]

Common Bile Duct

The junction of the common hepatic duct with the cystic duct forms the common bile duct. The length of the common duct is variable, reported in the adult to be as short as 1 cm and as long as 17 cm.[23] The upper limit of normal for the diameter of the common bile duct was formerly controversial. Increased use of ultrasonography has now defined the upper limit of normal for common bile duct diameter as 6 mm; the upper limit of normal for the entire width of the duct including the walls is 8 mm. These measurements are described as the 95% confidence limits of normal, so one still needs to consider normal in the differential of other ductal widths. After cholecystectomy, the normal common bile duct may dilate to 10 to 12 mm.

Once the common bile duct has formed by the junction of the cystic and common hepatic ducts, it is designated as the supraduodenal segment of the common bile duct. Subsequently, it becomes the retroduodenal portion

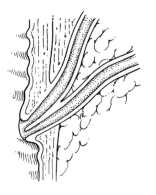
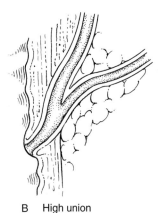
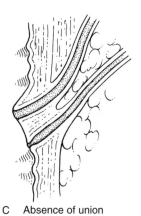

FIGURE 11.7. Typical configurations of the union of the common bile duct and the pancreatic duct: A. Low union. B. High union. C. Absence of union.

A Low union   B High union   C Absence of union

that in turn leads to the pancreatic and eventually the intraduodenal segments of the common bile duct. The supraduodenal segment is usually the longest portion of the common duct and lies in the hepatoduodenal ligament. Superior to the first portion of the duodenum, the common bile duct lies ventral to the epiploic foramen of Winslow. Classically, a stone in this segment of the common bile duct was often easily palpated during an open procedure. Multiple lymph nodes also lie close to the supraduodenal portion of the common bile duct. Most of these are on the portal (posterior) side of the duct. When enlarged, these occasionally may be mistaken for gallstones during palpation.

The retroduodenal segment of the duct varies in length from 2 to 4.5 cm. It lies dorsal to the middle aspect of the duodenum and slants obliquely as it runs from the superior to the inferior duodenal surface. To the left of the retroduodenal portion of the duct is the gastroduodenal artery. There, the common bile duct is sometimes involved in the inflammatory reaction associated with a posterior duodenal ulcer. The surgeon must also be careful not to divide or entrap the common bile duct while transecting or suturing the proximal portion of the duodenum.[14]

The pancreatic segment of the common bile duct is related to the head of the pancreas in either of two ways. It may be entirely retropancreatic, lying between the pancreas and areolar tissues of the retroperitoneum; or it may lie within the substance of the dorsal portion of the pancreatic head, covered dorsally by a thin layer of pancreatic tissue. This segment of the common bile duct has a gentle convex curve as it descends relatively close to the descending portion of the duodenum. About halfway along its pancreatic course, the common duct starts to curve gently to the right, then quite abruptly turns almost 90° in the same direction to enter the descending duodenum. The superior pancreaticoduodenal branch of the gastroduodenal artery crosses this segment of the common bile duct. The location of the artery and its multiple duodenal and pancreatic branches makes exposure of the common duct in this region challenging.[24]

The intraduodenal segment of the common bile duct passes through the duodenal wall tangentially for almost 2 cm. Most of its course lies in a submucosal plane. The classic anatomic position given for the site of penetration of the duodenum by the common bile duct is the posteromedial wall. Generally, this site is about 7 cm from the pylorus. The intraduodenal portion of the common bile duct forms the ampulla of Vater, usually as a consequence of the junction of the bile duct and major pancreatic duct. The length of the ampulla varies from 3 to 14 mm, depending to some degree on the location of the junction. This junction forms the ampulla in one of three ways. (1) Frequently there is an extraduodenal junction of the two ducts just external to the posteromedial duodenal wall (high union). In such instances, the two ducts run parallel to one another for a distance of 2 to 10 mm before they penetrate the duodenal wall. During this close extraduodenal association, the lumens of the two ducts join and form a single lumen entering the wall. (2) During the passage of the closely applied ducts through the duodenal wall, the septum between the two may be lost just at the ampulla (low union); this would form a true common channel that would open through a single ostium on the major duodenal papilla. (3) In about 20% of cases, the septum between the ducts persists throughout the entire passage. In this case there is no common channel proximal to the major duodenal papilla, and the two ducts empty by separate ostia (absence of union)[25] (Fig. 11.7). These three junctions are the most common types, but there are rare instances when the pancreatic and common bile duct share a long common channel before they reach the duodenum to form the ampulla. For example, as many as 90% of patients with a type III choledochal cyst have a supraduodenal junction of the pancreatic and biliary ducts leading to a lengthy single common duct.

As the common bile duct proceeds through the duodenal wall, it narrows markedly. In 50% of cases, it narrows just before emptying into the ampulla. In virtually all patients the ampulla also narrows just before it empties via the major duodenal papilla. These narrow areas are the most common sites for stone impaction in biliary calculus disease. These sites can also appear to form a ridge between the wide extraduodenal portion of the duct and the narrower intraduodenal segment. This ridge is important in the interpretation of endoscopic retrograde cholangiopancreatography (ERCPs) and during common duct explorations because it might be interpreted as a pathological mass or, unless care is taken when the intraduodenal junction is probed, a false passage might be created.

The circular smooth muscle fibers in the ampulla of Vater area constitute the sphincter of Oddi, which regulates flow of bile from the liver into the duodenum (Fig. 11.8). The sphincter of Oddi consists of three principal parts. The first part is the sphincter of the choledochus, the group of circular muscle fibers surrounding the intramural and submucosal bile duct that is responsible for gallbladder filling during fasting. The second portion is the pancreatic sphincter, which is the variable amuscular septum between the biliary and pancreatic ducts that laminates the secretions from these ducts. The final part is the ampullary sphincter, which is the most important component of the sphincter of Oddi.[26] The ampullary sphincter includes a layer of longitudinal muscle fibers that helps prevent reflux of intestinal contents into the ampulla. Relaxation of the ampullary sphincter also promotes reflux into the pancreatic duct.[27,28]

Arterial Supply

The hepatic artery supplies approximately 25% of the total blood flow to the liver; however, it provides up to 75% of the oxygenated blood and about 85% to 90% of the blood to the extrahepatic biliary system (Fig. 11.9). This extrahepatic arterial system does not parallel the portal channels, although the intrahepatic system does. More than 50% of the population has the same hepatic arterial pattern.[29] The hepatic artery arises from the celiac axis and passes along the upper part of the pancreas toward the liver. Posterior and superior to the duodenum it gives off the gastroduodenal artery. Within the hepatoduodenal ligament, the hepatic artery divides into right and left branches and subsequently into smaller branches corresponding to the portal venous system, segmental, or subsegmental anatomy. Often a third artery feeds portions of segment IV and the right lobe of the liver.

Because of abundant collaterals, ligation of the hepatic artery proximal to the gastroduodenal artery fails to damage the liver.

Ligation of the hepatic artery distal to the gastroduodenal artery occasionally produces hepatic necrosis. Usually, however, this does not result in serious consequences because there are also rich extrinsic collaterals to the hepatic artery beyond the gastroduodenal artery. Ligation of the right or left hepatic artery individually predictably results in marked elevation of hepatic enzyme levels but often still without severe clinical manifestations. A diffuse subcapsular arterial plexus may

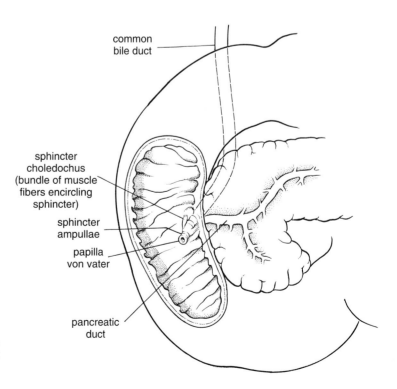

FIGURE 11.8. The ampulla of Vater including papilla, ampullary sphincter, and union of common bile duct and pancreatic duct.

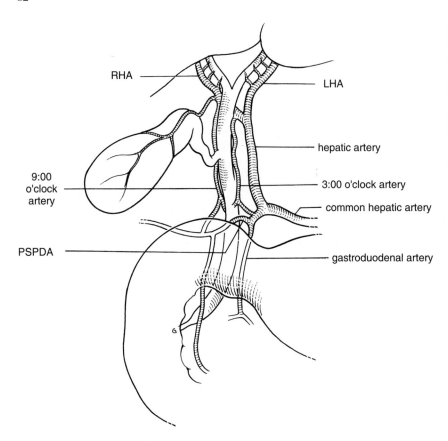

Figure 11.9. Blood supply to the extra-hepatic biliary tree. The distal portion is usually supplied by the retroduodenal artery (RDA) and the proximal portion by branches from the right and left hepatic arteries (RHA, LHA). The mid-portion of the biliary tree is usually dependent on the marginal anastomotic artery (MAA) and other fine axially arranged collaterals between the RDA and the RHA.

contribute significantly to the hepatic arterial collateral circulation, as well as supply from the celiac, superior mesenteric, and inferior phrenic artery. A recent angiographic study showed that rich collaterals can also develop in the liver's suspensory ligaments.[30]

The most important variations of the hepatic arterial system are a right hepatic artery arising from the superior mesenteric artery and a common hepatic artery arising from a superior mesenteric trunk ("replaced" hepatic artery). Other anomalies include the left hepatic artery arising from the left gastric artery and the right hepatic artery traveling anterior rather than posterior to the portal vein. In addition, the right hepatic artery often has a curved extrahepatic course, which may lead to inadvertent ligation during cholecystectomy. When significant hepatic arterial branches arise from the superior mesenteric artery, they usually pass behind and to the right of the portal vein.

The gallbladder receives its blood supply from the cystic artery. The cystic artery usually originates from the right hepatic artery shortly after it passes beneath the common hepatic duct. The site of origin of the cystic artery varies greatly, however. The more common variations are from an aberrant right hepatic artery, left hepatic artery, more proximal hepatic artery, gastroduodenal, or even another branch of the celiac artery. In about 10% of cases, a double cystic artery is present. In

most cases, the cystic artery branches near the neck of the gallbladder. If neither a superficial or deep branch of the cystic artery is found near that point, one should suspect double cystic arteries.

The blood supply of the common bile duct classically arises from the cystic artery or the posterior superior pancreaticoduodenal artery. Generally, the arterial vessels supplying the common bile duct are quite small, and easily disrupted. This characteristic, in combination with the great variation in the distribution of the arterial supply to the common bile duct and the extremely inconsistent anastomotic patterns of the vessels that supply it, probably account for the postoperative ischemic sequelae that follow extensive mobilization of long segments of the duct. Small branches from the cystic artery usually nourish the supraduodenal portion of the common bile duct. These vessels also supply the common hepatic duct and the lower part of the right hepatic duct. If ascending arterial branches from vessels supplying the lower segments of the common bile duct are not well developed, the cystic artery and occasionally the right hepatic artery will send off one or two descending branches to the first part of the duct.

The retroduodenal or second portion of the common bile duct is usually supplied by four to six branches from the posterior superior pancreaticoduodenal artery as this vessel loops around this segment of the common bile duct. One of these branches may ascend to become an accessory cystic artery. The supraduodenal branch of the gastroduodenal artery occasionally sends a tiny branch to the retroduodenal portion of the duct. Both the anterior and the posterior superior pancreaticoduodenal arteries supply the third and fourth portions of the common duct. These portions of the duct seem to have a better anastomotic arterial pattern than the first and second ductal segments. Despite the large variations in the extrinsic arterial supply of the common bile duct, there is an intrinsic arterial system that is generally consistent throughout the course of the duct. This intrinsic system is a plexus formed on the duct that provides two axial vessels, the 3 o'clock and 9 o'clock arteries, named for their positions relative to a cross section of the duct.[31]

Venous Drainage

Most of the hepatic venous effluent drains into the three major hepatic veins (right, middle, and left) (Fig. 11.10). Each of the three has only a short extrahepatic segment before draining into the inferior vena cava. These short extrahepatic segments make surgical accessibility difficult, particularly for control of traumatic bleeding. The right hepatic vein, the largest of the three, provides the principal drainage for the right lobe of the liver. The main trunk of the right hepatic vein follows an intrasegmental plane between the anterior and posterior segments.

Several small veins also normally drain directly from the right lobe into the vena cava. The middle hepatic vein lies in the lobar (portal) fissure draining the medial segment of the left lobe and a portion of the anterior segment of the right lobe. The middle hepatic vein joins the left hepatic vein in 80% of dissections.[32] The exact site of this junction varies considerably. The left hepatic vein provides the principal venous drainage of the left lateral segment. In addition, several small veins from the caudate lobe drain inferiorly directly into the vena cava. Following thrombosis of the major hepatic veins (Budd–Chiari syndrome), these small posterior caudate veins become important in the formation of collateral drainage. Venous obstruction can also lead to varying degrees of biliary varices.

There is no constant, single major venous trunk of the gallbladder. Venous return from the gallbladder occurs in multiple directions, via multiple small vessels running directly into the liver bed or toward the common duct. Venous drainage from the superior portion of the common bile duct ascends along the surface of the common duct and the hepatic and cystic ducts. It enters the liver directly rather than by joining branches of the portal vein. The venous drainage from the inferior portion of the common bile duct, however, flows into small radicals that directly enter the portal vein. The ventral surface of the common duct is marked by a constant ascending vein that can become a hindrance if bleeding from this vessel cannot be controlled during duct surgery.

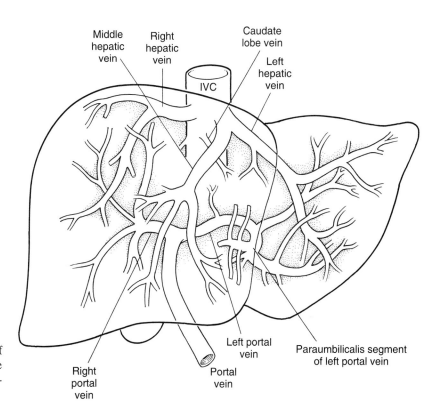

FIGURE 11.10. Schematic representation of the hepatic veins and their proximity to the portal venous system in the liver. *IVC*, inferior vena cava.

Lymphatics

Hepatic lymph forms in the perisinusoidal spaces of Disse and in the clefts of Mall to drain into larger lymphatics in the porta hepatis[33]; this subsequently drains into the cisterna chyli and eventually into the thoracic duct. Lymphatic vessels lie near the hepatic vein in Glisson's capsule and around the bile ducts. Lymphatics also pass through the diaphragm directly into the thoracic duct. Hepatic lymph nodes are found in the porta hepatis, celiac region, and near the inferior vena cava. The classic porta hepatis lymph node dissection involves a portal (posterior) as well as a celiac (anterior) dissection. Cirrhosis, venoocclusive disease, and glycogenosis can all lead to lymph vessel dilation. Alterations in the permeability of sinusoidal epithelial cells can alter lymph flow and protein content, an observation important in the pathogenesis of ascites.[34]

The lymphatic drainage of the gallbladder is into cystic duct nodes near the superior aspect of the cystic duct or directly into the hepatic parenchyma. Numerous lymphatics traverse the connective tissue between the gallbladder and its bed in the liver. This lymphatic (and adjacent venous) drainage accounts for the high rate of local invasion seen with gallbladder malignancies.

The lymphatic drainage from the common bile duct courses superiorly and inferiorly into nodes that lie along the course of the duct and finally into a group of 6 to 10 nodes in the porta hepatis. Some lymphatic drainage from the common duct reaches the deep pancreatic group of nodes, situated near the origin of the superior mesenteric artery, but usually the drainage reaches into the deep celiac nodal group. The drainage pattern of the extrahepatic ductal system accounts for the need to perform a posterior and deep portal node dissection when dealing with biliary malignancies. An important degree of drainage also occurs from the ductal confluence area directly posteriorly into the caudate lobe. For that reason, several hepatobiliary surgeons advocate routine caudate lobe resection in conjunction with cholangiocarcinoma resection.

Neural Supply

The portal and pericapsular regions harbor a complex system of nerves of unknown clinical importance. An anterior neural plexus consists primarily of sympathetic fibers derived bilaterally from ganglia T7 to T10 and synapse in the celiac plexus. Fibers from the right and left vagus nerves also contribute to this plexus. The anterior plexus surrounds the hepatic arteries. A posterior plexus that intercommunicates with the anterior plexus lies around the portal vein and bile ducts. The sympathetic nerves innervate the hepatic arteries. Distension of the liver capsule or gallbladder causes pain that is referred to the right shoulder or scapula via the third and fourth cervical nerves. Interruption of the anterior neural plexus can have various physiological effects including altering the accumulation of fat in the liver and changing the lipid composition of hepatic biliary secretions.

Anatomic Changes from Gallbladder and Biliary Pathology

In addition to the pathophysiological conditions that necessitate cholecystectomy, there are multiple diseases that can lead to significant anatomic changes important for the hepatobiliary surgeon. Many of these conditions were initially thought to be contraindications to laparoscopic cholecystectomy, but as the laparoscopic surgical experience has grown, so have the indications for laparoscopic cholecystectomy. These situations include acute and chronic cholecystitis, the Mirizzi syndrome, acute pancreatitis, cirrhosis, and other less frequently encountered pathological conditions. Because these diseases are addressed in greater detail further in this volume, the anatomic changes and their clinical significance are briefly mentioned here.

Cholecystitis, as the name suggests, is marked by acute and/or chronic forms of inflammation and fibrosing changes of the gallbladder wall. Both acute and chronic cholecystitis are notable for significant anatomic changes seen at the time of cholecystectomy. The most significant of these findings is the abundance of adhesions surrounding the gallbladder. These adhesions of the gallbladder fossa (and sometimes the entire right upper quadrant, often with omental involvement) make the surgical dissection difficult by obliterating the usually distinct tissue planes as well as making the anatomy in the all-important triangle of Calot difficult to define.[35,36] At times these adhesions, especially in chronic cholecystitis, can lead to adherence of the gallbladder to the colon, small bowel, or even the stomach. Cholecystoenteric, cholecystocolonic, and cholecystogastric fistulas can form in these conditions and potentially lead to the rare condition of gallstone ileus. This ileus is described as passage through a fistula of a large gallstone that would otherwise be unable to pass into the biliary tree from the gallbladder with subsequent bowel obstruction resulting from stone impaction in the distal ileum or ileocecal valve. In addition to the significance of the pathological adhesions, the friability of the gallbladder due to inflammatory changes (primarily notable in acute cholecystitis) can make retraction impossible and lead to significant incidental cholecystotomies with peritoneal soiling of bile and stones. Retraction difficulty is also seen in empyema with a gallbladder containing pus or in hydrops when the gallbladder distends with mucoid material secondary to outlet obstruction, both necessitating drainage of the gallbladder before it can be grasped for retraction.[37]

The Mirizzi syndrome shows similar anatomic changes due to inflammation as those seen in acute cholecystitis, and it often presents such a difficult problem to the laparoscopic surgeon that conversion to open cholecystectomy is usually necessary. Mirizzi, an Argentinean surgeon, described this syndrome in 1948 as jaundice (and sometimes cholangitis) caused by an impacted stone in the gallbladder neck or cystic duct leading to external compression and obstruction of the common hepatic duct.[38] This definition was expanded to two types in the 1980s. Type I is characterized by common hepatic duct obstruction by external compression (stone, tumor, lymphadenopathy, etc.) whereas type II is obstruction due to stone passage through a cholecystocholedochal fistula resulting from pressure necrosis between the gallbladder or cystic duct and common hepatic duct. Both are very rare, occurring in 0.7% to 1.4% of all cholecystectomies performed, but can have a high occurrence of gallbladder carcinoma (up to 28% of cases).[39] The nature of the condition in both types requires very close proximity of the gallbladder or cystic duct to the common hepatic duct. This proximity, in combination with the significant inflammatory changes in the triangle of Calot intrinsic to the syndrome, makes anatomic differentiation of the ducts difficult during surgical dissection.[40]

Pancreatitis is also known to create anatomic changes affecting the ability to perform laparoscopic cholecystectomy. The most notable anatomic changes do not involve the gallbladder itself but may distort the anatomy of surrounding structures instead.[41] The intense retroperitoneal inflammation and edema that can accompany pancreatitis can have a mass effect on adjacent structures, leading to widening of the duodenal C loop, anterior displacement of the stomach, and duodenal mucosal thickening. These changes in addition to possible intraperitoneal inflammation or fluid collections can make adequate exposure of the gallbladder fossa and Calot's triangle difficult.[42]

Cirrhosis and its anatomic changes may not directly affect the gallbladder but can make the surgical approach difficult. Associated portal hypertension can lead to the formation of varices leading to difficulty with exposure. Among these varices is the umbilical vein, which is open to create collaterals from the left portal vein to the epigastric vessels (caput medusa), and therefore presents a direct obstruction between the umbilical trocar site and the gallbladder during laparoscopic cholecystectomy.[43] The bleeding potential of these and other varices as well as from the gallbladder fossa is the most frequent intraoperative complication during cholecystectomy in cirrhotics. The bleeding risk is further potentiated by the coagulopathy characteristic of the protein synthesis dysfunction caused by the hepatocellular failure of cirrhosis.[44] Another anatomic change caused by the abnormal fibrosis and hepatocellular regeneration found in cirrhosis is the rigidity of the liver, making retraction of the gallbladder and surrounding tissue exceedingly difficult.

Other less common pathophysiological changes of the gallbladder can cause difficulty during cholecystectomy as well. Examples of these conditions include gallbladder diverticula and adenomyomatosis of the gallbladder. Diverticular disease of the gallbladder, similar to that of the colon, includes true and false diverticula. This complication can lead to trouble during resection caused by chronic scarring of the diverticulae to surrounding structures or even intrahepatic diverticulae, necessitating a subtotal cholecystectomy to avoid significant hepatic injury or bleeding.[45] Adenomyomatosis also leads to similar changes of scarring or intrahepatic extensions, making cholecystectomy challenging. It is an acquired disease characterized by localized or diffuse extensions of gallbladder mucosa into, and often beyond, the muscular layer of the wall. Invaginations of the epithelium externally lead to Rokitansky–Aschoff sinuses, also seen in diverticular disease of the gallbladder. Adenomyomatosis has a known increase in occurrence of gallbladder carcinoma[46] whereas no such relationship is noted with diverticular disease.

References

1. Lindner H. Embryology and anatomy of the biliary tree. In: Way LW, Pellegrini CA (eds) Surgery of the Gallbladder and Bile Ducts. Philadelphia: Saunders, 1987:3–4, 7–8.
2. Bismuth H. Surgical anatomy and anatomical surgery of the liver. In: Blumgart LH (ed) Surgery of the Liver and Biliary Tract, 2nd Ed. Edinburgh: Churchill Livingstone, 1994:3–7.
3. Rappaport AM. Anatomic considerations. In: Schiff L (ed) Diseases of the Liver, 4th Ed. Philadelphia: Lippincott, 1975.
4. Cantlie J. On a new arrangement of the right and left lobes of the liver. J Anat Physiol (Lond) 1898;32:iv.
5. Healy JE Jr. Clinical anatomic aspects of radical hepatic surgery. J Int Coll Surg 1954;22:542.
6. Chenderovitch J. Les conceptions actielles des mecanismes de la secrection biliarie. Presse Med 1963;71:2645.
7. Hicken NF, Coray QB, Franz B. Anatomic variations of the extrahepatic biliary system as seen by cholangiographic studies. Surg Gynecol Obstet 1949;88:577.
8. Rappaport AM. Hepatic blood flow: morphologic aspects and physiologic regulation. In: Javitt ND (ed) Liver and Biliary Tract Physiology. Int Rev Physiol 1980:21.
9. Anson BJ, McVay CB. Surgical Anatomy, 5th Ed. Philadelphia: Saunders, 1971:597.
10. Smadja C, Blumgart LH. The biliary tract and the anatomy of biliary exposure. In Blumgart LII (ed) Surgery of the Liver and Biliary Tract, 2nd Ed. Edinburgh: Churchill Livingstone, 1994:11–16.
11. McIndoe AH, Counseller VS. A report on the bilaterality of the liver. Arch Surg 1927;15:589.

12. Thaler MM, Way LW. The biliary tract. In: Sleisenger MH, Fordtran JS (eds) Gastrointestional Disease. Philadelphia: Saunders, 1978:1245.
13. Hjortsjo CH. The topography of the intrahepatic duct systems. Acta Anat (Basel) 1951;11:599.
14. Meyers WC, Jones RS. Anatomy. In: Textbook of Liver and Biliary Surgery. Philadelphia: Lippincott 1990;18.
15. Goss CM (ed). Gray's Anatomy, 29th American Ed. Philadelphia: Lea & Febiger, 1974.
16. Rex H. Beitrage zur Morphologie der Saugerleber. Morphol Jahrb 1888;14:517.
17. Higgins GM. The biliary tract of certain rodents with and those without a gallbladder. Anat Rec 1926;32:89.
18. Schulenberg CAR. Anomalies of the biliary tract as demonstrated by operative cholangiography. Med Proc 1970;16:351.
19. Muirhead WR, O'Leary JP. Calot's triangle: loose interpretation or respectful accuracy? Am Surg 1999;65(2):186–187.
20. Nahrwold DL. The biliary system. In: Sabiston DC (ed) Textbook of Surgery. Philadelphia: Saunders, 1968:1128.
21. Sekimoto M, Tomita N, Tamura S, et al. New retraction technique to allow better visualization of Calot's triangle during laparoscopic cholecystectomy. Surg Endosc 1998; 12:1439–1441.
22. Hugh TB, Kelly MD, Mekisic A. Rouviere's sulcus: a useful landmark in laparoscopic cholecystectomy. Br J Surg 1997; 84(9):1253–1254.
23. Jacobson JB, Brody PA. The transverse common duct. AJR 1981;136:91.
24. Hollinshead HW. The liver and the gallbladder. In: Anatomy for Surgeons, 3rd Ed. New York: Hoeber-Harper, 1982.
25. Job TT. The anatomy of the duodenal portion of the bile and pancreatic ducts. Anat Rec 1926;32:212.
26. Boyden EA. The sphincter of Oddi in man and certain representative mammals, Surgery (St. Louis) 1937;1:25.
27. Keddie NC, Taylor AW, Sykes PA. The termination of the common bile duct. Br J Surg 1974;61:623.
28. Linder HH, Pena VA, Ruggieri RA. A clinical and anatomical study of anomalous termination of the common bile duct into the duodenum. Ann Surg 1976;184:626.
29. Michels NA. Newer anatomy of the liver and its variant blood supply and collateral circulation. Am J Surg 1966; 112:337.
30. Charnsangavej C, Chuang VP. Angiography classification of hepatic arterial collaterals. Radiology 1982;144:485.
31. Johnston EV, Anson BJ. Variations in the formation and vascular relationships of the bile ducts. Surg Gynecol Obstet 1952;94:669.
32. Nakamura S, Tsuzuki T. Surgical anatomy of the hepatic veins and the inferior vena cava. Surg Gynecol Obstet 1981;152:43.
33. Mall FP. A study of the structural unit of the liver. Am J Anat 1906;5:227.
34. Mallet-Guy P, et al. Recherches experimentales sur la circulation lymphatique due fofie. I. Donnes immediates sur la permeabilite biliolymphatique. Lyon Chir 1962;58: 847.
35. Liu C, et al. Factors affecting conversion of laparoscopic cholecystectomy to open surgery. Arch Surg 1996;131:98–101.
36. Kum C, Eypasih E, Lefering R, et al. Laparoscopic cholecystectomy for acute cholecystitis: is it really safe? World J Surg 1996;20:43–49.
37. Nahrwold DL. Acute cholecystitis and chronic cholecystitis and cholelithiasis. In: Sabiston DC (ed) Textbook of Surgery, 15th Ed. Philadelphia: Saunders, 1997:1126–1139.
38. Mergener K, et al. Pseudo-Mirizzi syndrome in acute cholecystitis. Am J Gastroenterol 1998;93(12):2605–2606.
39. Redaelli CA, et al. High coincidence of Mirizzi syndrome and gallbladder carcinoma. Surgery (St. Louis) 1997;121(1): 58–63.
40. Posta CG. Unexpected Mirizzi anatomy: a major hazard to the common bile duct during laparoscopic cholecystectomy. Surg Laparosc Endosc 1995;5(5):412–414.
41. Tang S, et al. Timing of laparoscopic surgery in gallstone pancreatitis. Arch Surg 1995;130:496–500.
42. Yeo CJ, Cameron JL. The pancreas. In: Sabiston DC (ed) Textbook of Surgery, 15th Ed. Philadelphia: Saunders, 1997: 1156–1161.
43. Rikkers LF. Surgical complications of cirrhosis and portal hypertension. In: Sabiston DC (ed) Textbook of Surgery, 15th Ed. Philadelphia: Saunders, 1997:1088–1089.
44. Angrisani L, Lorenzo M, Corcione F, Vincenti R. Gallstones in cirrhotics revisited by a laparoscopic view. J Laparoendosc Adv Surg Tech 1997;7(4):213–220.
45. Kramer AJ, et al. Gallbladder diverticulum: a case report and review of the literature. Am Surg 1998;64(4):298–301.
46. Alberti D, et al. Adenomyomatosis of the gallbladder in childhood. J Pediatr Surg 1998;33(9):1411–1412.

12
Laparoscopic Cholecystectomy: The Technique

Douglas O. Olsen and Renee S. Wolfe

General Principles

The general principles of laparoscopic cholecystectomy are no different than those that have been established and followed for open cholecystectomy. These basic principles are the key to safe surgery:

1. Gaining safe access to the abdominal cavity.
2. Ensuring adequate exposure before proceeding with the operation.
3. Careful and meticulous dissection with maintenance of hemostasis. No blind clipping or cauterization of bleeding sites.
4. Positive identification of the anatomy before any structure is ligated or divided.

Safe Access

Multiple techniques exist for accessing the abdominal cavity for laparoscopic procedures. These techniques can generally be divided into those that rely on the blind insertion of either a Veress needle or a trocar and those which rely on a direct cutdown under visual control to access the abdominal cavity (open technique). Once the initial access is achieved, all secondary ports are placed under direct visual control and should be relatively risk-free with regards to hollow organ or major vessel injury. Although there has been much debate on the safety of one technique compared to another, the complication of trocar injury to the retroperitoneal structures, such as the great vessels, can be nearly eliminated by the routine use of an open technique. In special circumstances when an open technique is precluded by large amounts of scarring in the midabdomen, a Veress needle technique can be used to gain safe access in either the right or left upper quadrant.

Adequate Exposure

It is hard to match the exposure that can be achieved with the laparoscopic approach, and this is perhaps the reason that laparoscopic cholecystectomy was accepted by physicians as quickly as it was by their patients. The surgical dictum that you can only operate on what you can see remains a guiding principle of laparoscopic surgery. Once safe access to the abdominal cavity is achieved, the exposure obtained depends on certain techniques that will assure the surgeon the best possible view. Exposure is facilitated by the inherent 16× magnification of the laparoscope, the liberal use of angled laparoscopes, appropriate port positioning, optimal patient and table position, and familiarity with the relevant anatomy. Technical hindrances include an inadequate or dysfunctional light source, broken fiber optics, camera malfunction, inadequate insufflation, fogging, bleeding, and poorly placed ports.

Dissection and Maintenance of Hemostasis

Rigorous attention to hemostasis is paramount to good exposure because relatively small amounts of bleeding can obscure the laparoscopic view. Laparoscopy is a visual procedure, and what you cannot see you cannot safely dissect. The best way to maintain hemostasis is to prevent bleeding through careful dissection and judicious use of pressure, coagulation energy and vessel ligation. Electrocautery, argon beam coagulation, laser, bipolar cautery, and ultrasound (harmonic scalpel) are all forms of coagulation energy that have been used successfully during laparoscopic cholecystectomy. Occasionally, multiple forms of energy are used in the same operation when the need dictates. The type of energy utilized by the surgeon is a personal choice and is dictated by the availability of the technology and the familiarity of the

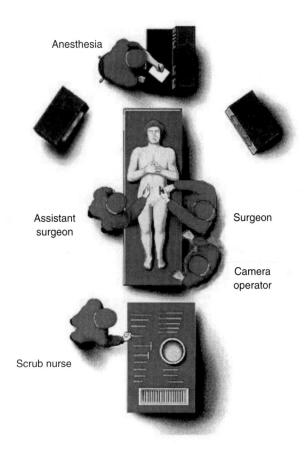

Anesthesia

Assistant
surgeon

Surgeon

Camera
operator

Scrub nurse

FIGURE 12.1. Typical operating room setup for laparoscopic cholecystectomy.

surgeon is obliged to convert the procedure to an open technique, wherein the addition of tactile sense can sometimes help in further dissection and identification of the anatomy. With cholangiography techniques, open conversion is rarely required but should be kept as an option for particularly challenging cases.

General Technique

The Workspace

The operating room is organized as shown in Figure 12.1. Preoperative setup should include ensuring the availability of potentially needed instruments, the use of a bed that permits either static films or real-time C-arm fluoroscopy for cholangiography, and a systems check of the video, insufflation, and cautery units. The value of the ability to recognize and solve or troubleshoot problems that arise with this equipment cannot be overstated. The patient can be in the supine or lithotomy position, per surgeon preference. The primary and slave monitors must be positioned accordingly to maintain a direct line of vision for the surgeon.

Access

Although many access techniques are still generally accepted, the routine use of an open technique should reduce the risk of major trocar injuries. Trocar injury to a hollow viscus or to major vessels are two of the more serious complications of laparoscopic access and remain the second and third most common reasons that a lawsuit is brought against a laparoscopic surgeon.[1-4] The major advantage of an open technique is the elimination of impaling injuries that occur when a sharp trocar is inserted too far and catches either bowel or a major retroperitoneal vessel between the sharp tip and the spine. These injuries are particularly treacherous, because they are more likely to be overlooked by the surgeon when gaining the initial access.

Open access is initiated with a 1.0 to 1.5-cm incision made in the vertical midline at the inferior border of the umbilicus. The subcutaneous tissues are separated with blunt dissection utilizing a hemostat. The umbilical raphe is identified as the thickened tissue extending down from the umbilicus to the anterior fascia. This raphe is grasped with a towel clamp as close to the anterior fascia as possible. With obese patients, a hand-over-hand technique with two towel clamps may be necessary to get down to this level. This maneuver will bring the anterior fascia up into the wound to give access for the surgeon to proceed with the fascial cutdown. A small incision in the fascia is made with a scalpel, just large enough to introduce the cannula to be used. Care should be used to try and

surgeon with that technology. If bleeding does occur, the source should be clearly identified before making any attempt to stop it. Blind clipping and coagulation should not be practiced because this can result in injury to important structures (i.e., common duct). Suction should be employed when needed, and irrigation should be used freely. Irrigating with a heparin-containing irrigation solution helps to clear a bloodstained field by keeping the blood fluid and therefore easy to aspirate.

Identification of the Anatomy

Biliary anatomy is consistent only in its variability. Even the routine, elective cholecystectomy can harbor a myriad of aberrancies in biliary anatomy. Further, the acutely inflamed gallbladder can result in gross distortion and contraction of the normal (or aberrant) anatomy. Absolute identification of the anatomy of the porta hepatis and triangle of Calot before ligation of any structure is the only safe way to reduce the risk of inadvertent injury, particularly to the common bile duct. No structure should be ligated or divided until it is clearly identified. If the anatomy cannot be clearly identified, then the catch the underlying peritoneum in the incision. Gentle spreading with a hemostat generally allows obvious access into the abdominal cavity under direct vision. If there is obvious tissue under the initial cutdown from underlying adhesion, then the surgeon has the option of abandoning this technique and utilizing a Veress needle technique in the right upper quadrant. The type of cannula that is chosen is the surgeon's preference. A classic Hasson-type trocar (Fig. 12.2) can be used, which allows a larger fascial incision to be made without compromising the seal around the cannula to maintain the pneumoperitoneum.

When using the Hasson-type trocar, a single, untied, 0-vicryl suture is placed through each side of the fascia. These sutures are used as fixation sutures for the Hasson trocar, which is equipped with anchoring sites for these sutures. If a larger fascial incision was created, resulting in a persistent air leak, the inferior and superior fascial edges can be sutured with a single interrupted stitch or with a figure-of-eight suture to reduce the diameter of the fascial defect through which the cannula passes. An alternative to the Hasson trocar is a standard trocar cannula, using fascial sutures to seal around the cannula. Personally, I begin by making a small fascial incision (less than 10 mm) and, after entering the abdominal cavity, insert a 5-mm cannula. Once the pneumoperitoneum is established, the secondary ports are placed with the aid of a 5-mm telescope. The telescope is then switched to one of the accessory ports, and the 5-mm cannula at the umbilicus is switched over to a 10-mm cannula under direct laparoscopic control. The larger 10-mm cannula seals the peritoneal incision.

Trocar Placement

The first step in adequate laparoscopic exposure is that of proper trocar position. Once initial safe trocar access is achieved at the umbilicus, the placement of the accessory trocars can make a significant difference in the surgeon's ability to see the tissues and area of dissection. The most critical of these trocar positions is the operating port, which is placed in the epigastrium. This trocar should be placed as high in the epigastrium as possible so that the angle between the instruments and the axis of the camera is at its maximum (Fig. 12.3); this allows the surgeon to see the tips of the dissecting instruments and clip applier much easier than if passed along the viewing axis.

Caution must be used to place the trocar at or below the edge of the liver. Because the falciform ligament fixes the liver at this location, elevating the liver will not compensate for a trocar that is placed too high, as is the case with the lateral trocars. This epigastric cannula can be either 5 or 10 mm, depending on the instrumentation available to the surgeon. Two 5-mm trocars are placed laterally just below the costal margin, one along the midclavicular line and the other along the anterior axillary line (Fig. 12.4). Even when the patient's liver extends below the costal margin, the edge of the liver is ultimately elevated, and with the high position of the 5-mm trocars, the surgeon has better leverage to manipulate the tissues for exposure. The placement of these lateral trocars is not as critical as the epigastric trocar, but the improved ability to manipulate and elevate the tissues does aid in gaining the best optimum exposure.

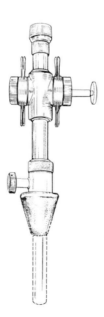

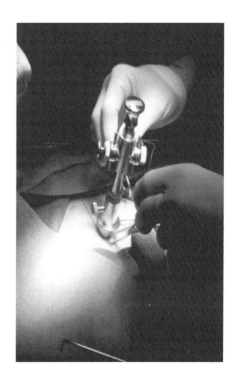

Figure 12.2. A Hasson trocar used for open laparoscopy.

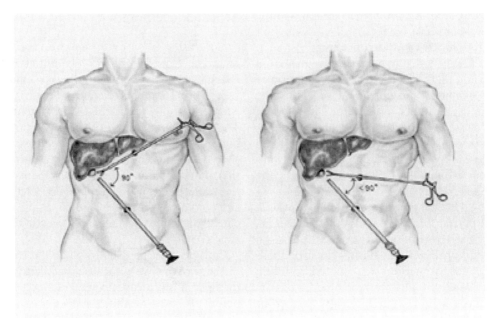

FIGURE 12.3. To facilitate instrumentation, the angle between the telescope and the operating instruments should be as close to 90° as possible.

Table Positioning

Gravity is the surgeon's friend during laparoscopic surgery. With the pneumoperitoneum that is created, elevating the head of the table in a steep reverse Trendelenburg position allows the omentum and transverse colon to fall down toward the pelvic cavity. Because the liver is attached to the diaphragm, the liver along with the biliary structures remain in the upper abdominal cavity. A slight rotation of the table to the left will further draw the organs away from the right upper quadrant. This rotation also allows the surgeon to operate in a more comfortable position.

Exposing the Porta Hepatis

The ultimate ability to gain exposure with laparoscopic cholecystectomy lies in the ability of the surgeon to grasp the gallbladder and elevate the right lobe of the liver, exposing the gallbladder and the porta hepatis. With a normal liver, the liver is literally folded back onto itself within the space created by the pneumoperitoneum, giving an exposure that is literally a textbook view; this is achieved by grasping the fundus of the gallbladder with an atraumatic grasper placed through the lateral 5-mm trocar cannula and lifting and elevating the fundus over the liver edge (Fig. 12.5). Care must be taken to release any adhesions to the gallbladder or liver that may prevent this elevation. Often the elevation needs to be achieved in steps. As the adhesions are released, additional traction is applied to gain successively more elevation, until

maximum exposure has been achieved. This end goal is best obtained by grasping the very tip of the fundus. If the liver is thickened from fatty infiltration, edema, or cirrhosis, and an effective folding over of the liver cannot be achieved, the surgeon must rely on the simple lifting of

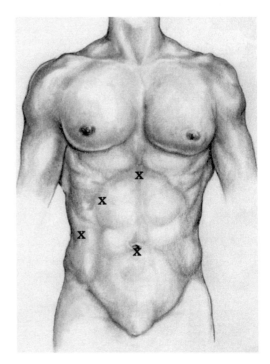

FIGURE 12.4. Typical trocar positions for laparoscopic cholecystectomy.

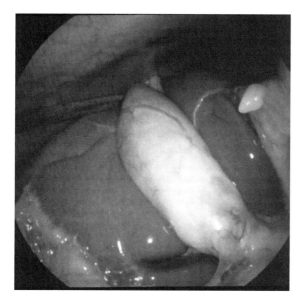

FIGURE 12.5. Exposure is facilitated by lifting the fundus of the gallbladder over the liver edge, causing the liver to fold over on itself.

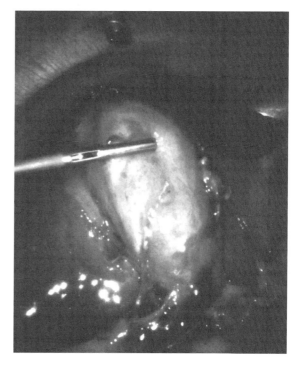

FIGURE 12.6. When the liver cannot be rolled over, the gallbladder is grasped midbody and simply lifted straight up.

the liver, best achieved by grasping the gallbladder more midbody and simply lifting straight up toward the anterior abdominal wall as opposed to up and toward the diaphragm (Fig. 12.6). The gallbladder is grasped down the body even more if additional lift is required.

With proper lift, exposure of the porta hepatis is completed by grasping Hartman's pouch and applying downward and lateral traction with a grasper placed through the midclavicular 5-mm trocar cannula. This maneuver helps to reestablish the normal angle between the cystic duct and the common bile duct that is closed with the upward traction applied to the gallbladder. Cephalad traction on the gallbladder distorts the normal anatomic relationship between the cystic duct and common bile duct and can lead to confusion in identification of the

anatomy. By reestablishing a more normal angle between the cystic duct and the common bile duct, the surgeon is more able to identify and correctly dissect out the neck of the gallbladder (Fig. 12.7). Care must be taken to not grab the gallbladder too close to the neck. If this occurs, the surgeon can pull the structures in the hepatoduodenal ligament into the operative field, causing tenting of the common bile duct and possibly leading to inadvertent dissection and transection of the common bile duct (Fig. 12.8). This inadvertent misidentification of the common bile duct as the cystic duct is the most common type of bile duct injury seen during laparoscopic cholecystectomy.[5,6]

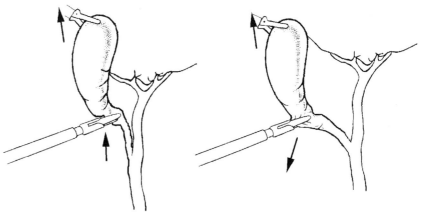

FIGURE 12.7. Proper traction on Hartman's pouch is outward and downward to open up the triangle of Calot. Upward traction into the liver will close the angle between the common hepatic duct and cystic duct, causing difficulty in identification.

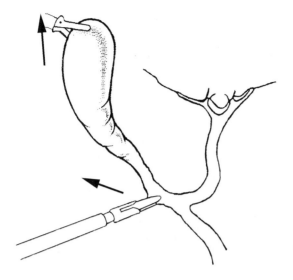

FIGURE 12.8. If too much traction is applied too close to the cystic duct–common bile duct junction, a tenting phenomenon can occur, causing a straightening of the common bile duct and putting it at risk.

Dissection of the Triangle of Calot

The triangle of Calot is defined by the cystic duct, the common hepatic duct, and the cystic artery. Proper dissection and exposure of these structures assures proper identification of the anatomy. A too vigorous dissection in the triangle of Calot can, however, lead to bleeding that is not only difficult to control laparoscopically but also dangerous. To avoid this possibility, the initial dissection is initiated on the lateral aspect of the triangle of Calot, that is, the cystic duct. Dividing the lateral peritoneal attachments of the infundibulum from the liver allows mobilization of the infundibulum. Dissection down the lateral aspect of the infundibulum allows identification of

the lateral margin of the cystic duct. With this landmark identified, dissection is then carried out on the medial margin of the infundibulum. As the infundibulum is further mobilized, the neck of the gallbladder will begin to appear. Blunt dissection at the neck allows the surgeon to encircle the cystic duct. The dissection is continued until clear demonstration of the infundibular–cystic duct junction is achieved (Fig. 12.9). This dissection must be circumferential and complete to ensure that no ductal structure is hidden in the tissues behind the area of dissection (Fig. 12.10A,B). With this landmark identified, the dissection is carried down the cystic duct a sufficient distance to allow instrumentation or ligation of the cystic duct. Isolation of the cystic artery is best achieved up on the infundibulum of the gallbladder. Not only does this minimize the risk of injury to an aberrant right hepatic artery, but if bleeding occurs during the dissection, the bleeding can be controlled with less risk to the ductal structures.

Although I generally ligate and divide the cystic artery after the cholangiogram and ligation/division of the cystic

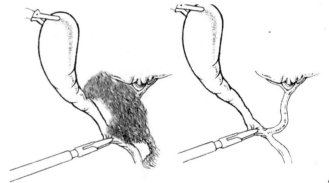

A

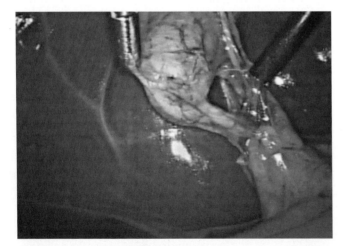

FIGURE 12.9. For absolute identification of the "gallbladder–cystic duct junction," the infundibulum of the gallbladder must be dissected out circumferentially.

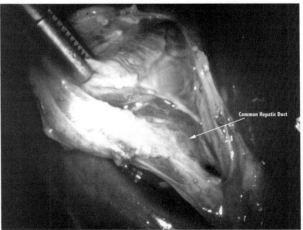

B

FIGURE 12.10. If incomplete dissection is accepted (A), posterior structures such as a tented common hepatic duct could be at risk (B).

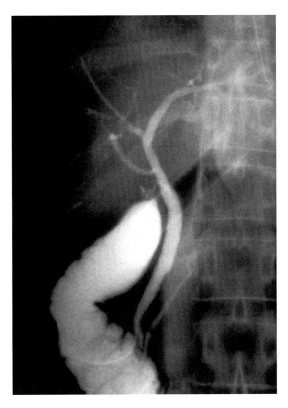

FIGURE 12.11. A cholangiogram not only aids in identifying common bile duct (CBD) stones but can greatly aid in the identification of the anatomy. In this cholangiogram, an accessory duct can be seen with an intact biliary tree.

duct, occasionally it must be divided early on if the anatomy dictates (i.e., the artery lies anterior to the cystic duct). In this case, however, the surgeon MUST be absolutely certain of all the anatomic relationships before dividing the presumed artery to minimize an injury to what might be aberrant ductal structures. By keeping the dissection and identification of the anatomy high up near the neck of the gallbladder, the surgeon can minimize possible injury to the biliary tree. Coagulation energy should be used to a minimum in this area to avoid inadvertent injury to adjacent structures. Careful, gentle blunt dissection can usually define the appropriate plane of dissection without significant bleeding. With the cystic duct exposed, a cholangiogram is performed if desired. Cholangiography can give full detail of the ductal anatomy, not only to help identify incidental common bile duct stones but also to aid in the identification of the anatomy (Fig. 12.11). Details of cholangiography are discussed in Chapter 13.

Ligation of the Cystic Duct and Artery

After the cholangiogram has been performed and the cholangiogram catheter is removed, the cystic duct is clipped with two proximal clips, placed just below the incision in the cystic duct used for the cholangiogram. The clip applier is placed through the epigastric port, and the clip should be inspected as it is placed to verify that it completely traverses the cystic duct before deployment. Once doubly clipped proximally and singly clipped distally, the cystic duct can be divided with scissors at the cholangiogram site. As with placement of the clips, it is important to visualize the tips of the scissors before cutting the duct to avoid inadvertent injury to structures behind the duct. With the cystic duct ligated and divided, upward traction on the neck of the gallbladder facilitates exposure of the cystic artery high on the neck of the gallbladder, making it quite easy to isolate, ligate, and divide (Fig. 12.12). Occasionally a posterior branch of the cystic artery must be ligated separately, particularly if it has a proximal site of origin. The artery must clearly be identified as supplying the gallbladder before ligation. Most cystic arteries can be seen not only to enter the gallbladder but also to branch along the gallbladder wall as they travel from the infundibulum to the fundus.

Mobilization and Removal of the Gallbladder

Mobilization of the gallbladder is accomplished with an appropriate energy source. The choice of the energy source is the surgeon's preference. The dissection proceeds from the infundibulum to the fundus. The assistant's grasper retracting the fundus upward, the remaining liver attachments holding the gallbladder

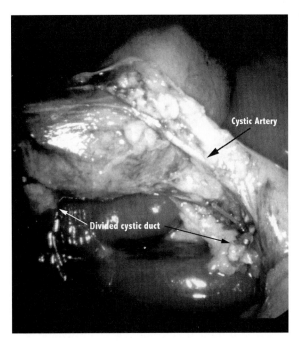

FIGURE 12.12. The cystic artery is best identified after the cystic duct has been identified, ligated, and divided. With upward traction on the neck, the cystic artery is easily found high up on the gallbladder.

inward, and a grasper placed on the infundibulum of the gallbladder retracting the neck outward away from the liver provide the essential traction and countertraction to facilitate the dissection. This traction–countertraction is of paramount importance in the mobilization of the gallbladder, by not only exposing the plane of dissection but also by placing those tissues that need to be divided under tension, facilitating their division. The left hand of the surgeon, which controls the infundibular grasper, retracts the infudibulum cephelad at first, exposing the posterior gallbladder wall as it lies in its bed. The infundibular retraction is then alternated between medial and lateral positions to expose and place the lateral and medial sides of the gallbladder under tension, respectively. The plane between the gallbladder and the gallbladder bed of the liver should be avascular in the uninflamed gallbladder. Bleeding in the routine cholecystectomy at this point often indicates departure from this plane. As the fundus is approached, it is often necessary to regrasp the fundus with the grasper that had been on the infundibulum. With two graspers on the fundus, one medial and one lateral, and the main portion of the gallbladder lying on the anterior surface of the liver, the remaining attachments of the fundus to the gallbladder bed can be divided.

Before dividing the final attachments of the gallbladder, the gallbladder bed should be inspected for hemostasis or bile leakage (from a duct of Luschka). The clips on the cystic duct and artery should be inspected, but not manipulated, to ensure they have not been dislodged during mobilization of the gallbladder. These inspections are facilitated by being performed before completely separating the gallbladder from its bed. Once the gallbladder has been detached, the liver will fall down to its more normal location and the exposure of the gallbladder bed and cystic duct and artery stumps will be obscured. Bleeding from the liver bed usually responds to electrocautery. The presence of biliary leakage from the hepatic bed may warrant placement of a drain.

When the final gallbladder attachments are divided, the gallbladder is placed over the liver. The laparoscope is changed from the umbilical port to the epigastric port, and with a toothed grasper placed through the umbilical port, the neck of the gallbladder is grasped. The gallbladder is brought into the umbilical trocar and the trocar and gallbladder are removed together, under direct vision. The fixation sutures must be released before removing the trocar if a Hasson cannula has been used. The gallbladder neck, once seen outside the abdomen, is grasped with a Kelly clamp to facilitate its complete extrusion. Alternatively, if there has been spillage of bile, or if the patient had acute cholecystitis with a tense or fragile gallbladder, the gallbladder can be placed in a retrieval bag before removal. The fascial incision may need to be extended if the gallbladder is thickened and

does not pass through the site comfortably. If there are multiple or large stones that preclude extraction of the gallbladder, they can be crushed within the gallbladder and removed with the aid of a stone forcep. The forcep can be passed through the neck of the gallbladder before removal of the gallbladder. With the gallbladder decompressed of the stones, it can usually then be extracted. If not, a fascial extension may be required. If a retrieval bag is used, the neck of the bag is brought through the fascial opening in a similar fashion with its opening exiting through the fascial defect. Ringed forceps can then be used to remove the gallbladder and stones.

Wound Closure

Once the gallbladder has been removed, either the trocar can be replaced in the umbilical site or, if the fascial defect is larger than the trocar, a finger can occlude the trocar site; this allows the pneumoperitoneum to be reestablished. With the laparoscope in the epigastric port, the operative site is inspected for hemostasis. The abdomen is irrigated, and the irrigant is drained with the patient supine and level. The 10-mm umbilical site can be closed at this point with a suture closure device. There is a benefit to making the fascial closure under laparoscopic guidance; not only does this ensure adequate closure but it minimizes inadvertent injury to bowel that can get in harm's way once the pneumoperitoneum is lost. The 5-mm trocars are removed under direct vision and their port sites inspected for hemostasis. If a trocar larger than 10 mm is used in the epigastrium, then this site also should be closed with a fascial stitch. The residual pneumoperitoneum is expelled from the abdomen before removing the last trocar cannula. The skin is closed with interrupted subcuticular 4-0 sutures at all sites.

The Difficult Gallbladder

Acute Inflammation

Acute cholecystitis was originally believed to be a relative contraindication to a laparoscopic approach to cholecystectomy.[7–11] Although the conversion rate is higher (25% compared to 2%), laparoscopic cholecystectomy can be performed safely in the face of acute inflammation.[12–14] It is important to differentiate between the patient with early acute cholecystitis (<24h) and the patient who has been symptomatic for more than 48 to 72h. Performing laparoscopic cholecystectomy in the early period greatly improves the chance for a successful, uncomplicated removal of the gallbladder. As the disease and the degree of inflammation progress, the technical difficulty increases. At greater than 48h, the amount of edema, adhesion formation, scar, distortion of the normal anatomy, and increased vascularity greatly increases the

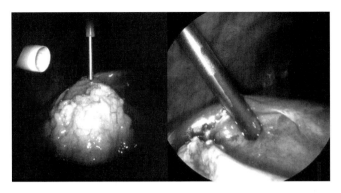

FIGURE 12.13. When the gallbladder is too terse or distended to be grasped, it can be decompressed either with an aspiration needle or by placing the midclavicular 5-mm trocar directly into the gallbladder for aspiration with a 5-mm suction device.

difficulty of the procedure. This greater difficulty forces the possibility for conversion to open cholecystectomy to avoid added risk of complications.

So long as the basic principles (as previously outlined) are followed, a safe laparoscopic cholecystectomy can be achieved. The problem arises when a surgeon is unable to adhere to these principles and does not know when the threshold for conversion to an open approach has been reached. The surgeon must know their own limitations. The basic technique of laparoscopic cholecystectomy with acute inflammation is the same as for an elective, nonacute cholecystectomy, with some modifications as detailed next.

Access

Safe access to the abdomen is usually not hindered by the presence of acute gallbladder inflammation. If the state of inflammation is advanced, the patient can have a degree of intestinal ileus, but safe access to the abdominal cavity should still be achievable without significant difficulty. The distended or tense gallbladder may be physically palpated and can often vary from its usual subhepatic location. Rarely does this finding prompt altering the trocar sites, or interfere with safe access so long as the surgeon avoids a right upper quadrant (RUQ) primary puncture.

Exposure

Adequate exposure may be hindered by a very distended gallbladder. Furthermore, a tense or thick-walled gallbladder may resist grasping or may be too fragile to be grasped safely. Such a gallbladder warrants decompression before exposure of the triangle of Calot. An aspirating needle can either be placed through the right upper lateral port or passed via a percutaneous approach to drain the gallbladder. The needle can be attached either directly to the suction tubing or to a syringe. The gallbladder is pierced with the aspirating needle in the

region of the top of the fundus. An assisting grasper may be required to provide stabilization or countertraction for the penetrating needle. If the contents of the gallbladder are too thick to be aspirated through this needle, an alternative approach is to insert the 5-mm RUQ midclavicular trocar into the fundus of the gallbladder so a 5-mm suction/irrigator can be advanced into the gallbladder (Fig. 12.13). Carefully, the gallbladder is gently irrigated and suctioned out. The hole in the fundus of the gallbladder is then closed with an endoscopic ligature before proceeding with the cholecystectomy. Additional trocars are rarely required, although the surgeon should never hesitate if their use means allowing adequate exposure to carry out a safe procedure. If the inflammation is exceptionally intense, an additional 5-mm port in the left flank can occasionally be of benefit to allow passage of an instrument to help retract a distended transverse colon with a thickened phlegmasous omentum (Fig. 12.14).

An exceptionally thick-walled gallbladder can be difficult to grasp with the usual laparoscopic grasper and often requires an aggressive toothed grasper (Fig. 12.15). If a 5-mm version of this instrument is not available, converting one of the lateral 5-mm trocars to a 10-mm port allows the use of larger, stronger instruments. Percutaneous sutures can also be used to retract the gallbladder by placing a suture (such as 2-0 prolene) transcutaneously, into the abdomen, and then laparoscopically through the area of the gallbladder to be retracted, then back through the abdominal wall. These sutures can be tightened and secured (untied) outside the abdomen with a hemostat.

Exposure of the triangle of Calot is often difficult in the setting of acute inflammation. The tissue planes are edematous, distorted, and often prone to bleeding. This inflammation causes scarring with contraction of the gallbladder and adjacent structures, distorting the anatomy and making the dissection treacherous and dangerous. Dissection must proceed deliberately and cautiously. All structures must be identified before manipulating, cauterizing, or ligation.

Hemostasis

Although hemostasis should always be meticulously maintained, the acute inflammation causes generalized bloody oozing that obscures exposure. The routine use of heparin (5000 units/liter) in the irrigating fluid allows the blood to be continuously irrigated clear and easily aspirated from the operative field, allowing for an unobstructed view. Bleeding points should be identified, grasped, retracted away from adjacent structures, and then cauterized, clipped, or sutured. Bleeding whose source cannot be clearly identified should not be subjected to blind cautery or clipping. Pressure can be applied by pressing the infundibulum of the gallbladder on the bleeding site either directly with a grasping forceps

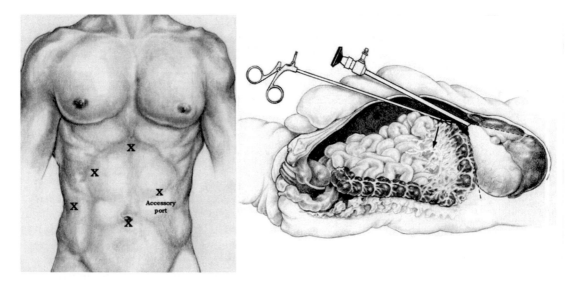

FIGURE 12.14. When the omentum is thickened and firm from inflammation, it can obscure the exposure of the porta hepatis. In this case, an additional instrument can be passed through a left flank 5-mm trocar to help depress and retract the omentum for exposure.

or with a 4 × 4 sponge introduced through one of the 10-mm ports. Pressure often controls the bleeding enough to allow proper exposure and identification of the source of bleeding. Bleeding that persists, that is excessive, or whose source cannot be clearly identified should prompt consideration of conversion to open cholecystectomy.

Identification of the Anatomy

Identification of the cystic duct and cystic artery can be difficult. Acute cholecystitis may be associated with enlargement of the node of Calot, which can serve as a landmark for identification of the cystic duct and artery (Fig. 12.16). This lymph node is located overlying the cystic artery, or duct, near the infundibulum of the gallbladder. Dissection in this region should always begin lateral to the node and close to the gallbladder, remaining high in the cystohepatic triangle. Early dissection near the junction of the cystic duct and the common bile duct should be avoided. Early cholangiography should be performed to provide a roadmap before extensive dissection and certainly before ligation of any structure. Misidentification of the common bile duct as the cystic duct is fre-

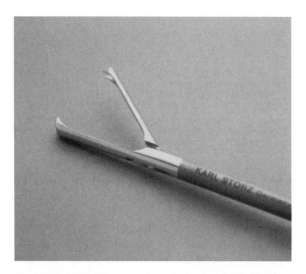

FIGURE 12.15. A 5-mm toothed grasper will hold onto any gallbladder, but the surgeon must keep in mind the likelihood of tearing the gallbladder, with subsequent spillage. For this reason, before using an aggressive grasper, decompression of the gallbladder is a must.

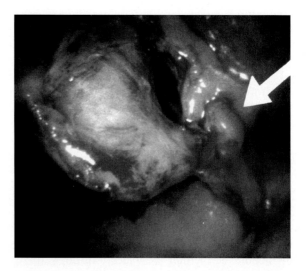

FIGURE 12.16. The enlarged cystic duct lymph node (*arrow*) can be a valuable landmark during the dissection of an acutely inflamed gallbladder. The node typically lies in the lateral angle of the triangle of Calot.

quently cited as a cause of inadvertent transection of the common bile duct.[11]

In those cases where clear identification of biliary ductal anatomy cannot be achieved either through an anatomic dissection or cholangiography, an attempt at removing the gallbladder in a retrograde fashion can be made before converting the patient to an open procedure. Occasionally, cholecystography can be helpful in delineating the neck of the gallbladder before further dissection in this area. The anatomic relationships of the cystic artery may be also be distorted and on occasion absent due to thromboses from the inflammation. It is therefore beneficial to leave the identification of the cystic artery until after the cystic duct has been identified, ligated, and divided. Upward traction on the neck of the gallbladder after the cystic duct has been divided allows identification of the cystic artery high up on the neck of the gallbladder. Taking this care helps avoid inadvertent injury to either a right hepatic artery that may have been pulled up into the triangle of Calot due to the inflammation or an aberrant right hepatic artery that lies naturally in this location but is obscured by the inflammation, making it difficult to identify. Both these situations are potentially hazardous and, therefore, only structures that clearly supply the gallbladder should be ligated. The presence of a posterior branch of the cystic artery should always be considered. Of utmost importance is a low threshold for conversion to open cholecystectomy if the anatomy cannot be identified.

Mobilization and Removal of the Gallbladder

Once the anatomy is identified and the cystic duct and cystic arteries ligated and divided, the gallbladder is excised from the liver bed. It is very beneficial to place all inflamed gallbladders in a specimen bag for removal. Not only is the inflamed gallbladder usually damaged by dissection and prone to spilling material during extraction, but as the gallbladder is involved with acute inflammation and likely infected its removal in a specimen bag reduces possible trocar site infection. Additionally, with the neck of the specimen bag exteriorized, morcellation of a thickened inflamed gallbladder can ease the extraction without extension of the fascial incision.

Morbid Obesity

The morbidly obese patient presents unique challenges. Morbid obesity is not a contraindication to laparoscopic cholecystectomy. In fact, obese patients benefit greatly from a laparoscopic approach.[15] The reduced size of the incisions relative to an open procedure in an obese patient is even greater than for a patient of normal weight. In addition, the surgical exposure possible with laparoscopy is usually much greater and easier than when approaching the same morbidly obese patient through an open incision. This overall reduction in the incision size leads to decreased postoperative pain, allowing earlier return to ambulation/activity; this advantage has special importance in morbidly obese patients who are at a higher risk of complications due to deep venous thrombosis and pulmonary atelectasis. The additional effort required is well worth offering the morbidly obese patient a laparoscopic approach. Learning to overcome the unique challenges of these patients allows the procedure to be performed safely and effectively.

Access

Alterations in abdominal habitus may call for adjustment in trocar positioning. In general the relationship of the trocars to each other is maintained, and it is only the positioning of the umbilical trocar with respect to the usual abdominal landmarks that may need adjustment. The 10-mm port for the laparoscope and camera may have to be placed above the umbilicus in the patient who has an extremely long and thick torso. The relationship of this port to the gallbladder is the prime determinant as to if and how far above the umbilicus it should be placed. Initial access can be achieved either with an open trocar technique or with a Veress needle technique. The open technique may require a slightly larger skin incision to allow visualization of the fascia, which can be a considerable distance from the skin. Following the umbilical raphe to identify the proper location on the fascia to make the initial fascial incision is of extreme importance in the morbidly obese patient. It is very easy to get lost in the thick panniculus present in most of these patients. This problem can cause the initial trocar to be placed too low in the abdomen and at an angle that precludes a normal-length trocar from gaining entrance into the abdominal cavity (Fig. 12.17). Using towel clamps on the umbilical raphe in a hand-over-hand technique to pull the fascia up into the wound simplifies the dissection compared to using blunt dissection with long clamps and S retractors to identify the fascia.

Once the fascia is exposed, entrance into the abdomen is then performed as in the nonobese patient. In most cases, extralong trocars are not required. Because of difficulty exposing the fascia, consider placing the sutures for fascial closure at this point, because at the end of the case this same exposure may not be as easy to achieve. Alternatively, a Veress needle technique can be used. To avoid the problems of the thick and distorted anatomy around the umbilicus, the initial placement of the Veress needle should be in the RUQ where the 5-mm midclavicular trocar is usually placed. After establishing the pneumoperitoneum, the 5-mm trocar is placed, followed by a 5-mm telescope connected to the video camera. Care

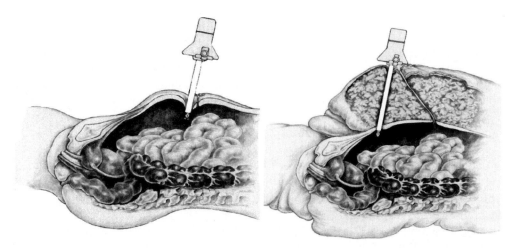

FIGURE 12.17. The large abdominal panniculus in the morbidly obese patient distorts the anatomy at the umbilicus and can make trocar insertion difficult unless the "true" fascial umbilicus is identified. This difficulty is seen here on cross section of a patient of normal weight (*left*) and an obese patient (*right*).

must be exercised to test the Veress needle with instillation of saline and aspiration before initiating gas flow to minimize the risk of air embolus, a real possibility if the Veress needle is inadvertently placed into the liver and instillation of CO_2 is started. This RUQ approach avoids the larger incision and sometimes difficult dissection that may be required with an open technique at the umbilicus. Once pneumoperitoneum is established, all other ports are placed under direct visual control.

Placement of these ports should take into account the thickened liver present in many of these patients because of fatty infiltration. A thickened liver can be difficult to lift and elevate and, for this reason, the ports must be placed below the liver edge. A surgeon cannot count on being able to lift and elevate a thickened liver as in the normal patient. Additional ports may be required to the left of the midline, below the epigastric port, to aid in omental or hepatic retraction.

Exposure

The table is placed in reverse Trendelenburg and left lateral decubitus position for gravitational reduction of the omentum, colon, and duodenum away from the gallbladder. It is very important to make sure the patient is properly secured to the table before manipulating table position. A large fatty omentum can be expected. Either a 30° or 45° angled laparoscope is often useful in seeing the cystohepatic triangle over the omentum (Fig. 12.18). The omentum can be retracted with additional graspers placed through additional trocars if necessary. The omentum can also be retracted transabdominally with an endoscopic ligature placed on a small part of the omentum. The tail of the ligature is left long and passed extrabdominally with a suture passer. The suture is then tightened with a clamp placed outside the abdomen. The degree of pull on the extrabdominal portion determines

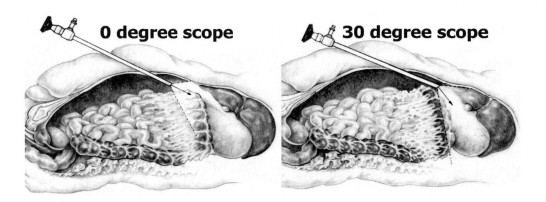

FIGURE 12.18. An alternative to using a fifth trocar to insert an additional instrument for retraction of an obscuring transverse colon is to use an angled laparoscope. The angled laparoscope allows the surgeon to look over the colon and view the porta hepatis.

the degree of pull on the omentum away from the gall-bladder. The increased visceral fat surrounding the gall-bladder as well as around the structures in the triangle of Calot requires meticulous dissection and hemostasis. Extra care must be given to full identification of anatomy before any structure is ligated or divided because this extra fat can also obscure and distort the normal anatomic landmarks.

Wound Closure

Extra care must be given to closure of the umbilical trocar site because these patients have a propensity to developing trocar site hernias, partly because of the larger amount of dissection required at the umbilicus for trocar placement and gallbladder extraction.

The Large Left Liver Lobe

A particularly large, floppy left lobe of the liver is a unique problem that can often be seen in thin, older, female patients. The floppiness of the liver often causes difficulty. As the liver is elevated in the usual fashion, the left lobe, which is not directly attached to the right lobe, falls down into the operative view obscuring vision. Even if vision can be restored using an angled scope, the left lobe is usually still in the way of the operative port, preventing direct surgical access to the portal structures. The easiest and most direct way of regaining exposure is to use torque on the liver to rotate the left lobe of the liver out of the way. The proper torque is gained by elevating the fundus of the gallbladder upward and medially; this will usually allow a slight rotation of the liver on its axis and allow the left lobe to fall out of the way. If this manuever is not successful, placing an additional 5-mm trocar in the left upper quadrant allows the surgeon to retract the left lobe of the liver.

The Porcelain Gallbladder

Deposition of calcium into the wall of a chronically inflamed gallbladder results in a porcelain gallbladder. The calcific outline of the gallbladder is often seen on plain films. The presence of a porcelain gallbladder is an indication for cholecystectomy, as a significant number of patients develop carcinoma of the gallbladder.

Originally considered a contraindication, laparoscopic management of this rare premalignant lesion is controversial. Laparoscopic cholecystectomy for the porcelain gallbladder has been performed safely. Special consideration must be paid to preoperative delineation of the biliary anatomy. The cystic duct is commonly shortened, and if it cannot be safely exposed or grasped, conversion to open cholecystectomy is warranted. Dense adhesions

and contraction similar to those seen in acute inflammation can be found, but with more scarring, fibrosis, and contraction. Difficulty with grasping and controlling the gallbladder because of the calcific nature of the organ can be overcome by placing traction sutures through the gallbladder wall. Strategically placing these sutures allows points of grasping that minimize disruption of the gallbladder that may occur using a more aggressive toothed grasper. Adherence to the principles of adequate exposure and identification of the anatomy improves the likelihood of successful laparoscopic removal of the gallbladder.

References

1. Deziel DJ, Millikan KW, Economou SG, et al. Complications of laparoscopic cholecystectomy: a national survey of 4292 hospitals and an analysis of 77,604 cases. Am J Surg 1993;165:9–14.
2. Deziel DJ. Complications of cholecystectomy; incidence, clinical manifestation and diagnosis. Surg Clin N Am 1994; 74(4):809–823.
3. SVMIC's 1998 Loss Prevention Seminar Series. State Volunteer Mutual Insurance Company, Brentwood, TN, 1998.
4. Physician Insurers Association of America Laparoscopic Procedure Study. Physician Insurers Association of America, Rockville, MD, 1994.
5. Olsen DO. Bile duct injuries during laparoscopic cholecystectomy. Surg Endosc 1997;11(2):133–138.
6. Davidoff A, Pappas T, Murray E, et al. Mechanisms of major biliary injury during laparoscopic cholecystectomy. Ann Surg 1992;215:196–202.
7. Soper N. Effect of nonbiliary problems on laparoscopic cholecystectomy. Am J Surg 1993;165:522–526.
8. Cameron JC, Gadaez TR. Laparoscopic cholecystectomy. Ann Surg 1991;213:1–2.
9. Soper N. Laparoscopic cholecystectomy. In: Wells S (ed) Current Problems in Surgery. St. Louis: Mosby-Year Book, 1991:583–655.
10. Baily R, Zucker K, et al. Laparoscopic cholecystectomy: experience with 375 consecutive patients. Ann Surg 1991; 214:531–541.
11. Cushieri A, Berci G, McSherry C. Laparoscopic cholecystectomy. Am J Surg 1990;159:273.
12. Olsen D, Asbun H, Reddick E, Spaw A. Laparoscopic cholecystectomy for acute cholecystitis. Probl Gen Surg 1991;8:426–431.
13. Cooperman AM. Laparoscopic cholecystectomy for severe, acute, gangrenous cholecystitis. J Laparoendosc Surg 1990;1: 37–40.
14. Unger S, Edelman D, Scott J, Hunger H. Laparoscopic treatment of acute cholecystitis. Surg Laparosc Endosc 1991; 1:14–16.
15. Unger S, Unger H, Edelman D, et al. Obesity: an indication rather than contraindication to laparoscopic cholecystectomy. Obesity Surg 1992;2:29–31.

13
Laparoscopic Cholangiography

Karen Draper-Stepanovich and William O. Richards

Few topics in general surgery generate as much heated discussion as routine versus selective cholangiography. Disagreement was present when open cholecystectomy was the standard of care, and the introduction of laparoscopic cholecystectomy has only fueled the debate as well as provided new technical challenges for the performance of the operative cholangiogram. There are proponents of both approaches and numerous arguments to support each opinion; however, most surgeons would agree that it is necessary for all surgeons who perform laparoscopic cholecystectomy to be familiar with the technique of operative cholangiography.

Absolute Indications

Indications for the performance of intraoperative cholangiogram include the presence of two cystic ducts, an accessory gallbladder, visual identification of ducts of Luschka, a history of gallstone pancreatitis, or evidence of common bile duct (CBD) stones by lab analysis, history, or radiographic exams.[1–3]

Surgical Techniques

Several techniques for laparoscopic cholangiogram exist, but there are two main types: via cystic duct cannulation and via gallbladder cannulation. Cystic duct cholangiogram is the most widely used technique, with success rates in recent reports ranging from 90% to 99%.[4–8] Several different catheters in different sizes and configurations are available for cannulation of the cystic duct. The catheters can either be introduced into the abdomen using one of the lateral cholecystectomy ports and held in place with a specialized cholangiography grasping forceps, such as the Olson clamp (Karl Storz Endoscopy), or can be introduced via a 14-gauge needle and sheath

inserted through the abdominal wall and held in place with an inflatable balloon tip or clip placement.[9–13]

The basic technique for cystic duct cholangiography begins with dissection of the neck of the gallbladder to identify the gallbladder–cystic duct junction. The cystic duct near the gallbladder is occluded with clips to prevent the introduction of contrast dye into the gallbladder. The cystic artery should also be identified and clipped proximally and distally so that placement of these clips without impingement on the common bile duct can be confirmed by the cholangiogram as well. The cystic duct is then opened anterolaterally and, using a blunt dissector, the duct is gently "milked" toward the gallbladder to extract any small stones from the cystic duct.

The catheter is then inserted into the cystic duct and held in place using clips, clamps or balloon inflation (Fig. 13.1). The catheter is attached to a three-way stopcock with two attached syringes, one containing contrast dye and one containing saline flush solution. After flushing the catheter with saline, 15 to 20 ml half-strength radiopaque contrast medium is injected and radiographic images are obtained of the entire biliary tree. Images are usually best obtained by tilting the table slightly with the patient's left side up to move the spine out from behind the biliary structures. Radiopaque ports and towel clips should be positioned out of the field. (One must also be sure that the patient is placed on a table that is compatible with radiographic imaging.) For optimal visualization of CBD stones, an initial injection of 5 ml dye should be performed so that small stones are not obscured by a heavy load of contrast. The catheter can then be flushed with small amounts of saline to dilute the intraductal dye, which can help reveal small stones. The remaining dye is then injected to fully outline the anatomy of the biliary tree.[10,14]

Cannulation of the gallbladder for cholangiography has been reported to be easier and faster than cystic duct cannulation.[6,15,16] No dissection of the cystic duct is required to perform the cholecystocholangiogram, and

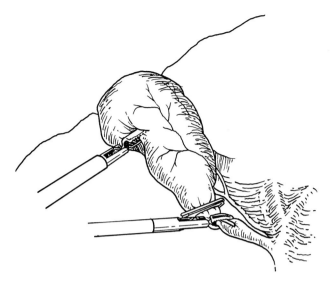

FIGURE 13.1. The catheter is held in place using clamps or clips that prevent extravasation of dye. (From Ref 10, with permission.)

the biliary anatomy is defined at the start of the procedure. There is therefore no risk of inadvertently cannulating the common bile duct (CBD) for the cholangiography. The disadvantages of cholecystocholangiography are that it does not indicate whether the surgeon has correctly identified the cystic duct, it does not

provide training in cystic duct cannulation, it requires filling of the entire gallbladder with contrast and subsequent flow into the biliary tree, and leakage from the puncture site may occur after catheter removal. The basic technique for performing cholecystocholangiography consists of puncturing the gallbladder using a cyst aspiration needle through the lateral port, aspirating bile from the gallbladder, and injecting about 30 ml contrast material for the radiographic images (Fig. 13.2). After removal of the needle, the gallbladder can be grasped and held at the puncture site or a loop of suture can be placed over this area to prevent leakage of the gallbladder contents into the peritoneal cavity. Although the technique is easier, success rates are reportedly lower than cystic duct cholangiography. In a comparison study of gallbladder versus cystic duct cholangiography,[5] the success rate for the cystic duct approach ($n = 38$) was 92% compared to 48% for the gallbladder approach ($n = 31$). Failure is usually a result of the presence of cystic duct stones.

We have reported a success rate of 83% ($n = 60$) using a specialized clamp (Kumar clamp; Nashville Surgical, Nashville, TN, USA) that isolates the infundibulum of the gallbladder so that filling of the entire gallbladder is unnecessary.[15] A side channel within the clamp allows introduction of a flexible catheter with a 19- to 23-gauge needle for injection of 5 to 15 ml contrast (Fig. 13.3). The technique does not require advanced laparoscopic skills, and the cholangiogram is obtained before any dissection or partial transection of ductal structures. Difficulty

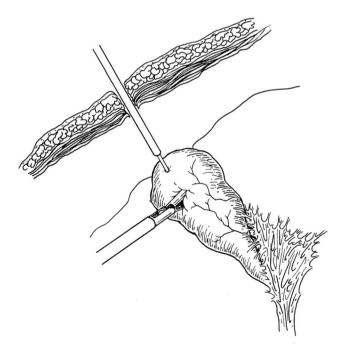

FIGURE 13.2. Bile is aspirated from the gallbladder using a cyst aspiration needle, and about 30 ml contrast is injected for radiographic imaging. (From Ref. 10, with permission.)

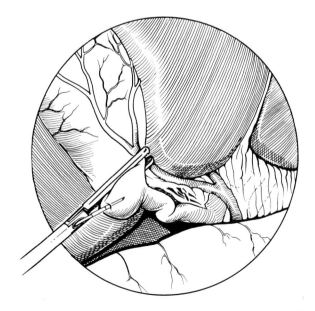

FIGURE 13.3. A Kumar clamp is applied across the infundibulum of the gallbladder. A side channel of the clamp allows insertion of sclerotherapy needle into the gallbladder for injection of contrast. (From Ref 15, with permission.)

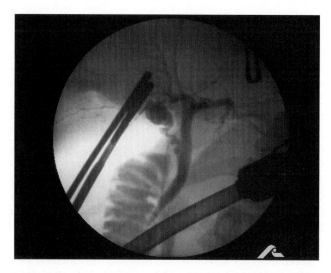

FIGURE 13.4. An adequate cholangiogram using Kumar clamp.

obtaining a seal across the gallbladder is encountered, however, when the gallbladder is very thick walled or is packed with gallstones.

Regardless of the technique chosen for cholangiography, it is essential that adequate images are obtained and correctly interpreted by the surgeon. Several studies have documented the use or absence of intraoperative cholangiogram in patients who subsequently suffered a CBD injury and have noted that in some instances a cholangiogram had been obtained but was then incorrectly interpreted by the surgeon.[4,17–19] An adequate cholangiogram must delineate the entire CBD, the proximal biliary tree, including both left and right branches, and flow into the duodenum[20,21] (Fig. 13.4). Opacification of the gallbladder during cholangiography can sometimes be seen, usually resulting from inadequate placement of the clips or clamps at the gallbladder–cystic duct junction. Opacification of the gallbladder after filling of the biliary

tree should alert the surgeon to the possibility of retrograde filling from accessory cystic ducts or ducts of Luschka.[1] On review of incorrectly interpreted cholangiograms, the most common mistake noted is failure of the surgeon to appreciate the significance of a nonopacified proximal biliary tree.[4,18,19] In many instances, this was attributed to "rapid emptying of the dye into the duodenum." Although it is common to have difficulty visualizing the proximal ducts on initial injection of contrast, the surgeon must be aware that this picture can be seen on the cholangiogram when the CBD is mistaken for the cystic duct and is inadvertently cannulated[18] (Fig. 13.5). If unrecognized, CBD transection or excision will result. The surgeon should assume that this is the cause until proven otherwise. The catheter can be repositioned in the cystic duct and/or the cholangiogram repeated with the patient in Trendelenburg position. Often, vigorous injection is needed to force the contrast proximally even in Trendelenburg position. If the entire proximal tree cannot be demonstrated using these maneuvers, however, exploration is warranted.

Fluoroscopic imaging of the cholangiogram is preferred over static films. Although fluoroscopic equipment is expensive to purchase initially, it can be used for many other types of studies such as orthopedic and vascular procedures. The fluoroscopic technique with image intensifying has been shown to be superior to static films in speed and image resolution of the cholangiogram.[5,7] In a report by Cuschieri et al. on fluoroscopic versus static imaging in 496 laparoscopic cholangiograms, 22% of the static images were inadequate and required repeat imaging. The mean time interval to complete the cholangiogram using static films was 23 min versus 4 min for fluoroscopy. No unsatisfactory images were noted on review of the fluoroscopic films.[5]

Allergic Reactions

Although allergic reactions during intravenous cholangiograms have been commonly reported, reports of serious allergic reactions during intraductal cholangiography are scarce.[22,23] Nonetheless, because all types of radiopaque contrast, ionic and nonionic, contain various amounts of iodine, patients who relate an allergic history to iodine should be premedicated. There are several drug regimens available for this (Table 13.1).[22] Iodinated contrast should probably be avoided altogether in

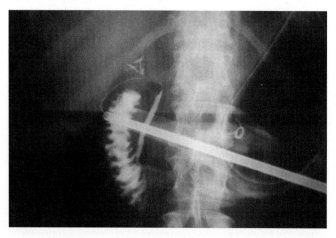

FIGURE 13.5. The common bile duct (CBD), mistaken for the cystic duct and inadvertently cannulated.

TABLE 13.1. Premedication for contrast allergy.

1. Prednisone 50 mg, 13, 7, and 1 h before procedure
2. Diphenhydramine 50 mg PO or IM, 1 h before procedure
3. Ephedrine 25 mg PO, 1 h before procedure

Source: From Ref. 22, with permission.

TABLE 13.2. Rate of common bile duct (CBD) injury during laparoscopic cholecystectomy and selective cholangiography.

Author	Total patients	IOC performed (%)	CBD injuries (%)
Newman et al.[28]	1525	165 (10%)	0
Robinson et al.[29]	495	161 (33%)	0
Lorimer et al.[26]	500	2 (0.4%)	0
Taylor et al.[27]	2038	0 (0)	7 (0.2%)
Dorazio[25]	1344	98 (7%)	1 (0.07%)
Barkun et al.[48]	1300	54 (4.2%)	5 (0.38%)

IOC, intraoperative cholangiography.

patients who relate a history of definite anaphylaxis to it. Alternative imaging could be obtained using intraoperative ultrasound or possibly by substituting gadolinium (used for MRI imaging) contrast for the iodinated contrast.

Selective Approach to Cholangiography

The selective approach to cholangiography is favored by many surgeons who argue that the extra time and expense is not justified in every patient. The criteria used to determine which patients undergo selective cholangiography differ slightly between surgeons, with some being more liberal in its use than others. The most common indications, however, are the same as the absolute criteria stated previously as well as delineation of the anatomy during a difficult dissection.[24–30] When the selective approach is used, the primary role for cholangiography is to delineate causes of CBD obstruction and to clarify any ambiguous biliary anatomy. Many patients who exhibit evidence of CBD stones now undergo preoperative endoscopic retrograde cholangiopancreatography (ERCP), which is greater than 90% successful in clearing the CBD of stones, eliminating the need for an intraoperative cholangiogram.[31,32] Cholangiograms in patients without signs and symptoms of CBD stones are argued to be of low yield, because these patients have been shown to have an incidence of only about 4% to 8% of choledocholithiasis during routine cholangiography.[4,5,7,33,34] Most of these unsuspected stones will pass without incident because the rate of postoperative symptomatic retained stones is less than 4% in patients undergoing laparoscopic cholecystectomy without cholangiogram.[24,25,29] There are data to suggest that common duct stones less than 4mm in diameter will pass spontaneously. Sauerbruch et al.[35] examined the success of CBD stone fragmentation by extracorporeal shockwave lithotripsy over a 5-year period. Of patients who underwent a cholangiogram to determine the presence and size of stone fragments following lithotripsy, 31 had fragments measuring less than 5mm, and spontaneous clearance of the fragments was seen in 22 of those

patients. Kondylis et al.[36] followed 10 patients with CBD stones measuring less than 4mm following laparoscopic cholecystectomy with intraoperative cholangiogram. None of the patients required readmission or interventional therapy during the 12-month follow-up period. Twelve patients with residual stones measuring more than 5mm were also followed for 12 months. Two patients of 12 required subsequent ERCP for symptoms.

Intraoperative cholangiography cannot be substituted for appropriate dissection and identification of the contents of Calot's triangle. The best way to avoid CBD injury is undoubtedly by careful identification of the gallbladder–cystic duct junction and its relationship to the common bile duct. In support of this argument, several large series of laparoscopic cholecystectomy without routine cholangiogram have been published showing CBD injury rates equal to or lower than the 0.1% to 0.2% incidence reported for open procedures (Table 13.2). The data also suggest that cholangiography does not prevent CBD injury, as incidences as high as 0.38% have been reported despite routine cholangiography (Table 13.3).

Besides adding time to and increasing the cost of a laparoscopic cholecystectomy, cholangiograms can be falsely positive, resulting in unnecessary CBD explorations. False-positive rates reported during routine use range from 0.4% to 4%[29,30,33,34] and are probably due to air bubbles in most cases. Defects secondary to air bubbles can be decreased by careful filling of the dye and saline syringes and by using real-time fluoroscopy to observe whether the defect disappears or moves upon repeat injections or repositioning of the table.

TABLE 13.3. Rate of CBD injury during laparoscopic cholecystectomy and routine cholangiograpy.

Author	Total patients	CBD injuries (%)
Khalili et al.[33]	1323	5 (0.38%)[a]
Sackier et al.[34]	464	1 (0.2%)
Corbitt et al.[4]	511	1 (0.2%)
Kullman et al.[37]	590	3 (0.5%)

[a] Two injuries during CBD exploration, one Mirizzi's syndrome.

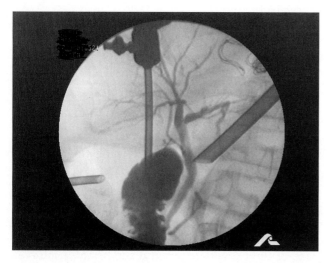

FIGURE 13.6. Accessory duct is identified through cholangiography.

Routine Use of Cholangiography

There are several points in support of routine use of intraoperative cholangiography during laparoscopic cholecystectomy. The presence of CBD stones cannot be definitively predicted with any laboratory test. Although elevated bilirubin or alkaline phosphatase, or a history of jaundice or pancreatitis, increases the probability that a patient has CBD stones,[2] unsuspected stones have been reported in about 4% to 8% of patients undergoing a routine cholangiogram.[4,5,33,34,37] Identification of CBD stones during laparoscopic cholecystectomy allows definitive treatment at the time of operation. Although some surgeons use preoperative ERCP for symptomatic patients or postoperative ERCP with spincterotomy to extract CBD stones, endoscopic sphincterotomy carries

with it a 1% to 3% risk of serious hemorrhage, a 1% risk of duodenal perforation, a 1% to 2% risk of moderate to severe pancreatitis, and a 1% to 2% mortality rate.[31,32] Success rates for ERCP vary with experience of the endoscopist, but on average 90% are successful.[31,32]

Performance of routine cholangiograms can increase proficiency in CBD cannulation, an important skill for the subsequent performance of laparoscopic CBD exploration. Routine use of cholangiography also increases the surgeon's familiarity with radiographic interpretation of the cholangiograms.

Clarification of the biliary anatomy is another important advantage of routine use of cholangiography. The selective approach cannot accurately predict which patients have anomalous biliary anatomy. Studies of laparoscopic cholecystectomy and routine cholangiography report a 2% to 19% incidence of abnormal biliary anatomy.[5,14,33,34,37,38] Anomalies that are of particular importance during cholecystectomy include accessory ducts (Fig. 13.6), anomalous insertion of the cystic duct into the right hepatic duct (Fig. 13.7), and a short cystic duct. Identification of a short cystic duct may necessitate ligation using fine suture or ties to avoid crowding of the CBD by clip placement. Cephalad traction employed during cholecystectomy may also result in "tenting" of the CBD at its junction with a short cystic duct (Fig. 13.8) which can result in injury to the CBD if not recognized.[14,19,39]

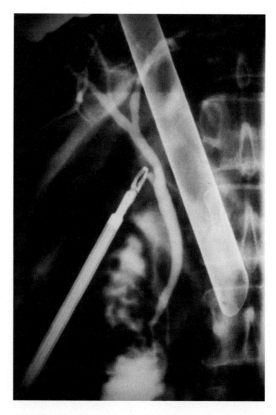

FIGURE 13.8. Cholangiography identifies a short cystic duct.

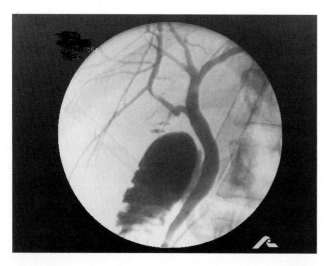

FIGURE 13.7. Anamolous insertion of cystic duct into the right hepatic duct.

TABLE 13.4. Bile duct injury series.

Author	Number of CBD Injuries	IOC performed (%)	Injury level >Bismuth 3	Recognized at initial operation
Moosa et al.[44]	6	0	4 (67%)	0
Larson et al.[49]	5	0	1 (20%)	0
Barkun et al.[48]	5	1 (20%)	1 (20%)	1 (20%)
Rossi et al.[50]	11	1 (9%)	6 (55%)	3 (28%)
Davidoff et al.[46]	12	3 (25%)	6 (50%)	0
Southern Surgeons[51]	7	4 (57%)	3 (43%)	4 (57%)
Woods et al.[43]	63	25 (40%)	N/A	27 (45%)
Carroll et al.[17]	12	12 (100%)	0	11 (92%)

Finally, the amount of operative time required for and the cost of cholangiography have been markedly reduced by the radiographic equipment that is now available. Previous studies reporting a cost of about $700 per cholangiogram and a mean time of 24 min to complete the cholangiogram were based on the use of static films.[40,41] Recent studies report that, with the use of real-time fluoroscopy, the time required to perform cholangiography has reduced significantly, to about 3 to 5 min.[7,41] At our institution, the charge to the patient for 1 h of fluoroscopy (regardless of actual time used) is $200. The cholangiogram catheter charge is $75, and the extra operating room time is $80 for 5 min. The total charge to the patient for intraoperative cholangiography is therefore about $315, similar to the charge reported by Khalili et al.[33]

Prevention of Common Bile Duct Injury

Common bile duct injury is one of the most serious complications of cholecystectomy, resulting in high rates of subsequent morbidity and mortality. Many patients require more than one operation over their lifetime following a major CBD injury.[42–44] The incidence of recurrent CBD stricture reported by Phillips ranges from 36% for a Bismuth type I injury to 90% for a Bismuth type IV injury.[45] It has been estimated that the average cost of a type III CBD injury is about $300,000.[46] The question of whether routine intraoperative cholangiography is superior to the selective approach in reducing the occurrence of CBD injury is still debated. Although a prospective randomized study comparing the two approaches would be ideal, the incidence of CBD injury in either group is so low that tens of thousands of patients would need to be recruited to prove a statistical difference. Although CBD injury rates range from 0% to 0.38% despite routine operative cholangiography, the injuries noted upon review of these cases are more likely to be minor and amenable to primary repair at the time of identification.[4,17,33,34,37] Several studies investigating

patients with CBD injuries reveal that in cases in which most of the patients did not undergo cholangiography at the time of cholecystectomy, a high percentage of them suffered Bismuth III level injuries or worse. In contrast, the series presented by Carroll et al.[17] reported 12 cases of CBD injury, all of which had undergone intraoperative cholangiogram. All but 1 patient had the injury recognized immediately, and only 1 patient required hepaticojejunostomy. None of the 12 patients had Bismuth III or greater injuries (Table 13.4).

Although sometimes presented as an argument against routine cholangiogram, inadvertent injury to the CBD during cholangiogram catheter insertion is not caused by the cholangiogram performance but rather is the result of misidentification of the CBD as the cystic duct by the surgeon. Recognition of this mistake by cholangiography prevents a major transection or excision of the CBD. Primary repair of a small CBD laceration sustained from catheter insertion has much less morbidity and mortality than a biliary–enteric anastamosis. In several studies reporting on routine use of cholangiography, in 83% to 100% of patients who suffered a CBD injury, the injury was recognized during the initial operation and primary repair of the duct was performed (Table 13.5). Because it has been shown that delayed diagnosis increases morbidity and mortality,[19,45,47] it is important for these injuries to be recognized during the initial procedure.

TABLE 13.5. Routine intraoperative cholangiogram and CBD injuries.

Author	Total patients	CBD injuries (%)	Primary repair
Khalili et al.[33]	1323	5 (0.38%)[a]	5
Sackier et al.[34]	464	1 (0.2%)	1
Corbitt et al.[4]	511	1 (0.2%)	1
Kullman et al.[37]	590	3 (0.5%)	3
Cuschieri et al.[5]	483	0	—
Carroll et al.[17]	3242	12 (0.37%)[b]	10

[a] Two injuries during CBD exploration, one Mirrizzi's syndrome.
[b] Three injuries during CBD exploration, one Mirrizzi's syndrome.

Conversely, a study of 1300 laparoscopic cholecystectomies with selective cholangiography by Barkun et al. reported only 5 CBD injuries, but 4 of the 5 occurred in patients who had not undergone cholangiography; only 1 duct of these 4 was primarily repaired at the same operation.[48] In a report by Asbun et al., the records of 21 patients who were referred for CBD injury were reviewed. Only 1 patient had undergone cholangiography during laparoscopic cholecystectomy; this single patient had had an incorrectly interpreted cholangiogram. Of the remaining 20 patients who had not undergone cholangiography, only 6 had had their injuries recognized at the initial operation. Nonetheless, 5 of the 6 required hepaticojejunostomy. Ultimately, 19 of the 21 patients required hepaticojejunostomy at least once.[42]

In conclusion, we believe that these studies show intraoperative cholangiography increases the rate of detection of injury during the initial procedure and also reduces the severity of injury by alerting the surgeon to the problem. Routine or selective cholangiography does not seem to reduce overall rates of injury.

References

1. Kellam L, Howerton R, Goco I, et al. Accessory bile duct and laparoscopic cholangiography: report of three cases. Am Surg 1996;62:270–273.
2. Onken JE, Brazer SR, Eisen GM, et al. Predicting the presence of choledocholithiasis in patients with symptomatic cholelithiasis. Am J Gastroenterol 1996;91(4):762–766.
3. Argov S, Schneider H. The major role of the operative cholangiogram within the indications for common bile duct exploration. Am Surg 1984;50(10):530–533.
4. Corbitt J Jr, Yusem S. Laparoscopic cholecystectomy with operative cholangiogram. Surg Endosc 1994;8:292–295.
5. Cuschieri A, Shimi S, Banting S, et al. Intraoperative cholangiograpy during laparoscopic cholecystectomy. Routine vs selective policy. Surg Endosc 1994;8:302–305.
6. Glattli A, Metzger A, Klaiber C, et al. Cholecystocholangiography vs cystic duct cholangiography during laparoscopic cholecystectomy. Surg Endosc 1994;8:299–301.
7. Lezoche E, Paganini A, Guerrieri M, et al. Technique and results of routine dynamic cholangiography during 528 consecutive laparoscopic cholecystectomies. Surg Endosc 1994;8:1443–1447.
8. Sabharwal A, Miniford E, Marson L, et al. Laparoscopic cholangiography: a prospective study. Br J Surg 1998;85:624–626.
9. Velanovich V, Kaufmann C. Two pitfalls of laparoscopic balloon cholangiography: recognition and correction. Am Surg 1993;5(5):290–292.
10. Olsen D. Laparoscopic intraoperative cholangiography. Probl Gen Surg 1996;12(3):23–33.
11. Karanjia N, Banerjee D, Dickson G. Angled metal cholangiography cannula for laparoscopic cholecystectomy. Br J Surg 1996;83:1441.
12. Howell HS. Operative cholangiogram: a simple, reliable, inexpensive method. Am Surg 1995;61(3):254–256.
13. Fretigny E. A simple device for laparoscopic cholangiography. Surg Endosc 1996;10:942–943.
14. Berci G. Biliary ductal anatomy and anomalies. The role of intraoperative cholangiography during laparoscopic cholecystectomy. Surg Clin N Am 1992;72(5):1069–1075.
15. Holzman M, Sharp K, Holcomb G, et al. An alternative technique for laparoscopic cholangiography. Surg Endosc 1994;8:927–930.
16. Baigrie R, Krahenbuhl L, Dowling B. Laproscopic cholangiography through the gallbladder. J Am Coll Surg 1994;178:175–176.
17. Carroll B, Friedman R, Liberman M, et al. Routine cholangiography reduces sequelae of common bile duct injuries. Surg Endosc 1996;10:1194–1197.
18. Carroll B. The laparoscopic cholangiogram of doom. Surg Endosc 1995;9:1029–1031.
19. Woods M, Traverso L, Kozarek R, et al. Characteristics of biliary tract complications during laparoscopic cholecystectomy: a multi-institutional study. Am J Surg 1994;167:27–34.
20. Willekes C, Edoga J, Castronuovo J, et al. Technical elements of successful laparoscopic cholangiography as defined by radiographic criteria. Arch Surg 1995;130:398–400.
21. Low V. The normal retrograde cholangiogram: a definition of normal caliber. Abdom Imaging 1997;22:509–512.
22. Greenberger P. Contrast media reactions. J Allergy Clin Immunol 1984;74(4):600–605.
23. Shehadi W, Giuseppe T. Adverse reactions to contrast media. Diagn Radiol 1980;136:299–302.
24. Clair D, Brooks D. Laparoscopic cholangiography: the case for a selective approach. Surg Clin N Am 1994;74(4):961–966.
25. Dorazio R. Selective operative cholangiography in laparoscopic cholecystectomy. Am Surg 1995;61(10):91–13.
26. Lorimer J, Fairfull-Smith R. Intraoperative cholangiography is not essential to avoid duct injuries during laparoscopic cholecystectomy. Am J Surg 1995;169:344–347.
27. Taylor O, Sedman P, Mancey Jones B, et al. Laparoscopic cholecystectomy without operative cholangiogram: 2038 cases over a 5-year period in two district general hospitals. Ann R Coll Surg Engl 1997;79:376–380.
28. Newman C, Wilson R, Newman L III, et al. 1525 laparoscopic cholecystectomies without biliary injury: a single institution's experience. Am Surg 1995;61:226–228.
29. Robinson B, Donohue J, Gunes S, et al. Selective operative cholangiography. Arch Surg 1995;130:625–631.
30. Gregg R. The case for selective cholangiography. Am J Surg 1988;155:540–545.
31. Sivak M Jr. Endoscopic management of bile duct stones. Am J Surg 1989;158:228–240.
32. Cotton P, Lehman G, Vennes J, et al. Endoscopic sphincterotomy complications and their management: an attempt at consensus. Gastrointest Endosc 1991;37(3):383–393.
33. Khalili T, Phillips E, Berci G, et al. Final score in laparoscopic cholecystectomy. Surg Endosc 1997;11:1095–1098.
34. Sackier J, Berci G, Phillips E, et al. The role of cholangiography in laparoscopic cholecystectomy. Arch Surg 1991;126:1021–1026.
35. Sauerbruch T, Holl J, Sackmann M, et al. Fragmentation of bile duct stones by extracorporeal shock-wave lithotripsy: a five-year experience. Hepatology 1992;15(2):208–350.

36. Kondylis PD, Simmons DR, Agarwal SK, et al. Abnormal intraoperative cholangiography. Treatment options and long-term follow-up. Arch Surg 1997;132:347–350.

37. Kullman E, Borch K, Lindstrom E, et al. Value of routine intraoperative cholangiography in detecting aberrant bile duct injuries during laparoscopic cholecystectomy. Br J Surg 1996;83:171–175.

38. Traverso L, Hauptmann E, Lynge D. Routine introperative cholangiography and its contribution to the selective cholangiographer. Am J Surg 1994;167:464–468.

39. Olsen D. Bile duct injury during laparoscopic cholecystectomy. Surg Endosc 1997;11(2):133–138.

40. Ladocsi L, Benitez L, Filippone D, et al. Intraoperative cholangiography in laparoscopic cholecystectomy: a review of 734 consecutive cases. Am Surg 1997;63(2):150–156.

41. Soper N, Dunnegan D. Routine versis selective intraoperative cholangiography during laparoscopic cholecystectomy. World J Surg 1992;16(6):1133–1140.

42. Asbun H, Rossi R, Lowell J, et al. Bile duct injury during laparoscopic cholecystectomy: mechanism of injury, prevention, and management. World J Surg 1993;17:547–552.

43. Woods M, Traverso L, Kozarek R, et al. Biliary tract complications of laparoscopic cholecystectomy are detected more frequently with routine intraoperative cholangiography. Surg Endosc 1995;9:1076–1080.

44. Moossa A, Easter D, VanSonnenberg E, et al. Laparoscopic injuries to the bile duct. Ann Surg 1992;215(3):203–208.

45. Phillips E. Routine versus selective intraoperative cholangiography. Am J Surg 1993;165:505–507.

46. Davidoff AM, Pappas TN, Murray EA, et al. Mechanisms of major biliary injury during laparoscopic cholecystectomy. Ann Surg 1992;215:196–202.

47. McSherry CH. Cholecystectomy: the golden standard. Am J Surg 1989;158:174–178.

48. Barkun J, Fried G, Barkun A, et al. Cholecystectomy without operative cholangiography. Ann Surg 1993;218(3):371–379.

49. Larson G, Vitale G, Casey J, et al. Multipractice analysis of laparoscopic cholecystectomy in 1983 patients. Am J Surg 1992;163:221–225.

50. Rossi R, Schimer W, Braasch J, et al. Laparoscopic common bile duct injuries. Arch Surg 1992;127:596–602.

51. Southern Surgeons' Club. A prospective analysis of 1518 laparoscopic cholecystectomies. N Engl J Med 1991;324(16):1075–1078.

14
Laparoscopic Cholecystectomy in Children and Adolescents

George W. Holcomb III

The first reported laparoscopic cholecystectomy in a child was performed in June 1990.[1] In the early 1990s, there were scattered reports of small series of children undergoing laparoscopic cholecystectomy.[2-4] Since these early publications, the laparoscopic approach for cholecystectomy has become the preferred method for removal of the gallbladder in infants and children. Although the application of laparoscopy for many abdominal conditions in children has lagged behind what has been seen in adult patients, most pediatric surgeons are proficient in performing a laparoscopic cholecystectomy. This chapter describes the etiology for the development of cholelithiasis in infants and children, the preoperative preparation of the pediatric patient, the operative technique, with necessary modifications for small patients, and a review of the experience at Vanderbilt Children's Hospital through 1998.

Cholelithiasis

Historically, cholelithiasis has not been considered a disease frequently found in children. However, in the past two decades, its frequency has increased significantly, and gallstones should be considered in the differential diagnosis of any child with vague or colicky abdominal pain. Moreover, certain children are predisposed to the development of cholelithiasis. Included in this group are children requiring prolonged total parenteral nutrition (TPN), especially in the absence of enteral feeding, gallbladder stasis, ileal resection from necrotizing enterocolitis or Crohn's disease, and hemolytic disease.

The incidence of hemolytic disease varies among institutions, depending on whether there is an active pediatric hematological department within each hospital. In the past, most series of children undergoing open cholecystectomy centered on hemolytic disease as the most common etiology for the development of gallstones. However, the growing incidence of nonhemolytic cholelithiasis has been emphasized from previous reports from our institution and has been reported by other investigators as well.[5-10]

Nonhemolytic Cholelithiasis

Infancy (Birth to 2 Years)

Cholelithiasis found in this age group is usually related to associated conditions, such as cystic fibrosis, ileal resection, or the prolonged use of TPN. The correct management for patients in this age group is not completely clear, as several authors have reported spontaneous resolution of neonatal cholelithiasis without treatment.[11,12] However, complications do occur, and choledochal obstruction has been reported.[11] Therefore, observation for up to 6 months, with the hope of spontaneous resolution, is not unreasonable. However, should the gallstones persist, calcification of the stones be observed, or symptoms be recognized, cholecystectomy is recommended and can be performed laparoscopically.[13]

Children (Age 2 to 12 Years)

Although symptoms related to biliary disease in this age group are usually vague and intermittent in frequency, management of these children is straightforward, in that spontaneous resolution is not expected. Therefore, once confirmation has been documented with ultrasound, laparoscopic cholecystectomy is recommended.

Teenagers (Age 13 to 19 Years)

Symptoms are more specific in this age group and quite similar to those found in adults. The pain is usually localized in the right upper abdomen, with radiation posteriorly to the subscapular region. Many of the teenagers complain of nausea with vomiting and intolerance to fatty foods. Etiological factors similar to those found in adults, such as pregnancy, oral contraception, and obesity, predominate in this age group. Choledocholithiasis definitely occurs in this age group, and these older children can present with jaundice or symptoms of pancreatitis. Management of these patients is identical to that of adults, with cholecystectomy recommended to prevent these associated complications from developing.

Hemolytic Cholelithiasis

Hereditary spherocytosis and sickle cell anemia are the two primary hemolytic diseases associated with cholelithiasis. In addition, thalassemia major has been found to be another hemolytic process associated with cholelithiasis in the past, but its incidence is decreasing because of the use of a hypertransfusion regimen.[14]

Up to 60% of patients with hereditary spherocytosis develop cholelithiasis.[15] Therefore, before laparoscopic splenectomy in children with spherocytosis, an ultrasound examination should be performed to determine whether concomitant laparoscopic cholecystectomy is also required.

Preoperative Preparation

Following confirmation of cholelithiasis by ultrasound, a thorough preoperative conference should be held with the parents, as well as the patient (if age appropriate), regarding the risks and benefits of laparoscopic cholecystectomy. The possibility of conversion, although small, should also be mentioned during these discussions. The most common reason for conversion will likely be concern regarding the correct identification of the common and cystic ducts.

The one group of patients undergoing cholecystectomy who require special treatment are those with sickle cell disease. Presently, these patients require transfusion to a hematocrit greater than 30% or hemoglobin greater than 10 g/dl; this can be accomplished on an outpatient basis within 2 weeks of the proposed cholecystectomy. Once these patients arrive for the scheduled surgery, an intravenous catheter is inserted and further hydration initiated. Preoperative admission for transfusion and hydration, although possible, is not necessary under our present outpatient transfusion protocol. However, these patients should certainly be observed in a hospital setting overnight and their hydration status monitored closely.

In our experience, 20% of the patients have presented initially to the emergency department with complications related to their cholelithiasis.[16] For such patients presenting with acute complications, medical management is initially indicated. Moreover, as in adult patients, preoperative testing with cholescintigraphy with technetium 99m-labeled iminodiacetic acid (IDA) or endoscopic retrograde cholangiopancreatography (ERCP)

may be required for evaluation of jaundice, acute cholecystitis, or choledocholithiasis. In the patient without complicating choledocholithiasis, once the acute inflammatory process has resolved, whether in the gallbladder or pancreas, laparoscopic cholecystectomy can be performed during the same admission or may be postponed for 4 to 6 weeks. The disadvantages of delaying the operation are the potential for recurrent symptoms or choledochal obstruction during the period of observation. However, the disadvantage of proceeding during the same admission is a more difficult procedure secondary to the acute inflammatory process. In our experience, most of the patients have undergone laparoscopic cholecystectomy during their initial admission without complications.[16] A few families have desired postponing the definitive operation until a more convenient time, and these wishes have been honored, also without adverse sequelae.

Special Concerns in Children

The smaller size of the pediatric patient offers several concerns particular to this age group. The bladder is an intraabdominal organ in infants and young children, and it is important to decompress it before placement of the initial cannula; this is even more important if the Veress needle technique is employed. However, iatrogenic urethral injury can occur with placement of a urinary catheter in a small infant. For this reason, manual pressure (Credé maneuver) is recommended, and is usually adequate to empty the bladder, especially for a relatively short procedure, such as a laparoscopic cholecystectomy.

The surface area of the abdominal cavity in an infant or child is much smaller than in the adult. Therefore, it is important to position the cannulas as widely as possible to allow adequate working space between them. If the ports are situated too close, an efficient procedure will not be possible. Moreover, the umbilical cutdown technique is recommended in infants and children to prevent iatrogenic injury with the Veress needle technique.

The abdominal wall of the infant and young child is very pliable. For this reason, it is quite easy to injure the abdominal viscera upon insertion of a sharp trocar. Therefore, use of the Step System (Innerdyne, Sunnyvale, CA, USA) is especially recommended for those surgeons who infrequently introduce cannulas in children. With this technique, a Veress needle with sheath is introduced into the abdominal cavity, the needle is removed, and a blunt-tipped cannula is inserted through the sheath. With this approach, it is unlikely that visceral injury will occur.

Another concern is rapid intestinal insufflation with anesthetic induction. It is quite easy to rapidly force anesthetic gas and air into the small intestine with vigorous mask induction in small children. Such small bowel distension can make the laparoscopic procedure more difficult. Therefore, it is important to discuss this concern with your anesthesia colleagues and avoid prolonged mask ventilation at anesthetic induction.

A final concern regards closure of the fascial incisions. Umbilical fascial incisions should be closed with either 2-0 or 3-0 absorbable suture. In infants and small children, it is also recommended to close the anterior fascia of 5-mm incisions. However, this is not necessary in older children, as the incidence of postoperative hernias should be very small in the older age group.

Surgical Techniques

Port Placement

Placement of the monitors and operating personnel for laparoscopic cholecystectomy in an infant or a child mirrors that seen in adults. Two video monitors are positioned at the head of the table on each side of the patient. The surgeon typically stands to the patient's left, with the camera operator to the surgeon's left. The first assistant usually is positioned opposite the surgeon with the scrub nurse to the assistant's right, opposite the camera operator.

Following initiation of general endotracheal anesthesia, an orogastric tube is introduced for gastric decompression. The bladder can be decompressed nicely with manual pressure (Credé maneuver). The pediatric patient is then prepped and draped widely, especially in the suprapubic region, as it may be necessary to place cannulas in the lower abdomen in smaller children. As in the adult patient, four ports are utilized, but the location of these ports is so important that their position should be individualized according to the patient's age and body habitus.

Infants

A 5-mm port is placed in the umbilicus following umbilical cutdown. Another 5-mm port is located in the right inguinal area. A third 5-mm port is placed to the left of the midline, over the rectus muscle. The final port is 3 mm in size and placed in the right upper abdomen (Fig. 14.1). As mentioned, the smaller the patient, the more critical it is to widely space the cannulas for adequate working space.

Ages 2 to 12 Years

Unlike infants, a 10-mm port is usually required to extract the gallbladder through the umbilicus, although a 5-mm port may be satisfactory in the younger members of this age group. Therefore, after introducing either a 10-mm or 5-mm port through an umbilical cutdown, three additional ports are placed. Again, a 5-mm right lower abdominal port can be positioned either in the inguinal region or in the midabdomen, depending on the body

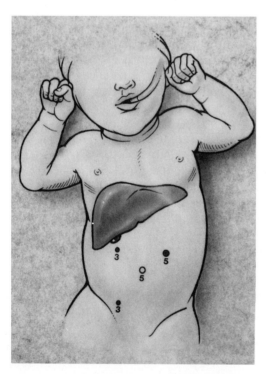

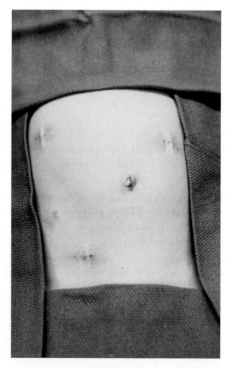

FIGURE 14.1. In infants, it is important to space the cannulas widely to create adequate working distance between instruments. Note how the right lower port is situated in the inguinal crease region. The gallbladder can easily be extracted through a 5-mm umbilical incision in these small patients.

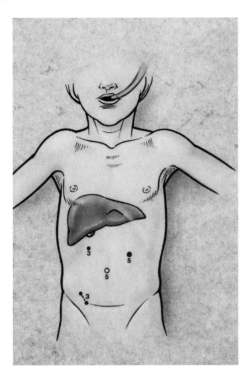 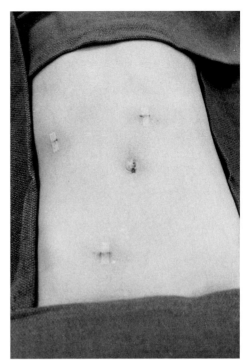

FIGURE 14.2. In children between the ages of 3 and 12 years, placement of the ports varies widely depending on the child's body habitus. Note that the epigastric incision is to the patient's left of the falciform ligament and the right lower incision is situated near the inguinal region. Such spacing allows for an efficient operation in young children.

habitus. Similarly, the epigastric port is still placed to the left of the midline to achieve an adequate working space. A 3-mm port in the right upper abdomen is adequate, as this port is used for retraction of the infundibulum (Fig. 14.2). In this age group and in infants, 5-mm endoscopic clips are certainly adequate, and the clip applier is introduced through the 5-mm left epigastric cannula.

Teenagers

The location of ports for laparoscopic cholecystectomy in teenagers is similar to that seen in the adult, especially those teenagers who are overweight. The epigastric port can be placed near the midline, either just to the right or left of the midline. The lower abdominal port is positioned at the same level as the umbilicus. A 3-mm port can be used in the right upper abdomen for retraction of the infundibulum (Fig. 14.3). In older patients, a 10-mm umbilical port is usually needed for extraction of acutely inflamed gallbladders, gallbladders with large stones, or gallbladders with a significant number of stones.

Laparoscopic Cholecystectomy

Following introduction of the four cannulas, the laparoscopic cholecystectomy is performed in a fashion similar to that in adults. The fundus of the gallbladder is grasped by a forceps introduced through the right lower abdom-inal port, and the gallbladder rotated superiorly and ventrally over the liver. A 3-mm forceps is placed through the right upper abdominal port and the infundibulum is retracted laterally to expose the triangle of Calot. Lateral infundibular retraction creates a 90° angle between the cystic and common ducts, which helps to prevent misidentification of these two structures. Adhesions between the cystic duct, gallbladder, and portal triad are gently divided, and the cystic duct is isolated. At this point, cholangiography should be performed if there are concerns about the anatomy or possible choledocholithiasis. Cholangiography in children is most easily performed using the Kumar clamp[17] (Fig. 14.4) (see Chapter 13). If cholangiography is performed, the sclerotherapy needle and clamp are then removed. The cystic duct is ligated with two clips placed near the origin of the cystic and common ducts and one clip on the cystic duct near the infundibulum. The duct is then divided between the second and third clips, leaving two clips remaining on the cystic duct stump. In a similar fashion, the cystic artery is clipped and divided.

The gallbladder is then removed in a retrograde fashion, using either the hook or spatula cautery. Following almost complete detachment of the gallbladder from the liver, the area of previous dissection is carefully inspected for hemostasis. Once hemostasis is assured, the gallbladder is completely separated from the liver and extracted. As the telescope was positioned through the

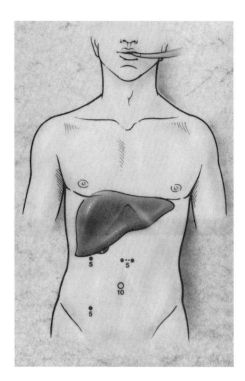 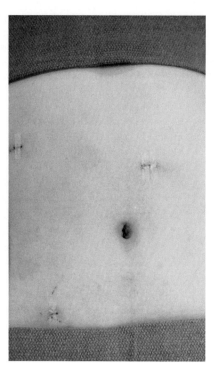

FIGURE 14.3. In teenagers, positioning of the ports is similar to that for adults. In this particular patient, the epigastric incision is situated to the left of the falciform ligament. Also, a 10-mm umbilical incision is usually required for extraction of the gallbladder.

umbilical port for the operation, it is rotated to the right upper abdominal port, and the gallbladder extracted through either the umbilical port or the umbilicus after the cannula is removed.

Once the gallbladder is exteriorized, the area of previous dissection is carefully inspected and hemostasis assured. Following removal of the cannulas, bupivacaine (0.25%) is instilled in the incisions for postoperative analgesia. The umbilical fascia is closed with either a 2-0 or 3-0 absorbable suture. The skin of the other incisions is closed with 5-0 absorbable suture. Sterile dressings are applied, and the orogastric tube is removed.

Postoperatively, a clear liquid diet is initiated on the night of the surgery and advanced to a regular diet the next morning. The patients are usually discharged the day following the procedure, with postoperative pain controlled well with either acetaminophen with codeine or oxycodone. An occasional nonsickle cell patient can be discharged on the day of the surgery, if desired by the patient and family and if the patient lives relatively close to the hospital. Patients are usually evaluated 2 weeks postoperatively and thereafter as needed. Routine ultrasound or laboratory evaluations are not necessary, unless specifically indicated.

Choledocholithiasis

As previously mentioned, a number of children have been seen at Vanderbilt Children's Hospital with complications related to their cholelithiasis, including choledo-

cholithiasis with jaundice or gallstone pancreatitis.[16] The management of preoperatively recognized choledocholithiasis varies depending on institutional capabilities. During preoperative evaluation with ultrasound, if choledocholithiasis is documented, several options exist.[18] If an experienced endoscopist (adult or pediatric) is avail-

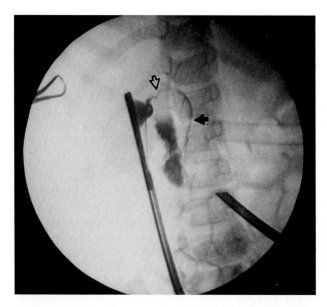

FIGURE 14.4. This cholangiogram was performed in a 7-year-old patient using the Kumar clamp. Note the small cystic (*open arrow*) and common bile ducts (*closed arrow*). It would be very difficult to cannulate this small cystic duct using traditional techniques.

able, preoperative ERCP with sphincterotomy and stone extraction is recommended. If choledocholithiasis is found unexpectedly at the time of laparoscopic cholecystectomy, and an experienced endoscopist is available, then completion of the laparoscopic cholecystectomy with postoperative ERCP and sphincterotomy is certainly a reasonable approach. Moreover, if the surgeon is experienced with laparoscopic choledocholithotomy, this approach is also reasonable when stones are found unexpectedly in the common bile duct on cholangiography. In addition, conversion to an open operation is always an option.

The foregoing above recommendations are made generally for the teenage patient whose size and body habitus mirrors that seen in the adult patient. In general, for children less than 10 years of age with choledocholithiasis noted preoperatively, referral to a children's hospital is recommended. If choledocholithiasis is found unexpectedly at laparoscopic cholecystectomy, completion of the laparoscopic cholecystectomy with postoperative referral to a children's hospital is also recommended.

Complications

Over the past 10 years, it is estimated that close to 1000 children have undergone laparoscopic cholecystectomy in this country. Major complications are rare but have occurred. Although small in incidence, the most common major complication has been misidentification of the cystic and common bile ducts with transection or injury to the common bile duct, requiring choledochojejunostomy. Therefore, with each operation, it is important to correctly identify the cystic and common bile ducts. Cholangiography can aid in this differentiation if the anatomy is unclear.

A biliary leak, which is also a problem, has been reported to occur in 1.5% to 2% of adult series.[19–21] Although the incidence of this complication in children is not known, it is believed to be small, and probably occurs in less than 1% of operations.

Vanderbilt Experience

From June 1990, through December 1998, 120 infants and children have undergone laparoscopic cholecystectomy at Vanderbilt Children's Hospital (Table 14.1). Two of the patients required cholecystectomy because of biliary dyskinesia, and the remainder had gallstones. Eighty-four patients were female, and 89 were Caucasian. The patients ranged in age from 25 to 230 months (mean, 105 months) and weight from 10 to 122 kg (mean, 49.6 kg) Risk factors for gallstone development included hemolytic disease (sickle cell, 17; spherocytosis, 5; pyruvate

TABLE 14.1. Summary data on 120 children undergoing laparoscopic cholecystectomy at Vanderbilt Children's Hospital from June 1990 to December 1998.

Mean age, 9.9 years
Mean weight, 49.6 kg
Risk factors:
Hemolytic disease, 24
Obesity, 17
Pregnancy/oral contraceptives, 8
Elective operations (97):
Operative time (mean):
Cholangiography (53), 112 min (±18)
No cholangiography (44), 86 min (±19)
Postoperative hospitalization, 1.10 days (±0.4)
Urgent Operations (23):
Presenting complications
Acute cholecystitis, 8
Jaundice/pain, 6
Gallstone/pancreatitis, 5
Biliary colic, 4
Operative time (mean):
Cholangiography (16), 149 min (±44)
No cholangiography (7), 131 minutes (±41)
Postoperative hospitalization (Mean): 1.68 days (±1.2)
Laparoscopic choledocholithotomy, 2

kinase deficiency, 1; hemolytic anemia, 1), obesity (in 17), and pregnancy/oral contraceptive use (in 8).

Four patients had previously undergone chemotherapy for malignancies and 2 had required extracorporal membrane oxygenation (ECMO) as neonates. Seven patients had previously undergone abdominal operations: insertion of ventriculoperitoneal shunt (3), open gastrostomy (3), and excision of a pelvic rhabdomyosarcoma (1). In addition, four children underwent laparoscopic splenectomy at the time of their laparoscopic cholecystectomy due to the diagnosis of hereditary spherocytosis. In the total group of 120 patients, 23 children required hospitalization as the initial presentation for a complication of their cholelithiasis. Reasons for admission included acute cholecystitis (8), jaundice and abdominal pain (6), gallstone pancreatitis (5), and biliary colic (4). The differentiation between acute cholecystitis and acute biliary colic was made according to the ultrasound examination. Patients with acute cholecystitis had gallbladder wall thickening or pericholecystic fluid on ultrasound, whereas children with similar symptoms but without ultrasound findings of acute cholecystitis were placed in the acute biliary colic category. Patients who presented with jaundice, abdominal pain, and a normal amylase were classified as jaundice/pain, whereas patients who presented with pain and elevated bilirubin and amylase were categorized as having gallstone pancreatitis.

The mean operative time for patients undergoing elective cholecystectomy (97 patients) with cholangiography was 112 (±18.6) min and 86 min (±19.3). The mean operative time for complicated cholelithiasis (23 patients) was

149 min (±44.1) if cholangiography was performed and 131 mm (±41.5) if cholangiography was not performed. The mean postoperative hospitalization for all elective patients was 1.10 days (±0.4), compared with 1.68 (±1.2) days if complications initially developed ($p = 0.0005$). Other than a single wound infection, there have been no significant complications, such as the need for reoperation, injury to the choledochus during the operation or to other viscera with introduction of the cannulas, bile leak, or retained choledocholithiasis.

References

1. Holcomb GW III, Olsen DO, Sharp KW. Laparoscopic cholecystectomy in the pediatric patient. J Pediatr Surg 1991;26:1186–1109.

2. Newman KD, Marmon LM, Attori R, et al. Laparoscopic cholecystectomy in pediatric patients. J Pediatr Surg 1991; 26:1184–1185.

3. Sigman HH, Laberge JM, Croitoru D, et al. Laparoscopic cholecystectomy: a treatment option of gallbladder disease in children. J Pediatr Surg 1991;26:1181–1183.

4. Rescorla FJ, Grosfeld JL. Cholecystitis and cholelithiasis in children. Semin Pediatr Surg 1992;1:98–106.

5. Kirtley JA, Holcomb GW Jr Surgical management of diseases of the gallbladder and common duct in children and adolescents. Am J Surg 1996;111:39–46.

6. Holcomb GW Jr, O'Neil JA Jr, Holcomb GW III. Cholecystitis, cholelithiasis, and common duct stenosis in children and adolescents. Ann Surg 1980;191:626–635.

7. Frexes M, Neblett WW III, Holcomb GW Jr. Spectrum of biliary disease in childhood. South Med J 1986;79:1342–1349.

8. Holcomb GW Jr, Holcomb GW III. Cholelithiasis in infants, children and adolescents. Pediatr Rev 1990;11:268–274.

9. Reif S, Sloven DG, Lebenthal E. Gallstones in children: characterization by age, etiology and outcome. Am J Dis Child 1991;145:105–108.

10. Bailey PV, Connors RH, Tracy TF Jr, et al. Changing spectrum of cholelithiasis and cholecystitis in infants and children. Am J Surg 1989;158:585–586.

11. St-Vil D, Yazbeck S, Luks FI, et al. Cholelithiasis in newborn and infants. J Pediatr Surg 1992;27:1305–1307.

12. Jacir NN, Anderson KD, Eichleberger M, et al. Cholelithiasis in infancy: resolution of gallstones in three of four infants. J Pediatr Surg 1986;21:567–569.

13. Holcomb GW III, Naffis D. Laparoscopic cholecystectomy in infants. J Pediatr Surg 1994;29:86–87.

14. Borgna-Pignatti C, DeStafano P, Pajno D, et al. Cholelithiasis in children with thalassemia major: an ultrasonographic study. J Pediatr 1981;99:243–244.

15. Bates GC, Brown CH. Incidence of gallbladder disease in chronic hemolytic anemia (spherocytosis). Gastroenterology 1952;21:104–109.

16. Holcomb GW III, Morgan WM, Neblett WW, et al. Laparoscopic cholecystectomy in children: lessons learned from the first 100 patients. J Pediatr Surg 1999;34(8):1236–1240.

17. Holzman MD, Sharp K, Holcomb GW III, Frexes-Steed M, Richards WO. An alternative technique for laparoscopic cholangiography. Surg Endosc 1994;8:927–930.

18. Newman KD, Powell DM, Holcomb GW III. The management of choledocholithiasis in children in the era of laparoscopic cholecystectomy. J Pediatr Surg 1997;32:1116–1119.

19. Peters JH, Gibbons GD, Innes JT, et al. Complications of laparoscopic cholecystectomy. Surgery (St. Louis) 1991;110:769–778.

20. Schirmer BD, Edge SB, Dix J, et al. Endoscopic cholecystectomy: treatment choice for symptomatic cholelithiasis. Ann Surg 1991;213:665–667.

21. Wolfe BM, Gardiner BN, Leary BF, et al. Endoscopic cholecystectomy: an analysis of complications. Arch Surg 1991;126:1192–1198.

15
Complications of Laparoscopic Cholecystectomy

Jonathan A. Cohen and Kenneth W. Sharp

The hallmark of any boom is unbridled confidence, which conceals and condones practices that—in a less giddy climate—would seem sloppy, unethical or illegal.[1]
—Robert J. Samuelson

When Heuer reviewed the results of cholecystectomy leading up to the 1930s, he observed that mortality was usually related to chronic liver disease and surgical technique; perioperative mortality was 6.6%.[2] In the 1930s and 1940s, Glenn, McSherry, and Hays determined that hepatic failure had become the prime culprit.[3,4] In the 1950s, cardiovascular complications contributed most to the perioperative mortality, which was now down to 0.6%.[3,4] The 1970s and 1980s witnessed notable improvements in critical care and coronary interventions, and mortality following cholecystectomy fell to 0.2%.[5] Then, in the 1990s, something remarkable happened: surgical technique again became a major factor in the morbidity and mortality of cholecystectomy. This time, however, the gallbladder was being removed without a laparotomy.

Thousands of patients with symptomatic cholelithiasis have benefited from the advent of therapeutic laparoscopy; however, the development and popularization of laparoscopic cholecystectomy have not been without accompanying tribulations. From the frivolous prosecution of Dr. Erich Muhe in connection with a respiratory complication following the first laparoscopic cholecystectomy, to the concerning realization in the early 1990s that this technological miracle was fraught with danger, laparoscopic cholecystectomy has been at once euphoric and dysphoric for surgeons and patients.[6] Consequently, the media and the American justice system have scrutinized the procedure and become expert in dissecting its complications, some of which are almost exclusive to this procedure.

Unfortunately, academic study of complications is difficult and often flawed. For example, true numerators and denominators for rates of complications and results are occasionally indeterminate because of systematic under-reporting in some sectors. Also, although a self-limited cystic duct leak and an inadvertent excision of the common bile duct share very little in common in terms of presentation, management, and consequence, they are frequently grouped together under the umbrella of ductal injury for purposes of study. Furthermore, a complication such as a lateral cautery injury to a duct may not manifest as a complication until years after the procedure, making the injury rate a truly unknown figure. Finally, the literature is filled with retrospective reports with inherent selection bias, with very few prospective studies that provide true insight.

Nonetheless, it is the aim of this chapter to provide a review of the literature concerning laparoscopic cholecystectomy, with an emphasis on the more common complications of bile duct injury, vascular injury, and visceral injury. In addition, we discuss associated complications of stone loss as well as issues related to gallbladder carcinoma and laparoscopic cholecystectomy. Finally, we examine some unusual complications, of which the practitioner should be aware.

Bile Duct Injury and Leak

The most feared complication of laparoscopic cholecystectomy is a bile duct injury. Due to the tenuous axial blood supply of the extrahepatic biliary tree, injury in this area carries significant morbidity.[7,8] In addition, complex and variable anatomy often makes recognition of an injury difficult, especially for many general surgeons who infrequently explore the porta hepatis and hepatic hilum. Furthermore, the public's high expectations for rapid discharge and recovery make these complications particularly distressing in light of their possible long-term implications. The bile duct injury during laparoscopic cholecystectomy has forced surgeons to rethink the idea of minimally invasive surgery and has tested their conceptions of informed consent.

General Considerations

Successful management of bile duct injuries depends on the type of injury, prompt recognition of a problem, complete definition of the anatomy, and multidisciplinary expert intervention. When an injury is recognized in the operating room, several principles should be followed: (1) conversion to an open procedure, (2) hepatobiliary consultation, (3) close attention to anastomotic tension and blood supply, and (4) drainage or exclusion of the repair. If a patient appears ill or fails to completely recover following what appeared to have been a routine laparoscopic cholecystectomy, the surgeon should obtain blood work and perform appropriate imaging studies. Interventionists from gastroenterology and radiology should be involved early and recognized as an integral part of the treatment team; percutaneous and endoscopic methods of defining biliary and vascular anatomy and accomplishing drainage are paramount to successful outcome. Surgeons practicing in communities without specialist support or extensive experience in complex biliary surgery certainly should consider transfer of the patient to a tertiary referral center.

Epidemiology and Classification

Before the laparoscopic era, cholecystectomy was associated with a low rate of bile duct injury.[5,9,10] Multiple large studies estimated the rate of bile duct injury during an open cholecystectomy to be from 0.053% to 0.6%, but the accepted standard is a rate of 0.1% to 0.2%.[9,11,12] Laparoscopic cholecystectomy, in contrast, is associated with a bile duct injury rate in the range of 0.2% to 2%.[13–19] A "learning curve" phenomenon has been described and disputed, with a significant proportion of injuries occurring before a given surgeon's 13th,[19] 30th[20] or even the 100th case,[21,22] depending on the study. Another report demonstrated that 91% of bile duct injuries occurred in the first 50 cases of a surgeon's experience.[23] Although the mortality associated with laparoscopic cholecystectomy is perhaps as low as 0.04%, these deaths are often related to bile duct injuries.[17,18] Rutledge and colleagues did a population-based study of laparoscopic cholecystectomy covering the rate of bile duct injury during the first 4 years of the procedure in their state. The injury rate in this study fell drastically from 1.5% in 1990 to 0.36% in 1993; consequently, the proportion of bile duct repairs to all biliary disease admissions has remained relatively constant even though the laparoscopic approach is now far more prevalent than the open procedure.[24] Optimistically, a 1996 report by Richardson et al. and a 1999 report by Kramling and colleagues seemed to indicate that the peak incidence of bile duct injuries has come and gone.[14,25]

Injury is broadly defined and includes everything from cystic bile duct leaks to proximal segmental hepatic duct ligation and excision. Bismuth classified bile duct strictures on the basis of their location with respect to the hepatic duct confluence.[26] The utility of this classification scheme is based upon the high correlation between cholangiography and findings at surgical exploration (Fig. 15.1). However, biliary leaks (choledochal, hepatocystic, or sectoral) and isolated sectoral duct occlusions are not included in this classification scheme, and these account for a large proportion of the injuries following laparoscopic cholecystectomy.

Strasberg's classification scheme, proposed in 1995, reflects the diversity of biliary injuries and their management[27] (Fig. 15.2). This scheme includes Bismuth's classification of strictures as its highest injury category. This newer scheme has not replaced Bismuth's despite its superior specificity, perhaps because it has not proven to be practical in actual practice.

Presentation, Mechanism and Management

Strasberg type A injuries include leaks from the cystic duct stump or a minor duct on the liver bed, but biliary–enteric continuity is intact (Fig. 15.3). Leakage from the cystic duct occurs secondary to clip failure or a burst phenomenon in the presence of retained common duct stones; it may also be seen when the cystic duct stump necroses, strangulated by clips that are simply too tight. In one survey of experienced laparoscopic surgeons, cystic duct leakage complicated laparoscopic cholecystectomy in 0.26% of cases, and was associated with acute cholecystitis and a cystic duct described as short, thick, or dilated.[28,29] This finding underscores the importance of visualizing the tips of the clips before application, and learning to use ties or preformed loops on such ducts, which may decrease the incidence of cystic duct leak.[30] Minor duct leaks are usually caused by separating the gallbladder from the gallbladder fossa in a plane that is too deep, that is, excising a rim of liver with the specimen, thus injuring a subvesical duct or a hepatocystic duct of Luschka.[31]

Patients with this type of injury present with symptoms related to the presence of intraperitoneal bile: abdominal pain, anorexia, ileus, nausea, or bile peritonitis with sepsis; the latter presentation may mandate laparotomy. These leaks are often treated with endoscopic transampullary stenting or sphincterotomy to decrease endobiliary pressure and percutaneous drainage of localized bile collections; success with endoscopic management approaches 90%.[32,33] An elegant animal study by Marks et al. demonstrated that stenting resolved cystic duct leaks faster than sphincterotomy.[34] Alternatively, a nasobiliary drain may be used.[33,35,36] Common duct stones, present in 10% of patients with gallbladder disease, should be removed to facilitate closure of the fistula.[37,38] The decision to drain a peritoneal bile collection should be based upon the

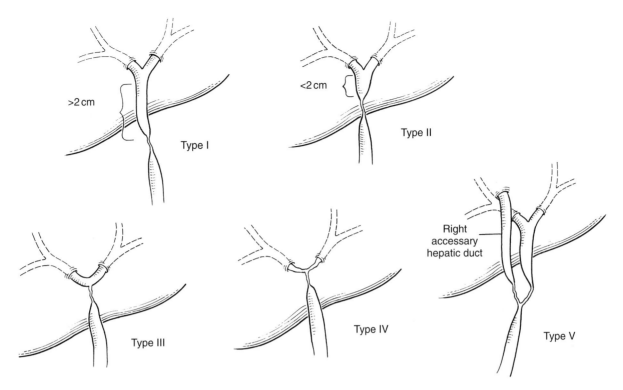

FIGURE 15.1. Bismuth's classification of bile duct injuries is based on the level of the stricture resulting from an injury as it relates to the confluence of the hepatic ducts. Levels I though IV relate to progressively higher levels of injury; a level IV

(Type IV) injury involves not only the common hepatic duct but also the confluence of the right and left ducts. A level V injury is a unique injury that involves an aberrant right hepatic duct with its confluence to the common duct.

patient's clinical status and size of the collection. When bile is noted to be leaking from the gallbladder fossa at the time of surgery, a cholangiogram should be performed. If this demonstrates peripheral extravasation from the fossa with normal intra- and extrahepatic ductal anatomy, a sutured repair may be attempted. Should this fail, a closed-suction drain should be placed, with the understanding that postoperative stenting may be required.

It should be stressed that postoperative fluid collections are very common but rarely clinically significant. Almost 10% of patients who undergo laparoscopic cholecystectomy are found postoperatively to have intraperitoneal bile,[39–41] yet less than 1% of all laparoscopic cholecystectomies are complicated by a clinically detectable leak.[16,19,42]

Type B injuries occlude a portion of the biliary tree and may occur when the cystic duct drains into the right hepatic duct rather than the common duct, as is seen in a small segment of the population.[23] The right hepatic duct or an aberrant right hepatic duct is then mistaken for the cystic duct, ligated, divided, and partially resected with the gallbladder. An "accessory cystic duct," often described in the operative note, represents a more proximal part of the right hepatic duct. Therefore, if a second ductal structure is seen entering the gallbladder, a cholangiogram should be obtained. This anatomic var-

iant underscores the importance of identifying not only the cystic duct–common duct junction but also the entire path of the cystic duct and its entrance into the gallbladder. Patients with type B injuries may remain asymptomatic as the obstructed lobe or segment atrophies and the remaining liver hypertrophies; alternatively, they may present with pain or cholangitis in the occluded area. If the patient is symptomatic, management includes completely defining the anatomy with percutaneous and endoscopic cholangiograms, placement of drains for the control of sepsis, and subsequent Roux-en-Y hepaticojejunostomy by experienced operators. Timing of operation depends upon when the injury was recognized. An injury recognized intraoperatively should be repaired immediately if the expert resources are available; if appropriate hepatobiliary expertise is not immediately available, a drain should be secured in the proximal limb of the ligated duct, the patient should be closed, and transfer to a tertiary care facility arranged. Injuries recognized postoperatively should be repaired only after accompanying sepsis has resolved. If hepaticojejunostomy is indicated but cannot be accomplished, a limited resection of the liver parenchymal proximal to the injury may be warranted.

A type C injury is a leak from a duct not in continuity with the common duct, that is, a sectoral duct injury.[27] As

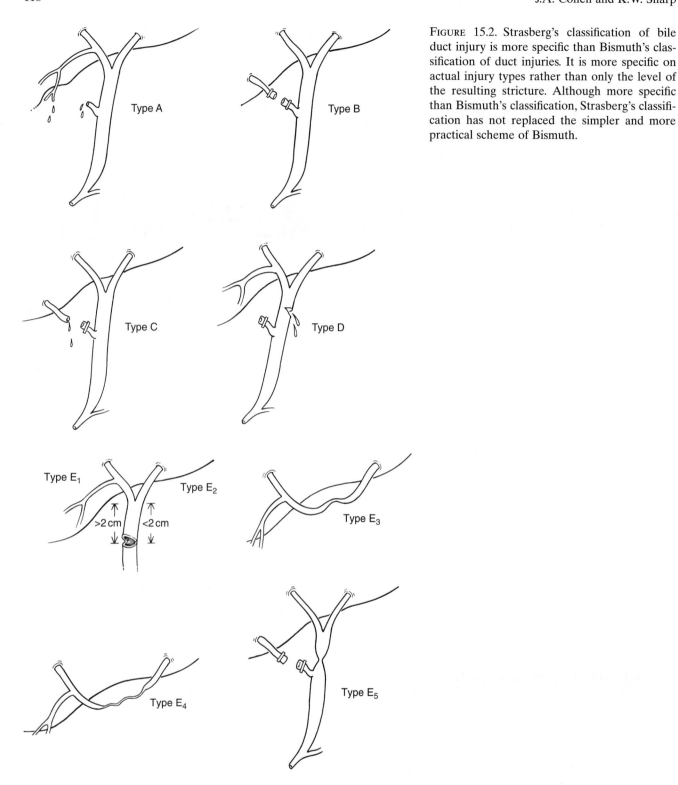

FIGURE 15.2. Strasberg's classification of bile duct injury is more specific than Bismuth's classification of duct injuries. It is more specific on actual injury types rather than only the level of the resulting stricture. Although more specific than Bismuth's classification, Strasberg's classification has not replaced the simpler and more practical scheme of Bismuth.

with type A injuries, patients become symptomatic secondary to the presence of a peritoneal bile collection, with pain, ileus, nausea, peritoneal irritation, and signs of sepsis. However, because the portion of the biliary tree draining into the peritoneum is not in communication with the common duct, distal stenting for this type of injury is inappropriate; this is in contradistinction to the type A injury in which the injury is still in continuity with the common bile duct. Again, the control of sepsis and complete imaging are of paramount importance in the decision for definitive management, which may require Roux-en-Y hepaticojejunostomy if the leaking duct is large (i.e., draining two or more segments), or ligation if the duct is small. If the leak seals by itself or is ligated, cholangitis may ensue, thus requiring bypass; alternatively, the dependent portion of liver may simply atrophy.

The type D injury is a lateral injury (not a complete transection) to any extrahepatic duct, and, like many injuries, may be caused by cautery, scissors, or improper placement of clips. The severity and location of the injury determine its presentation. A clip or scissor injury to the right hepatic duct, for example, might present as a leak with biliary–enteric continuity intact, much like a type A injury. Stenting across the injury or distally may be helpful, but if a stricture develops, repair may be necessary. A common duct leak may be repaired over a T-tube, in end-to-end fashion, or by Roux-en-Y hepaticojejunostomy, but the end-to-end repair is commonly plagued by tension on the anastomosis. Results tend to favor the bypass approach, but most data have serious selection bias and probably underestimate the rate of injuries treated successfully with the more conservative measures. A type D injury may be asymptomatic, as when a cautery injury to the common duct does not cause a leak; a patient with such an injury may present years postoperatively with a stricture, with or without jaundice, cholangitis, or liver failure.[43]

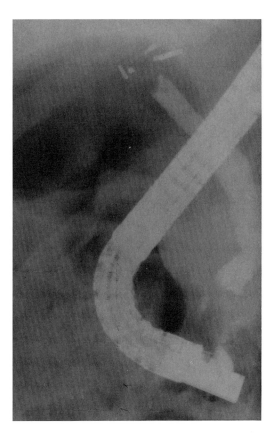

FIGURE 15.4. Endoscopic retrograde cholangiogram demonstrates a type E injury, with total disruption of biliary–enteric continuity.

A type E injury is an excision or complete occlusion of the common hepatic or common bile duct that totally disrupts biliary–enteric communication (Figs. 15.4 15.5).Eighty percent of such injuries are seen following cholecystectomy, but they also occur during operations on the stomach, duodenum, and pancreas[43–46] (Figs. 15.6, 15.7). The injuries occur during laparoscopic cholecystectomy when major ducts are misidentified as the cystic duct, with subsequent ligation, division, and excision; when there is a severe cautery injury to a major duct or its blood supply; or when the cystic duct is ligated too close to the common duct. In Davidoff's 1992 review, the most frequent mechanism of injury occurred when the common duct was mistaken for the cystic duct, with subsequent excision.[47] The poor prognosis of a type E injury is thought to be related to injury to the bile duct's fragile axial blood supply, described next. Subsequent repairs are therefore at risk for ischemia, which complicates management.

Type E injuries most commonly present with jaundice, recurrent cholangitis, pain, and sepsis. Presentation may be subtle, as only 10% of postcholecystectomy strictures are detected within a week of the initial operation. Although

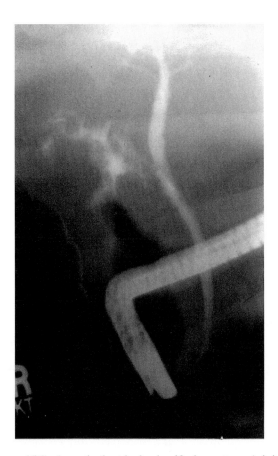

FIGURE 15.3. A cystic duct leak, classified as a type A injury.

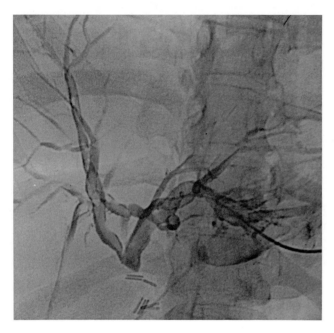

FIGURE 15.5. Percutaneous transhepatic cholangiogram demonstrates a type E injury.

80% are detected within the first year, a stricture may not become evident for several years following the injury; this not only complicates efforts to determine the incidence of such injuries, but, more important, puts the patient at risk for cirrhosis and portal hypertension.[44,48]

The management goal in treating a type E injury is to reestablish biliary–enteric continuity in a fashion that minimizes the chance of restricture with subsequent cholangitis and liver failure (Fig. 15.8). Successful management of the type E injury must include (1) completely defining the nature of the injury with cholangiography from above and below, (2) percutaneously draining the entire biliary system, (3) treating sepsis and periportal inflammation with antibiotics and drainage of collections, and (4) appropriately timing an expert, definitive repair. The focus should be on preventing the need for future rerepair. We discuss here both operative and nonoperative options for repair, but in-depth technical aspects are beyond the scope of this chapter.

Surgical management of the stenotic or occluded bile duct is determined primarily by three factors. The first factor is the anatomy of the injury and the need to preserve blood supply and minimize tension on a repair. For example, an immediately recognized, nonthermal transection and ligation, with less than 1 cm of ductal tissue loss, may be repaired in end-to-end fashion over a T-tube. In contrast, thermal injuries, injuries unrecognized at operation, and injuries involving tissue loss should be repaired with an end-to-side Roux-en-Y hepaticojejunostomy or choledochojejunostomy after appropriate debridement.[44,45,49,50] Although it may be tempting to perform a hepaticoduodenostomy or a non-Roux hepaticojejunostomy, leakage from a defunctionalized Roux limb will not result in a duodenal fistula, and this type of repair (with a 40- to 60-cm Roux limb) minimizes reflux of enteric contents into the biliary tree. The second factor determining management is the condition of the patient and the right upper quadrant when the injury is recognized. It should be emphasized that once sepsis is controlled and the biliary system is drained, there is no urgency to perform the definitive repair.[27,50] Periportal inflammation can make it nearly impossible to expose healthy ductal mucosa suitable for anastomosis, so immediate repair of an injury discovered postoperatively may

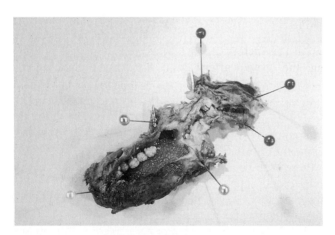

FIGURE 15.6. Gross specimen following laparoscopic cholecystectomy in which a type E injury occurred. Note gallbladder, cystic duct, and excised common bile duct.

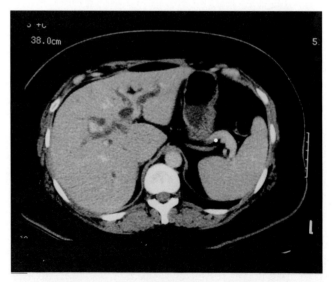

FIGURE 15.7. CT scan demonstrates dilated intrahepatic bile ducts following a bile duct injury during laparoscopic cholecystectomy.

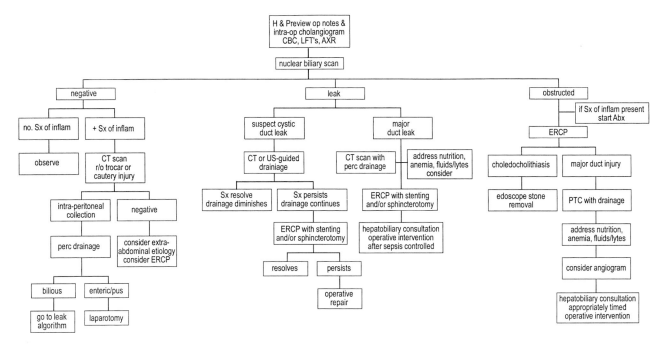

FIGURE 15.8. Treatment algorithm for patients with vague abdominal complaints following laparoscopic cholecystectomy.

not be advisable. In addition, malnutrition and anemia must be addressed, and fluids and electrolytes should be corrected before repair. The final factor is the operator's experience; if an inexperienced surgeon recognizes a proximal injury and expert assistance is unavailable, he should open the patient, perform a cholangiogram, place intraductal drains, close, and refer the patient for hepatobiliary consultation. *The first repair has the greatest chance of success.*

Nonoperative definitive interventions such as percutaneous balloon dilation and endoscopic dilation for the type E injuries are possible only when there is an occluded stenosis through which a wire can be passed; this obviously precludes their use following a ligation or excision of a duct. These techniques are extremely valuable when a patient is too ill to undergo laparotomy; however, like biliary reconstruction, they are difficult and require a high level of expertise. They are associated with significant postintervention morbidity, including hemorrhage, hemobilia, pancreatitis, and sepsis. Furthermore, they often need to be performed multiple times, making the total hospital stay for nonoperative treatment similar to that for surgical repair.[45] It should be noted that many surgeons believe that any type E injury is by definition not amenable to nonoperative repair.

Whichever method is chosen to treat a ductal injury, long-term frequent follow-up examinations are necessary to quickly detect restenosis, which can occur as long as years after a repair. The examinations should include serum bilirubin, alkaline phosphatase, and transaminases, as well as imaging with biliary scintigraphy and ultra-

sound to demonstrate the free flow of bile and normal-sized intrahepatic ducts.[45]

Biliary Injuries with Associated Vascular Injury

The right hepatic artery is at risk during laparoscopic cholecystectomy, as it appears in the triangle of Calot 82% of the time and may therefore be mistaken for the cystic artery and thus ligated[51] (Figs. 15.9, 15.10, 15.11). It may also be inadvertently injured while attempting to control hemorrhage during the course of dissection. Bleeding encountered during laparoscopic surgery should be addressed by tamponade, the isolation of the bleeding vessel, and precise clip or ligature placement; if these maneuvers are unsuccessful, conversion is indicated. This factor emphasizes the importance of identifying the cystic artery, following its course to the gallbladder wall, and ligating it close to the gallbladder, even if this entails ligating anterior and posterior branches of the cystic artery separately. The right hepatic artery, in addition to supplying well-oxygenated blood to the right lobe of the liver, perfuses the common duct from above whereas the gastroduodenal or right gastric artery supplies the duct from below.[8] Therefore, a transection of the common duct in conjunction with a right hepatic artery injury may create ischemia in the proximal common or hepatic duct. This compound injury makes primary repair of a duct injury particularly hazardous and supports a generous proximal debridement before an anastomosis of any kind.

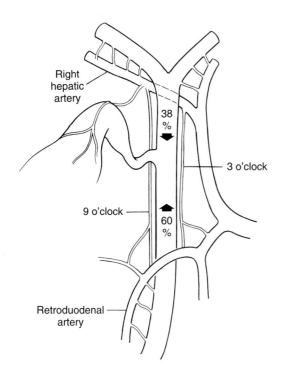

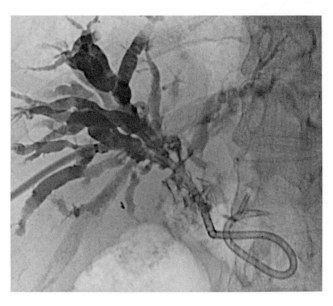

FIGURE 15.11. Cholangiogram in same patient, demonstrating multiple ischemic strictures.

FIGURE 15.9. Arterial supply of the extrahepatic biliary system. Note the axial nature of the supraduodenal bile duct vasculature, with vessels at the 3 and 9 o'clock positions. Note also the dominance of the blood supply from below. The *retroduodenal artery* originates from the gastroduodenal artery.

In addition to the possibility of duct leakage and stricture formation after such an injury, the portion of liver drained by this duct is also at risk for necrosis and abscess formation, which may necessitate hepatic resection or even transplantation in extremely rare circumstances.[52] Alternatively, patients may present with hemobilia.[53] Surgeons who are referred patients for biliary reconstruction with stricture, hepatic necrosis, or abscess should review prior operative notes and query the primary surgeon specifically with regard to intraoperative bleeding. Preoperative angiography is indicated if there is suspicion of vascular injury,[54,55] whether by history, chart review, or the presence of multiple clips in a "shotgun" pattern on X-ray (Fig. 15.12).

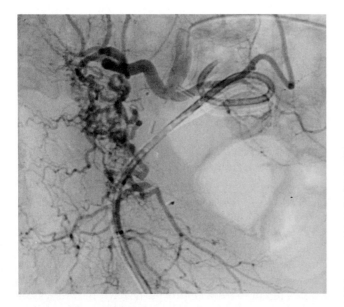

FIGURE 15.10. Angiogram demonstrates injury to the right hepatic artery incurred during laparoscopic cholecystectomy.

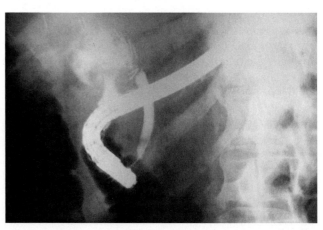

FIGURE 15.12. Cholangiogram reveals "shotgun" pattern of hemostatic clips applied to control bleeding during laparoscopic cholecystectomy. One should suspect a concurrent major vascular injury when viewing such a cholangiogram.

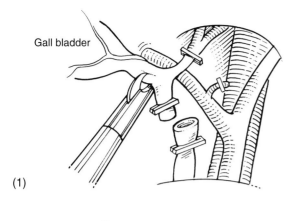

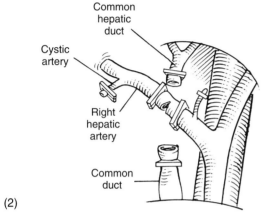

FIGURE 15.13. Davidoff's "classic laparoscopic biliary injury." Note normal portal anatomy, misidentification of the common duct as the cystic duct with ligation and excision (1), and simultaneous injury/ligation to the right hepatic artery (2).

Risk Factors and Prevention of Injury During Laparoscopic Cholecystectomy

Several studies have documented risk factors to assess the likelihood that a biliary injury will occur. While "no surgeon is immune and no case should be considered routine,"[22] considering these factors could help surgeons determine what additional maneuvers can to lessen risk. Risk factors for biliary injury during laparoscopic cholecystectomy include aberrant anatomy, adhesions, acute or chronic inflammation, hemorrhage, and perhaps inexperience of the surgeon.[23] Obesity, a predictor for conversion to laparotomy, does not appear to be a risk factor for bile duct injury,[28,56] though this has been argued.[57]

Dissection in the triangle of Calot is dangerous if aberrant anatomy of the extrahepatic biliary system and vasculature is not considered. More than two-thirds of biliary complications of laparoscopic cholecystectomy result from a misinterpretation of the anatomy with or without a cholangiogram[58] (Fig. 15.13). This finding indicates that emphasis has been placed on identifying the cystic duct–common duct junction but not on defining the

entire course of the cystic duct and its entrance into the gallbladder; in fact, visualizing the cystic duct–common duct junction is not entirely necessary.[59] Several anatomic variants deserve mention in discussing injury potential during laparoscopic cholecystectomy. First, as previously mentioned, is the cystic duct that drains into the right hepatic duct; this variant should be considered every time the cystic duct–common duct junction is identified to avoid injury to the right hepatic duct. A second variation is the cystic duct that parallels and is attached to a main duct. Traction on the Hartman pouch toward the right lower quadrant, correctly used to "open the angle" between the cystic and hepatic ducts, can "tent" such a duct and lead to injury.[60] A cholangiogram can be helpful, and cautery should be avoided. The third variant is a cystic duct that travels posterior to the common duct before joining it on the left side; therefore, one cannot assume, when two ducts are visualized, that the one on the right is the cystic duct. Dissecting close to the gallbladder and staying away from the porta hepatis is the rule; a retained stone in a long cystic duct remnant is rarely problematic. Finally, the presence of a "sessile" gallbladder or short cystic duct can lead to injury, as can the situation in which the gallbladder is fibrosed to the common bile duct or common hepatic duct. In such situations, clips or loops may not be appropriate and may end up impinging upon the common duct; an endoscopic stapling device has been advocated for this use,[61] but this is an extremely dangerous anatomic variant, and unless the stapler can be placed clearly away from the common duct, laparotomy is warranted.

Another risky anatomic situation is found with Mirizzi's syndrome, seen in less than 1% of laparoscopic cholecystectomies.[62,63] Extrinsic compression of the hepatic duct by a cystic duct calculus with associated inflammation puts the hepatic duct at tremendous risk of injury during dissection of the triangle of Calot, especially if a fistula between the ducts has formed. Therefore, dissection of this triangle is contraindicated when this syndrome is present.[64] Because the syndrome is often not recognized (preoperatively or intraoperatively), a high index of suspicion is required to institute preventive measures. If the syndrome is recognized preoperatively (shrunken, atrophic gallbladder; jaundice; dilated duct; suggestion of compression on cholangiogram), initial therapy should be endoscopic, and definitive therapy should be via laparotomy. If the syndrome is recognized intraoperatively, the surgeon should strongly consider converting to laparotomy. Also, a cholangiogram should be performed (through the gallbladder if possible), and if this is nondiagnostic, intraoperative ultrasound may aid in delineating the anatomy. Furthermore, the fundus-down technique should be considered, as should opening the gallbladder to extract the stone. Moreover, a partial cholecystectomy may be necessary, leaving behind a densely adherent portion of the gallbladder wall; rarely, a biliary–enteric bypass may be indicated.[62,64]

Adhesions and inflammation can also add to the difficulty in performing a safe laparoscopic cholecystectomy. Much has been written about optimal timing of cholecystectomy in a patient with acute cholecystitis, and it has been shown that laparoscopic cholecystectomy can be performed safely in the setting of acute cholecystitis, particularly if it is done early in the course of the disease.[29,65–68] There is probably an increased rate of bile duct injury in this setting, however, and the threshold to perform a cholangiogram or convert to open surgery must be adjusted accordingly.[23,69]

The performance of routine or selective intraoerative cholangiography is addressed in a separate chapter. Here, let it suffice to say that surgeons who perform laparoscopic cholecystectomy should be comfortable with performing and interpreting cholangiograms. It has been shown, however, that in the setting of bile duct injury, misinterpretation of cholangiograms is commonly found to have occurred.[22] In the context of litigation, misinterpretation of an X-ray by a surgeon is often the salient factor that has led to the delay in diagnosis and treatment.

As with any dissection, there is a time and place for electrosurgery. Although most bowel injuries incurred during laparoscopic surgery are caused by trocars, electrical burns also account for many injuries. Several points are to be considered in decreasing the incidence of electrical injury. First, before use, instruments should be inspected for defects in insulation (courts have not exonerated surgeons for equipment failures).[70] Second, electrosurgery should never be used outside the visual field, and only those electrosurgical generators equipped with a return electrode monitoring system should be used. Third, laparoscopic port cannulas should be either all metal or all plastic to prevent capacitive coupling of energy to surrounding structures, and other metal instruments should be kept clear of the cautery to prevent arcing[71] (Fig. 15.14). Finally, to minimize the potential for capacitive coupling when performing electrosurgical dissection, one should favor the use of "cutting" current, reserving "coagulation" current for surfaces requiring electrical fulguration. Pulling clear adhesions and peritoneum off the body of the gallbladder after brief pulses of current is acceptable, whereas simultaneous dissection and coagulation is not. Monopolar cautery should be discouraged in the triangle of Calot and should never be used near unidentified structures. Alternative devices such as bipolar and harmonic instruments are less convenient and sometimes more expensive but may lessen the risk of certain injuries.

Immediate inspection of the specimen upon removal has traditionally been done during operation for neoplastic disease, when confirmation of appropriate margins determines whether the surgeon is prepared to institute the reconstructive phase of the operation. Similarly, inspection of a gallbladder extracted through a laparoscopic port is the surgeon's last chance to confirm the removal of only a gallbladder and a cystic duct and the absence of carcinoma. Obviously, discovery of a branching duct or a mucosal mass would prompt a cholangiogram or conversion to laparotomy.

Ideally, all laparoscopic operations would be performed just as they would be performed in the open setting; that is, the identical "tried and true" operation would be performed but without an incision. In the era of open cholecystectomy, for example, one technique was to identify and isolate the cystic duct and artery, dissect the gallbladder off the liver from the fundus downward, confirm the identification of the cystic structures, and divide. This technique, described by Glenn, reduced the rate of ductal injuries during open cholecystectomy and was historically a great leap forward for biliary surgeons, especially for cholecystectomy in the setting of inflammation.[72–74]

The technique of laparoscopic cholecystectomy most commonly employed in the United States is somewhat altered, however, in that the cystic structures are often divided before complete dissection of the gallbladder from the liver. This method imparts two advantages: first, the gallbladder is kept up and away from the triangle of Calot during dissection, and second, early ligation of the cystic artery leads to better hemostasis with subsequent dissection. Several centers have reported a laparoscopic "fundus first" technique in which there is less traction applied to the common duct; presumably, less tenting of the common duct would lead to fewer cases of clip impingement and other duct injuries.[75–77] It seems reasonable to keep the fundus and body of the gallbladder attached to the liver *so long as the infundibulum is completely detached from the liver and the neck is seen "funneling down" to the completely exposed cystic duct before division.* Perhaps history shall repeat itself.

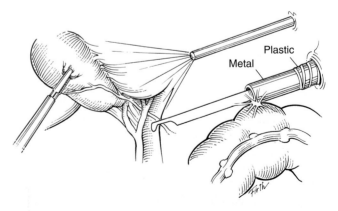

FIGURE 15.14. Capacitive coupling. A metal trocar sheath and a plastic anchoring device do not allow current to flow to the abdominal wall. Instead, current flows to adjacent viscera.

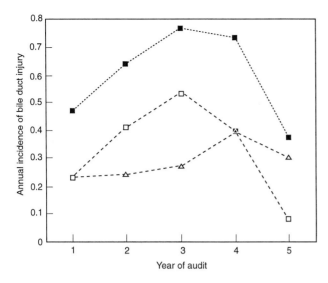

FIGURE 15.15. Annual incidence of bile duct injuries as reported by Richardson et al. from Scotland, 1990 to 1995. *Closed squares,* overall injuries; *open squares,* major duct injuries; *triangles,* minor duct injuries.

Medicolegal Aspects of Bile Duct Injuries

Fortunately, several population-based studies have indicated that the rate of biliary injuries incurred during laparoscopic cholecystectomy is falling[14,24,25] (Figs. 15.15, 15.16). Laparoscopic cholecystectomy, however, is still associated with more complications than any other laparoscopic procedure, and, as would be expected, it is the most common case found in litigation against general surgeons. Kern has written extensively on the topic of malpractice and how its study can be highly educational for surgeons, much like the weekly morbidity-mortality conference. He lists four general criteria that link complications with malpractice claims.[58,78,79] First is economic loss; given the chronic nature of biliary stricture and the convalescence following repair, a patient with a bile duct injury may miss weeks of work or may never be able to work again. In addition, hospital and physician fees may influence the patient's insurance company to litigate. Second is profound disability or death; clearly, liver failure and recurrent cholangitis are highly morbid conditions that predispose to these negative outcomes. Similarly, delayed peritonitis as a consequence of an unrecognized bowel injury has a mortality that approaches 25%. Third is the likelihood of a large indemnity payout; average verdict and settlement costs for an injury incurred during laparoscopic cholecystectomy are between $200,000 and $500,000. Finally is the patient's belief that negligence has occurred; delay in diagnosis, multiple reoperations, and the comments of the consulting hepatobiliary surgeon contribute to this belief. It is this fourth category over which physicians have the most control in avoiding litigation. Still, a claim is several times

more likely to be filed when a bile duct injury has occurred in comparison with most other adverse events.[80]

Kern also points out that although biliary anatomic variants occur in almost a fifth of the population, these are rarely involved in bile duct injuries. He recommends to surgeons performing laparoscopic cholecystectomy several strategies for risk management, which are essentially three policies that will minimize risk of a plaintiff settlement. (1) Warn patients of the risks and include nationally recognized complication rates. Documentation of such a discussion prevents allegations of "a failure to warn properly of operative risk," which can compound a reward for substandard care related to the complication. This discussion should specifically address bile duct injuries and injuries related to the use of electrosurgical devices. (2) Recognize injuries promptly to avoid multiple reoperations. Again, litigation is most likely to result when an injury is unrecognized, requires multiple operations to repair, or results in chronic morbidity. (3) Choose the appropriate repair; that is, do not let a common duct repair over a T-tube suffice when a Roux-en-Y hepaticojejunostomy is necessary. The repair should be done only by operators experienced in biliary reconstruction.

Traumatic Vascular Complications During Laparoscopic Cholecystectomy

Serious hemorrhagic complications during laparoscopic cholecystectomy account for 7% to 21% of conversions to laparotomy and occur in less than 1% of all laparo-

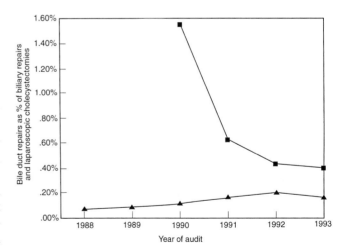

FIGURE 15.16. Study from North Carolina by Rutledge et al. shows decrease in bile duct repairs as a proportion of laparoscopic cholecystectomies and leveling off of proportion of bile duct repairs per total admissions for biliary tract disease from 1988 to 1993. *Squares,* bile duct repairs per number of laparoscopic cholecystectomies; *diamonds,* bile duct repairs per number of biliary disease admissions.

scopic cholecystectomies.[16–19,21,23,30,57,81,82] These complications occur by three mechanisms: (1) trocar or Veress needle injury to an intraabdominal, abdominal wall, or major retroperitoneal vessel; (2) liver laceration or bleeding from the gallbladder fossa; and (3) dissection injury to the cystic artery or a portal vessel such as the hepatic artery or portal vein. In one large series, injury to the cystic artery or bleeding from the gallbladder fossa accounted for 81% of intraoperative bleeding complications.[16] Here, we focus on injury during peritoneal access and liver lacerations; vascular injury associated with biliary tract injury has already been addressed. We also discuss the inherent danger of gas insufflation in the presence of a venous injury.

Trocar and Veress needle vascular injuries are certainly not exclusive to laparoscopic cholecystectomy, but they account for significant morbidity related to this procedure and, as such, are included herein. Generally occurring during the "blind" technique of establishing pneumoperitoneum, the vessels involved are the aorta, vena cava, and the iliac arteries and veins. Although the incidence of this type of injury is between 0.10% and 0.25% of all laparoscopies, mortality may approach 10%.[17,18,56,83,87] For this reason, using an open technique to access the peritoneum is encouraged.[88] If a closed method is employed, directing the Veress needle and primary trocar toward the pelvis with the patient in the Trendelenburg position, using conical-tipped needles, and strongly elevating the abdominal wall before insertion are techniques that enhance safety.[87,89] Furthermore, in thin patients, the aortic bifurcation can often be palpated before Veress needle insertion and can therefore be avoided.[90] Early recognition of hypotension, blood return in the Veress needle, or an expanding retroperitoneal hematoma with prompt conversion to laparotomy are keys to successful management. Once a trocar injury is recognized, the trocar that has struck the vessel should be left in place as the abdomen is opened, for the dual purposes of tamponade and localization of the injury. The injured vessel should be fully mobilized to rule out injury to its posterior wall.[91]

In addition to the obvious problem of bleeding from Veress needle injury, a real danger exists if the needle has been placed into a vein unknowingly, with subsequent carbon dioxide insufflation; fatal carbon dioxide emboli have been reported because this injury was not recognized.[92] Vascular injuries occurring during dissection can also allow gas to enter the vasculature, as has been seen in one report of a cardiac arrest following exposure of a hepatic sinusoid as the gallbladder was being dissected from the liver.[93] Having a high index of suspicion, promptly releasing the pneumoperitoneum, and placing the patient in the left lateral position (Durant's maneuver) may increase the chance of survival.

Injury to an abdominal wall vessel (usually an epigastric artery or vein; rarely, a patent umbilical artery) may be recognized following trocar insertion as continuous dripping of blood from a trocar or an expanding hematoma around a trocar site. This problem can be avoided by placing trocars lateral to the rectus sheath; also, transilluminating the abdominal wall with the laparoscope before insertion of trocars occasionally reveals abdominal wall vessels. Once such an injury is recognized, the surgeon has three options in controlling the hemorrhage: (1) tamponade can be accomplished by inserting a Foley catheter through the trocar and putting it on tension; (2) full-thickness abdominal wall sutures can be placed under direct laparoscopic visualization; or (3) the wound may be explored with direct ligation of the bleeder. The disastrous potential of these injuries is not to be downplayed; not recognizing a lacerated deep epigastric vessel or a disrupted umbilical artery in a cirrhotic can be fatal.[85]

Liver lacerations during laparoscopic cholecystectomy are usually caused while performing one of three maneuvers: (1) placing trocars, (2) applying cephalad traction to the gallbladder fundus, or (3) dissecting the gallbladder from its fossa.[94] The placement of trocars under direct vision can virtually eliminate the first mechanism of injury. The second mechanism can be avoided simply by not applying excessive traction, which tends to avulse the gallbladder off the liver. Also, by avoiding the falciform ligament when inserting the epigastric trocar, the liver is not fixed to the abdominal wall, allowing better mobility when cephalad traction is applied. The ligament can be avoided by retracting it to the left using a grasper placed through the midclavicular port. Additionally, the ligament can be divided if tension is encountered, thus releasing the liver from the abdominal wall. Meticulous dissection in the correct plane between liver and gallbladder avoids the final mechanism of injury to the liver and is accomplished by continually adjusting the direction of traction on the body of the gallbladder, allowing better exposure and avoiding "working in a hole." One additional mechanism of hemorrhage from the liver may involve the ever-increasing use of intravenous nonsteroidal antiinflammatory drugs in the perioperative period; subcapsular hematomas have been reported following the use of these agents during laparoscopic cholecystectomy.[95]

Traditional surgical principles apply to the management of hepatic trauma incurred during laparoscopic cholecystectomy. For this reason, an exhaustive discussion of the treatment of liver injury is beyond the scope of this chapter. Liver injuries incurred during laparoscopic cholecystectomy can usually be managed with electrocautery or argon beam coagulation. Endoscopic devices for the deployment of hemostatic agents are also available.

Bowel Injury During Laparoscopic Cholecystectomy

Injury to the alimentary tract can occur during trocar insertion or dissection in the right upper quadrant, especially when using electrosurgical devices. The jejunum, ileum, and colon are susceptible to Veress needle and trocar injury, whereas the duodenum is more likely injured while exploring the triangle of Calot.[96] Meckel's diverticula and urachal remnants that remain fixed to the umbilicus are particularly susceptible to injury during peritoneal access.[97,98] The rate of bowel injury is between 0% and 0.4% in reported series,[13,16–19,23,82,99,100] but this incidence appears to be decreasing.[99] Series reporting 0% incidence of bowel injury used the open technique in obtaining peritoneal access. In contrast, the enterotomy rate in a series of 1200 consecutive open cholecystectomies by Morgenstern et al. in the 1980s was 0.17%.[9]

As with bile duct injuries, bowel injury may not be detected at the time of the injury, leading to higher mortality. The mechanism of bowel injury may be thermal or mechanical; thermal injury in particular may go unnoticed, until several days following operation, when the bowel wall necroses and the patient returns with complaints of nausea, malaise, or signs of sepsis or peritonitis. Mortality following all bowel injuries during laparoscopic cholecystectomy was 4.6% in the retrospective analysis by Deziel et al., whereas duodenal injuries had an associated mortality of 8.3%.[17,18] This study, which demonstrated only 0.14% incidence of bowel injury, underscored the lethality of such an event, especially when not detected immediately. It should also be noted, however, that a Veress needle injury to the alimentary tract may remain completely asymptomatic and in fact may heal spontaneously.

Perforation of the Gallbladder and Dropped Stones

During mobilization of the gallbladder from the liver and again during extraction, there is a risk of perforation of the gallbladder with the possibility of stone spillage and loss. Perforation is common, occurring in 10% to 40% of laparoscopic cholecystectomies, but the rate of stone loss is unknown.[101,102] The risk of perforation appears to be increased in the setting of acute cholecystitis (almost 50%), despite the thickening of the gallbladder wall. DeSimone and colleagues recently retrospectively reviewed 350 consecutive laparoscopic cholecystectomies and found that evidence of inflammation (with a thickened gallbladder wall on preoperative ultrasound), previous laparotomy, and gallbladder hydrops were predictors of perforation.[103] Stone loss, although common, rarely leads to serious complication. In a Swiss review of more than 10,000 laparoscopic cholecystectomies with a 5.7% rate of stone spillage, only 8 patients had serious complications due to lost gallstones, representing 1.5% of those in whom stones were spilled.[101]

Although it was once thought that stones left in the peritoneum were innocuous or caused only adhesions, it is now known that stones on occasion may act unpredictably as a nidus for infection or erode through somatic and visceral structures. Reported sequelae of lost stones are protean and include intraabdominal, abdominal wall, and port site abscess formation; the development of peritoneal–cutaneous sinus tracks; and perforation into the intestine, uterus, and even the thorax with resulting obstructive pneumonia.[104–115] In addition, stones that erode into the intestine may cause obstruction.[116] These sequelae may present well beyond a year following the cholecystectomy with complaints of fever, pain, or a palpable mass.[117] Cultures of an associated inflammatory mass or fluid collection may be negative; that is, infection need not be present for a complication to occur. However, as shown by Johnston and colleagues using an animal model, complications of stone loss may be compounded when stones are left in the presence of bile, which is contaminated in 60% of patients with a previous history of cholecystitis.[118]

Preventing gallbladder perforation and stone loss during mobilization is accomplished by dissecting with proper countertraction and minimizing damage once a perforation has occurred. When bile is first noted escaping from a torn gallbladder, its contents should be aspirated and the wall should be repaired with a prepared loop tie, clips, or sutures. The prepared loop ties and clips are best suited for soft gallbladders with small perforations, whereas suturing is better for thick-walled gallbladders or those with large tears. Spilled stones should be removed with spoon forceps or placed in an endoscopic specimen bag. Copious irrigation of the subhepatic and subphrenic areas should follow. Perforation occurring during extraction of a large gallbladder should be prevented by enlarging the fascial incision or using an endoscopic specimen bag; enlarging the fascial incision incurs no additional morbidity.[119]

If it is known or suspected that stones have been lost, the surgeon must decide whether to perform a laparotomy. In the Swiss study just mentioned, converting to a laparotomy after stone loss halved the local complication rate and virtually eliminated the rate of reoperation. As would be expected, however, laparotomy was associated with a higher rate of systemic complications. Given the extraordinarily low risk of having a complication from a lost stone, it is generally agreed that laparotomy is not indicated for stone retrieval, though a short course of postoperative antibiotics is prudent. The patient should be made aware of the situation, and the discussion should be documented.

Treatment of the patient who presents with a late complication of stone loss usually entails percutaneous or surgical drainage of inflammatory collections and debridement of any sinus track, with removal of stone debris. Failure to completely remove the debris leads to recurrence of symptoms. The patient's clinical status and the results of wound cultures dictate the use of antibiotics.

Cancer of the Gallbladder and Laparoscopic Cholecystectomy

Background and Epidemiology

Metastatic spread of gallbladder carcinoma is an unexpected and unusual complication of laparoscopic cholecystectomy. After all, carcinoma of the gallbladder is rare, representing only 0.57% of all malignancies in the United States, and is seen in only 0.5% to 3% of all patients with gallstone disease.[120–122] However, there are markers that may alert surgeons to the presence of gallbladder carcinoma. For example, up to 90% of patients with gallbladder carcinoma have stones, so there is (in theory) a crude radiologic marker for this cancer. In contrast, a calcified gallbladder wall (the so-called porcelain gallbladder) is a more specific marker for carcinoma, successfully predicting carcinoma 25% to 60% of the time. Women are afflicted three times as often as men, and the mean age at diagnosis is 65. It is seen in Southwest Native Americans, Alaskans, Mexicans, and American Hispanics five to six times more often than in the general population, whereas African-Americans are rarely affected. Its incidence is markedly increased in patients with gallstones larger than 3 cm, and is also seen more often in chronic typhoid carriers.[122,123] Given this epidemiology, it is now possible to construct a typical case in which a patient presents with symptomatic cholelithiasis that results in disseminated gallbladder carcinoma following laparoscopic cholecystectomy.

> A 65-year-old Hispanic woman complained of right upper quadrant pain, which had worsened over the past month. As a young woman, she was told she had gallstones after a workup for abdominal pain during a pregnancy. Because her complaints at that time were mild, she was treated expectantly. Ultrasound examination now confirmed the presence of cholelithiasis, including a 3-cm stone, as well as signs of acute cholecystitis. After fluid resuscitation and administration of antibiotics, laparoscopic cholecystectomy was performed, during which the gallbladder was ruptured, with spillage of bile during dissection and again at extraction from the umbilical port site. Pathological examination revealed a stage III carcinoma, and she was treated with adjuvant therapy on research protocol. Three months later she presented with a

painful periumbilical nodule, and a biopsy demonstrated metastatic adenocarcinoma. The site was widely excised, but 4 months later she died of widespread disease.

Incidental gallbladder carcinoma is found at operation in 1% to 2% of all open cholecystectomies,[124–126] but in the Southern Surgeons Club's prospective study carcinoma was detected in only 0.1% of the laparoscopic cholecystectomies. Thus, it appears gallbladder carcinoma is now being diagnosed more often postoperatively, perhaps because tactile sensation is lost during the laparoscopic procedure.[19,127]

Ideally, gallbladder carcinoma would always be diagnosed preoperatively and at an early stage of invasion. An open cholecystectomy with an appropriate negative margin and lymphadenectomy would then be performed without violation of the gallbladder wall. In reality, however, gallbladder carcinoma is diagnosed preoperatively in only one-third of cases.[128–131] Furthermore, in a large retrospective review of 928 laparoscopic cholecystectomies in which nine carcinomas were identified, three were grossly normal; in fact, a pathological finding of cholecystitis was not associated with the presence of a carcinoma.[132]

Laparoscopic cholecystectomy is by no means a "cancer operation." Therefore, if a mass, polyp, or focal thickening is discovered by ultrasound or CT scan preoperatively, an open procedure for the definitive therapy is appropriate, especially when the diameter of a polyp exceeds 1 cm, when its likelihood of harboring a cancer approaches 90%.[133–135] One exception may be the cholesterol polyp; if there is a high suspicion of this type of polyp (the most common type of gallbladder polyp), laparoscopy is not necessarily contraindicated.[134,136] It has been proposed that laparoscopic cholecystectomy may be appropriate for early T-stage gallbladder carcinoma, but rarely can this be determined preoperatively[124]; it should be noted that even in situ carcinomas have been disseminated when the gallbladder has been perforated during dissection.[132,137]

The Problem of Port Site Metastases

It remains unclear whether wound metastases occur more often after laparoscopic cholecystectomies for cancer than after open cholecystectomies (Fig. 15.17). The difficulty in studying this important question is severalfold. First, when a carcinoma is suspected preoperatively, an open procedure is performed; in such a case the wound also would undoubtedly be protected during the operation, and water or even povidone-iodine might be used to irrigate the wound after the specimen is removed. Second, the rarity of this cancer makes it difficult to draw statistical conclusions; as was discussed, less than 1% of excised gallbladders are found to harbor a carcinoma. Finally, these tumors tend to appear at an advanced stage, and it

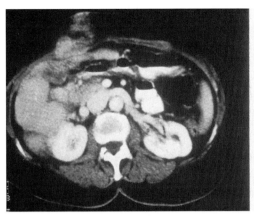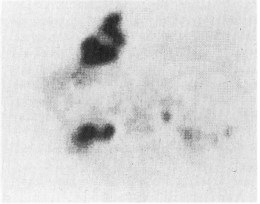

FIGURE 15.17. CT scan and PET scan show a port site metastasis of a gallbladder carcinoma in a patient who had undergone laparoscopic cholecystectomy.

cannot be said whether port site metastases are due to direct implantation of tumor cells or simply represent a more readily apparent manifestation of already disseminated disease. For these reasons and others, no prospective, randomized study has addressed this issue.

Metastases may develop rapidly at the extraction port, appearing as umbilical incisional hernias.[138,139] Although the extraction port is more often the site of recurrence, other ports are certainly not immune.[140] Theories regarding the mechanism of port site metastases center on the effect of positive pressure insufflation with carbon dioxide, as well as the more traumatic handling of tissues with laparoscopic instruments.[137,141] The rate of port site metastases in one prospective study was 14% of patients with carcinoma who had undergone laparoscopic cholecystectomy, representing 0.05% of all 10,925 laparoscopic cholecystectomies in the series.[121] Gallbladder rupture or conversion to an open cholecystectomy did not influence the rate of port site metastases, but there was a trend toward perforation, leading to a higher port site recurrence rate. Currently, it is recommended that laparoscopic cholecystectomy not be performed when there is preoperative suspicion or knowledge of carcinoma; rather, the patient should be referred for definitive therapy without laparoscopy, laparotomy, or percutaneous biopsy.[133] The consistent use of nonporous bags when extracting the specimen during laparoscopic cholecystectomy may decrease the rate of extraction port site metastases but will likely not affect recurrence at other port sites.[139,142] When gallbladder carcinoma is diagnosed following laparoscopic cholecystectomy, wide excision of all port sites is recommended, although it has not been shown that this will increase survival or disease-free interval. All patients with port site metastases in the Z'graggen series subsequently developed other distant metastases. When studying port site metastasis of colon cancer in rats, one group recently demonstrated that

irrigation of the port sites with 5-fluorouracil (5-FU) decreased the incidence of the incisional metastases when compared to irrigation with water, saline, or heparin.[143] How this step relates to gallbladder carcinoma in humans is unknown, but it merits investigation.

In conclusion, gallbladder carcinoma is a rare but unforgiving tumor that can be disseminated to laparoscopic port sites and peritoneal surfaces by unclear mechanisms if it is a lesion of adequate thickness or if the gallbladder is perforated. A clinical suspicion of gallbladder carcinoma based upon history and imaging may therefore warrant laparotomy. The use of a nonporous specimen bag may decrease the incidence of umbilical port site metastases when unsuspected carcinomatous gallbladders are removed laparoscopically.

Miscellaneous Complications

Atraumatic Vascular Complications of Laparoscopic Cholecystectomy

Laparoscopic cholecystectomy is most commonly performed under general anesthesia in the reverse Trendelenburg position, with carbon dioxide insufflation of the abdomen to 10 to 15 mmHg; these factors all affect lower extremity and splanchnic blood flow and are therefore implicated in thrombotic complications of the procedure.[144–146] In addition, hypercoagulability and vascular endothelial damage following laparoscopic cholecystectomy may play a role in the development of lower extremity deep-vein thrombosis (DVT).[147,148] With adequate prophylaxis, however, the rate of DVT is probably less than 1%,[147,152] and the risk of death from a pulmonary embolus is between 4 and 25 per 100,000 procedures.[17,153] For these reasons, all patients undergoing laparoscopic cholecystectomy should be given some form of perioperative DVT protection, whether pharmacological, mechanical, or both; preoperative risk stratification may aid in determining the method(s) employed. There appears to be no difference in plasma fibrinolytic activity when comparing laparoscopic cholecystectomy with open inguinal herniorrhaphy in the perioperative period.[154]

In addition to DVT, mesenteric arterial complications following laparoscopic cholecystectomy have been reported.[155–157] These complications have led to bowel resection and even perioperative death, but the case reports of such complications usually describe some underlying condition, with risk factors for atherosclerotic disease, or active inflammatory bowel disease. In an elegant study using an animal model, Ishizaki and colleagues demonstrated decreased cardiac output, increased systemic vascular resistance, and decreased superior mesenteric arterial blood flow during peritoneal carbon dioxide insufflation to 16mmHg.[145] Again, preoperative risk stratification for mesenteric ischemia may lead to appropriate use of gasless laparoscopy, pulmonary artery catheters, intermittent release of the pneumoperitoneum, or even conventional open cholecystectomy.

Superficial Wound Infection and Incisional Hernia

The main advantage of the laparoscopic approach relates to the lack of a large wound; however, the wounds left from a laparoscopy are subject to the same complications as those following traditional laparotomy. It follows that laparoscopic wound management should be no different than laparotomy wound management, with the goals of preventing infection and herniation. Similarly, risk factors for wound problems are the same, namely, obesity, bronchitis, smoking, and perhaps steroid use.[158]

Reviews on the topic of wound infection do not always distinguish between superficial wound infection, deep wound infection, hematoma, seroma, and hernia and thus direct comparisons are often not possible. In addition, as acute cholecystitis became less of a contraindication to the laparoscopic approach, the samples changed and the risks increased. The risk of a wound infection following laparoscopic cholecystectomy is probably less than 1%, and the risk of incisional hernia is likely to be about 0.5%.[16,19,23,30,42,100,159,160] Compared with open cholecystectomy, one retrospective report was unable to demonstrate a significant difference in the rate of incisional hernia between the two procedures,[158] and a review of 1200 open procedures showed a "wound problem" rate of 0.75%.[9]

Most wound problems following laparoscopic cholecystectomy occur at the umbilical port site, usually a 10-mm incision where the gallbladder was extracted. Smaller port sites rarely become infected or become the sites of clinical hernias, although this has been described in pediatric and adult populations.[161–164] It is generally agreed that fascial defects greater than 8mm should be closed, whereas smaller incisions may be left open. Many surgeons do not close the fascia of the epigastric port, preferring instead to insert the trocar using a Z-shaped path or using the falciform ligament as a shield in preventing future herniation; however, the falciform ligament may house a patent vessel that may be exceedingly difficult to control once lacerated. Again, the use of a specimen bag for extraction may decrease the rate of infection, but this has not been substantiated in a randomized prospective study.

Subcutaneous Emphysema and Hypercarbia

Subcutaneous emphysema forms either when Veress needle insufflation is performed superficial to the fascia, or after pneumoperitoneum is established and carbon dioxide escapes through trocar sites into the subcutaneous space. Subcutaneous emphysema can track cephalad to the head and neck, or it may track to the feet and perineum. Subcutaneous emphysema was seen in 0.3% of patients in the prospective study by the Southern Surgeons Club and in 0.55% of patients in the Canadian study by Litwin and colleagues.[16,19] In almost all cases, subcutaneous emphysema is little more than an annoyance, and it generally resolves spontaneously; however, it can be associated with startlingly severe hypercarbia and acidosis.[165] Patients with significant subcutaneous emphysema should have blood gas analysis and should be hyperventilated as appropriate. In addition, pneumothorax should always be ruled out (clinically, then radiologically). Subcutaneous emphysema can be prevented by not making the fascial incisions too big and by angling the trocars as they penetrate the abdominal wall; these maneuvers minimize the movement of the ports in and out of their intraperitoneal location. Also, an open technique of peritoneal access virtually eliminates the possibility of initially insufflating into the wrong plane.[166] Hypercarbia and respiratory acidosis secondary to pneumoperitoneum are uniformly observed and are easily overcome by increasing the minute ventilation. Animal studies have suggested that this acid–base abnormality may be transmitted through placental circulation; therefore, special attention should be given to blood gas analysis when performing laparoscopic cholecystectomy in pregnant women.[61]

Diaphragmatic Injury

There are two reports of diaphragmatic injury associated with laparoscopic cholecystectomy. One case was that of a full-thickness 4-cm laceration to the diaphragm that occurred when the hook cautery slipped free of the gallbladder as it was being detached from the liver. Strong traction was being applied to the tissues and instruments at the time. The repair was immediately performed laparoscopically and a chest tube was placed; there were no hemodynamic effects of the pneumothorax during the procedure.[167] The second reported diaphragmatic injury was not recognized at the time of surgery; the patient returned 6 weeks postoperatively with pain, and, after an extensive evaluation including consultation by pain specialists and psychiatrists, a CT scan demonstrated a diaphragmatic hernia, which was repaired via thoracotomy. The authors posit that the diaphragm was either burned by the cautery or punctured with the sucker tip (during irrigation) or grasper (while retracting the gallbladder cephalad).[168] The obvious recommendation is that the diaphragm should be inspected before closing; an angled laparoscope will facilitate this maneuver.

Conclusion

Laparoscopic cholecystectomy incurs the same risks as conventional cholecystectomy, in addition to the risks associated with laparoscopy. However, because cholecystectomy was really the "boom" for therapeutic laparoscopy, its complications have always been highly publicized and scrutinized. As unconscionable as it may seem, learning curves are all too real, and some patients undoubtedly suffer as technology advances to help the masses. For the individual surgeon, however, the learning curve should have nothing to do with the safety or soundness of the procedure, for these are absolute and can never be compromised. Rather, the learning curve should only determine how long it takes to perform the task and the circumstances under which the surgeon requests assistance. Optimistically, the steep portion of the collective laparoscopic cholecystectomy learning curve appears to be in the past.

Whether an open technique is used to gain peritoneal access, whether a cholangiogram is performed routinely, or whether a gallbladder is removed from the fundus down, understanding the complications of laparoscopic cholecystectomy will facilitate a safer procedure. Although pioneering minimally invasive techniques demands creativity, surgeons should strive to duplicate the excellent results claimed by history's champions of open cholecystectomy.

Medicolegal attention has forced many surgeons to practice "defensive" medicine when it comes to managing patients with pain or unexplained fever following laparoscopic cholecystectomy. However, a high index of suspicion for injury, a low threshold to perform diagnostic tests, and liberal use of expert consultation may lead to earlier recognition of injury and improved outcome.

References

1. Samuelson R. A high-tech accounting? Newsweek 2000:37.
2. Heuer G. The factors leading to death in operations upon the gall bladder and bile ducts. Ann Surg 1934;99:881.
3. Glenn F, Hays D. The causes of death following biliary tract surgery for nonmalignant disease. Surg Gynecol Obstet 1952;94:283–296.
4. Glenn F, McSherry C. Etiological factors in fatal complications following operations upon the biliary tract. Ann Surg 1963;157:695–704.
5. McSherry C. Cholecystectomy: the gold standard. Am J Surg 1989;158:174–178.
6. Muhe E. The 1999 Karl Storz Lecture in New Technology. The first laparoscopic cholecystectomy: overcoming the roadblocks on the road to the future. SAGES Scientific Session, San Antonio, TX, March 26, 1999.
7. Vellar I. The blood supply of the biliary ductal system and its relevance to vasculobiliary injuries following cholecystectomy. Aust NZ J Surg 1999;69:816–820.
8. Terblanche J, Allison H, Northover J. An ischemic basis for biliary strictures. Surgery (St. Louis) 1983;94:52–57.
9. Morgenstern L, Wong L, Berci G. Twelve hundred open cholecystectomies before the laparoscopic era: a standard for comparison. Arch Surg 1992;127:400–403.
10. Glenn F. Trends in surgical treatment of calculous disease of the biliary tract. Surg Gynecol Obstet 1975;40.
11. Pickleman J, Gonzales R. The improving results of cholecystectomy. Arch Surg 1986;121:930–934.
12. Roslyn J, Tompkins R. Reoperation for biliary strictures. Surg Clin N Am 1991;71:109–116.
13. Huang X, Feng Y, Huang Z. Complications of laparoscopic cholecystectomy in China: an analysis of 39,238 cases. Chin Med J 1997;110:704–706.
14. Richardson M, Bell G, Fullarton G, Group TWoSLCA. Incidence and nature of bile duct injuries following laparoscopic cholecystectomy: an audit of 5913 cases. Br J Surg 1996;83:1356–1360.
15. Regoly-Merei J, Ihasz M, Szeberin Z, Sandor J, Mate M. Biliary tract complications in laparoscopic cholecystectomy: a multicenter study of 148 biliary tract injuries in 26,440 operations. Surg Endosc 1998;12:294–300.
16. Litwin D, Girotti M, Poulin E, Mamazza J, Nagy A. Laparoscopic cholecystectomy: trans-Canada experience with 2201 cases. Can J Surg 1992;35:291–296.
17. Deziel D, Millikan K, Economou S, Doolas A, Ko S-T, Airan M. Complications of laparoscopic cholecystectomy: a national survey of 4292 hospitals and an analysis of 77,604 cases. Am J Surg 1993;165:9–14.
18. Deziel D. Complications of cholecystectomy. Incidence, clinical manifestations, and diagnosis. Surg Clin N Am 1994; 74:809–823.
19. Southern Surgeons Club. A prospective analysis of 1518 laparoscopic cholecystectomies. N Engl J Med 1991;324: 1073–1078.
20. Cagir B, Rangraj M, Maffuci L, Herz B. The learning curve for laparoscopic cholecystectomy. J Laparoendosc Surg 1994;4:419–427.
21. Z'graggen K, Wehrli H, Metzger A, Buehler M, Frei E, Klaiber C. Complications of laparoscopic cholecystectomy

in Switzerland: a prospective 3-year study of 10,174 patients. Surg Endosc 1998;12:1303–1310.

22. Carroll B, Birth M, Phillips E. Common bile duct injuries during laparoscopic cholecystectomy that result in litigation. Surg Endosc 1998;12:310–314.

23. Vecchio R, MacFadyen B, Latteri S. Laparoscopic cholecystectomy: an analysis on 114,005 cases of United States series. Int Surg 1998;83:215–219.

24. Rutledge R, Fakhry S, Baker C, Meyer A. The impact of laparoscopic cholecystectomy on the management and outcome of biliary tract disease in North Carolina: a statewide, population-based, time-series analysis. J Am Coll Surg 1996;183:31–45.

25. Kramling H, Huttl T, Heberer G. Development of gallstone surgery in Germany. Surg Endosc 1999;13:909–913.

26. Bismuth H. Postoperative strictures of the bile duct. In: Blumgart L (ed) Clinical Surgery International, vol 5. The Biliary Tract. Edinburgh: Churchill Livingstone, 1982:209–218.

27. Strasberg S, Hertl M, Soper N. An analysis of the problem of biliary injury during laparoscopic cholecystectomy. J Am Coll Surg 1995;180:101–125.

28. Wise-Unger S, Glick G, Landeros M, Group CDLS. Cystic duct leak after laparoscopic cholecystectomy. Surg Endosc 1996;10:1189–1193.

29. Willsher P, Sanabria J-R, Gallinger S, Rossi L, Strasberg S, Litwin D. Early laparoscopic cholecystectomy for acute cholecystitis: a safe procedure. J Gastrointest Surg 1999;3:50–53.

30. Baird D, Wilson J, Mason E, et al. An early review of 800 laparoscopic cholecystectomies at a university-affiliated community teaching hospital. Am Surg 1992;58:206–210.

31. Roberts R, Pettigrew R, Van Rij A. Bile leakage after laparoscopic cholecystectomy: biliary anatomy revisited. Aust NZ J Surg 1994;64:254–257.

32. Davids P, Rauws E, Tytgat G. Post-operative bile leakage: endoscopic management. Gut 1992;33:1118–1122.

33. Liguory C, Vitale G, Lefebre F, Bonnel D, Cornud F. Endoscopic treatment of postoperative biliary fistulae. Surgery (St. Louis) 1991;110:779–784.

34. Marks J, Ponsky J, Shillingstad R, Singh J. Biliary stenting is more effective than sphincterotomy in the resolution of biliary leaks. Surg Endosc 1998;12:327–330.

35. Raijman I, Catalano M, Hirsch G, et al. Endoscopic treatment of biliary leakage after laparoscopic cholecystectomy. Endoscopy 1994;26:741–744.

36. Ryan M, Geenen J, Lehman G, et al. Endoscopic intervention for biliary leaks after laparoscopic cholecystectomy: a multicenter review. Gastrointest Endosc 1998;47:261–266.

37. Liberman M, Phillips E, Carroll B, Fallas M, Rosenthal R, Hiatt J. Cost-effective management of complicated choledocholithiasis: laparoscopic transcystic duct exploration or endoscopic sphincterotomy. J Am Coll Surg 1996;182:488–494.

38. Voyles C, Sanders D, Hogan R. Common bile duct evaluation in the era of laparoscopic cholecystectomy. Ann Surg 1994;219:744–752.

39. Elboim C, Goldman L, Hahn L, Palestrant A, Silen W. Significance of post-cholecystectomy subhepatic fluid collections. Ann Surg 1983;198:137–141.

40. Gilsdorf J, Phillips M, McLeod M, et al. Radionuclide evaluation of bile leakage and the use of subhepatic drains after cholecystectomy. Am J Surg 1986;151:259–262.

41. Rayter Z, Tonge C, Bennett C, Robinson P, Thomas M. Bile leaks after simple cholecystectomy. Br J Surg 1989;76:1046–1048.

42. Spaw A, Reddick E, Olsen D. Laparoscopic laser cholecystectomy: analysis of 500 procedures. Surg Laparosc Endosc 1991;1:2–7.

43. Parks R, Spencer E, McIlrath E, Johnston G. A review of the management of iatrogenic bile duct injuries. Ir J Med Sci 1994;163:571–575.

44. Lillemoe K, Pitt H, Cameron J. Postoperative bile duct strictures. Surg Clin N Am 1990;70:1355–1380.

45. Lillemoe K, Martin S, Cameron J, et al. Major bile duct injuries during laparoscopic cholecystectomy: follow-up after combined surgical and radiologic management. Ann Surg 1997;225:459–471.

46. Lindenauer S. Surgical treatment of bile duct strictures. Surgery (St. Louis) 1973;73:875–880.

47. Davidoff A, Pappas T, Murray E, et al. Mechanisms of major biliary injury during laparoscopic cholecystectomy. Ann Surg 1992;215:196–202.

48. Pitt H, Miyamoto T, Parapatis S. Factors influencing outcome in patients with postoperative biliary strictures. Am J Surg 1982;144:14–21.

49. Jarnagin W, Blumgart L. Operative repair of bile duct injuries involving the hepatic duct confluence. Arch Surg 1999;134:769–775.

50. Chapman W, Halevy A, Blumgart L, Benjamin I. Postcholecystectomy bile duct strictures: management and outcome in 130 patients. Arch Surg 1995;130:597–602.

51. Gray S, Skandalakis J. Atlas of Surgical Anatomy for General Surgeons. Baltimore: Williams & Wilkins, 1985.

52. Bacha E, Stieber A, Galloway J, Hunter J. Non-biliary complication of laparoscopic cholecystectomy. Lancet 1994;344:896–897.

53. Zilberstein B, Cecconello I, Cardoso Ramos A, Alfonso Sallet J, Andersen Pinheiro E. Hemobilia as a complication of laparoscopic cholecystectomy. Surg Laparosc Endosc 1994;4:301–303.

54. Gupta N, Solomon H, Fairchild R, Kaminski D. Management and outcome of patients with combined bile duct and hepatic artery injuries. Arch Surg 1998;133:176–181.

55. Balsara K, Dubash C, Shah C. Pseudoaneurysm of the hepatic artery along with common bile duct injury following laparoscopic cholecystectomy. Surg Endosc 1998;12:276–277.

56. Fried G, Barkun J, Sigman H, et al. Factors determining conversion to laparotomy in patients undergoing laparoscopic cholecystectomy. Am J Surg 1994;167:35–41.

57. Vincent-Hamelin E, Pallares A, Felipe J, et al. National survey on laparoscopic cholecystectomy in Spain: results of a multiinstitutional study conducted by the Committee for Endoscopic Surgery. Surg Endosc 1994;8:770–776.

58. Kern K. Medicolegal analysis of bile duct injury during open cholecystectomy and abdominal surgery. Am J Surg 1994;168:217–222.

59. Asbun H, Rossi R. Techniques of laparoscopic cholecystectomy. The difficult operation. Surg Clin N Am 1994;74: 755–775.

60. Ress A, Sarr M, Nagorney D, Farnell M, Donohue J, McIlrath D. Spectrum and management of major complications of laparoscopic cholecystectomy. Am J Surg 1993; 165:655–662.

61. Hunter J, Swanstrom L, Thornburg K. Carbon dioxide pneumoperitoneum induces fetal acidosis in a pregnant ewe model. Surg Endosc 1995;9:272–279.

62. Baer H, Matthews J, Schweizer W, Gertsch P, Blumgart L. Management of the Mirizzi syndrome and the surgical implications of cholecystodochal fistula. Br J Surg 1990;77: 743–752.

63. Bower C, Nagorney D. Mirizzi syndrome. Hepatopancreatobiliary Surg 1988;1:67–76.

64. Contini S, Dalla Valle R, Zinicola R, Botta G. Undiagnosed Mirizzi's syndrome: a word of caution for laparoscopic surgeons—a report of three cases and review of the literature. J Laparoendosc Adv Surg Tech 1999; 9:197–203.

65. Flowers J, Bailey R, Scovill W, Zucker K. The Baltimore experience with laparoscopic management of acute cholecystitis. Am Surg 1991;161:388–392.

66. Cooperman A. Laparoscopic cholecystectomy for severe acute, embedded, and gangrenous cholecystitis. J Laparoendosc Surg 1990;1:37–40.

67. Unger S, Rosenbaum G, Unger H, Edelman D. A comparison of laparoscopic and open treatment of acute cholecystitis. Surg Endosc 1993;7:408–411.

68. Wilson R, Macintyre I, Nixon S, Saunders J, Varma J, King P. Laparoscopic cholecystectomy as a safe and effective treatment for severe acute cholecystitis. Br Med J 1992;305: 394–396.

69. Kum C-K, Eypasch E, Lefering R, Paul A, Neugebauer E, Troidl H. Laparoscopic cholecystectomy for acute cholecystitis: is it really safe? World J Surg 1996;20:43–49.

70. Perantinides P, Tsarouhas A, Katzman V. The medicolegal risks of thermal injury during laparoscopic monopolar electrosurgery. J Healthcare Risk Manag 1998:47–55.

71. Voyles C, Tucker R. Education and engineering solutions for potential problems with laparoscopic monopolar electrosurgery. Am J Surg 1992;164:57–62.

72. Glenn F. Atlas of Biliary Tract Surgery. New York: Macmillan, 1963.

73. Moosa A, Mayer A, Stabile B. Iatrogenic injury to the bile duct. Arch Surg 1990;125:1028–1031.

74. Herman R. A plea for a safer technique of cholecystectomy. Surgery (St. Louis) 1976;79:609–611.

75. Cox M, Wilson T, Jeans P, Padbury R, Toouli J. Minimizing the risk of bile duct injury at laparoscopic cholecystectomy. World J Surg 1994;18:422–427.

76. Kato K, Matsuda M, Onodera K, Kobayashi T, Kasai S, Mito M. Laparoscopic cholecystectomy from fundus downward. Surg Laparosc Endosc 1994;4:373–374.

77. Martin I, Dexter S, Marton J, et al. Fundus-first laparoscopic cholecystectomy. Surg Endosc 1995;9:203–206.

78. Kern K. Risk management goals involving injury to the common bile duct during laparoscopic cholecystectomy. Am J Surg 1992;163:551–552.

79. Kern K. Malpractice litigation involving laparoscopic cholecystectomy. Arch Surg 1997;132:392–396.

80. Weiler P, Newhouse J, Hiatt H. Proposal for medical liability reform. JAMA 1992;267:2355–2358.

81. Perissat J, Collet D, Belliard R, Desplantez J, Magne E. Laparoscopic cholecystectomy: the state of the art. A report on 700 consecutive cases. World J Surg 1992;16: 1074–1082.

82. Trondsen E, Ruud T, Nilsen B, et al. Complications during the introduction of laparoscopic cholecystectomy in Norway. Eur J Surg 1994;160:145–151.

83. Wherry D, Marohn M, Malanoski M, Hetz S, Rich N. An external audit of laparoscopic cholecystectomy in the steady state performed in medical treatment facilities of the Department of Defense. Ann Surg 1996;224:145–154.

84. AJ P. How to prevent complications of open laparoscopy. J Reprod Med 1985;30:660–663.

85. Nordestgaard A, Bodily K, Osborne R Jr, Buttorff J. Major vascular injuries during laparoscopic procedures. Am J Surg 1995;169:543–545.

86. Saville L, Woods M. Laparoscopy and major retroperitoneal vascular injuries. Surg Endosc 1995;9:1096–1100.

87. Geers J, Holden C. Major vascular injury as a complication of laparoscopic surgery: a report of three cases and review of the literature. Am Surg 1996;62:377–379.

88. McKernan J, Champion J. Access techniques: Veress needle—initial blind trocar insertion versus open laparoscopy with the Hasson trocar. Endosc Surg Allied Technol 1995;3:35–38.

89. Hurd W, Wang L, Schemmel M. A comparison of the relative risk of vessel injury with conical versus pyramidal laparoscopic trocars in a rabbit model. Am J Obstet Gynecol 1995;173:1731–1733.

90. Apelgren K, Scheeres D. Aortic injury: a catastrophic complication of laparoscopic cholecystectomy. Surg Endosc 1994;8:689–691.

91. Usal H, Sayad P, Hayek N, Hallak A, Huie F, Ferzli G. Major vascular injuries during laparoscopic cholecystectomy. Surg Endosc 1998;12:960–962.

92. Lantz P, Smith J. Fatal carbon dioxide embolism complicating attempted laparoscopic cholecystectomy—case report and literature review. J Forensic Sci 1994;39: 1468–1480.

93. Khan A, Pandya K, Clifton M. Near fatal gas embolism during laparoscopic cholecystectomy. Ann R Coll Surg Engl 1995;77:67–68.

94. Fusco M, Scott T, Paluzzi M. Traction injury to the liver during laparoscopic cholecystectomy. Surg Laparosc Endosc 1994;4:454–456.

95. Erstad B, Rappaport W. Subcapsular hematoma after laparoscopic cholecystectomy, associated with ketorolac administration. Pharmacotherapy 1994;14:613–615.

96. Berry S, Ose K, Bell R, Fink A. Thermal injury of the posterior duodenum during laparoscopic cholecystectomy. Surg Endosc 1994;8:197–200.

97. McLucas B, March C. Urachal sinus perforation during laparoscopy. A case report. J Reprod Med 1990;35:573–574.

98. Westcott C, Westcott R, Kerstein M. Perforation of a Meckel's diverticulum during laparoscopic cholecystectomy. South Med J 1995;88:661.

99. Hashizume M, Sugimachi K, Study Group of Endoscopic Surgery in Kyushu J. Needle and trocar injury during laparoscopic surgery in Japan. Surg Endosc 1997;11:1198–1201.

100. Wolfe B, Gardiner B, Leary B, Frey C. Endoscopic cholecystectomy: an analysis of complications. Arch Surg 1991;126:1192–1198.

101. Schafer M, Suter C, Klaiber C, Wehrli H, Frei E, Krahenbuhl L. Spilled gallstones after laparoscopic cholecystectomy. Surg Endosc 1998;12:305–309.

102. Jones D, Dunnegan D, Soper N. The influence of intraoperative gallbladder perforation on long-term outcome after laparoscopic cholecystectomy. Surg Endosc 1995;9:977–980.

103. De Simone P, Donadio R, Urbano D. The risk of gallbladder perforation at laparoscopic cholecystectomy. Surg Endosc 1999;13:1099–1102.

104. Preciado A, Matthews B, Scarborough T, et al. Transdiaphragmatic abscess: late thoracic complication of laparoscopic cholecystectomy. J Laparoendosc Adv Surg Tech 1999;9:517–521.

105. Golub R, Nwogu C, Cantu R, Stein H. Gallstone shrapnel contamination during laparoscopic cholecystectomy. Surg Endosc 1994;8:898–900.

106. Carlin C, Kent R Jr, Laws H. Spilled gallstones—complications of abdominal wall abscesses (sic): case report and review of the literature. Surg Endosc 1995;9:341–343.

107. Memon M, Deeik R, Maffi T, Fitzgibbons R Jr. The outcome of unretrieved gallstones in the peritoneal cavity during laparoscopic cholecystectomy: a prospective analysis. Surg Endosc 1999;13:848–857.

108. Bour E, Gifford R. Gallstone umbilical sinus tract formation following laparoscopic cholecystectomy. Arch Surg 1995;130:1007–1008.

109. Steerman P. Delayed peritoneal-cutaneous sinus from unretrieved gallstones. Surg Laparosc Endosc 1994;4:452–453.

110. Gallinaro R, Miller F. The lost gallstone: complication after laparoscopic cholecystectomy. Surg Endosc 1994;8:913–914.

111. Van Brunt P, Lanzafame R. Subhepatic inflammatory mass after laparoscopic cholecystectomy: a delayed complication of spilled gallstones. Arch Surg 1994;129:882–883.

112. Janu N, Donnellan M. Chronic sinus after laparoscopic cholecystectomy. Aust NZ J Surg 1995;65:361–362.

113. Mellinger J, Elridge T, Eddelmon E, Crabbe M. Delayed gallstone abscess following laparoscopic cholecystectomy. Surg Endosc 1994;8(11):1332–1334.

114. Benhamou G, Opsahl S, Le Goff J-Y. Can gallstones be left in the peritoneal cavity? Surg Endosc 1998;12:1452.

115. Noda S, Soybel D, Sampson B, DeCamp M Jr. Broncholithiasis and thoracoabdominal actinomycosis from dropped gallstones. Ann Thorac Surg 1998;65:1465–1467.

116. Paul A, Eypasch E, Holthausen U, Troidl H. Bowel obstruction caused by a free intraperitoneal gallstone—a late complication after laparoscopic cholecystectomy. Surgery (St. Louis) 1995;117:595–596.

117. Zamir G, Lyass S, Pertsemlidis D, Katz B. The fate of the dropped gallstones during laparoscopic cholecystectomy. Surg Endosc 1999;13:68–70.

118. Johnston S, O'Malley K, McEntee G, Grace P, Bouchier-Hayes D. The need to retrieve the dropped stone during laparoscopic cholecystectomy. Am J Surg 1994;167:608–610.

119. Bickel A, Szabo A, Shtamler B. A safe simple method for removal of the gallbladder through the umbilical trocar site during laparoscopic cholecystectomy. J Laparorendosc Surg 1993;3:485–487.

120. Greenlee R, Murray T, Bolden S, Wingo P. Cancer statistics, 2000. CA Cancer J Clin 2000;50:7–33.

121. Z'graggen K, Birrer S, Maurer C, Wehrli H, Klaiber C, Baer H. Incidence of port site recurrence after laparoscopic cholecystectomy for preoperatively unsuspected gallbladder carcinoma. Surgery (St. Louis) 1998;124:831–838.

122. Piehler J, Crichlow R. Primary carcinoma of the gallbladder. Surg Gynecol Obstet 1978;147:929–942.

123. Morrow C, Sutherland D, Florack G, Eisenberg M, Grage T. Primary gallbladder carcinoma: significance of subserosal lesions and results of aggressive surgical treatment and adjuvant chemotherapy. Surgery (St. Louis) 1983;94:709–714.

124. Yamaguchi K, Chijiiwa K, Ichimiya H, et al. Gallbladder carcinoma in the era of laparoscopic cholecystectomy. Arch Surg 1996;131:981–984.

125. Bergdahl L. Gallbladder carcinoma first diagnosed at microscopic examination of gallbladders removed for presumed benign disease. Ann Surg 1980;191:19–22.

126. Frank S, Spjut H. Inapparent carcinoma of the gallbladder. Ann Surg 1967;33:367–372.

127. Targarona E, Pons M, Viella P, Trias M. Unsuspected carcinoma of the gallbladder: a laparoscopic dilemma. Surg Endosc 1994;8:211–213.

128. Donohue J, Nagorney D, Grant C, Tsushima K, Ilstrup D, Adson M. Carcinoma of the gallbladder. Does radical resection improve outcome? Arch Surg 1990;125:237–241.

129. Shirai Y, Yoshida K, Tsukada K, Muto T, Watanabe H. Radical surgery for gallbladder carcinoma. Long-term results. Ann Surg 1992;216:565–568.

130. Bartlett D, Fong Y, Fortner J, Brennan M, Blumgart L. Long-term results after resection for gallbladder cancer. Implications for staging and management. Ann Surg 1996;224:639–646.

131. Wanebo H, Castle W, Fechner R. Is carcinoma of the gallbladder a curable lesion? Ann Surg 1982;195:624–631.

132. Wibbenmeyer L, Wade T, Chen R, Meyer R, Turgeon R, Andrus C. Laparoscopic cholecystectomy can disseminate in situ carcinoma of the gallbladder. J Am Coll Surg 1995;181:504–510.

133. Fong Y, Brennan M, Turnbull A, Colt D, Blumgart L. Gallbladder cancer discovered during laparoscopic surgery. Arch Surg 1993;128:1054–1056.

134. Koga A, Watanabe K, Fukuyama T, Takiguchi S, Nakayama F. Diagnosis and operative indications for polypoid lesions of the gallbladder. Arch Surg 1988;123:26–29.

135. Edelman D. Carcinoma of a gallbladder polyp: treated by laparoscopic laser cholecystectomy. Surg Laparosc Endosc 1993;3:142–143.

136. Kubota K, Bandai Y, Otomo Y, et al. Role of laparoscopic cholecystectomy in treating gallbladder polyps. Surg Endosc 1994;8:42–46.

137. Texler M, King G, Hewett P. From inside out: microperforation of the gallbladder during laparoscopic surgery may liberate mucosal cells. Surg Endosc 1998;12:1297–1299.

138. Clair D, Lautz D, Brooks D. Rapid development of umbilical metastases after laparoscopic cholecystectomy for unsuspected gallbladder carcinoma. Surgery (St. Louis) 1993;113:355–358.

139. Nally C, Preshaw R. Tumour implantation at umbilicus after laparoscopic cholecystectomy for unsuspected gallbladder carcinoma. Can J Surg 1994;37:243–244.

140. Jacobi C, Keller H, Monig S, Said S. Implantation metastasis of unsuspected gallbladder carcinoma after laparoscopy. Surg Endosc 1995;9:351–352.

141. Bouvy N, Guiffrida M, Tseng L, et al. Effects of carbon dioxide pneumoperitoneum, air pneumoperitoneum, and gasless laparoscopy on body weight and tumor growth. Arch Surg 1998;133:652–656.

142. Weiss S, Wengert P, Harkavy S. Incisional recurrence of gallbladder cancer after laparoscopic cholecystectomy. Gastrointest Endosc 1994;40:244–246.

143. Eshraghi N, Swanstrom L, Bax T, et al. Topical treatments of laparoscopic port sites can decrease the incidence of incision metastasis. Surg Endosc 1999;13:1121–1124.

144. Lord R, Ling J, Hugh T, Coleman M, Doust B, Nivison-Smith I. Incidence of deep vein thrombosis after laparoscopic vs minilaparotomy cholecystectomy. Arch Surg 1998;133:967–973.

145. Ishizaki Y, Bandai Y, Shimomura K, Abe H, Ohtomo Y, Idezuki Y. Changes in splanchnic blood flow and cardiovascular effects following peritoneal insufflation of carbon dioxide. Surg Endosc 1993;7:420–423.

146. Ido K, Suzuki T, Kimura K, et al. Lower-extremity venous stasis during laparoscopic cholecystectomy as assessed using color Doppler ultrasound. Surg Endosc 1995;9:310–313.

147. Caprini J, Arcelus J. Prevention of postoperative venous thromboembolism following laparoscopic cholecystectomy. Surg Endosc 1994;8:741–747.

148. Caprini J, Arcelus J, Laubach M, et al. Postoperative hypercoagulability and deep-vein thrombosis after laparoscopic cholecystectomy. Surg Endosc 1995;9:304–309.

149. Bonatsos G, Leandros E, Dourakis N, Birbas C, Delibaltadakis G, Golematis B. Laparoscopic cholecystectomy. Intraoperative findings and postoperative complications. Surg Endosc 1995;9:889–893.

150. Bond G, De Costa A. Laparoscopic cholecystectomy: the experience of community hospital. Aust N Z J Surg 1996;66:14–17.

151. Dubois F, Levard H, Berthelot G, Mouro J, Karayel M. Complications of celioscopic cholecystectomy in 2006 patients. Ann Chir 1994;48:899–904.

152. Mayol J, Vincent-Hamelin E, Sarmiento J, et al. Pulmonary embolism following laparoscopic cholecystectomy: report of two cases and review of the literature. Surg Endosc 1994;8:214–217.

153. Scott T, Zucker K, Bailey R. Laparoscopic cholecystomy: a review of 12,397 patients. Surg Laparosc Endosc 1992;2:191–198.

154. Martinez-Ramos C, Lopez-Pastor A, Nunez-Pena J, et al. Changes in hemostasis after laparoscopic cholecystectomy. Surg Endosc 1999;13:476–479.

155. Sternberg A, Alfici R, Bronek S, Kimmel B. Laparoscopic surgery and splanchnic vessel thrombosis. J Laparoendosc Adv Surg Tech 1998;8:65–68.

156. Paul A, Troidl H, Peters S, Stuttmann R. Fatal intestinal ischaemia following laparoscopic cholecystectomy. Br J Surg 1994;81:1207.

157. Dwerryhouse S, Melsom D, Burton P, Thompson M. Acute intestinal ischaemia after laparoscopic cholecystectomy. Br J Surg 1995;82:1413.

158. Sanz-Lopez R, Martinez-Ramos C, Nunez-Pena J, Ruiz de Gopegui M, Pastor-Sierra L, Tamames-Escobar S. Incisional hernias after laparoscopic vs open cholecystectomy. Surg Endosc 1999;13:922–924.

159. Cuschieri A, Dubois F, Mouiel J, et al. The European experience with laparoscopic cholecystectomy. Am J Surg 1991;161:385–387.

160. Larson G, Vitale G, Casey J, et al. Multipractice analysis of laparoscopic cholecystectomy in 1983 patients. Am J Surg 1992;163:221–226.

161. Walhausen J. Incisional hernia in a 5mm trocar site following pediatric laparoscopy. J Laparoendosc Surg 1996;6:S89–S90.

162. Kopelman D, Schein M, Assalia A, Hashmonai M. Small bowel obstruction following laparoscopic cholecystectomy: diagnosis of incisional hernia by computed tomography. Surg Laparosc Endosc 1994;4:325–326.

163. Wagner M, Farley G. Incarcerated hernia with intestinal obstruction after laparoscopic cholecystectomy. Wis Med J 1993;93:169–171.

164. Reardon P, Preciado A, Scarborough T, Matthews B, Marti J. Hernia at 5-mm laparoscopic port site presenting as early postoperative small bowel obstruction. J Laparoendosc Adv Surg Tech A 1999;9:523–525.

165. Holzman M, Sharp K, Richards W. Hypercarbia during carbon dioxide gas insufflation for therapeutic laparoscopy: a note of caution. Surg Laparosc Endosc 1992;2:11–14.

166. Kent R III. Subcutaneous emphysema and hypercarbia following laparoscopic cholecystectomy. Arch Surg 1991;126:1154–1156.

167. Seiler C, Glattli A, Metzger A, Czerniak A. Injury to the diaphragm and its repair during laparoscopic cholecystectomy. Surg Endosc 1995;9:193–194.

168. Armstrong P, Miller S, Brown G. Diaphragmatic hernia seen as a late complication of laparoscopic cholecystectomy. Surg Endosc 1999;13:817–818.

Section III
Common Bile Duct

Lee L. Swanström, MD
Section Editor

16
Historical Overview of Surgical Treatment of Biliary Stone Disease

George Berci

Gallstones have been found in the gallbladders of Egyptian mummies dating back to 1000 B.C.[1] Paracelsus, in 1500, commented on the theory that "chemical disturbances in the body initiated the precipitation of impurities in the biliary ducts."[2] In 1863, Thudichum described stones of the biliary tract very well in his "Treatise of the History of Gallstones."[3] Another classical study was published in 1892 by Naunyn, "The Clinical Picture of Cholelithiasis."[4] At that time, prolonged bile stasis was thought to be the cause of stone formation. Naunyn also mentioned infection of bile as a secondary factor in the creation of stones.

Prevalence

Many factors impact the incidence of gallstones and common duct stones. One is the various genetic traits of the population, such as sex, ethnicity, and inheritance. Of males in the United States between the ages of 55 and 65 who have had a routine health screening, 10% have an abnormal ultrasound or cholecystogram.[5] In the Scandinavian population, where autopsies are performed more frequently, an even higher occurrence rate has been reported.[6] This rate is exceeded by the Pima Indians of Arizona, where 70% of the women have gallstones by the age of 30 and 70% of men by the age of 60.[7] In contrast, in Japan the prevalence is lower, and in certain parts of East Africa no gallstones have been found.[8–10]

Risk Factors

Heredity

In some families, an increased frequency of cholelithiasis is found, which can be either environmental or genetic. Obesity is a well-described risk factor for developing gallstones. Because dietary habits leading to obesity are acquired in the family milieu, it is not unusual to find multiple family members with biliary stones.[11] Young patients with sickle cell disease display a high frequency of stone disease. Calculi that result from hemolytic disease consist primarily of calcium and bilirubinate_components. For sickle cell patients, the prevalence is around 50% by the age of 20 and with increasing age it becomes even higher. It is sometimes difficult to differentiate the abdominal crisis of sickle cell disease or other hemolytic diseases from symptomatic gallstones.[12]

Age

Gallstones and common duct stones are more common in older age groups. The reasons for this may be decreased food intake, chronic dehydration, decreased total bile secretion by the liver, a greater concentration of serum cholesterol, absence of regulating influence of sex hormones, or simply an increase in the average lifespan.[13,14]

Pregnancy

The increased frequency of gallstones in women of childbearing age or during pregnancy is well documented. The changes in cholesterol metabolism have long been thought to be the major factor that explains the increased frequency of cholelithiasis in pregnant women.[15–18]

Other

Many other risk factors are also associated with a high incidence of biliary tract stones, including infection, immunoglobulin deficiency, liver disease, diabetes, pancreatitis, stricture of the common bile duct, and terminal illness.[19–22] Another cause is rapid weight loss in obese people.[15]

Asymptotic Bile Duct and Gallstones

The asymptomatic patient with biliary stones represents an interesting problem for surgeons. Is surgical intervention appropriate for these patients, or should they be observed until symptomatic? In this regard it is interesting to consider the Scandinavian study where all the inhabitants of Malmo underwent cholecystograms and were followed for 11 years. Of the positive cases, 49% remained asymptotic, 33% experienced biliary colic, and 18% developed acute cholecystitis. Choledocholithiasis was discovered in 27%.[6]

In the United States, the reported incidence of asymptomatic stones is lower. A widely reported study, which included only white males, followed 123 patients with gallstones for 11 to 24 years. Some of the study patients developed symptoms and underwent cholecystectomies; others died of nonbiliary disease. There were 58 patients with no previous history of symptoms; 28% of these eventually developed biliary colic. The symptoms were severe in only 5% of the 58 patients. The study drew the conclusion that, for the U.S. male with stones and no symptoms, surgery was not warranted. However, this conclusion was predicated on a relatively small number of cases.[23] For calcified or porcelain gallbladders, surgery should be considered because the chance of eventually developing cancer is approximately 20%.[24]

Indications for surgical intervention for biliary tract stones have broadened as the morbidity of the surgery, risk of anesthesia, and tolerance of discomfort by the symptomatic patient has decreased. Today, with the development of laparoscopic cholecystectomy (LC) and laparoscopic common duct exploration techniques, patients with diabetes, calcified gallbladder, generalized arteriosclerosis, and even the "silent" stone can be considered candidates for LC.

Short History of Surgical Treatment of Cholelithiasis and Choledocholithiasis

John Bobbs from Indiana reported the first details of a case of "lithotomy of the gallbladder" in 1868. The operation (cholecystostomy) was performed under chloroform anesthesia on the third floor of a wholesale drug company in downtown Indianapolis. The patient lived for 45 years.[11]

James Sims, a surgeon at the Women's Hospital in New York City, described an operative removal of gallstones in his article "Remarks on cholecystectomy in dropsy of the gallbladder" in the *British Medial Journal* in 1878. This procedure was the first planned cholecystostomy.[12]

Karl Langenbuch performed the first planned cholecystectomy in 1882 in Berlin. He was perhaps the first surgeon who practiced cholecystectomy on animals and cadavers. He recommended definitive surgery for cholelithiasis and did not recommend cholecystostomy. "The gallbladder should be removed not because it contains stones but because it forms them."[13]

Ludwig Courvoisier practiced surgery and fulfilled his teaching interest in Reihen (Switzerland). The first successful choledocholithotomy, performed in 1886, is credited to him. The condition called Courvoisier's gallbladder was named for him.

Theodore Kocher was the first surgeon to be awarded the Nobel Prize in 1909 for his contribution to the physiology and surgery of the thyroid. He spent his entire life in Berne (Switzerland). He popularized the right subcostal incision for surgery to the biliary tract and standardized the mobilization of the second portion of the duodenum for the examination and exploration of the distal common bile duct. He introduced spincteroplasty in 1911.

Hans Kehr devoted himself solely to the surgery of the biliary tract. He is known for the introduction of the T-tube, the Kehr incision, and reconstructive surgery of the bile ducts. In 1913 he published the first textbook on biliary surgery, based on 2600 biliary tract procedures.

William J. Mayo performed the first gallbladder operation in the United States in 1890. He organized the concept of teamwork in biliary surgery, and in 1919 he published 2147 operations for cholecystitis and cholelithiasis.

Among his major contributions in thoracic surgery, in 1923 Evarts A. Graham with Warren Cole, introduced cholecystography. He published their first experience in 1928.

Other surgeons who made significant contributions to the surgical treatment of bile duct and gallbladder stones include William Halstedt, Frank Leahy, Kenneth Warren, Frank Glenn, and Charles McSherry.

Open Choledocholithotomy

Over the past eight decades, open common duct exploration (CBDE) and other surgical therapies for common duct stones (sphincteroplasty, biliary–enteric bypass, etc.) have became quite well standardized. Indications, operative technique, treatment of complications, and morbidity and mortality rates were approximately the same for experienced surgeons. Major developments during the past 50 years that have improved the outcomes of open biliary tract surgery include the following:

1. The introduction of antibiotics and intensive care units
2. The use of operative cholangiography and, later, fluorocholangiography
3. Choledochoscopy
4. Endoscopic retrograde cholangiopancreatography (ERCP) and endoscopic papillotomy (ES)

ERCP and Endoscopic Sphincterotomy

Endoscopic retrograde cholangiopancreatography (ERCP) and endoscopic sphincterotomy (ES) and stone extraction techniques, first described in the mid-1970s, quickly became an important component of the diagnostic or therapeutic options for biliary stone disease.[25] The success of all these endoscopic techniques is dependent on the expertise of the performing endoscopist who, in the majority of cases in this country, is a gastroenterologist. ERCP is important in the preoperative period, particularly in elderly high-risk patients with severe cholangitis or septicemia who represent a very high risk group for surgical intervention. The role of ERCP in this situation is to establish the diagnosis, drain the common bile duct (CBD), or remove the stone; this approach has made it possible to operate on these very ill patients later, as a controlled elective procedure. Another major role of ERCP is in the postoperative period if symptoms and signs of retained stones develop. The morbidity of ERCP varies between 5% and 10%, and mortality is usually cited as being between 0.5% and 1%. In 5%, the CBD cannot be cannulated because of technical difficulties.[26] ERCP has also assumed a primary role in the treatment of postsurgical complications such as bile leaks, retained stones, and strictures.

Laparoscopy Choledocholithotomy

Laparoscopic cholecystectomy (LC) was introduced in 1987, and laparoscopic choledocholithotomy (LCL) was described shortly after. These minimally invasive surgical options have revolutionized the treatment of biliary tract stones, in both good ways and bad. Laparoscopy offers a truly less invasive option compared to traditional open surgery. Less tissue destruction means less pain, less immunosuppression, and, therefore, a shorter, more pleasant recovery for the patient. The technical difficulty and newness of laparoscopic CBDE has led to slow acceptance of this procedure by many surgeons who find it easier to leave common duct stones behind in hopes that the endoscopist can salvage the situation with a postoperative ERCP. This approach is a poor choice as it subjects the patient to the costs and risks of a second procedure and has a 5% risk of failure, which may necessitate a third operation.[27]

The evolving techniques of laparoscopic common duct exploration should be the preferred current choice as it offers the opportunity of clearing the duct of stones in one session.

References

1. Womack NA, Zeppa R, Irvin GL. Anatomy of gallstones. Ann Surg 1963;157:670.
2. Hoppe-Seyler G. In: Nothnagel's Encyclopedia of Practical Medicine (American translation). Philadelphia: Saunders, 1905.
3. Thudichum JLW. Treatise on Gall-Stones, Their Chemistry, Pathology and Treatment. London: Churchill, 1863.
4. Naunyn B. Die Klinik der Cholelithiasis. Leipzig, Germany, 1892.
5. Wilbur RS, Bolt RJ. Incidence of gallbladder disease in "normal" man. Gastroenterology 1959;36:251.
6. Wenchert A, Robertson B. The natural course of gallstone disease. Eleven years review of 781 non-operated cases. Gastroenterology 1966;50:376.
7. Sampliner RE, Bennett PH, Commess LJ, et al. Gallbladder disease in Pima Indians: demonstrations of high prevalence and early onset by cholecystography. N Engl J Med 1970; 283:1358.
8. Maki T, Saito T, Yamaguchi I, et al. Autopsy incidence of gallstones in Japan. Tohoku J Exp Med 1964;84:37.
9. Nakayama F, Miyake H Jr. Changing state of gallstone disease in Japan: composition of the stones and treatment of the condition. Am J Surg 1970;120:794.
10. Biss K, Hank-Jey H, Mikkelson B, et al. Some biologic characteristics of the Masai of East Africa. Afr Med 1971;284: 694.
11. Danzinger RG, Gordon H, Schoenfield LJ, et al. Lithogenic bile in siblings of young women with cholelithiasis. Mayo Clin Proc 1972;47:762.
12. Cameron JL, Maddoy WL, Zuidema GD. Biliary tract disease in sickle cell anemia: surgical considerations. Ann Surg 1971;174:702.
13. Kozoll D, Dwyer G, Meyer KA. Pathologic correlation of gallstones: a review of 1874 autopsies of patients with gallstones. Arch Surg 1959;79:514.
14. Torvik A, Hoivik B. Gallstones in an autopsy series. Acta Chir Scand 1960;120:168.
15. Kleeberg J. Experimental studies on the colloid-chemical mechanism of gall-stone formation. Gastroenterologia 1953; 80:336.
16. Bockus HL, Willard JH, Metzger HN. Role of infection and of disturbed cholesterol metabolism in gallstones genesis. Pa Med J 1935;39:482.
17. Admirand WH, Small DM. The physicochemical basis of cholesterol gallstone formation in man. J Clin Investig 1968; 47:1043.
18. Gerdes MM, Boyden EA. Rate of emptying of human gallbladder in pregnancy. Surg Gynecol Obstet 1938;66: 145.
19. Diaz-Buxo JA, Hermans PE, Elveback LR. Prevalence of cholelithiasis in idiopathic late-onset immunoglobulin deficiency. Ann Intern Med 1975;82:213.
20. Herfort K, Keclik M, Kovaurova M. Hepatitis and the origin of cholelithiasis. Am J Dig Dis 1962;7:907.
21. Bouchier IAD. Postmortem study of frequency of gallstones in patients with cirrhosis of the liver. Gut 1969;10: 705.
22. Twiss JR, Carter F. The relationship of biliary tract disorders to diabetes mellitus. Am J Med Sci 1952;224:263.
23. Gracie WA, Ransohoff DF. The natural history of silent gallstones: the innocent gallstone is not a myth. N Engl J Med 1982;307:798.

24. Ashur H, Siegel B, Oland Y, Adam YG, Calcified gallblad-
    der (porcelain gallbladder). Arch Surg 1978;118:594.
25. McCune WS, Shorb PE, Moscovitz H. Endoscopic cannula-
    tion of the ampulla of Vater: a preliminary report. Ann Surg
    1968;167:752.
26. Cotton PB. Cannulation of the papilla of Vater by endoscopy
    and retrograde cholangiopancretography (ERCP). Gut
    1972;13:1014.
27. Urbach DR, Khajanchee YS, Jobe BA, Standage BA,
    Hansen PD, Swanstrom LL. Cost-effective management of
    common bile duct stones: a decision analysis of the use of
    endoscopic retrograde cholangiopancreatography (ERCP),
    intraoperative cholangiography, and laparoscopic bile duct
    exploration. Surg Endosc 2001;15:4–13.

17
Operative Cholangiography

George Berci and Carl Westcott

Operative Cholangiography

Mirizzi first described operative cholangiography (OC) in 1932.[1] He postulated its usefulness for assessing the anatomy of the biliary tract during difficult cases. Hicken et al., in the United States, recommended the routine use of intraoperative cholangiograms in 1936.[2] Despite these strong early advocates and the documented advantages of its use, OC has never been universally accepted by the surgical community. Several points of view regarding cholangiography have emerged over the years.[3] One group uniformly rejects the use of OC because of technical problems such as the following:

1. Unsharp images resulting from the use of a static mobile X-ray machine, especially for the obese patient where required exposure times are too long.
2. Important anatomy missing on the final film, which happens because of difficulty in aiming static films or poor X-ray equipment.
3. High rates of false-negative or false-positive findings.
4. Films that are sometimes underexposed or overexposed because no scout film was made at the start of surgery to adjust the exposure.
5. Unnecessary delays of the operation; it is very frustrating to wait in sterile attire for 15 to 20 min until an X-ray technician is located or while one to three films are exposed, processed, and returned.
6. If the films are not informative, the whole process must be repeated, which further delays the operative process.

It is clear however, that never using OC can lead to higher rates of bile duct injuries and retained bile duct stones.

The second group recommends the selective use of OC, thereby balancing the difficulty and cost of obtaining the cholangiogram with the advantages of the clinical information obtained. Effective use of this approach requires the development of treatment algorithms that spell out when the OC should be obtained. The most commonly accepted indications are listed in Table 17.1.

Problems with the selective approach to OC include the poor preoperative predictive value of imaging or laboratory studies; this deficiency may lead to a higher rate of retained duct stones, which, however, can usually be treated by postoperative ERCP if they become symptomatic. Many common duct stones are asymptomatic, and some patients with clear-cut signs of choledocholithiasis may have already passed their stones at the time of surgery. Finally, anatomic variations are asymptomatic and may not be detected operatively until a bile duct injury has already occurred.

A third group of surgeons has postulated the advantages of routine application of OC. These surgeons claim that the costs and difficulty of the cholangiogram are outweighed by increased patient safety and because common duct stones can be detected and managed at one time. An additional benefit is that the OR crew and X-ray department are always set up and ready for the case as there is no "last minute" decision to obtain the film. Obtaining OC routinely also allows the surgeon to maintain a high skill level in performing this procedure, which is sometimes technically difficult.

The introduction of digitized intraoperative fluorocholangiography (IOF) in 1978[4] into the operating room and later in the form of mobile units[5] was a large step forward in resolving some of the problems with standard OC. The possibility that a surgeon could immediately observe the injection of the contrast material was unique. If there were problems of positioning or aiming, they could be immediately corrected. The detail and contrast of the image are usually excellent, and the ability to obtain magnified spot films and real-time videotape records make the accuracy of this technique much higher than that of static films. The digital format is also conducive to cable, or even Internet and teleconferencing

TABLE 17.1. Indications for selectively obtaining intraoperative cholangiograms.

Preoperative indicators
   History of jaundice
   History of pancreatitis
   Elevated liver function tests
   Common duct dilatation
   Multiple small stones
   Visualized common duct stone

Intraoperative indicators
   Obscured anatomy
   Identified aberrant anatomy
   Palpation or discovery of cystic or common duct stones

Equipment and Technology

A C-arm fluoroscope consists of a vacuum tube generator covered with a fluorscein layer. The X-rays fan out and penetrate the patient; the patient absorbs and filters most of the radiation. A small proportion of the generated beam passes through the patient and contacts the image intensifier. The image generated by this device from the filtered beam of X-rays is then projected onto the phosphor screen and amplified. The final image is transferred to a television screen for display.[3] (Fig. 17.1).

There are several settings on a standard fluoroscopy unit; knowledge of their importance helps in both image quality and radiation safety. Tube current, the rate at which electrons are produced in the X-ray tube, is expressed as milliamperes (mA); the higher the tube current, the higher the X-ray intensity. During conventional fluoroscopy, tube currents of 5 mA are rarely exceeded. Voltage of the electron beam, another important property of medical X-rays, is expressed as kilovolt peak (kVp). This setting effects the speed (energy per electron) and thus the penetration of the X-rays. The usual range for this setting is 60 to 125 kVp. Because higher-voltage X-rays penetrate better, lower tube currents can be used (mA) and the total exposure and scatter reduced. The drawback to a higher-voltage X-ray beam is the loss of image contrast. The best settings for these two properties depend on patient size, image quality required, and patient dose. In addition to current and voltage, patient dose is related to the time of exposure.

connections, which can allow rapid second opinions on difficult images. Fluorocholangiography has changed OC from a tedious and, on many occasions, inaccurate technique to a fast, accurate process typically requiring 5 min or less. To a large degree, this capability resolves the criticism of standard OC that it unduly extends the time spent in the operating room. The ability of IOF to detect intraluminal filling defects, anatomic anomalies, stoppage of contrast material, or extravasation allows immediate recognition and treatment of these problems. Routine intraoperative IOF can also eliminate a large number of unnecessary postoperative ERCP/ES, thereby minimizing the added cost, morbidity, and even mortality of this endoscopic procedure.

Despite the advantages of fluorocholangiography, there are times where a static image is needed. One of these instances concerns patients of extreme weight. Most operating room tables have weight restrictions, and a fluoroscope-compatible bed for obese patients is not universally available. In addition, a thick patient requires more energy to penetrate, and fluoroscope tube distances from the patient may have to be decreased to the point of possible skin overexposure to attain a good image. Another example of a useful static cholangiogram is when a patient is not positioned properly on the operating room (OR) table for the large fluoroscope tube to be placed underneath. This situation may result from OR personnel error or occur in a setting where a cholangiogram was not planned but circumstances encountered during surgery made it necessary. In addition, fluoroscopes are used by other services such as orthopedics and vascular surgery; a machine may not always be available or functional when a biliary procedure is being performed. Portable static X-ray devices are less expensive and durable and more often available on short notice. Also, financial restraints in many parts of the world as well as in parts of the most developed countries may limit the availability of fluoroscopy.[6]

Radiation Safety

The medical utility and dangers of fluoroscopy have been known for more than a century. Although rare, radiation burns to patients and physicians occur and have been documented by the FDA. A U.S. FDA advisory committee recommended in 1994 that hospitals and other patient care facilities assure proper credentialing and training for physicians who use fluoroscopy.[7] Several specific recommendations were made by this advisory, which are essentially a federal standard of care. Any physician who uses fluoroscopy, with or without a technician, needs to understand and follow them. This said, most cholangiograms are achieved with minimal patient exposure. One exception to this occurs in obese patients where high tube currents and a short tube distance from the skin is necessary to attain a good image. The other exception is where cholangiography is used for a prolonged period as in a fluoroscope-assisted common bile duct exploration. There are two alternatives for protection from X-ray radiation: (1) surgeons and scrubbed personnel, including anesthesiologists, should wear lead aprons or (2) personnel can be shielded behind a translucent mobile X-ray

FIGURE 17.1. Mobile digitized C-arm fluoroscopy equipment. The left screen shows a real-time, full-size fluoroscopic image; the right screen shows stored images (frames) to be selected and printed. The functions for a cholangiogram are preprogrammed, and only one button needs to be pushed. A foot switch activates modes and the VHS record. (Courtesy of OEC Co., Salt Lake City, UT, USA.)

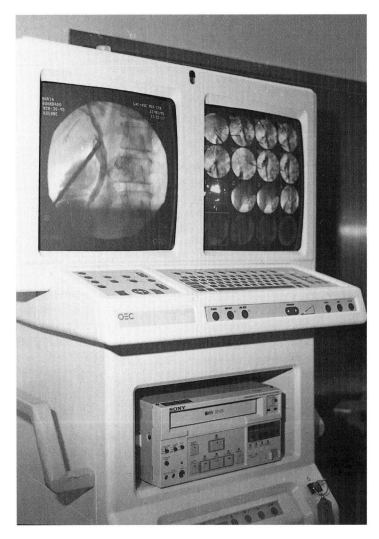

protection screen during the X-ray cholangiogram.[7,8] Surgeons should always be aware of these issues when performing X-ray cholangiograms of any type.

Aside from the X-ray device, little equipment is needed to perform laparoscopic cholangiography. A sharp pair of endosurgical scissors is essential to make a clean cystic ductotomy. Standard endosurgical clips are needed for proximal cystic duct control. There is an array of cholangiogram catheters and catheter systems on the market.

The catheters can be classified in two broad categories, self-retaining catheters and catheters that must be secured in place with clips or other devices such as a special reusable nonocclusive clamp ("Olson clamp") (Fig. 17.2) or endosurgical clips. Clip-secured catheters are effective but are more prone to leakage at the introduction site. It is prudent to have the more expensive self-retaining catheters, which rely on a balloon or flange at the tip for fixation, available for dilated and or short

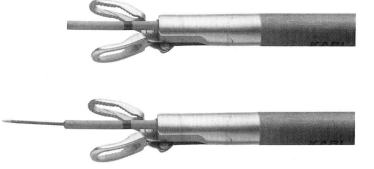

FIGURE 17.2. Close-up of cholangiograsper with protruding ureteral catheter (*top*). For difficult introductions, a guidewire is advanced and introduced into the cystic duct, followed by the catheter (*bottom*).

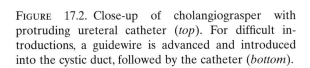

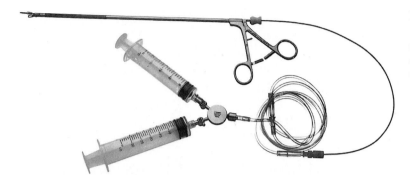

FIGURE 17.3. Cholangiograsper with 4-French (4F) ureteral catheter inserted, extension tubing, Y-shaped adapter, and two syringes of different sizes. (Courtesy of Karl Storz, Endoscopy-America, Culver City, CA, USA.)

cystic ducts where a good seal cannot be achieved with a clip system. Necessary extension tubing, stopcocks, and syringes should be available (Fig. 17.3). The contrast agent used should be relatively dilute so as to not obscure fine detail on the cholangiogram; renografin 30 or an equivalent is typical. Patients should be asked about possible allergies to iodinated contrast media before performing a cholangiogram and, if a patient is allergic, another technique or noniodinated contrast media should be used. Finally, a sterile drape or cover for the X-ray machine should be available to prevent contamination of the surgery field.

Technique

It is important when performing a cholecystectomy to circumferencially identify the gallbladder–cystic duct junction. In the laparoscopic approach, this is accomplished by mobilization of the gallbladder outflow tract followed by a progression from known to unknown toward the gallbladder–cystic duct junction. Freeing the distal gallbladder on both sides at the peritoneal interface with the liver helps achieve lateral and inferior retraction of the gallbladder infundibulum for definition of the cystic duct from its surroundings. Once isolated, a clip is placed on the cystic duct–gallbladder junction and an incision in the proximal cystic duct is made for introduction of the cholangiocatheter. Sharp microscissors are useful for the ductotomy but need to be visualized during their introduction because of their sharp tips. The cystic duct incision is made via the subziphoid port, so the initial cut is on the right lateral side of the proximal cystic duct. Once the duct is cut and bile visualized, the back blade of the microscissors can be placed inside the cystic duct and the anterior wall incision lengthened. This maneuver preserves the back wall of the cystic duct, providing a backstop or channel for anterior introduction of the cholangiocatheter.

The catheter is then placed through the anterior abdominal wall in a right subcostal position. The catheter is preflushed to avoid air introduction into the biliary system. It is best to position this introduction site away

from the other ports to optimize the angle between the catheter and the manipulating instruments. The catheter can be manipulated with an instrument inserted in the subziphoid or medial right abdominal port. Using a two-handed technique speeds up catheter introduction and is far more efficient than having both the surgeon and assistant collaborate on the placement.

There is often a close match in size between the catheter and the cystic duct incision, which can make catheter placement difficult. A well-positioned 30° telescope can help to visualize both the catheter tip and cystic duct incision at the same time. One hand is used to control the distal gallbladder and set the cystic duct at a favorable angle for introduction; the other hand is used to grasp the catheter. The catheter is best grasped about 1 cm behind the tip and introduced at an angle to match the cystic duct angle. Once the tip is introduced, the catheter can be released and regrasped for further introduction. The catheters are usually marked and should only be introduced about 1 cm because inserting it further can result in a common duct injection that often fails to show the cystic duct/common duct anatomy and may result in visualization of the distal common duct only. Fixation of the catheter is achieved according to the type of catheter. The retraction instruments are then removed from the operative field with care not to dislodge the catheter. The table is placed flat or in a slight headdown position to facilitate intrahepatic duct filling; this is more important if a static film is to be taken as the number of repeat exposures necessary to visualize the intrahepatic system will be reduced. Diluted renographin contrast is used in the static film cholangiogram. The static film usually has good penetration, and full-strength contrast could obscure a small filling defect. Then, 12 to 20 ml contrast is injected and the film exposed under radiation exposure precautions. Dilated ducts need more contrast, and reexposures are sometimes needed.

If a fluoroscopic cholangiogram is being attained, the fluoroscope is positioned and activated before injecting contrast. Contrast is then injected and the ducts filled. The machine is positioned to visualize the cystic duct, common duct, and duodenum first. After duodenal filling, the scope is moved toward the head to see hepatic and intrahepatic filling. Headdown positioning may be needed to opacify these structures and it can help to deinsufflate the abdomen and decrease pressure on the hepatic.

The majority of cholangiograms are easy to obtain, but there are situations where additional maneuvers are needed to obtain a quality image.

- The cholangiocatheter will not pass into the cystic duct after the tip is successfully introduced. The first step for this common problem is to eliminate the possibility of a cystic duct stone. The cystic duct should be gently "milked" with an atraumatic grasper from the bottom to top; this should move any lodged stones up to the duct incision. If a stone is palpated with this maneuver but not dislodged, distal mobilization of the cystic duct may be needed. Another reason for difficulty inserting the catheter is that the spiral valves of the cystic duct may be blocking its passage. To address this problem, a fine tapered dissector can be introduced into the cystic duct and the valves spread open. Another maneuver is gentle irrigation through the catheter during introduction to "float" the duct and valves open. In addition, this flushing can be used to clean the duct incision of stone debris, blood, or bile, improving visualization during cannulation. Finally, the use of a hydrophilic guide wire protruding 1 to 1.5 in. from the catheter and introduced first, followed by the catheter, may enable cannulation.
- Inability to fill the intrahepatic system with contrast. Gravity can help with this problem particularly in filling the left hepatic duct, which comes off the main hepatic duct in a anterior direction. Placing the patient in a headdown position will allow the "heavy" contrast media to flow into the intrahepatic ducts. Another trick is to give the patient a dose of IV morphine, which will cause a transient sphincter of Oddi spasm and allow the contrast to backflow into the hepatic tree. Another explanation for this problem is that the catheter has been introduced into the distal common duct. In this case, the catheter can be pulled back under fluoroscopic guidance, but often reinsertion of the laparoscope is necessary for repositioning. Overfilling of a balloon-type catheter, or insertion into the common duct, may compress the common duct; partially deflating the balloon may eliminate this problem. Another cause of poor proximal duct filling may be that dilated or chronically obstructed ducts may take as much as 60 to 70 ml contrast to see both duodenal and intrahepatic filling. Last, a clip may have been placed across the common duct or some other ductal injury may be present (Fig. 17.4). If this is a concern, open inspection of the anatomy is mandatory before any other dissection.
- Failure to document contrast flow into the duodenum represents another problem. This finding may be a result of an obstructing stone or lesion or spasm of the sphincter of Oddi. In the latter case, IV administration of 1 to 2 mg glucagon will relax the sphincter and allow contrast to flow into the duodenum. If this fails and, after repeated attempts, the appearance does not change, the surgeon should perform an open or laparoscopic common duct exploration.
- It can be difficult to distinguish between common duct air bubbles and stones. In general, stones are rarely round and bubbles are always round. One should look for irregular edges on the filling defects that indicate a stone. Second, because air floats in water while stones sink, the patient can be tilted; air bubbles tend to move up and stones down. Air bubbles also are easily flushed through into the duodenum with a brisk injection. An attempt should always be made to clear the duct by injecting the duct with warm saline and reinjecting contrast material slowly. If the lucency is still there, withdraw the plunger and inject again slowly. If the lucency moves freely with your maneuvers, it is likely to be an air bubble. If still undetermined, a choledochoscopy can easily differentiate this phenomenon in a more accurate manner. Last, realizing that air is compressible and stones are not, a brisk injection may show a round filling defect that moves easily and shrinks under pressure, which would be unlikely to be a stone. These maneuvers also speak to the advantages of fluoroscopy for cholangiography.
- True filling defects can be difficult to discern from overlying bone and bowel gas. This problem is more frequent in larger patients where the image tends to be poor. The fluoroscope can be tilted, which may eliminate confusion by changing the angle and eliminating overlaying anatomic structures. A larger patient also can have skin overexposure as high kphs, the generator positioned close to the skin, and long "fluoro-ON"

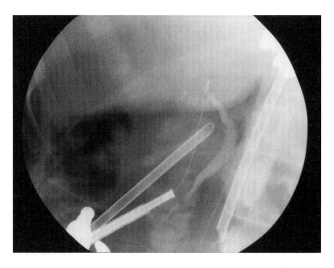

FIGURE 17.4. Stoppage of contrast in the proximal (hepatic) duct. Note the *clip* above the contrast cuttoff.

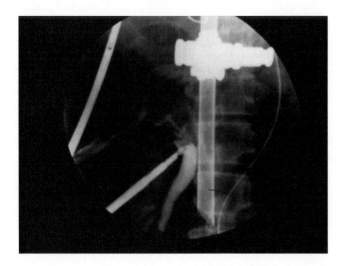

FIGURE 17.5. Extravasation above the site of cannulation (transection).

times may be needed to obtain a good image. An alternative would be a single static image if a good fluoroscopic image cannot be attained after a few attempts.

- If there is an extravasation, this needs immediate attention (Fig. 17.5).

Interpretation

Not only must surgeons be skilled in performing cholangiograms, they must also be adept at interpreting the resulting films. Little is gained by obtaining a film but then misreading it. Surgeons must be especially cognizant of anatomic variations of the extrahepatic biliary tree because these account for a percentage of surgical bile duct injuries. Extrahepatic biliary anatomy is defined more by variation than norm. In fact, the textbook

configuration of ducts and gallbladder occurs rarely. It is common surgical knowledge that in 75% of cases the cystic duct enters from the lateral side to the extrahepatic biliary system. Between 1978 and 1989, more than 3500 open cholecystectomies with routine fluorocholangiographies were performed at Cedars-Sinai Medical Center in Los Angeles, obtaining an average of 6 films per patient. Analyzing these more than 20,000 films has shown that in 41% the cystic duct enters the common duct posteriorly, 35% are spiral, 7% parallel, and in only 17% is the entry lateral (Fig. 17.6). This variability should be foremost in the mind of the surgeons who routinely perform cholecystectomy. Failure to define anatomy is the primary cause of iatrogenic bile duct injury. Respect for this variation often arises from first-hand experience with frequent or routine cholangiography. Other interpretation problems arise when the drainage into the common bile duct (CBD) [or common hepatic duct (CHD)] cannot be identified because of overlapping contrast of the junction and cystic duct. Overfilling of the duct can also lead to missing small calculi that are covered by two layers of contrast (the "sandwich" phenomenon).

During laparoscopic cholecystectomy (LC) procedures or laparoscopic common duct explorations, it is crucial to know where the cystic duct enters the CBD and the size and localization of stones to select the most appropriate surgical approach (Fig. 17.7). When the cystic duct is abnormally short, inadvertent but devastating injuries can occur (Fig. 17.5). The incidence of a truly short cystic duct is about 8% to 10%, of which 2% can drain into the right hepatic duct, posing another risk factor for ductal injuries if unrecognized (Figs. 17.8 and 17.9). If, on the cholangiogram, a clip, cholangiocatheter grasper, or any other tool appears too near the CBD, the surgeon should

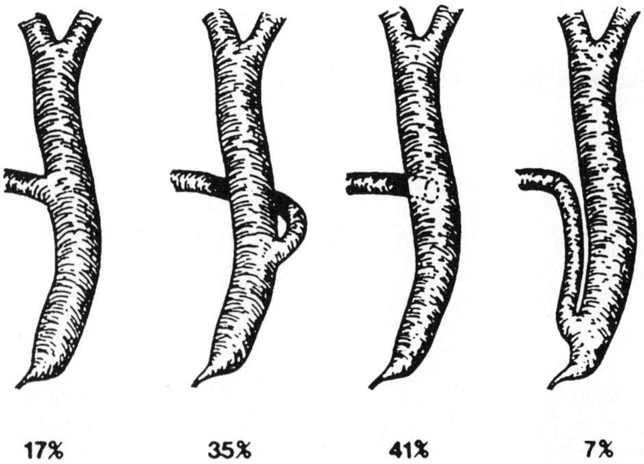

17%   35%   41%   7%

FIGURE 17.6. Only 17% of cystic ducts drain laterally into the common bile duct (CBD); 35% enter it in a spiral configuration, 41% enter posteriorly, and 7% have a close parallel run.

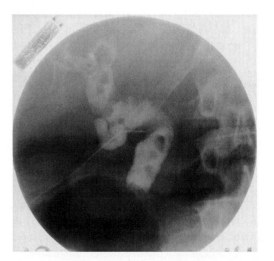

FIGURE 17.7. Diameter of the duct, number and size of stones, and ductal anatomy are important to determine which type of choledochotomy should be selected.

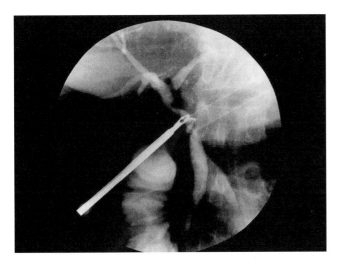

FIGURE 17.8. A short cystic duct can easily lead to an inadvertent ductal injury.

initiate further careful dissection. Another indication of possible bile duct injury is the presence of extravasation or an abrupt cutoff of the contrast on the cholangiogram. Some examples are shown in Figures 17.4 and 17.5.

Conclusion

Contemporary data strongly support the use of an operative cholangiogram for difficult cases, where it plays an important role in the recognition of anatomic anomalies of surgical importance (encountered in as many as 10% of cases) and has a great role in avoiding or identifying the majority of bile duct injuries. The advantages of identifying the inevitable accidental bile duct injury at the time of the laparoscopic surgery cannot be overstated. If an inadvertent injury occurs but is immediately repaired, the patient has a better chance to avoid further complications in the form of such problems as strictures and cholangitis. If the surgeon has minimal experience in biliary reconstructive surgery, the intraoperative identification of a bile duct injury allows the patient to be drained and, after general improvement of their condition, referred to an expert team with experience with these difficult cases. Without an intraoperative cholangiogram, the majority of ductal injuries are, unfortunately, recognized only in the postoperative period when the patient has bile peritonitis and is deathly ill, which contributes to a higher morbidity and mortality (Fig. 17.10). This point is well illustrated by the Cedars-Sinai experience where 2500 LCs were performed by residents and staff over a period of 4 years (1991–1995). During this time, 13 bile leakages were discovered (0.52%), of which 4 had complete transections. All but 1 injury was detected with IOF at the time of initial surgery; which permitted the 12 patients to have a primary intraoperative repair with good results. Only 1 patient returned a few days later with symptoms requiring exploration and repair.

It takes only a few minutes of operative time to obtain an IOF. If you prevent only 1 injury for 200 normal cholangiograms, or if an inadvertent injury is discovered but immediately repaired, this 1 in 200 cases was worth the total time, effort, and financial investment. The recognition of common bile duct stones at the time of surgery also allows preventative treatment, either surgical or endoscopic, avoiding the cost and inconvenience of unplanned procedures for symptomatic retained stones. There is no question that laparoscopic biliary tract surgery is a tremendous advance for patients. There are, however, some ethical issues regarding the identification and treatment of common duct stones and prevention of bile duct injuries that need to be considered by the surgeons who perform laparoscopic biliary surgery.[9]

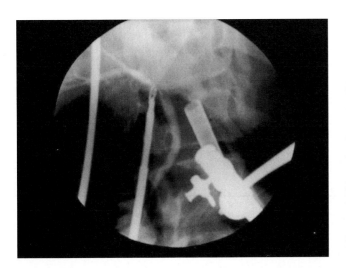

FIGURE 17.9. Short cystic duct entering the right hepatic duct.

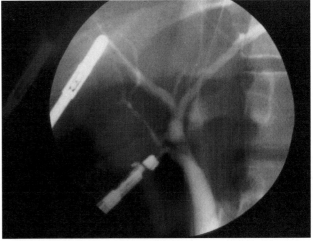

FIGURE 17.10. Accessory duct entering the cystic duct.

Epilogue: Fluorocholangiography

Although laparoscopic cholecystectomy was the first chapter in the laparoscopic revolution, the laparoscopic common bile duct exploration (LCBDE) has lagged far behind.

Advanced laparoscopic technique has achieved widespread use in such procedures as antireflux (Nissen) splenectomy, colectomy, adrenalectomy, nephrectomy, and recently bariatric mini-invasive approaches (all previously performed by open techniques). These new and more complex procedures are more difficult and time-consuming than LCBDE. Why have surgeons neglected to learn it and to do it?

In high-risk patients, with cholangitis, or septicemia in case of CBD stones, preoperative ERCP is indicated. However, in the majority of elective CBD stone carriers, it could be performed during the first procedure. Today, the patient has to undergo two sessions with added morbidity, mortality, and significant increase in cost. Fluoro-cholangiography is an organic part of LCBDE, and it is time that the younger generation of surgeons considered the laparoscopic removal of CBD stones as part of laparoscopic cholecystectomy with our final goal of improving patient care.

References

1. Mirizzi PL. La Cholangiografia durante las Operaciones de las vias Biliares. Bol Soc Cir Buenos Aires 1932;16:1133.
2. Hicken NF, Best RR, Hunt HB. Cholangiography. Ann Surg 1936;103:210.
3. Berci G, Sackier JM, Paz-Partlow M. Routine or selected intraoperative cholangiography during laparoscopic cholecystectomy. Am J Surg 1991;161(3):355–360.
4. Berci G, Hamlin JA, Morgenstern L, et al. Modern operative fluorocholangiography. Gastrointest Radiol 1978;3:401.
5. Berci G, Cuschieri A. Techniques of laparoscopic cholangiography. In: Berci G, Cuschieri A (eds) Bile Ducts and Ductal Stones. Philadelphia: Saunders, 1997:60–77.
6. Berci G. Static cholangiography vs digital flouroscopy. Intraoperative cholangiography: benefit and cost ratio. Surg Endosc 1995;9:1244.
7. U.S. Food and Drug Administration. Avoidance of serious x-ray induced skin injuries to patients during fluoroscopically guided procedures. Public health advisory, Sept. 30, 1994.
8. Earley D. Radiation hazard. In: Berci G, Hamlin JA (eds) Interoperative Biliary Radiology. Williams and Wilkins, Baltimore: 1981:27–35.
9. Morgenstern L. Ethical considerations in laparoscopic choledocholithotomy. In: Berci G, Cuschieri A (eds) Bile Ducts and Ductal Stones. Philadelphia: Saunders, 1997:161–166.

18
Laparoscopic Ultrasound for Assessment of the Common Bile Duct

Nathaniel J. Soper

The most appropriate means for evaluating the common bile duct during cholecystectomy has been debated for years. During the early 1900s, assessment of the common bile duct was limited to visual inspection and palpation. Mirizzi described intraoperative cholangiography in the 1930s,[1] which has become the gold standard method for screening of the bile duct. The relative merits of routine versus selective cholangiography have been debated almost endlessly since then, continuing into the laparoscopic era.[2–7] The use of ultrasound for screening the common bile duct during open cholecystectomy was also championed in the 1980s; it was shown to be equally as accurate as cholangiography[8–10] but was utilized infrequently by most practicing surgeons.

The emergence of laparoscopic cholecystectomy a decade ago rekindled the debate regarding the appropriate means of evaluating the common bile duct during cholecystectomy. It was initially thought that cholangiography was a difficult technical feat during laparoscopic cholecystectomy.[11–14] Many surgeons rarely, if ever, performed cholangiography during laparoscopic cholecystectomy, instead relegating the evaluation of the common bile duct to retrograde endoscopic evaluation. Numerous studies have subsequently demonstrated that cholangiography can be performed successfully in most laparoscopic cholecystectomies and that cholangiography is useful not only to screen the common bile duct for stones[15] but also to display biliary anatomy and perhaps help minimize the extent of common bile duct injuries.[7] Here, we discuss the relative value of techniques for evaluating the common bile duct during laparoscopic cholecystectomy, primarily in relation to screening the common bile duct for gross anomalies or dissection pertinent anatomy and for the presence or absence of common bile duct stones.

Recently, intracorporeal ultrasonography has been reported during laparoscopic cholecystectomy for assessing the biliary tree.[16–20] As a contact probe is used rather than imaging through the body wall, higher-frequency transducers can be utilized than for transabdominal ultrasonography, resulting in higher-resolution images with less depth of field. Several trials have been reported that compared ultrasound to cholangiography during laparoscopic cholecystectomy for screening of the common bile duct.[21–23] These studies generally have shown ultrasound to be performed more rapidly than cholangiography and that ultrasound may be more sensitive than cholangiography for the discovery of common bile duct stones. However, cholangiography often demonstrates ductal anatomy better. Therefore, several authors have considered cholangiography and ultrasound to be complementary for evaluating the bile duct.[17]

Ultrasound Physics and Instrumentation

Ultrasonography may be performed using both extracorporeal and intracorporeal techniques. Miniaturization of ultrasound transducers opened the way for development of both flexible endoscopic and laparoscopic imaging methods. This union of endoscopic and ultrasound technology has expanded the potential for clinical application of ultrasonography, which may grow in importance as laparoscopic surgical techniques evolve.

Ultrasound consists of mechanical sound waves that propagate through a medium. Medical ultrasound waves oscillate at frequencies from 1 to 30 megahertz (MHz; millions of cycles per second). The velocity of ultrasound waves depends upon the medium in which they are propagated. Soft tissue of the human body (like water) is an excellent medium for ultrasound transmission.

Ultrasound images are produced using the pulse-echo principle of sonar and radar. A transducer transmits and then receives the ultrasound waves (pulses) reflected back to it. During passage through tissue, some of the ultrasound pulse is lost (attenuated) by absorption and scattering. A portion of the energy (called an echo) is reflected back to the transducer, which measures the time since transmission and the amplitude of the received echo. Energy attenuation is dependent on the tissue impedance, a factor related primarily to tissue density. An interface is the boundary between two media with differing impedances. Ultrasound waves are either transmitted through or reflected or refracted at an interface.

The amplitude of the ultrasound echo received back by the transducer is represented by shades of gray on a video monitor (gray scale). Specular echoes arise from bright reflectors and have large amplitudes (e.g., the diaphragm or liver capsule). Diffuse echoes originate from small point reflectors and have low amplitudes due to scatter of the ultrasound pulse (e.g., liver parenchyma). Specular echoes define boundaries of large organ masses. Focal disease or areas of differing acoustic properties (stones, cysts, surgical clips) present echo amplitudes higher (hyperechoic) or lower (hypoechoic) than the surrounding tissue.

The ultrasound transducer produces a planar, two-dimensional image that may be transverse, longitudinal, or oblique in orientation. The active element inside a transducer is a piezoelectric disk. Electric voltages are converted into changes in the disk thickness, resulting in ultrasound waves. When an echo is received back at the disc, changes in disk conformation caused by the incoming echo produce electrical voltage changes that are proportional to the pressure amplitude of the echo. Modern ultrasound transducers are capable of producing 25 frames (images) or more per second and can thus present anatomical information in "real time."

Several transducer configurations are used clinically for real-time ultrasonography. The simplest is the mechanical sector scanner in which a single element is oscillated to and fro and renders a pie-shaped image. Alternatively, several elements can be mounted on a wheel that rotates around the axis. These radial transducers scan a plane perpendicular to the axis of the transducer and produce a 360° image. Multiple transducers may also be configured in longitudinal arrays of single elements. These linear array transducers use groups of neighboring elements to produce parallel beams by firing and receiving sequentially along the array producing a rectangular image. Bending the transducer array onto a convex surface increases the field of view. Phased array transducers consist of transducer heads constructed with a number of elements placed side by side. Slight time delays, or phase differences, allow for control of the direction of the resultant ultrasound beam. A small stationary transducer head may thus be used to view a large anatomic area or avoid an anatomic acoustic obstruction.

Small parts scanners produce images of limited depth for visualizing specific structures. Limited requirements for depth penetration permit the use of higher frequencies, which enhances resolution and image detail. Intraoperative ultrasonography places transducers in close proximity to the area of interest. Such scanners are designed to incorporate the benefits associated with small parts scanners.

Most medical ultrasound techniques employ the same method of collecting anatomic information. Variation is only found in the way the acoustic beam is directed into the body or in the presentation of the signals on a display. Real-time or B-mode imaging is a method of displaying the amplitude of an echo by varying the brightness of a dot on an image to correspond to the echo strength. B-mode imaging is the most common display technique used clinically. Real-time processing of images is possible because of the high speed of ultrasound transmission in soft tissue. More than 25 images may be generated per second. Below this rate of processing, the image will appear to flicker. B-mode imaging allows the observation of motion of organs within the body and allows the scanning plane to be changed quickly to scan through anatomy.

Doppler ultrasound measures the dependence of the observed frequency of sound reflected back to the transducer on the motion of the source of the reflection. The observed frequency of the sound reflected from flowing fluid, such as blood, is higher if the blood is moving toward the receiver than when flow is moving away. Two transducer elements are necessary for Doppler imaging: one continuously generates ultrasound waves that a second receives. The combination of Doppler ultrasound with B-mode ultrasound scanning is called duplex imaging. Regions of blood flow are either depicted by changes in audible tone of pulses or by color flow imaging techniques, with red representing movement of blood toward the probe and blue representing movement away from the probe.

Ultrasound is a useful, inexpensive, and safe imaging method. The accuracy and utility of extracorporeal, flexible endoscopic intraluminal, and conventional intraoperative ultrasound examinations done at laparotomy have been established. Laparoscopic ultrasonography is particularly valuable in that it allows the surgeon to "see beyond the visible surface" during laparoscopic operations. Also, using a transducer that is placed directly on the area of interest, a transducer with higher frequency and less penetration but greater resolution can be used. Therefore, laparoscopic ultrasonography should be much more accurate than ultrasonography performed across the body surfaces. Laparoscopic ultrasonography can be used for many purposes. It is particularly helpful for assessing the parenchyma of solid organs (such as the liver, spleen, kidney or adrenal), viewing retroperitoneal structures, and may be useful for identifying abnormalities in the walls of hollow viscera. However, we have found the greatest utility of laparoscopic ultrasonography to be for screening the common bile duct during laparoscopic cholecystectomy and, combined with laparoscopic exploration, to improve the staging of patients with hepatobiliary-pancreatic cancers before laparotomy.[24]

Laparoscopic Ultrasound Technology

Laparoscopic transducers utilize varying frequencies, ranging from 5 to 10 MHz, using various configurations of the electronic transducers (linear, sector, convex array, etc.). Most laparoscopic ultrasound probes also incorporate a doppler function that assists in the differentiation of vascular and nonvascular structures which are being imaged. Some probes are rigid whereas others are flexible with varying degrees of articulation, controlled by a rotating knob similar to that used for flexible endoscopy (Fig. 18.1). The diameter of most laparoscopic ultrasound probes is 10 mm, thereby allowing insertion of the probe through standard 10- to 11-mm trocars. Although the rigid probes are acceptable when screening the common bile duct in most cases, flexible probes allow additional freedom of movement and more even contact with the surfaces of convex tissue, such as the liver surface. The probe that we currently employ is flexible, allowing articulation in one plane, and has a combined linear array-convex probe design at its tip (B & K Medical Systems, North Billerica, MA, USA).

Indications and Contraindications of Laparoscopic Ultrasonography for Screening the Common Bile Duct

The indications for laparoscopic ultrasonography are very broad. Laparoscopic ultrasonography can be utilized during nearly any laparoscopic case, depending on the imaging needs. During laparoscopic cholecystectomy, we routinely perform ultrasonography to assess the common bile duct for stones and to ascertain dissection-pertinent anatomic details. In most cases of laparoscopic cholecystectomy, the detailed anatomy of the proximal biliary tree is not critical, but the location of the junction of cystic duct with common bile duct is useful and can be readily displayed in most cases. It is possible to assess the more proximal biliary tree, but this often requires the sequential insertion of the probe through multiple ports, which is more time consuming. Laparoscopic ultrasound also displays anatomy outside of the biliary tree, such as aberrant hepatic arteries, enlarged lymph nodes, or abnormalities in the head of the pancreas. In cases with severe inflammation or other anatomic abnormalities interfering with the dissection, it is possible to perform the examination early in the case to assist with decision

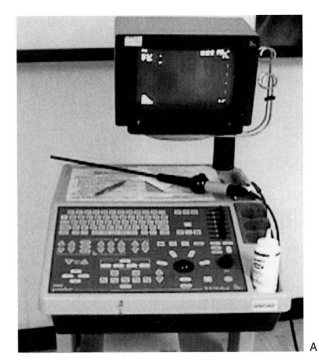

A

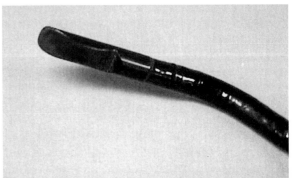

B

FIGURE 18.1. Example of laparoscopic ultrasound machine (A) and flexible probe with combined linear array and convex probe tip design (B).

making. In cases where gallbladder polyps have been demonstrated preoperatively, it is also possible to assess the wall of the gallbladder for evidence of invasion, which would suggest the presence of a gallbladder carcinoma (Fig. 18.2).

There are virtually no contraindications to the use of laparoscopic ultrasonography during laparoscopic cholecystectomy. The examination may be made difficult at the extremes of body weight; excessive amounts of adipose tissue in the region of the porta hepatis may interfere with ultrasound penetration, whereas thin patients may have inadequate soft tissue to use as an acoustic interface. In these patients, the examination may be facilitated by instilling water in the right upper quadrant to be used as an acoustic coupler.

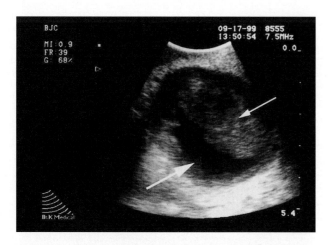

FIGURE 18.2. Laparoscopic ultrasound image of gallbladder carcinoma. *Large arrow* indicates gallbladder lumen; *small arrow* displays intraluminal polypoid mass.

the ultrasound transducer directly through the tract of the trocar into the abdominal cavity. The technique of scanning the bile duct in a transverse orientation with the ultrasound transducer inserted through the epigastric port site is as follows. A video mixer is used so that the laparoscopic view and ultrasound view can be seen simultaneously on the video screen. The grasping forceps on the fundus of the gallbladder is used to elevate the gallbladder and roll the right lobe of the liver superiorly for exposure of the gallbladder and porta hepatis. The transducer is initially placed in contact with the gallbladder itself, which is scanned from fundus to infundibulum. This step allows rapid assessment of the thickness and morphology of the gallbladder wall and the size and number of stones while familiarizing the surgeon with the ultrasound appearance; fine tuning of the image (changing the gain or depth enhancement) can be performed at this time. The transducer is then placed into gentle contact

Technique

For assessing the common bile duct during laparoscopic cholecystectomy, the ultrasound transducer can be introduced through any 10-mm port location. Using the "American technique" of laparoscopic cholecystectomy, many surgeons use 10-mm ports at the umbilicus and in the epigastrium. With introduction of the transducer through the epigastric port, the orientation of the probe and scan is generally transverse or perpendicular to the axis of the porta hepatis (Fig. 18.3). With the insertion of the ultrasound transducer through the umbilical port, longitudinal scans are obtained of the porta hepatis and bile duct. Because the laparoscope is generally positioned at the umbilical port site, transverse scanning of the porta hepatis using a laparoscopic ultrasound probe placed through the epigastric port site is our preferred mode of scanning. When using this technique, the usual image of the operative field is maintained, the laparoscope does not need to be removed and reinserted at a second port, mirror imaging of the transducer is not a problem, and reliable images of the entire common bile duct can be obtained. The disadvantage of scanning through the epigastric port is that the proximal bile ducts are not reliably imaged well. The majority of bile duct stones reside in the distal bile duct, however, and dissection-pertinent biliary anatomy can almost always be displayed using this approach.

The ultrasound transducer probe is sheathed with a plastic or rubber coating; if this sheath is damaged, images cannot be obtained, and replacement of the sheathing is quite expensive (approximately $5000). Particularly when using older reusable laparoscopic trocars, the valves may catch on the sheathing and strip it during insertion and removal of the transducer probe. Thus, our practice is to remove the laparoscopic trocar and reinsert

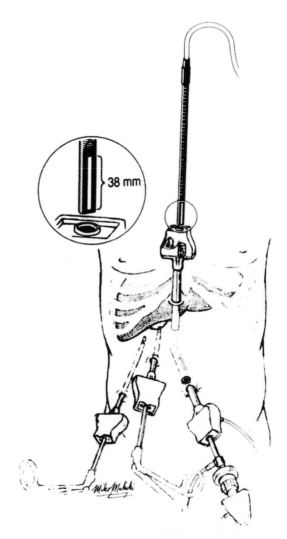

FIGURE 18.3. Introduction of the laparoscopic ultrasound probe into the epigastric (subxiphoid) trocar. (From Machi et al.,[16] with permission.)

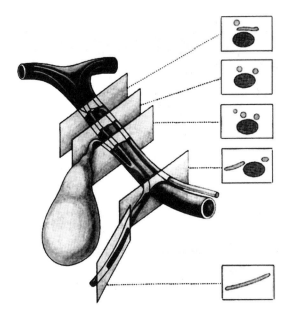

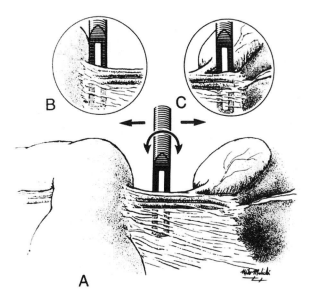

FIGURE 18.4. Schematic view of the structures of the hepato-duodenal ligament illustrates the normal anatomy and the characteristic views of laparoscopic sonography using a probe inserted through the epigastric trocar. (From Rothlin and Largiader,[19] with permission.)

FIGURE 18.5. Transverse imaging of the porta hepatis using the epigastric trocar. The probe is positioned inferior to the cystic–hepatic duct junction (A), superior to the duodenum (B), in which the probe is rotated clockwise to facilitate imaging of the intrapancreatic bile duct), and superior to the cystic–hepatic duct junction (C). (From Machi et al.,[16] with permission.)

with the surface of the porta hepatis. The "Mickey Mouse" appearance of the portal anatomy can usually be readily appreciated; the portal vein lies posterior and resembles "Mickey's head," whereas the common bile duct and hepatic artery make up the anteriorly situated right and left "ears," respectively (Fig. 18.4).

When it is difficult to maintain adequate contact with the tissue without compressing the bile duct, the operative field is flooded with sterile irrigant and the scan performed again using the water as an acoustic coupler. If the vascular and biliary structures of the porta hepatis cannot be differentiated, the doppler function should clearly distinguish the portal vein and hepatic artery (with flow) from the common bile duct, which does not exhibit internal flow. After precisely identifying the bile duct, the transducer is gently slid inferiorly along the anterior surface of the bile duct while maintaining adequate contact. In so doing, the orientation of the scan becomes slightly more oblique to that of the common bile duct (Fig. 18.4), and the sliding motion continues until the transducer tip is wedged at the junction of the porta hepatis with the antimesenteric wall of the duodenum. The transducer tip is then slowly rotated in a clockwise direction to image posterior to the duodenum through the head of the pancreas and visualize the distal common bile duct as it enters the medial wall of the duodenum (Fig. 18.5). Usually, the junction of the common bile duct and pancreatic duct can be visualized as well as the hypoechoic ring of ampullary muscles. If the distal bile

duct is not well imaged using this technique, the transducer is lifted away from the tissue and repositioned on the duodenal wall itself. The duodenum is gently compressed to squeeze the air from the duodenal segment being imaged, as air causes bright reflections and many artifacts. The distal bile duct and its entry into the duodenum can almost always be seen using this technique (Fig. 18.6). After imaging the distal bile duct, the transducer is once again rotated into an axis perpendicular to that of the common duct and slid back up along the porta

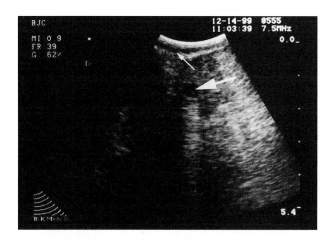

FIGURE 18.6. Laparoscopic image of the intrapancreatic portion of the bile duct obtained by transduodenal imaging. *Small arrow* depicts the duodenal wall; *large arrow* displays the distal common bile duct.

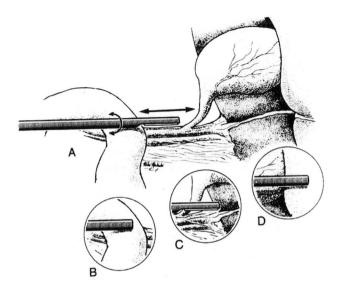

FIGURE 18.7. Placement of the probe via the umbilical port to obtain longitudinal and oblique sections of the bile duct. The probe is positioned at the center of the hepatoduodenal ligament (A), on the duodenum (B), and inferior to the hepatic hilum (C). The probe is also placed on the superior surface of the liver to image the intrahepatic ducts (D). (From Machi et al.,[16] with permission.)

hepatis until the takeoff of the cystic duct can be seen. The cystic duct is then imaged up to its junction with the neck of the gallbladder. The cystic duct–common bile duct junction is reliably imaged, but the more proximal cystic duct may be difficult to see due to its small size, superficial location, and relative lack of investing tissue to use as an acoustic interface.

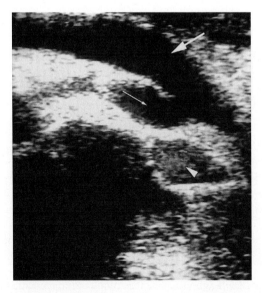

FIGURE 18.8. Longitudinal image of the common hepatic duct–cystic duct junction. *Large arrow*, common hepatic duct; *small arrow*, cystic duct; *arrowhead*, lymph node.

To obtain a longitudinal view of the biliary system, the videolaparoscope is repositioned at the epigastric port site and the ultrasound probe is inserted through the umbilical port. The probe is advanced up onto the surface of the porta hepatis (Fig. 18.7); unfortunately, this requires "mirror image" viewing and requires practice to be performed adeptly. The ultrasound probe is positioned over the hepatoduodenal ligament and dragged distally along its course while maintaining the bile duct in view (Fig. 18.8). To visualize the most distal part of the bile duct, transduodenal imaging is required. If access to the proximal ducts is not acceptable using this technique and imaging of this area is imperative, the gallbladder is released and the liver is allowed to roll inferiorly to its normal position. The probe is then placed over the anterosuperior aspect of segment IV of the liver so that the intrahepatic ducts and proximal common hepatic duct can be seen through the hepatic parenchyma window.

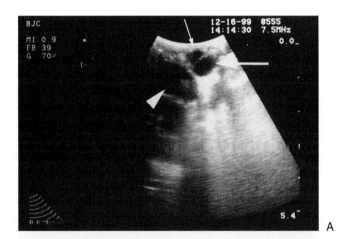

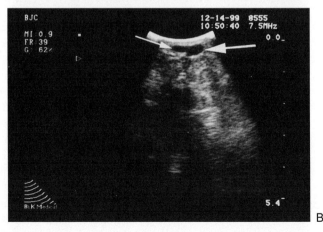

FIGURE 18.9. Transverse laparoscopic ultrasound image obtained just proximal to junction of cystic duct (*small arrow*) with common hepatic duct (*large arrow*). The portal vein is indicated by the *arrowhead* (A); the site of insertion of cystic duct (*small arrow*) into the common hepatic duct (*large arrow*) is clearly seen in (B).

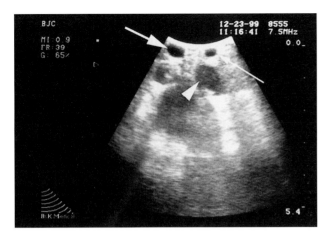

FIGURE 18.10. "Mickey Mouse" appearance obtained by transverse laparoscopic ultrasound imaging via the epigastric port just proximal to cystic duct–hepatic duct junction. *Large arrow*, common bile duct; *small arrow*, hepatic artery; *arrowhead*, portal vein.

Laparoscopic Ultrasound Images

Examples of laparoscopic ultrasound scans of the porta hepatis obtained using a transducer placed through the epigastric port site are shown in Figures 18.9 to 18.12. The junction of cystic duct and common duct can be clearly seen well removed from the area of dissection (Fig. 18.9). The diameter of the bile duct is approximately 4 mm, and there are no visible echogenic filling defects. The typical "Mickey Mouse" view just distal to the cystic–common duct junction is seen in Figure 18.10. The presence of a common bile duct stone is evidenced by an echogenic filling defect that casts an acoustic shadow (Fig. 18.11). As opposed to stones, when sludge is present in the

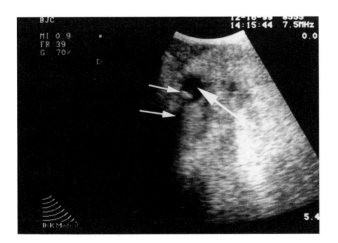

FIGURE 18.11. Laparoscopic ultrasound image of a stone casting an acoustic shadow (*small arrows*) contained within the distal intrapancreatic portion of the common bile duct (*large arrow*).

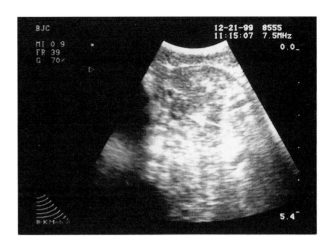

FIGURE 18.12. Echogenic sludge seen in the distal common bile duct (*arrow*) that does not cast an acoustic shadow.

common bile duct, it is seen as echogenic material that does not shadow and usually moves freely (Fig. 18.12).

Results

Surgeons at our institution initially evaluated laparoscopic intracorporeal ultrasound by performing a prospective trial in which 95 consecutive patients undergoing elective laparoscopic cholecystectomy first underwent ultrasonography, followed immediately by fluoroscopic cholangiography.[23] The images were reviewed independently by radiologists and surgeons. In this trial, 93 of the 95 ultrasound examinations successfully visualized the common bile duct, compared to 90 of 95 cholangiograms. Performance time was significantly less for ultrasonography (mean ± SEM, 8 ± 3 min) than for cholangiography (14 ± 6 min; $p < 0.05$). Choledocholithiasis was demonstrated in 12 of the 93 patients in the ultrasound group compared to 5 of those undergoing cholangiography; this discrepancy likely represented small stones being flushed into the duodenum during cholangiography. In two individuals, cholangiography attempts were unsuccessful and laparoscopic ultrasound demonstrated common duct stones, thereby markedly altering their operative management. Ductal anomalies were not visualized by ultrasonography and were seen on 13 of the 90 cholangiograms; however, these ductal anomalies did not influence the performance of the cholecystectomy, and most anomalies involved the proximal hepatic ducts, an area that is not well visualized using the transducer placed through the epigastric port.

After becoming familiar with the ultrasound techniques, we began performing ultrasonography preferentially to cholangiography during laparoscopic cholecystectomy. Since that time, more than 600 patients have undergone laparoscopic cholecystectomy with ultra-

TABLE 18.1. Results of ultrasonography (U/S) versus intraoperative cholangiography (IOC) for diagnosing bile duct stones during laparoscopic cholecystectomy.

Author	Number	Stones	U/S (%)			IOC (%)		
			Sensitivity	Specificity	Accuracy	Sensitivity	Specificity	Accuracy
Barteau et al.[22]	236	—	83	97	—	96	99	—
Orda et al.[26]	117	12	92	98	97	100	87	89
Stiegmann et al.[21]	209	19	89	100	99	53	100	96
Birth et al.[25]	518	24	83	100	99	96	99	99

sonography. The findings from the first 200 patients were compared to 407 consecutive patients undergoing laparoscopic cholecystectomy with routine fluoroscopic cholangiography just before the introduction of laparoscopic ultrasound.[15] Demographics of the patients and indications for surgery were similar in the two groups. Early in our experience with ultrasonography, several patients with a high likelihood of common bile duct stones went directly to fluoroscopic cholangiography, as it was our impression that cholangiography remained the gold standard. Excluding patients who were converted to open surgery and those who did not undergo the respective screening modalities, 381 patients were screened by cholangiography and 172 were screened by ultrasonography. The common bile duct was adequately visualized in 97% of those undergoing cholangiography and in 100% of those undergoing ultrasonography ($p < 0.05$). The mean time to perform cholangiography was 15 min compared to 5 min for ultrasonography ($p < 0.001$). In the cholangiography group, 7% of patients were found to have duct stones compared to 13% of those undergoing ultrasonography ($p < 0.05$). Another 6% of patients undergoing ultrasonography were found to have sludge in the common bile duct; this finding was never demonstrated by cholangiography. Of the patients with common bile duct stones, most patients (77%) in the ultrasonography group were able to have their stones cleared by simple flushing techniques as opposed to more invasive maneuvers. In the ultrasound group, the mean diameter of common duct stones successfully cleared by flushing was 1.6 mm compared to 2.7 mm for stones that required more invasive techniques for removal. Stones less than 2 mm in diameter were always able to be flushed and cleared. A cost analysis of the two techniques revealed fluoroscopic cholangiography to cost $150 more per case than ultrasonography.[23]

Other Reported Results with Laparoscopic Ultrasonography

A number of trials have been reported comparing laparoscopic ultrasonography to intraoperative cholangiography for the assessment of the common bile duct during laparoscopic cholecystectomy. The sensitivity, specificity, and accuracy of the two techniques for establishing the diagnosis of common bile duct stones are both greater than 90%, with intraoperative ultrasound being slightly more accurate in most series (Table 18.1).[21,22,25,26]

Results Using Ultrasound Compared to Cholangiography

There are numerous advantages and disadvantages to both ultrasound and cholangiography for evaluating the common bile duct during laparoscopic cholecystectomy (Table 18.2). Laparoscopic ultrasonography requires novel equipment in the operating room that must be purchased and maintained appropriately. There is a learning curve of approximately 20 cases to attain technical proficiency.[27] The ability to see detailed and precise anatomic anatomy of the proximal biliary tree is not so good as that for cholangiography. In contrast, laparoscopic ultrasonography can be repeated at will throughout the operation without exposing the patient or the operative team to ionizing radiation. The cystic duct does not need to be dissected or cannulated, and consumable supplies such as catheters and radiographic contrast media are not required. Scanning of the common bile duct can be performed much more rapidly with ultrasound than by cholangiography, and the technique seems to be even more sensitive than cholangiography for showing stones and sludge within the distal common bile duct. Cost accounting is somewhat less clear given the large expen-

TABLE 18.2. Relative merits of laparoscopic ultrasound (U/S) and intraoperative cholangiography (IOC) for assessing the common bile duct during laparoscopic cholecystectomy.

	U/S	IOC
Repeatability	++	+/−
X-ray exposure	+	−
Time of examination	+	+/−
Cost	+/−	+/−
Sensitivity for detecting common bile duct (CBD) stones	++	+
Detailed assessment of biliary anatomy	+/−	++
Flexibility/value for other procedures	++	−
Dissection required to perform examination	+	−

+, positive attribute; −, negative attribute.

diture required to buy a dedicated ultrasound machine and probe, especially if the probes are mishandled, requiring replacement of the transducer sheath. However, on a per case basis, ultrasound examination of the common bile duct costs approximately $150 less than cholangiography in our hands. Given the various advantages of both techniques, we consider them to be complementary methods to evaluate the common bile duct during laparoscopic cholecystectomy.

Conclusion

Laparoscopic ultrasonography has been dubbed the "stethoscope of the surgeon in the era of endoscopic surgery"[28] and has been shown to be invaluable in settings other than during cholecystectomy. This advantage occurs because laparoscopy images the surfaces of structures, whereas ultrasonography allows visualization of structures deep to the visible surface. Most general surgeons are unfamiliar with ultrasound principles and practice. Given the large numbers of laparoscopic cholecystectomies performed on an annual basis, this procedure is the ideal springboard for learning laparoscopic ultrasound techniques. During laparoscopic cholecystectomy, intraoperative ultrasonography is a rapid, inexpensive, and reliable means of assessing the common bile duct for stones and dissection-pertinent anatomy. Ultrasonography and cholangiography are complementary techniques for screening the common bile duct during laparoscopic cholecystectomy. Both techniques should be available and used when indicated. Residency programs should expose trainees to both techniques to maximize the flexibility of the laparoscopic surgeon in coming years.

References

1. Mirizzi PL. Operative cholangiography. Surg Gynecol Obstet 1932;65:702–710.
2. Robinson BL, Donohue JH, Gunes S, et al. Selective operative cholangiography: appropriate management for laparoscopic cholecystectomy. Arch Surg 1995;130:625–631.
3. Lorimer JW, Fairfull-Smith RJ. Intraoperative cholangiography is not essential to avoid duct injuries during laparoscopic cholecystectomy. Am J Surg 1995;169:344–347.
4. Berci G, Sackier JM, Paz-Partlow M. Routine or selected intraoperative cholangiography during laparoscopic cholecystectomy? Am J Surg 1991;161:355–360.
5. Soper NJ, Dunnegan DL. Routine versus selective intraoperative cholangiography during laparoscopic cholecystectomy. World J Surg 1992;16:1133–1140.
6. Cuscheri A, Shili S, Banting S, Nathanson LK, Pietrabissa A. Intraoperative cholangiography during laparoscopic cholecystectomy: routine versus selective policy. Surg Endosc 1994;8:302–305.
7. Carroll BJ, Fiedman RL, Liberman MA, Phillips EH. Routine cholangiography reduces sequelae of common bile duct injuries. Surg Endosc 1996;10:1194–1197.
8. Lane RJ, Coupland GAE. Ultrasonic indications to explore the common bile duct. Surgery (St. Louis) 1982;91:268–274.
9. Sigel B, Machi J, Beitler JC, et al. Comparative accuracy of operative ultrasonography and cholangiography in detecting common duct calculi. Surgery (St. Louis) 1983;94:715–720.
10. Jakimowicz JJ, Rutten H, Jurgens PJ, Carol EJ. Comparison of operative ultrasonography and radiography in screening of the common bile duct for calculi. World J Surg 1987;11:628–634.
11. Clair DG, Carr-Locke DL, Ecker JM, Brooks DC. Routine cholangiography is not warranted during laparoscopic cholecystectomy. Arch Surg 1993;128:551–555.
12. Voiles CR, Sanders DL, Hogan R. Common bile duct evaluation in era of laparoscopic cholecystectomy: 1050 cases later. Ann Surg 1994;219:744–752.
13. Lillemoe KD, Yeo CJ, Talamini MA, Wang BH, Pitt HA, Gadacz TR. Selective cholangiography: current role in laparoscopic cholecystectomy. Ann Surg 1992;215:669–674.
14. Flowers JL, Zucker KA, Graham SM, Scovill WA, Imbembo AL, Bailey RW. Laparoscopic cholangiography: results and indications. Ann Surg 1992;215:209–216.
15. Jones DB, Soper NJ. Results of the change to routine fluorocholangiography during laparoscopic cholecystectomy. Surgery (St. Louis) 1995;118:693–702.
16. Machi J, Schwartz HAH, Zaren HA, Noritomi T, Sigel B. Technique of laparoscopic ultrasound examination of the liver and pancreas. Surg Endosc 1996;10:684–689.
17. Yamashita Y, Kurohiji T, Hayashi J, et al. Intrasoperative ultrasonography during laparoscopic cholecystectomy. Surg Laparosc Endosc 1993;3:167–171.
18. Machi J, Sigel B, Zaren HA, et al. Technique of ultrasound examination during laparoscopic cholecystectomy. Surg Endosc 1993;7:544–549.
19. Rothlin M, Largiade RF. The anatomy of the hepatoduodenal ligament in laparoscopic sonography. Surg Endosc 1994;8:173–180.
20. Wu JS, Dunnegan DL, Soper NJ. The ultility of intracorporeal ultrasonography for screening of the bile duct during laparoscopic cholecystectomy. J Gastrointest Surg 1998;2:50–59.
21. Stiegmann GV, Soper NJ, Filipi CJ, McIntyre RC, Callery MP, Cordova JF. Laparoscopic ultrasonography as compared with static or dynamic cholangiography in laparoscopic cholecystectomy: a prospective multi-center trial. Surg Endosc 1995;9:1269–1273.
22. Barteau JA, Castro D, Arregui ME, Tetik C. A comparison of ultrasound versus cholangiography in the evaluation of the common bile duct during laparoscopc cholecystectomy. Surg Endosc 1995;9:490–496.
23. Teefey SA, Soper NJ, Middleton WD, et al. Imaging of the common bile duct during laparoscopic cholecystectomy: sonography versus video fluoroscopic cholangiography. AJR Am J Roentgenol 1995;165:847–851.
24. Callery MP, Strasberg SM, Doherty GM, Soper NJ, Norton JA. Staging laparoscopy with laparoscopic ultrasonography: optimizing resectability in hepatobiliary and hepato-

biliary and pancreatic malignancy. J Am Coll Surg 1997;
185:33–39.

25. Birth M, Ehlers KU, Delinikolas K, Weiser H-F. Prospective randomized comparison of laparoscopic ultrasonography using a flexible-tip ultrasound probe and intraoperative dynamic cholangiography during laparoscopic cholecystectomy. Surg Endosc 1998;12:30–36.

26. Orda R, Sayfan J, Levy Y. Routine laparoscopic ultrasonography in biliary surgery. Endosc Surg 1994;8:1239–1242.

27. Falcohn RA, Fegelman EJ, Nussbaum MS, et al. A prospective comparison of laparoscopic ultrasound versus intraoperative cholangiogram during laparoscopic cholecystectomy. Surg Endosc 1999;13:784–788.

28. Holthausen U, Troidl H, Paul A. Ultrasonography—the stethoscope of the surgeon in the era of endoscopic surgery. Surg Endosc 1994;8:1163–1164.

19
Endoscopic Management of Common Duct Stones

John R. Craig and Aaron S. Fink

Twenty years ago, laparotomy provided the primary access by which common bile duct (CBD) stones were diagnosed and removed. Open cholecystectomy was accompanied by intraoperative cholangiography and common bile duct exploration. Since that time, several less invasive modalities have been introduced, including endoscopic retrograde cholangiopancreatography (ERCP) and endoscopic sphincterotomy (ES). These newer techniques have become quite popular, despite limited long-term outcome data. Although patients have benefited from these developments, choice of the most appropriate procedures is often complicated and controversial. Certainly, the appropriate therapy for CBD stones must be based upon locally available expertise, disease-specific factors, and patient comorbidities. This chapter discusses the numerous methods for diagnosing and managing CBD stones, focusing on the role of ERCP and ES and their best utilization in various clinical settings.

Diagnostic Modalities

As many as 50% of patients with CBD stones develop symptoms that lead to treatment.[1] CBD obstruction leads to increases in intraductal pressure and blockage of normal excretion of conjugated bilirubin. Increased serum bilirubin leads to jaundice and dark urine, whereas its absence in the GI tract leads to clay-colored stools. Should infection develop, the patient may present with right upper quadrant pain, jaundice, and fever (Charcot's triad), diagnostic of cholangitis. Additional findings of mental status deterioration and hypotension (Reynold's pentad) often signify suppurative cholangitis, a more serious, life-threatening infection. The latter condition usually mandates emergent decompression of the biliary system. Patients may also present with biliary pancreatitis, usually manifested by midabdominal pain, nausea, vomiting, and elevated serum amylase.

Although these conditions usually lead to the diagnosis of CBD stone disease, common bile duct stones may also be asymptomatic. Indeed, as many as 10% to 15% of patients presenting with acute cholecystitis are found to harbor CBD stones.[2] Although the natural history of such asymptomatic stones is unknown, their potential threat usually justifies their removal when intervening for symptomatic cholelithiasis. Laboratory measurements should be performed routinely in evaluating patients with suspected biliary tract disease. Although not specific, elevations of serum bilirubin (conjugated and unconjugated), aspartate transaminase (AST), and alkaline phosphatase may raise suspicion of posthepatic biliary obstruction caused by CBD stones.

Ultrasound and Computed Tomography

Ultrasonography, the most frequently performed diagnostic modality, offers moderate diagnostic sensitivity for CBD stones. Periampullary masses are the most common lesions that must be distinguished from stones of the common bile duct. Unfortunately, visualization of stones within the CBD is not uniform.

Although not specific, dilation of the intra- and extrahepatic ducts is the most reliable ultrasonographic abnormality. As a general rule, a CBD diameter less than 3 to 4mm rules out stones in the common duct, whereas diameters of 10mm or more, in the proper clinical setting, are highly suggestive of ductal stones.[3] The level of biliary obstruction is identified in 90% of cases, although the cause of obstruction is determined in only 71%.

CT scanning is also an accurate method for diagnosing CBD stones (Fig. 19.1). This modality is better than transabdominal ultrasound, particularly in those patients whole body habitus or bowel gas pattern limits the application of ultrasound. The sensitivity and specificity are 76% and 98%, respectively.[3]

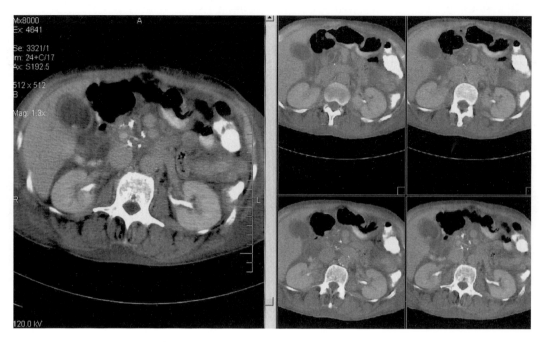

FIGURE 19.1. CT scan shows dilated common bile duct and common bile duct stones. (Courtesy of Dr. Randy Ernst, Dept. of Radiology, Emory University School of Medicine, Atlanta, GA, USA.)

Magnetic Resonance Cholangiopancreatography (MRCP)

MRCP is a relatively new diagnostic modality that produces images of the biliary tree similar to those obtained by direct cholangiographic techniques. MRCP is of particular interest because of its ability to generate images without exogenous contrast administration.

MRCP is based upon the principle that body fluids such as bile appear white (high signal intensity) whereas background tissues appear dark (minimal signal intensity) on heavily T_2-weighted magnetic resonance imaging (MRI). Background signal is further decreased by magnetic resonance techniques that selectively suppress signal from fat, a major source of residual background signal in abdominal MRI. Because respiratory motion degrades image quality during abdominal MRI, images are preferentially obtained during a single breath hold; respiratory triggering can be used in those patients unable to suspend their respiration. Various fast spin-echo scanning sequences are utilized, depending on the specific scanner.

Images are usually obtained with multislice techniques, which create a data set amenable to computer processing. The data set is then subjected to a maximal intensity-projection (MIP) algorithm in which only the pixel with the highest intensity along a ray perpendicular to the projection plane is displayed. This algorithm creates a three-dimensional image similar in appearance to that obtained during ERCP. Alternatively, with the single-slice technique, only one thick slice of data is obtained. Data acquired with the latter technique need not be processed using maximal intensity-projection algorithms; the resultant images represent the average of the data contained within the entire tissue volume imaged and are complementary to those obtained using maximal intensity-projection.

MRCP images are interpreted as with ERCP. Bile duct caliber may be more accurately reflected by MRCP because the bile ducts are displayed in the resting state. Biliary stones appear as areas of signal void within the high signal intensity bile on MRCP (Fig. 19.2). Each of the multiple slices through the biliary tree must be carefully reviewed not to overlook CBD stones obscured on maximal intensity-projection reconstructions. MRCP can detect choledocholithiasis with remarkably high sensitivity (81%–100%) and specificity (85%–100%), with positive and negative predictive values between 90% and 100%.[4-7] False positives have been reported in other series and are due to air bubbles or surgical clips in the region of the CBD. It is notable that while these results are similar to those obtained with ERCP, this non-invasive technique allows visualization of extraductal anatomy that may be important in the complete evaluation of the jaundiced patient. Obviously, a disadvantage is that MRCP is purely diagnostic and does not allow for therapeutic intervention.

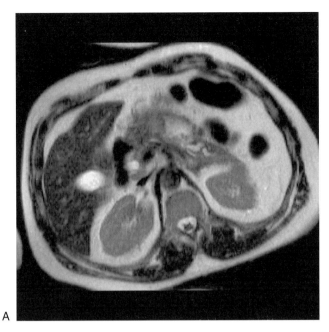

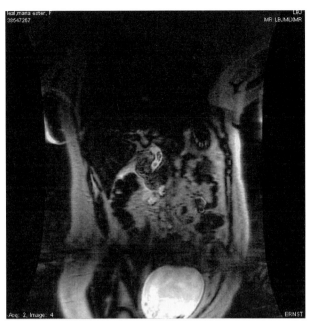

FIGURE 19.2. Heavily T$_2$-weighted magnetic resonance cholangiopancreatography (MRCP) image shows (A) cholelithiasis and (B) common bile duct stone. (Courtesy of Dr. Randy Ernst, Dept. of Radiology, Emory University School of Medicine, Atlanta, GA, USA.)

Endoscopic Management of Common Bile Duct Stones

Endoscopic Retrograde Cholangiopancreatography (ERCP)

Since the original description of endoscopic sphincterotomy (ES) in 1974 by Classen and Demling and by Kawai,[8,9] use of ERCP and papillotomy have come to play vital roles in the diagnosis and therapy of CBD stones. By 1984, 10 years after its introduction, 50,000 cases had been reported in the world literature.[10]

ERCP is a sophisticated procedure requiring the cooperation of a skilled endoscopist and an interested radiologist. Indeed, it is essentially a radiologic procedure driven by an endoscopist. After the patient is appropriately prepared, the long, side-viewing endoscope is passed into the upper esophagus through the cricopharyngeus. The scope is rapidly passed into the proximal stomach where any residual secretions are aspirated. As the scope is passed to and through the pylorus, it is vital to keep the scope within the central axis of the antrum; such a position is ensured by maintaining the scope perpendicular to the incisura.

The endoscope is then passed into the descending duodenum. This maneuver requires "corkscrewing" the endoscope around the superior duodenal angle. The endoscope is usually withdrawn during this maneuver, ideally leaving the scope in the short scope position, 60 to 70 cm from the incisors, facing the medial duodenal wall (Fig. 19.3). If the endoscope is passed into the duodenum by continually advancing, steering, and rotating, the long scope position usually results (Fig. 19.4). This position is not preferred; it is not only uncomfortable to the patient but it also reduces control of the endoscope tip.

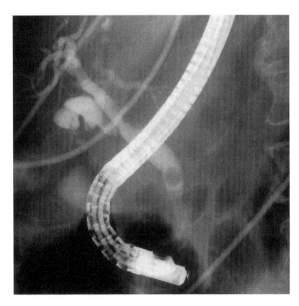

FIGURE 19.3. Side-viewing duodenoscope in the "short scope" position in the duodenum. The cholangiogram demonstrates a large common duct stone. A sphincterotome has been placed through the ampulla into the common bile duct in preparation for endoscopic sphincterotomy.

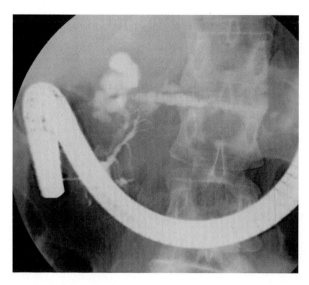

FIGURE 19.4. Duodenoscope in the "long scope" position. This position is suboptimal because it is uncomfortable for the patient and reduces control at the endoscope tip. The pancreatogram demonstrates chronic pancreatitis, primarily involving the dorsal pancreatic duct.

In the short scope position, the papilla will frequently be directly in view along the medial duodenal wall. If not, the papilla can usually be located at the apex of one or several longitudinal folds arising from the inferior duodenal angle. Once located, intermittent boluses of glucagon (0.25mg) should be administered to induce and maintain duodenal paralysis. A scout radiograph is obtained to verify adequate radiologic technique, as well

as to identify calcifications or other findings present before contrast injection. The papilla is then cannulated using one of the various catheters available (Fig. 19.5). Catheters with radiopaque tips are often preferred because the radiologic marker facilitates radiologic identification of the catheter tip. Once the papilla has been successfully cannulated, contrast is injected under radiologic control to avoid overfilling the biliary and the pancreatic ductal systems. If dilated ducts are encountered, use of diluted (half-strength) contrast may prevent obscuring small stones. Attention to radiologic technique is critical because diagnostic information is only as good as the quality of the radiologic images obtained.

Selective cannulation of the biliary and pancreatic ducts is the key to successful ERCP, as well as to therapeutic intervention. Although various maneuvers are available (e.g., cannulation with taper-tipped catheters, guidewires, sphincterotomes), all aim to successfully manipulate the catheter into the correct ductal axis. The pancreatic duct tends to enter the papilla in a relatively perpendicular fashion. In contrast, the bile duct runs toward 11 o'clock from the lower right aspect of the papilla.

As already mentioned, attention to proper radiologic technique is critical to obtaining interpretable radiographs. Artifacts such as air bubbles, streaming and layering of contrast, and contrast spillage into the duodenum should be recognized and corrected with proper technique. With the expertise currently available, the greatest risk that ERCP poses may well be misinterpretation.[11]

If endoscopic sphincterotomy is indicated, the diagnostic cannula is removed and replaced with a sphincterotome (Fig. 19.6). The latter consists of a standard

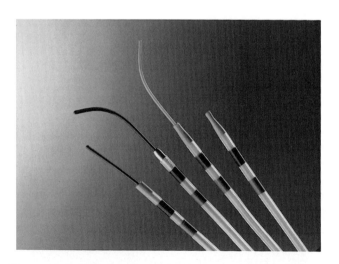

FIGURE 19.5. Selection of endoscopic retrograde cholangiopancreatography (ERCP) catheters demonstrating several of the different tips available. Many of the catheter tips are radiopaque, which facilitates location of the catheter during fluoroscopic imaging. Note that most of the catheters allow passage of 0.035 in. guidewires. (Courtesy of Microvasive, Boston Scientific Corporation, Watertown, MA, USA.)

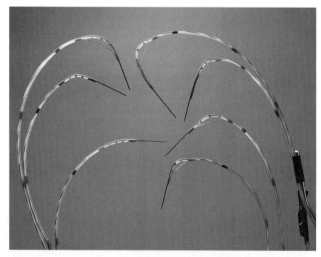

FIGURE 19.6. Examples of different types of endoscopic sphincterotomes currently available. (Courtesy of Microvasive, Boston Scientific Corporation, Watertown, MA, USA.)

cannula containing a continuous wire loop, 20 to 30 cm of which is exposed near the tip. Initially, the tip is inserted well into the bile duct (see Fig. 19.3); sphincterotomy must not be attempted until the sphincterotome has been clearly demonstrated to be within the bile duct and not the pancreatic duct.

Once proper ductal cannulation is verified, the sphincterotome is withdrawn until approximately half the wire is visible outside the papilla, pointing toward 11 or 12 o'clock. The wire is then tightened, bowing it against the papillary roof. Current is then applied in short bursts while maintaining gentle upward force on the wire, making the incision in small increments. It is important to ensure that the sphincterotomy length is adequate but not excessive. Incision lengths should be based on the size of the largest stone.

Large series from expert centers report that following sphincterotomy 85% to 90% of CBD stones can be extracted successfully with Dormia baskets or balloon catheters.[12,13] Complications include hemorrhage, perforation, cholangitis, and pancreatitis. Although experienced centers report morbidity and mortality rates of 6.5% and 1.0%, respectively,[14,16] less experienced operators have reported disturbingly high failure and morbidity rates.[14,17] Approximately 75% to 80% of complications can be managed without surgery.

Hemorrhage is the most common complication seen after endoscopic sphincterotomy and can be avoided by slow, controlled incisions.[14] Epinephrine injection or balloon tamponade may be useful if the bleeding allows adequate endoscopic vision. If surgical intervention is necessary, it is probably best to include ligation of the feeding vessel.

Perforation, the least common complication, most often leads to surgical intervention and mortality.[14] The diagnosis is usually made upon discovering air or contrast in the retroperitoneal space. A CT scan may also be helpful if differentiation from postsphincterotomy pancreatitis proves difficult. If perforation is diagnosed early and the bile duct has been cleared, many patients can be managed with nasobiliary decompression, nasogastric suction, and intravenous antibiotics.[14] However, if stones remain in the common bile duct or if the patient deteriorates after attempted conservative management, surgical intervention is indicated. The latter should include clearance and decompression of the bile duct and retroperitoneal drainage.

Pancreatitis and cholangitis can also occur after endoscopic sphincterotomy. The former may be decreased by minimizing trauma during cannulation and avoiding coagulation near the pancreatic duct. Cholangitis should be extremely uncommon if adequate biliary drainage has been achieved.

It is recommended that ductal clearance be attempted at the time of endoscopic sphincterotomy, because relying on spontaneous stone passage increases the risk of cholangitis, pancreatitis, and stone impaction, as well as the need for repeated endoscopic interventions.[14] Adequate ductal drainage must be ensured if all stones cannot be removed. The latter can be accomplished with nasobiliary drainage or endoprosthesis insertion[18–20]; the choice depends on the clinical setting (e.g., need for repeat cholangiogram, planned solvent infusion, residual stone burden, patient risk factors).

Operative Cholangiography

Mirizzi developed operative cholangiography in 1931, hoping to improve on the 50% rate of negative CBD explorations (CBDE) and the 25% incidence of retained stones in those who underwent CBDE. This procedure reduced the rates to 6% and 11%, respectively.[21] The technique of open transcystic cholangiography has changed little over time. Catheters specifically designed for this purpose have made the technique easier. With the increased use of laparoscopy, techniques have evolved to allow the performance of laparoscopic transcystic cholangiography.

Debate persists regarding whether intraoperative cholangiography (IOC) should be used routinely or selectively during laparoscopic cholecystectomy (Fig. 19.7). Some have suggested that IOC is never indicated.[22] The opponents to IOC claim poor image quality, false-positive exams, prolonged operative time, and increased costs, as well as the reliability of ERCP and sphincterotomy for removal of any remaining ductal stones. Proponents suggest that, in experienced hands, IOC can be performed in less then 7 min with minimal morbidity, thereby saving the patient the potential morbidity, increased cost, and inconvenience of postoperative ERCP.[23]

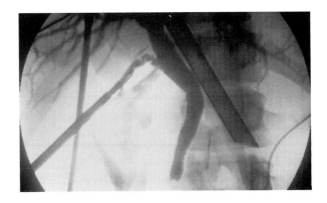

FIGURE 19.7. A laparoscopic cholangiogram shows a common duct stone.

Other Techniques

On occasion it is not possible, or not in the patient's best interest, to depend upon ERCP or ES for stone extraction. Such instances can include failure of an attempted preoperative ERCP resulting from anatomic (duodenal diverticulum, previous gastric surgery) or technical factors. Also, if the stone is recognized during surgery, a second procedure can be avoided if the surgeon has methods to handle the problem during surgery.

Intraoperative ERCP

Intraoperative ERCP has been reported to solve the problem of stones found during an open or laparoscopic surgery. In this scenario, the endoscopist inserts a therapeutic duodenoscope into the duodenum and visualizes the ampulla. The identification and cannulation of the sphincter can be greatly facilitated by having the surgeon advance a guidewire or, in some cases, a transcystic cholangiogram catheter through the cystic duct across the sphincter. Special hydrophilic guidewires can help pass distal duct strictures or impacted stones. The ampulla is cannulated with a standard sphincterotome and ES performed. Stones and debris can be flushed out by the surgeon by injecting saline through the cholangiocatheter.

The main problem with intraoperative ERCP is the technical difficulty posed by performing the endoscopy on an anesthetized, supine patient. The crowded conditions of the OR and the needed to protect the sterile operating field also contribute to the challenge for the endoscopist and the frustration for the operating team.

Laparoscopic Transcystic Antegrade Sphincterotomy

In 1993, DePaula et al.[24] described their technique, which combines features of laparoscopic common bile duct exploration and endoscopic sphincterotomy. Although recommended for numerous indications by the authors,[24] most would resort to this technique only when laparoscopic transcystic CBD exploration and laparoscopic choledochotomy have failed.

In this technique, access to the CBD is obtained via the cystic or common duct, depending on the maneuvers performed previously. A standard endoscopic sphincterotome is passed into the common bile duct and through the ampulla into the duodenum. As the sphincterotome is being passed, a side-viewing video endoscope is passed through the patient's mouth into the duodenum. Using the image provided by the endoscope, the surgeon manipulates the bowed sphincterotome until it is aligned at the 12 o'clock position. Traction on the sphincterotome while applying electrocautery current completes the sphincterotomy, allowing CBD clearance by flushing or pushing residual stones into the duodenum through the widened ampulla.

This technique is rather technologically demanding and is usually best performed by those with experience in pancreaticobiliary endoscopy. However, once the equipment is assembled, the procedure can usually be performed fairly quickly. In addition, it does eliminate or minimize many of the major risks of endoscopic sphincterotomy, including pancreatitis, duodenal perforation, and entrapment.

Percutaneous Transhepatic Cholangioscopy

Percutaneous transhepatic catheter drainage (PTC) of the CBD is performed under fluoroscopy in an interventional radiology suite. A spinal needle is passed under local anesthesia into the right side of the abdomen, usually in the midaxillary line, and aspirated until bile return is obtained. Guidewire techniques are then used to pass a drainage catheter into the biliary system, allowing decompression of the biliary tree proximal to an obstruction. The success of this procedure is variable. Coagulopathy may be present in many patients and is a contraindication to PTC placement. However, if successful, PTC allows resuscitation and interval therapy for stone extraction following resolution of sepsis. This procedure can be rapidly followed with transhepatic cholangioscopy, in which the tract is dilated and an endoscope is inserted directly into the biliary ductal system. Stones can be removed or fragmented via this approach.[25] This procedure is usually reserved for debilitated patients at poor risk for anesthesia.

Management Decisions

Preoperative Decisions

Management decisions in the preoperative phase are most often based on the clinical condition and stability of the patient. Most patients will require admission to the hospital for management of dehydration. Intravenous antibiotics are given for evidence of systemic infection or to debilitated patients who may not manifest signs of systemic toxicity (immunosuppressed, diabetic, elderly). Medical conditions should be managed aggressively if the patient's hemodynamic condition will tolerate such a delay in definitive treatment.

Emergent ERCP, if available, is indicated in those patients with severe cholangitis. The success of ERCP is very high and carries less morbidity than open procedures. Lai et al. compared ERCP to urgent surgical decompression in 82 patients suffering severe acute cholangitis; their study demonstrated significantly less mortality in patients treated endoscopically (10% versus 32%).[26] Interval laparoscopic cholecystectomy should be performed before discharge, once the sepsis has resolved. For severely debilitated patients who may not tolerate general anesthesia, observation after ERCP and stone extraction may be adequate.[1] If ERCP cannot be performed, the alternatives are open biliary drainage or percutaneous transhepatic drainage. Open drainage may involve only placement of a T-tube proximal to the obstructing stone or thorough CBD exploration, stone extraction, and T-tube placement, depending on the patient's hemodynamic stability. If the patient is unstable, T-tube drainage alone may be all that is necessary in the acute phase, allowing resolution of sepsis, resuscitation, and definitive stone extraction at a later time. In either case, when definitive surgery is performed to clear the CBD, cholecystectomy should also be performed to eliminate a potential source of recurrent ductal stones. ERCP also appears to be indicated for severe biliary pancreatitis. Several randomized prospective trials suggest this procedure to be of benefit if performed early by experienced endoscopists.[27,28]

In hemodynamically stable patients with suspected CBD stones, preoperative ERCP and subsequent laparoscopic cholecystectomy has long been the standard approach. However, as surgeons gain experience in laparoscopic CBDE and stone extraction, the necessity of preoperative ERCP is diminishing. Such patients may require brief (24–48h) rehydration and antibiotic therapy. Laparoscopic or open cholecystectomy follows, with intraoperative cholangiography and CBD exploration if stones are detected. Such an approach eliminates routine use of ERCP in stable patients with only "soft signs" of CBD stones, in which more than 50% of ERCP cases will be negative.[29,30] A recent randomized trial supports selective use of ERCP preoperatively in these situations.[31] Similarly, routine use of preoperative ERCP in patients without suggestion of CBD stones by clinical, radiographic, or laboratory evaluation is not justified.[32–34]

Intraoperative Decisions

Ductal exploration is most clearly indicated when common duct stones are identified either by palpation or by intraoperative cholangiography during open or laparoscopic cholecystectomy. During laparoscopic cholecystectomy, the options include CBD exploration (CBDE) for stone removal or completion of the laparoscopic cholecystectomy and post-operative ERCP and sphincterotomy. As noted, experience and success with laparoscopic CBDE continue to increase. ERCP in the postoperative period does expose the patient to an additional procedure but carries a 90% to 95% success rate. It is an attractive

option, when laparoscopic CBDE is not available, for those patients and surgeons who wish to adhere to the goals of minimally invasive surgery. Such an approach seems reasonable if experienced endoscopy is available. Indeed, recent adjuncts such as laparoscopic CBD stenting may improve success of postoperative ERCP.[35]

When laparoscopic CBD exploration or postoperative ERCP are not available or not desirable, conversion to open laparotomy and open CBDE with stone extraction is a reliable alternative. Open CBDE and stone extraction is 90% to 100% successful but is clearly more invasive than endoscopic therapy. In addition, the mortality of open CBDE ranges from under 1% in the young patient to almost 4% in the elderly or debilitated patient. For stones larger than 1.5cm, open extraction should be strongly considered because ERCP with sphincterotomy is more likely to fail in the postoperative period with larger stones.[2,13,36] Retained stones after open CBDE are reported in 2% to 10% but can often be managed via Burhenne T-tube extraction techniques.

Debate continues whether failed laparoscopic CBDE should be managed with laparoscopic transcystic antegrade sphincterotomy, conversion to open laparotomy, or postoperative ERCP and sphincterotomy. As experience grows with laparoscopic transcystic and transcholedochal CBD exploration, the need for postoperative ERCP or conversion to laparotomy and open CBDE will clearly diminish.

Postoperative Decisions

Ideally, few patients will have CBD stones detected only in the postoperative period. Asymptomatic patients may be observed initially in expectation of spontaneous passage of small stones. However, these circumstances are undoubtedly quite rare, as most stones found postoperatively will be in symptomatic patients with either left liver function test (LFT) abnormalities, jaundice, or pancreatitis. ERCP and sphincterotomy is the procedure of choice for stable, symptomatic patients. Failure of ERCP in symptomatic patients warrants operative exploration.

Retained stones detected on postoperative T-tube cholangiograms are usually managed by retaining the T-tube for 6 to 8 weeks to allow a fibrous tract to develop. Percutaneous access to the CBD then allows stone extraction with baskets, balloons, or lithotripsy devices.[1]

Conclusion

Flexible endoscopy has become an important method to manage CBD stones in all phases of patient management. ERCP and ES can stabilize the patient acutely ill with cholangitis, help remove stones during surgery, and salvage symptomatic retained stones postoperatively.

References

1. Jones D, Soper N. Current management of common bile duct stones. Adv Surg 1996;29:271–289.
2. Fink A. Current dilemmas in the management of CBD stones. Surg Endosc 1993;7:285–291.
3. Sharp K, Peach S. Common bile duct stones. In: Cameron J (ed) Current Surgical Therapy. St. Louis: Mosby, 1998: 410–415.
4. Ledinghen V, Lecesne R, et al. Diagnosis of choledocholithiasis: EUS or MRC? A prospective controlled study. GI Endoscopy 1999;49:26–31.
5. Guibaud L, Bret PM, et al. Bile duct obstruction and choledocholithiasis: diagnosis with MR cholangiography. Radiology 1995;197:109–115.
6. Reinhold C, Bret PM, Current status of MR cholangiography. AJR 1996;166:1285–1295.
7. Coakley F, Schwartz L. Magnetic resonance cholangiopancreatography. Magn Reson Imaging 1999;9:157–162.
8. Classen M, Demling L. Endoskopische Sphikterotomie der Papilla Vateri und Steinextraktion aus dem Ductus Choledochus. Dtsch Med Wochenschr 1974;99:496.
9. Kawai K, Akasaka Y, Murakami K. Endoscopic sphincterotomy of the ampulla of Vater. GI Endoscopy 1974;20: 148.
10. Cotton P. Endoscopic management of bile duct stones (apples and oranges). Gut 1984;25:587.
11. Fink AS, Valle PA, Chapman M, Cotton PB. Radiological pitfalls in endoscopic retrograde pancreatography. Pancreas 1987;1:180–187.
12. Seitz U, Bapaye A, Bohnacker S. Advances in therapeutic endoscopic treatment of CBD stones. World J Surg 1998; 22:1133–1144.
13. Cotton P. Non-operative removal of bile duct stones with duodenoscopic sphincterotomy. Br J Surg 1980;67:1.
14. Cotton P, Lehman G, Vennes J, et al. Endoscopic sphincterotomy complications and their management. An attempt at consensus. GI Endoscopy 1991;37:383–393.
15. Leese T, Neoptolemos J, Carr-Locke D. Successes, failures, early complications and their management following endoscopic sphincterotomy: results in 394 consecutive patients from a single center. Br J Surg 1985;72:215–219.
16. Freeman M, Nelson D, Sherman S. Complications of endoscopic biliary sphincterotomy. N Engl J Med 1996;335:909–918.
17. Cotton PB, Baillie J, Pappas TN, et al. Laparoscopic cholecystectomy and the biliary endoscopist. GI Endoscopy 1991; 37:94–97.
18. Cotton PB, Forbes A, Leung JWC, et al. Endoscopic stenting for long-term treatment of large bile duct stones with a biliary endoprosthesis: 2 to 5 year follow-up. GI Endoscopy 1987;33:411.
19. Bergman J, Rauwa E, Tijssen J, et al. Biliary endoprostheses in elderly patients with endoscopically irretrievable bile duct stones: report on 117 patients. GI Endoscopy 1995; 42:195.
20. Maxton DG, Tweedle DE, Martin DF. Retained common bile duct stones after endoscopic sphincterotomy: temporary and long-term treatment with biliary stenting. Gut 1995;36:446.
21. Mirizzi P. La colangiograffia durante las operaciones de las vias biliares. Bol Trab Soc Ciruj Buenos Aires 1932;30: 1413.
22. Rosenthal RJ, Steigerwald SD, Imig R, Bockhorn H. Role of intraoperative cholangiography during endoscopic cholecystectomy. Surg Laparosc Endosc 1994;4:171.
23. Carroll B, Phillips E, Rosenthal R, Gleishman S, Bray J. One hundred consecutive laparoscopic cholangiograms: results and conclusions. Surg Endosc 1996;10:319.
24. De Paula AL, Hashiba K, Bafutto M. Laparoscopic management of choledocholithiasis. Surg Endosc 1994;8:1399.
25. Simon T, Fink A. Experience with percutaneous transhepatic cholangioscopy in the management of biliary tract disease. Surg Endosc 1999;13:1199–1202.
26. Lai E, Mok F, Tan E, et al. Endoscopic biliary drainage for severe acute cholangitis. N Engl J Med 1992;326:1582–1586.
27. Neoptolemos JP, Carr-Locke DL, London NJ, et al. Controlled trial of urgent ERCP vs. conservative treatment for acute pancreatitis due to gallstones. Lancet 1988;2:979–983.
28. Fan S, Lai EC, Mok FP, et al. Early treatment of acute biliary pancreatitis by endoscopic papillotomy. N Engl J Med 1993;328:228–232.
29. Surick B, Washington M, Ghazi A. ERCP in conjunction with laparoscopic cholecystectomy. Surg Endosc 1992;7: 388–392.
30. Stiegmann G, Pearlman, Goff J. Endoscopic cholangiography and stone removal prior to cholecystectomy. Arch Surg 1989;124:787–790.
31. Chang L, Lo S, Stabile BE, et al. Preoperative versus postoperative endoscopic retrograde cholangiography in mild to moderate gallstone pancreatitis. Ann Surg 2000;231:82–87.
32. Berci G, Morgenstern L. Laparoscopic management of CBD stones: a multi-institutional SAGES study. Surg Endosc 1994;8:1168–1175.
33. Neuhaus H, Hoffman W, Feussner H, et al. Prospective evaluation of the utility and safety of ERC before laparoscopic cholecystectomy. GI Endoscopy 1992;38:257A.
34. Sackmann M, Beuers U, Helmberger T. Biliary imaging: MRC vs. ERC. J Hepatol 1999;30:334–338.
35. Fanelli, RD, Gersin KS, Mainella, MT. Laparoscopic endobiliary stenting significantly improves success of postoperative endoscopic retrograde cholangiopancreatography in low-volume centers. Surg Endosc 2002;16:487–491.
36. Hunter J, Soper N. Laparoscopic management of bile duct stones. Surg Clin N Am 1992;72(5):1077–1097.

20
Transcystic Fluoroscopic-Guided Common Bile Duct Exploration

Matthew F. Hansman and L. William Traverso

Before laparoscopic cholecystectomy, surgeons were comfortable removing common bile duct stones during open cholecystectomy using well-established techniques. As the techniques for removing the gallbladder have changed in the era of laparoscopic surgery, the techniques for exploring the common bile duct have also changed. In an effort to maintain the minimally invasive nature of laparoscopic cholecystectomy, surgeons have relied more frequently on postoperative endoscopic retrograde cholangiopancreatography (ERCP) to remove common bile duct (CBD) stones discovered during laparoscopic cholecystectomy. This approach is inherently not cost-effective and subjects the patient to increased morbidity. To reverse this trend, new technology has evolved that allows treatment of gallbladder and CBD stones during laparoscopic surgery. A very simple methodology, fluoroscopic transcystic duct stone retrieval, has been developed that requires minimal additional training and which can remove most CBD stones discovered during laparoscopic cholecystectomy. It is the goal of this chapter to outline this simple and effective technique.

CBD stones are observed in 10% of cases in which intraoperative cholangiography (IOC) is routinely performed during laparoscopic cholecystectomy.[1] Because no preoperative chemical or imaging studies can reliably predict the presence of choledocholithiasis during surgery,[2] the only way to determine the presence of a CBD stone during laparoscopic cholecystectomy is to actively look for stones using IOC or intraoperative ultrasound. Successful intraoperative CBD stone removal avoids postponing the treatment until postoperative symptoms develop and avoids subsequent ERCP with endoscopic papillotomy. It is more cost-effective and patient friendly to use fluoroscopic-guided transcystic CBD exploration, which can easily remove most of these stones,[3] before attempting transcystic choledochoscopy

or other more advanced laparoscopic techniques such as choledochotomy.

Routine Intraoperative Cholangiography

There are no preoperative tests that can reliably predict the presence or absence of CBD stones. Therefore, it is unlikely that a surgeon can accurately select patients to perform IOC.[2] For the purposes of this chapter, we assume that the surgeon accepts the long-standing dictum that a detected CBD stone should be removed at surgery to prevent the potential complications of residual or retained stones in the CBD. Such postoperative complications include cholangitis, pancreatitis, or simply postoperative pain. Once a CBD stone is detected at surgery, there are no definitive studies to guide the surgeon's judgment whether to observe the stone or stones, to obtain postoperative ERCP, or to attempt intraoperative removal of the CBD stones.

If the surgeon elects to defer intraoperative treatment of a detected CBD stone, the patient usually requires an ERCP with or without endoscopic papillotomy. The patient is then exposed to the risks of both the disease and the additional procedure. Also, the surgeon must realize that there are situations where the endoscopist will not wish to attempt removal of common bile duct stones, either before or after cholecystectomy. These situations vary with the expertise of the endoscopist and include multiple stones greater than 2 cm in size, stones above a stricture, difficult access to the ampulla of Vater (such as history of Billroth II gastrectomy or Roux-en-Y gastrojejunostomy), and young age. The reluctance to perform endoscopic papillotomy in a young person is derived from the multiple studies

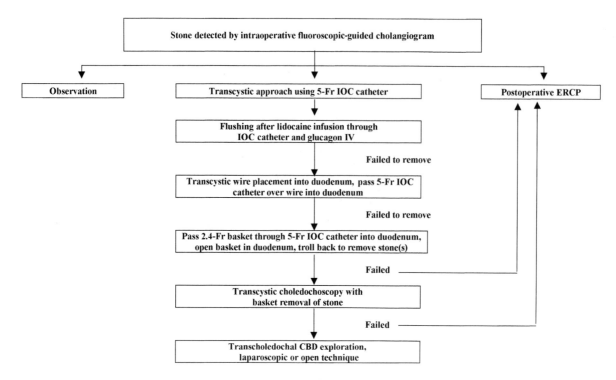

FIGURE 20.1. Algorithm after discovery of common bile duct (CBD) stones using the simplest techniques first. If the simplest technique fails, the next step is more complicated. Equipment listed is explained more fully in the text or outlined in Table 20.1.

showing a persistent stenosis rate after endoscopic papillotomy in young patients *without obstructive biliary tract disease*, for example, biliary dyskinesia. In young people with choledocholithiasis, this perceived stenosis rate may be as high as 10% over a 5- to 10-year period.

It is therefore optimal, from an ethical standpoint and for clinical efficacy, for the operating surgeon to remove the stones during the operation, either laparoscopically or by open techniques. Of course, this is not always practical. Relative contraindications to transcystic common bile duct exploration include a left-sided cystic duct, entrance of the cystic duct near the ampulla of Vater, proximal common bile duct stones that cannot be approached through the cystic duct junction, a diminutive biliary tree (diameter <3 mm), an extremely short or absent cystic duct (extremely rare in our experience), inability to pass a hydrophilic wire into the duodenum, large (>2 cm) impacted CBD stones, or the technical inability of the surgeon to perform the basic maneuvers listed next.

An algorithm for the management of common bile duct stones discovered during laparoscopic cholecystectomy is presented in Figure 20.1. Note the importance of ERCP in this algorithm. Although ERCP is associated with some risk, it is a useful technique with a high success rate for specific indications.

Knowledge and Equipment

The following elements are needed for successful IOC, the first step in transcystic fluoroscopic-guided common bile duct exploration (TFCBDE). First, an experienced team to perform IOC must be in place. In addition to the surgeon, this includes the circulating and scrub nurses plus the radiology technicians. Second, a common bile duct stone cart must be available with all the equipment listed here. Third, a modern digital fluoroscope unit must be available; these units, commonly used in orthopedic surgery, usually contain digital storage capacity. In addition to the fluoroscope, radiation protection must be available: either the independent sterile hanging variety or the lightweight personal lead apron. Fourth, all cholangiography and stone retrieval equipment should be engineered to function together, that is, the catheters must accept the guidewires and baskets used even when the catheters are angled as they pass through the cystic duct into the duodenum (Table 20.1). Fifth, the operating surgeon must have a thorough knowledge of the patterns of biliary tract anatomy that could be encountered. The surgeon cannot rely on the radiologist for this information and must be able to interpret cholangiograms accurately. Sixth, the frequency and site of observed CBD stones in the biliary tree should be well known to the operating surgeon.[1]

TABLE 20.1. Equipment list for successful laparoscopic transcystic common bile duct (CBD) exploration.

Cholangiogram catheter: 5 F, flexible tip, Luer-Lok hub, distal marks every 1 cm

Contrast infusion system that allows remote infusion away from the radiation source: two intravenous extension tubes connected by a three-way stopcock connected to two 20-ml syringes, one for saline flushing solution and the other for a 50% contrast solution

Olsen–Berci cholangiocatheter clamp to support the IOC 5 F cholangiocatheter and to increase the successful cannulation rate by allowing leakfree cholangiography with a shallow (<1 cm) insertion into the cystic ductotomy

Flexible Martin arm to stabilize the cholangiocatheter clamp; this multiple-articulated arm is attached to the side rail of the operating table on the right side of the patient

Contents of the CBD stone cart:
1. Hydrophilic "slime" guidewire: 0.035-in. with flexible terminal segment
2. Variety of stone baskets: begin with a 2.4 F size, then use a 3- and then a 4-wire basket; first use a flat wire and then a helical basket
3. 1% lidocaine (10 ml) for infusion into the CBD throught the IOC
4. 1 mg intravenous glucagon for administration by the anesthesiologist

Specific Equipment for Transcystic Fluoroscopically Guided Common Bile Duct Exploration

The cholangiocatheter described in the Techniques section is a 5 F catheter and has a flexible tip; it is very helpful for the distal end of the catheter to be marked every 1 cm. Also helpful during insertion of fine wires through the proximal end of the catheter is a friction lock-type hub, tapered for this purpose. A catheter with these characteristics is user friendly and allows successful cannulation in almost every attempt. We use a catheter modified from a 5 F ureteral catheter (Cook Surgical, Inc., Bloomington, IN, USA). Infusion of contrast material through this catheter is provided by connecting two 20-ml syringes (one for 50% dilution of contrast solution and one for normal saline flushing solution) via a stopcock connected to an IV extension tube. The connecting tubing should allow the surgeon to be well out of the radiation field during fluoroscopy. Once the cystic duct is cannulated and a stone detected, the friction lock hub of the cholangiocatheter can be disconnected and used as access for CBD exploration. When the surgeon can use both hands for manipulation of wires and catheters into the hub, the CBD exploration is greatly facilitated. We accomplish this by suspending the IOC catheter to allow a hands-free approach. The IOC cholangiocatheter is mechanically supported using the Olsen–Berci IOC clamp held by the Martin Arm (Fig. 20.2 A,B).

The Olsen–Berci cholangiocatheter clamp stabilizes the catheter but also allows the cystic duct to be cannulated successfully after only a shallow insertion (<1 cm) of the catheter (Fig. 20.3). The jaws of the cholangiocatheter clamp allow occlusion of the cystic ductotomy over the catheter, which prevents contrast extravasation. Because the IOC catheter need not be placed deeply into the cystic duct, cannulation success rate approaches 100%. This type of clamp does not occlude the catheter for passage of wires and baskets. The proximal end of the cholangiocatheter clamp allows the IOC catheter to be stabilized in a hands-free manner so that the CBD can be explored through the disconnected hub of the proximal end of the catheter. The Olsen–Berci clamp is itself stabilized with a flexible articulated arm attached to the side rail of the operating table on the right side of the patient (Fig. 20.2B).

Both the Olsen–Berci clamp and the retraction arm are reusable. We use all this equipment for every IOC. However, when a CBD stone is detected, several inexpensive disposable items must be retrieved from the CBD stone cart. First, flush through the biliary tree after inducing a flaccid sphincter of Oddi, accomplished pharmaceutically with intravenous glucagon (1 mg IV) and an intra-CBD infusion of 1% lidocaine through the IOC cholangiocatheter. If this flushing maneuver fails, a guidewire and a basket are obtained from the CBD stone cart (see Table 20.1); a 0.035-in. hydrophilic guidewire with a flexible terminal segment and one of various stone baskets are needed. All these must be pretested to ensure they will pass through the 5F cholangiocatheter. We begin with a 2.4F flat four-wire Segura basket; if this fails to engage the stone, we then use a 2.4F helical four-wire basket.

Description of Technique: The Transcystic Fluoroscopic-Guided Approach

This approach mimics the successful procedures developed by urologists, endoscopists, and interventional radiologists. The transcystic approach avoids a choledochotomy and eliminates subsequent need for a T-tube. The fluoroscopic transcystic technique does not require the surgeon to be skilled in laparoscopic suturing. Use of intraoperative real-time fluoroscopy is, however, mandatory. All necessary equipment is available in most modern operating rooms. The technique assumes the cholangiocatheter described previously has been placed in the cystic duct and yielded a quality cholangiogram. Note that the cystic duct should have been cannulated for about 1 cm. The flexible tip of the IOC catheter allows a shallow cannulation and avoids puncturing the opposite

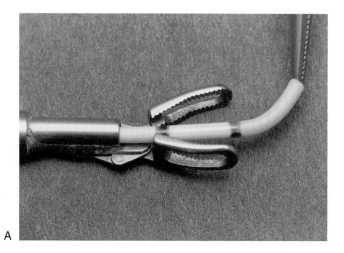

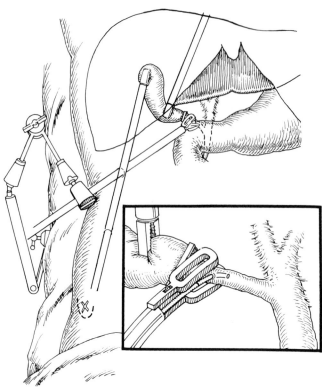

FIGURE 20.2. A. Close-up view of tip of the Olsen–Berci cholangiocatheter clamp as the tip of the Cook 5F ureteral catheter with its flexible tip emerging from the channel (Karl Storz Company, Los Angeles, CA, or Olympus Corp., San Jose, CA, USA.). The jaw paddles are open. A 0.035-in. hydrophilic wire can be advanced through the catheter using the catheter as a sheath. This maneuver is required only if there is difficulty inserting the catheter for less than 1 cm as required to accomplish a leakfree infusion during IOC. The wire is also used if the catheter must be advanced into the duodenum over the wire using fluoroscopic control, as described in the text. B. Artist's drawing of positioning of the Olsen–Berci cholangiocatheter clamp with a multi-articulated Martin arm (Elmed, Inc., Addison, IL, USA). The Martin arm is attached to the railing of the operating room table on the right side of the patient. Note the more lateral position of the right subcostal trocar than usual. This position places the axis of the cystic duct and the trocar in a more parallel position and facilitates placement of the catheter through the ductotomy.

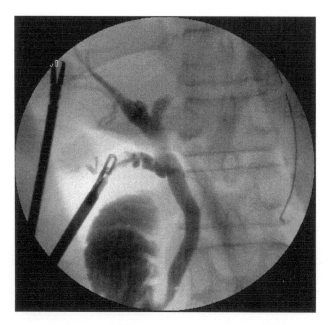

FIGURE 20.3. Intraoperative cholangiogram shows the Olsen–Berci cholangiocather clamp and how the clamp allows for shallow cannulation of the cystic duct <1 cm to obtain a leakfree infusion during IOC. The shallow cannulation avoids negotiating the spiral valves of Heister, making the success rate for IOC almost 100% in the author's experience.

wall of the cystic duct (see Fig. 20.2A). The Olsen-Berci clamp jaws are lightly clamped over the cystic ductotomy to yield the IOC without crushing the flexible tip. Crushing the tip can compromise the catheter's lumen enough to prohibit a stone basket from passing through into the common duct. Once the catheter clamp has been successfully applied, adjust the end of the clamp so that there is no tension on the cystic duct–CBD junction (to avoid avulsion). Securing the tip of the cholangiocatheter clamp without tension on the cystic duct–CBD junction is accomplished using a multiarticulated retractor holder arm, allowing the end of the clamp to be placed accurately and to remain within 1 mm of that position. Using this technique, we have never experienced an inadvertent avulsion of the cystic duct or caused other inadvertent damage to the duct.

Radiation protection for the surgical team is mandatory; we prefer a hanging lead apron with sterile drapes on the left side of the patient. The surgeon stands behind this sterile lead apron during the IOC as the fluoroscope is brought in from the patient's right side. When a CBD stone is observed during real-time fluoroscopic cholangiography, the surgeon will scrub out, put on a lead apron, and rescrub into the operation on the patient's right side. During this delay, 10 ml 1% lidocaine solution is instilled into the CBD through the cholangiocatheter and the stopcock is closed. Simultaneously, the anesthesiologist administers 1 mg IV glucagon. Full sphincter of Oddi relaxation requires only a few minutes. When the surgeon rejoins the operative team, the CBD is rapidly irrigated with 20-ml aliquots of normal saline during fluoroscopic observation, which successfully irrigates stones from the CBD into the duodenum in approximately one-half of cases.[3] We have not observed any complications of injection-induced pancreatitis; these results are contingent on hand flushing with a 20-ml syringe. We do not recommend mechanical pressure irrigation systems that can achieve much higher pressures while attempting to flush a stone from the CBD as this may induce postoperative pancreatitis. It should be remembered that more than 30% of patients during routine IOC have a radiographic common channel with the main pancreatic duct; that is, a portion of the pancreatic duct will fill with contrast during IOC, which should highlight the potential for iatrogenic pancreatitis.[1]

If stones are still present after these maneuvers, other methods should be used to retrieve them (see Fig. 20.1). First, a 0.035-in. hydrophilic "slime" wire is moistened and placed through the hub of the cholangiocatheter, which is stationary because of the table-mounted retractor arm. The 5F catheter size ensures an adequate internal lumen for passing this wire. Under fluoroscopic control, the wire is passed into the duodenum and the cholangiocatheter is advanced over the wire until it also is safely in the duodenum. The cholangiocatheter clamp allows the surgeon to use both hands to manipulate the wire, catheter, and basket. The wire can now be replaced through the catheter with a 2.4F flat four-wire basket. The basket is also advanced under fluoroscopic control through the IOC catheter into the duodenum. If the IOC catheter bends too much as it passes through the cystic duct and then curves down into the CBD, the 2.4F basket may have difficulty in passing through the catheter at the bend. The rule of thumb is to prevent an acute bend in the catheter and, instead, to try to achieve a smaller curve such as than would occur if the catheter followed the border of a silver dollar.

The basket is advanced beyond the tip of the catheter and, under fluoroscopic observation, opened in the duodenum. The open basket is trolled backward through the ampulla until it nears the stone, which is usually easily observed by the residual radiographic contrast. Some catheter systems use a side port to administer contrast during this manipulation; however, we have found that the residual contrast is almost always sufficient to see the stone. The basket is jiggled up and down adjacent to the stone until the stone enters the open basket. The basket–stone combination is either pushed back into the duodenum and the stone released by rotating and shaking the basket or the basket is pulled back through the cystic duct. Concern has been expressed that a stone cannot fit through a small-diameter cystic duct; however, remember that this stone probably originated in the gallbladder and passed into the bile duct through the tiny but elastic cystic duct.

Technical Aids

Transcystic techniques all begin with an IOC. Performance of IOC depends, of course, on successful cannulation of the cystic duct. To make canulation easy, the axis of the Olsen–Berci IOC clamp should parallel the axis of the cystic duct. To accomplish this, the right subcostal trocar should be placed last, once the unique axis of the cystic duct for each patient has been observed. Stated in another way, the gallbladder should be grasped and retracted upward by the right lateral port to allow determining the new axis of the cystic duct. The optimal placement site of the right subcostal trocar is then chosen; this trocar site is usually lateral to the usual position (Fig. 20.2B). Using the right subcostal trocar for the IOC clamp and catheter avoids a falsely negative IOC, for example, obliterating portions of the CBD with radiodense equipment during fluoroscopy as occurs when the subxiphoid port is used for the IOC.

Hydrophilic guidewires negotiate the spiral valves of Heister in almost all cases, especially when using the support of the cholangiocatheter. The IOC catheter is first placed no more than 1 cm through the cystic ducto-

TABLE 20.2. Success of transcystic laparoscopic technique during our learning curve.

	No. of patients	Single stone	Multiple stones	Flushing[a]	Basket retrieval[b]	Overall
At discharge	32	87% (13/15)	35% (6/17)	62% (8/13)	58% (11/19)	59% (19/32)
Long-term follow-up	29	77% (10/13)	25% (4/16)	54% (7/13)	44% (7/16)	48% (14/29)

[a]Flushing after infusion of 10 ml 1% lidocaine into CBD and intravenous administration of 1 mg glucagon.
[b]Basket retrieval after failure of flushing irrigation.

tomy, followed by passing the guidewire through the catheter. We have never observed the flexible terminal end of the hydrophilic wire to puncture the cystic duct or the CBD. A distal impacted CBD stone can be troublesome if either the slime wire or the IOC catheter cannot be passed beyond the stone. As shown in the algorithm of Figure 20.1, if the basket attempt fails (a minority of cases), the options are transcystic choledochoscopy, laparoscopic or open choledochotomy, or, if the surgeon chooses, postoperative ERCP.

The proximal CBD stone above the cystic duct junction also presents a challenge but can often be successfully approached by changing the angle of the operating table. Some stones float while others are heavier than bile or saline. Observation of which way the stones move with respect to gravity may be important to determine correct positioning of the OR table. In many cases, with fluroscopic manipulation, the hydrophilic wire can be placed proximally in the biliary tree, but this is not usual. If CBD stones can be repositioned distal to the cystic duct junction by gravity, clearance of the duct is possible. Of course, this assumes that the patient's cystic duct can be repetitively accessed. Occasionally, the patient's cystic duct does not allow for multiple cannulations and the procedure must be consequently abandoned.

If there is too much bend in the cholangiocatheter, it can be very difficult to pass the basket through the resistance of this point. Thus, we use the smallest diameter basket possible, usually a 2.4F. This small diameter has some disadvantages. The space between the wires of the basket can become a limiting factor, as a four-wire basket has less space between the wires than a three-wire Segura basket. A four-wire basket in a small ductal system may not allow adequate expansion of the basket for stone entrance. In this case, the three-wire Segura basket may have the advantage as the larger space between the wires offers more potential for engaging the stone. It is therefore advisable to have both four-wire and three-wire baskets available.

Balloon-tipped catheters can be helpful in laparoscopic exploration of the bile duct. We use baskets preferentially because balloons can only remove a stone from the CBD by pushing it through the ampulla into the duodenum. However, the balloon may efficiently pull back an impacted common duct stone to the level of the cystic

duct–CBD junction. Once the stone is dislodged distally, a basket can engage the free-floating stone. Unfortunately, most balloon-tipped catheters do not have a channel for insertion of a catheter over a guidewire, and they are frequently not long enough to use through a stabilizing IOC clamp.

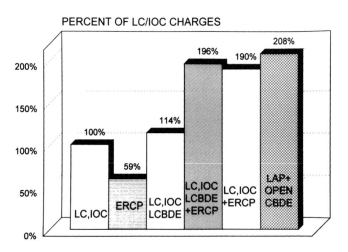

FIGURE 20.4. Proportional cost comparison for each type of CBD stone treatment. These total estimated charges include professional fees, length of hospital stay, and the facility charges of the GI lab and OR. The charge of an uncomplicated LC with a negative IOC is represented as 100% in this graph on the left bar labeled "LC,IOC." When the IOC is positive for stones, the cost implications are readily apparent for each option available to the surgeon. If the surgeon successfully clears the CBD with transcystic techniques then the increase over LC with negative IOC is only 14%, but if the surgeon chooses to go directly to ERCP without attempting transcystic methods, then the increase will be 90%. *LC*, laparoscopic cholecystectomy; *IOC*, intraoperative cholangiogram; *ERCP*, endoscopic papillotomy with stone retrieval; *LCBDE*, laparoscopic transcystic removal of CBD stones with either flushing or basket; *LAP + OPEN CBDE*, diagnostic laparoscopy with cholangiogram and then open cholecystectomy with open common bile duct exploration. (From Traverso LW, Hargrave K, Kozarek RA. A cost-effective approach to the treatment of common bile duct stones with surgical versus endoscopic techniques. In: Berci G, Cuschieri A (eds) *Bile ducts and Bile Duct Stones*. Philadelphia: Saunders, 1997:154–160, with permission.)

Results

There are only a few reports of short- and long-term follow-up of transcystic fluoroscopic-guided basket exploration of the biliary tree for intraoperatively discovered CBD stones.[3] Our study, reported in 1995, included our learning curve between 1990 and 1994 and involved 55 patients with positive IOC. The results, according to technique of exploration or number of stones present, are summarized in Table 20.2. The major reason for failure of transcystic exploration was inability to clear multiple stones, whether they were in the proximal or distal duct. When single stones were present, the only reasons for failure were cystic duct anomalies (low-lying insertion of the cystic duct into the common bile duct or a cystic duct entering into the right hepatic duct) or abandonment of the technique by the surgeon after irrigation failed.

The average fluoroscopy time during these procedures was 306 seconds; average time for the entire laparoscopic operation, including cholecystectomy, was 166 min. For those who did not undergo transcystic exploration, operative time was 122 min. Mean length of stay for patients undergoing transcystic exploration was 1.7 days; it was 3.3 days in those undergoing ERCP and papillotomy after laparoscopic cholecystectomy. There were no cases of posttranscystic exploration complications, particularly pancreatitis. However, 2 of 10 patients who underwent postcholecystectomy ERCP developed pancreatitis and required hospitalization.[3] Initial success rate for duct clearance was 59%, but this improved to 100% over the final 6-month period of the study. Concern has been expressed that IOC itself may cause postoperative pancreatitis and the flushing method could therefore also result in pancreatitis. In a subsequent study reviewing 435 consecutive cases of routine IOC, CBD stones were found in 14%. Regardless of the presence of CBD stones or use of CBD exploration, we found no instances of pancreatitis from IOC in these 435 cases.[4]

In summary, using the transcystic technique, 87% of single stones can be removed at the time of surgery; those that cannot are usually above the cystic junction with the CBD. In our initial series, only 35% of multiple stones were successfully cleared. These data included our learning curve, and more recently almost all single stones have been cleared from the CBD.

A subsequent cost analysis compared open, laparoscopic, and ERCP techniques of CBD exploration to a standard laparoscopic cholecystectomy with negative IOC (Fig. 20.4). If transcystic laparoscopic CBD exploration was successful, the surgeon spent only 14% more than the cost of a laparoscopic cholecystectomy with negative IOC. In cases referred for postcholecystectomy ERCP, even if a transcystic laparoscopic CBD exploration had been unsuccessful, the cost was at least 90% more because of the added procedure and hospitalization.[5] Therefore, an attempt at intraoperative treatment of the CBD stone can be justified on a cost basis alone.

Conclusion

Laparoscopic cholecystectomy is one of the most common operations performed by general surgeons today. Approximately 10% of the patients undergoing this operation have CBD stones that are noted on a routine intraoperative cholangiogram. The minimally invasive laparoscopic procedure can be maintained and the CBD stone removed by utilizing a fluoroscopic-guided transcystic CBD exploration. This procedure is a relatively simple method for clearing CBD stones in the majority of cases and requires no additional training. The method is safe and cost-effective and decreases the need, risks, and expense of postoperative ERCP.

References

1. Traverso LW, Hauptmann EM, Lynge DC. Routine intraoperative cholangiography and its contribution to the selective cholangiographer. Am J Surg 1994;167:464–468.
2. Koo KP, Traverso LW. Do preoperative indicators predict the presence of common bile duct stones during laparoscopic cholecystectomy. Am J Surg 1996;171:495–499.
3. Roush TS, Traverso LW. Management and long-term follow up of patients with positive cholangiograms during laparoscopic cholecystectomy. Am J Surg 1995;169:484–487.
4. Morgan S, Traverso LW. Intraoperative cholangiography and postoperative pancreatitis. Surg Endosc 2000;14:264–266.
5. Traverso LW, Hargrave K, Kozarek RA. A cost effective approach to the treatment of common bile duct stones with surgical versus endoscopic techniques. In: Berci G, Cuschieri A (eds) Laparoscopic Diagnosis and Treatment of Common Bile Duct Stones. Philadelphia: Saunders, 1997:154–160.

21
Laparoscopic Transcystic Duct Choledochoscopy

Kristín H. Haraldsdóttir, Sigurdur Blondal, and Margret Oddsdottir

Laparoscopic cholecystectomy was quickly accepted after its introduction in 1987 as the treatment of choice for cholelithiasis. Cholangiography during laparoscopic cholecystectomy was first performed in 1989; shortly thereafter, several successful laparoscopic common bile duct explorations (LCBDE) for common bile duct stones were reported.[1-4] Over the years, the technique and instrumentation for LCBDE have evolved and the safety and efficacy of the procedure have been proven and well documented.[5-11] Several studies, both retrospective reports and prospective randomized trials, have shown the advantage of the single-stage laparoscopic approach (laparoscopic cholecystectomy and LCBDE) over the two-stage approach [laparoscopic cholecystectomy and pre- or postoperative endoscopic retrograde cholangiography (ERC) and ductal clearance].[8,12-14] The single-stage approach offers patients a single, less costly procedure for their biliary calculi and a shorter hospital stay.[14,15] The duct clearance rate for LCBDE and ERC and stone removal does depend on the skills of the surgeon and of the endoscopist, but the reported success rate is similar.[11,12,16] However, the single-stage laparoscopic approach leaves the sphincter mechanism intact and carries lower overall morbidity and mortality.[8,12,13,17,18]

Choledocholithiasis is present in about 8% to 15% of patients with cholelithiasis.[12,13,19] The presence of choledocholithiasis increases the morbidity and mortality of biliary surgery about fourfold.[4] Therefore, evaluation and treatment of common bile duct (CBD) stones is essential in the management of patients with gallstone disease. The preoperative diagnosis of choledocholithiasis is imprecise unless invasive methods such as ERC are employed.[3,13,16,20] However, subjecting all patients with suspected choledocholithiasis to a preoperative ERC would lead to unneccesary intervention in more than 50% of patients and still miss about 5% of patients with choledocholithiasis who were asymptomatic and not suspected to have CBD stones at the time of surgery.[6,12,21,22] Routine intraoperative cholangiography detects suspected and unsuspected choledocholithiasis, is quick and simple, and has not been reoprted to cause morbidity.[6,23] Other arguments for routine intraoperative cholangiography are training of residents and detection of bile duct injury. Additionally, by performing intraoperative cholangiography on a routine basis, the surgeon and staff acquire experience in accessing the duct and using fluoroscopy. If CBD stones are identified in about 10% of cases, the average general surgeon (doing 50–75 cholecystectomies a year) will see 5 to 7 cases of CBD stones a year. Therefore, a routine intraoperative cholangiogram is an important practice for the surgeon who plans to perform laparoscopic transcystic CBDE because many of the maneuvers are the same for both.

Three approaches have evolved for LCBDE[8]: laparoscopic transcystic-CBDE, laparoscopic choledochotomy, and laparoscopic antegrade sphincterotomy. Each approach has its specific indications, but in many instances the surgeon has a choice. The transcystic-CBDE is the first choice of most laparoscopic surgeons when faced with choledocholithiasis that seem feasible for the transcystic approach (see indications). It requires no cutting and suturing of the CBD (with the theoretical risk of stricture formation), biliary drainage is rarely required, and patient satisfaction is high.[8,13,24] Transcystic-CBDE is associated with lower morbidity and mortality than laparoscopic choledochotomy as well as quicker recovery.[8,13] The laparoscopic antegrade sphincterotomy has not been widely used, because it requires a side-viewing gastroscope in the room and an additional surgeon or gastroenterologist.[25,26]

This chapter focuses on the laparoscopic, transcystic choledochoscopic approach for CBD exploration.

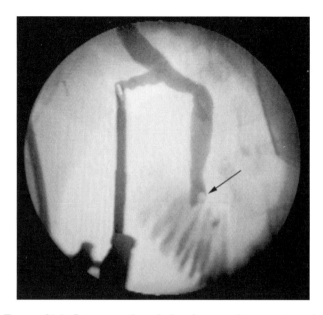

FIGURE 21.1. Intraoperative cholangiogram shows a stone in the distal common bile duct (*arrow*).

Indications and Contraindications

When an intraoperative cholangiogram shows a common bile stone(s), the surgeon must evaluate which therapeutic alternative is best for the patient (Fig. 21.1). If the tools for LCBDE are not available or the surgeon is not skilled or trained in LCBDE, the choice is either to convert to an open procedure or to refer the patient for a postoperative ERC and stone removal. If LCBDE is an option, the surgeon has the choice of a transcystic approach or a choledochotomy. However, before making that choice, the likelihood of a successful transcystic exploration must be assessed (Fig. 21.2). The cholangiogram gives most of the information needed.

Large stones (more than 8 mm in diameter) and multiple stones (5 or more) probably will not be successfully removed by the transcystic approach. Stones in the hepatic ducts are difficult, if not impossible, for the tran-

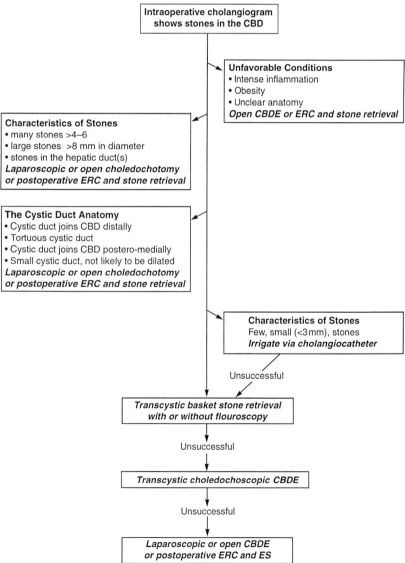

FIGURE 21.2. Algorithm for stones in the common bile duct. *CBD*, common bile duct; *CBDE*, common bile duct exploration; *ERC*, endoscopic retrograde cholangiography; *ES*, endoscopic sphincterotomy.

scystic approach. Second, the anatomy and the course of the cystic duct must be studied. A very narrow cystic duct may not dilate enough to accept the 3-mm choledochoscope or the stones. A long cystic duct entering the CBD very distally or a cystic duct that curves around the CBD and enters it posteromedially is often not feasible for a transcystic CBD exploration. Other features that make the transcystic approach difficult include severe cholecystitis with gangrene of the cystic duct and the proximal gallbladder, obesity, and intense inflammation in the porta hepatis with poor definition of the anatomy of the triangle of Calot.

Patients who present with gallstones and cholangitis or moderate to severe pancreatitis are not candidates for LCBDE and are better treated by an ERC with sphincterotomy and stone removal.[14,27] Laparoscopic cholecystectomy can be performed when their clinical and chemical parameters improve. Elderly or unstable patients with gallstones and severe comorbid diseases who present with jaundice (or recent history of jaundice), abnormal liver function tests, and a dilated CBD on an ultrasonography should also be considered for an ERC and ductal clearance. Frequently, ERC and sphincterotomy with stone retrieval are all that is necessary for these patients. The need for a subsequent cholecystectomy depends on their general condition as well as their gallstone disease. If unsuspected CBD stones are discovered on a routine intraoperative cholangiogram in an elderly or a poor-risk patient, a postoperative ERC with sphincterotomy and stone removal is indicated instead of a prolonged procedure.[1,14]

Instruments

Embarking on laparoscopic CBDE is prohibitively frustrating and time consuming if the instruments and equipment are not available, labeled, and ready in the operating room area. The needed items should be together on a trolley or in a specific cabin. In addition to a regular laparoscopic cholecystectomy instrument tray with a cholangiocatheter and a setup for cholangiogram, the following items are needed for the laparoscopic transcystic CBDE:

1. Glucagon 1 mg IV injection, for sphincter relaxation
2. Digital C-arm fluoroscopy unit and sterile coverings
3. A percutaneous introducer sheath with an airtight gasket, 12F (4 mm) in diameter and 10–15 cm long, with a needle, introducer, and a guidewire for percutaneous placement; alternatively, an additional 5-mm trocar without mechanical valve can be used
4. A floppy hydrophilic guidewire 0.0035 in. (0.89 mm) in diameter, at least 90 cm long
5. A straight, 2.4F or 3F flat wire basket of the Segura type (Fig. 21.3B)
6. A cystic duct dilator (Fig. 21.3C); an over-the-wire balloon angioplasty catheter, with a 4-cm-long balloon and a maximum inflated outer diameter of 0.8 cm (available, 0.4–0.8 cm); mechanical over-the-wire dilators, 7–14 French, are an alternative
7. A fiberoptic choledochoscope with an outer diameter of 3.2 mm or less and at least 1.2-mm working channel and a tip deflection (Fig. 21.3A)

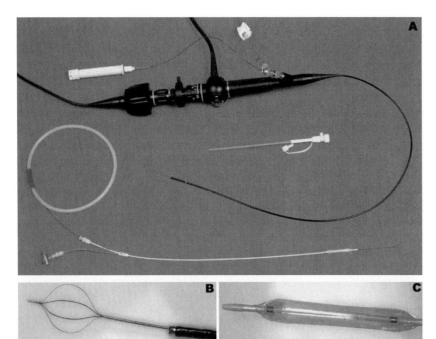

FIGURE 21.3. A. The choledoscope with a basket inserted through the working channel. *Bottom*, balloon angioplasty catheter passed over a guidewire; *middle*, percutaneous introducer sheath. B. Close up-view of an open, straight, flat, four-wire basket. C. Close-up view of inflated balloon of balloon angioplasty catheter for cystic duct dilation. Note the two black, radiopaque markers on each end of the balloon.

8. A light source for the choledochoscope

9. A camera for the choledochoscope

10. A second monitor for the choledochoscope or a video mixer for a simultaneous same-monitor display (a picture in picture image)

11. Saline irrigation, warm, pressurized to 50–100 mmHg, for use through the working channel of the choledochoscope

12. Intravenous tubing for the saline irrigation

13. Atraumatic grasping forceps to manipulate the choledochoscope

14. Cystic duct drainage tube or a 5F pediatric feeding tube for biliary drainage

15. A pretied loop-tie or a suture to ligate the cystic duct

(The following may be useful but are not always needed:)

16. Fogarty biliary catheters, 3–5

17. A lithotripter, either a pulsed dye or an electrohydrolic unit with long probes that will pass through the working channel of the choledochoscope

Technique

When the cholangiogram shows stones in the CBD that seem feasible for a transcystic approach, the instruments and tools for LCBDE are brought into the operating room (see Fig. 21.3). Before any manipulation of the bile ducts, intravenous glucagon 1 mg should be given by the anesthesiologist to induce relaxation of the sphincter of Oddi. Because of its short half-life, glucagon administration must be given approximately every 20 to 30 min so long as the CBD exploration is in process. If the stones are not large or impacted, it is worth trying to flush the duct with normal saline via the cholangiocatheter while waiting for the CBD exploration items to be collected and set up. Small stones can often be flushed into the duodenum.

If, on the cholangiogram, the cystic duct stump is long proximal to the common duct entrance, it should be dissected up toward the cystic duct–CBD junction. A new ductotomy is then made approximately 1 cm from the junction. At this point, the triangle of Calot should already be dissected out with the cystic artery clipped and cut and the peritoneum between the infundibulum of the gallbladder and the liver divided. A percutaneous introducer sheath or an additional trocar is then placed for the passage of the choledochoscope and the baskets. For a free passage of the scope, the trocar needs to be without a mechanical valve and have no sharp edges. Usually the best location for the introducer is subcostal, a few centimeters medial to the midclavicular port (Fig. 21.4). One needs to place and direct the introducer so it will guide the scope by the shortest and the most direct route to the cystic duct.

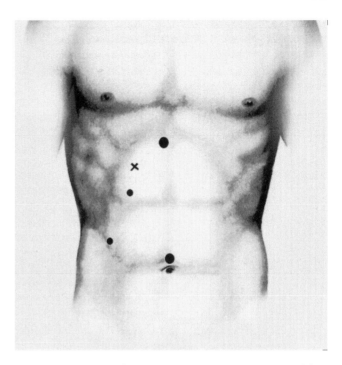

FIGURE 21.4. Trocar placement. *Dots* represent trocar positioning for laparoscopic cholecystectomy. The best place for the percutaneous introducer is usually a few centimeters medial to the midclavicular port, marked with an X.

In most cases, free passage of a wire basket under fluoroscopic guidance should be tried next as this will successfully clear the duct in about 30% of nonimpacted CBD stones (see Chapter 20). If there still are stones in the duct, a transcystic choledochoscopy is the next step.

The choledochoscope is connected to a separate light source and a camera. If a video mixer is not being used, the additional monitor should be positioned close to the main monitor so the operating surgeon can easily observe both screens. The warm normal saline for infusion through the scope (to distend the bile duct and improve visualization) is connected to the scope. The operative area will be quite cluttered, so it is a good idea to have a separate sterile stand for the scope and its cables and tubing. Before the scope is passed, the size of the cystic duct needs to be assessed and dilated if it is too small for the scope. The cystic duct requires dilation in approximately 50% of cases.

The duct can be dilated with either balloon dilators or mechanical graduated dilators. For both, a long hydrophilic guidewire is first inserted through the sheath, through the cystic duct, and into the common duct. The balloon catheter is advanced over the wire so that the distal end of the balloon is past the cystic duct–CBD junction, but the proximal end is outside the ductotomy (Fig. 21.5). Balloon dilation should be performed for at least 5 min; it works with a radially directing force and is thought to be safer and more effective than graduated

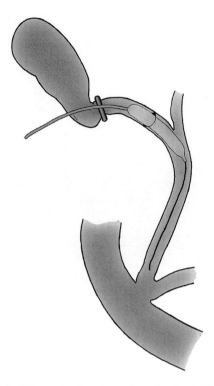

FIGURE 21.5. Schematic drawing of cystic duct dilation. The balloon catheter has been passed over a wire. The distal end of the balloon is past the cystic duct–common duct junction but the proximal end is outside the ductotomy.

dilators. However, it can still tear the cystic duct and the cystic duct–common duct junction if not applied correctly. If the graduated dilators are used, a 9F dilator is usually the first to be passed, then in sequence up to a 12F. It is imperative to watch the monitor as the cystic duct is being dilated; the graduated dilators work by a shearing force and can easily cause avulsion of the cystic duct.

The dilators are then removed but the guidewire is left in place. The guidewire is then inserted into the working port of the choledochoscope and the scope passed over the wire and into the cystic duct. Atraumatic forceps, designed to handle the scope, are placed through the epigastric port. The scope needs careful handling; the outer coat is easily torn, and the fibers can break. The scope is advanced into the CBD, the guidewire withdrawn into its sheath, and normal saline irrigation is turned on. If there is difficulty in advancing the scope passed the cystic duct–CBD junction, further dissection of the cystic duct may be necessary.

The surgeon uses one hand on the head of the scope and controls the deflection lever; the other hand manipulates the scope just outside the trocar/introducer sheath by twisting it. Thus, the scope is advanced into the distal CBD under direct vision. When a stone is found, the scope is placed in a direct view of the stone. A basket is

now inserted through the working channel of the scope and past the stone; there, the basket is opened and then withdrawn back to the stone (Fig. 21.6). The basket may need to be manipulated back and forth before it captures the stone. In some cases it may be necessary to twist and manipulate the scope as well to catch the stone in the wire basket.

Once the stone is inside the basket, it is closed slowly around the stone and advanced a little out of the scope at the same time (the basket withdraws itself into the choledochoscope as it is being closed, and the stone can be lost). The closed basket is pulled back against the choledochoscope, and together the choledochoscope with the basket and the stone (Fig. 21.7) are now withdrawn from the bile duct. The stone is deposited either onto the omentum where it can be retrieved with a grasper via the epigastric port or placed in a small collection bag that is removed at the end of the operation. The basket is removed and the scope advanced again into the duct. Usually the guidewire is not needed this time. If there is any resistance to the advancement of the scope, however, the guidewire should be used again.

The same process is repeated until all stones have been removed. If there are many stones and the scope and the baskets are being passed several times, small debris and gravel can be seen floating in the duct or attached to the duct wall; this will usually pass spontaneously or by flushing the duct with normal saline. When a stone is impacted and has not moved despite flushing manipulations with a guidewire a balloon tip catheter, or a lithotripter, if

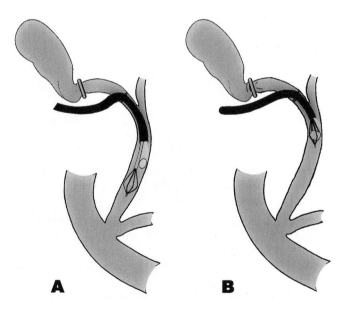

FIGURE 21.6. A. A choledochoscope in the common bile duct with the basket open and a stone lined up be entrapped. B. The basket, closed around the stone, has been pulled back against the choledochoscope. The choledochoscope with the basket and stone are being withdrawn from the duct.

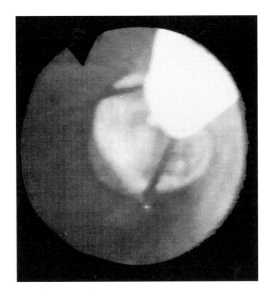

FIGURE 21.7. View through the choledochoscope of a stone entrapped in a basket.

available, could be applied. Either an electrohydrolic or a pulse dye laser lithotripter can be used. The lithotripter probes are passed through the working channel of the choledochoscope and tip of the probe placed on the stone and lithotriptic energy applied with the stone and the probe under direct vision. Care must be taken with the use of a lithotripter as they can cause ductal damage if the tip of the probe is not accurately applied to the stone. Large fragments can now be captured with a basket and the smaller ones flushed into the duodenum.

Once the duct seems cleared of stones, a completion cholangiogram is obtained. If no stones are seen, the cystic duct stump is either clipped, tied off with a pretied loop tie, or suture ligated. If postoperative sphincter spasms or edema of the ampulla are of concern, a tube can be left in the cystic duct; either a special cystic duct tube or a pediatric feeding tube (5F) can be used. The entire tube is brought into the abdomen; the end is placed into the cystic duct and secured with a tie. The end is brought out through one of the trocar sites at the completion of the cholecystectomy, connected to a bag and placed to a passive drainage for 2 to 3 weeks.

If there are residual stones on the completion cholangiogram, the surgeon must decide whether they seem likely to be caught with the aforementioned technique, whether a choledochotomy (laparoscopic or with conversion to an open procedure) is needed, or whether to rely on a postoperative ERC and sphincterotomy for ductal clearance. The decision depends not only on the size and the location of the stone(s) and the patient's condition, but also on the skills of the surgeon and the available endoscopic expertise.

Drains are usually not required after a transcystic common duct exploration. If needed, a closed suction drainage is used. A drain should be considered if the gallbladder was severely inflamed or infected and if the tissue integrity of the cystic duct is questionable. Some surgeons also leave a drain if a tube is left in the cystic duct, to catch any leak of bile when the cystic duct tube is removed, or if a retained stone is left after transcystic exploration for a postoperative ERC.

Postoperative Course

After a successful transcystic CBD exploration and stone removal, with no tubes or drains in place, the postoperative course is the same as that for a laparoscopic cholecystectomy without a common duct exploration. If only a closed-suction drain was placed because of severe cholecystits, it can usually be removed on the first or second postoperative day.

The patient with a tube in the cystic duct who had a clear completion cholangiogram can usually have the drain removed without a repeat cholangiogram if the liver function tests are normal and the drainage via the tube is low (<50 ml/24 h). A limited small bile leak is frequently associated with the removal of the tube. The patient may need pain medication and rest for a few hours after the drain is removed.

Perioperative Problems

Intense inflammation in the porta hepatis can make identification of the anatomy difficult. Although laparoscopic transcystic CBD exploration is probably safer than a laparoscopic choldochotomy when dealing with inflammation in the area, it can still be very difficult to perform. An intraoperative cholangiogram gives valuable information about the location and configuration of the biliary tree and should, in the case of significant inflammation, be done before any significant dissection of the bile ducts. Even so, when the area is very inflamed, dissection of the proximal cystic duct and cystic duct–CBD junction will be difficult in the best of hands. The tissue planes can be obscure and the tissue integrity poor. There is also an increased risk of injuring the CBD under these conditions when passing the scope and instruments. When faced with severe inflammation in the porta hepatis, the surgeon must assess the risks of proceeding with laparoscopic transcystic exploration versus that of conversion to an open procedure or a postoperative ERC and duct clearance. Other reasons for inability to perform a transcystic CBD exploration include obesity, intrahepatic stones, and equipment problems.[8,27]

Tearing of the proximal cystic duct and cystic duct–CBD junction can occur during the dissection or the dilation of the duct and when passing the scope or withdrawing it with a stone in the basket. The tear can usually be closed with an absorbable suture followed by ligation of the cystic duct. A closed-suction drain is placed in the area in case of a bile leak. Injury to the CBD can also occur when using baskets and when applying electrohydraulic lithotripsy to stones in the duct. The best time to recognize ductal injury is at the time of surgery, when it can be either repaired or bypassed. When doing the completion cholangiogram one must look for ductal injury in addition to retained stones.

Bile leaks specifically related to transcystic CBD exploration, may be from the cystic duct orifice, the cystic duct–CBD junction, or the common duct itself. At the completion of the transcystic CBD exploration, the cystic duct should be secured adequately. A suture ligation may be required, in particular when the cystic duct is short, thickened, large, or partly gangrenous and when manipulation of the distal CBD may cause temporary ductal hypertension. Also, if a postoperative ERC is anticipated, a suture ligation of the duct should be considered. When a bile leak is suspected postoperatively, a radionuclide scan may confirm the leak as well as demonstrating a distal obstruction. An abdominal ultrasound or CT scan will help localize possible bile collection and direct the placement of a drain, if necessary. Postoperative ERC is indicated if a relative obstruction of the sphincter of Oddi is suspected, to prevent spontaneous closure of the leak. A stent placed across the sphincter will relieve an obstruction caused by a stone, spasm, or debris. If the leak still does not seal itself or if the patient condition deteriorates and peritonitis is suspected, a surgical exploration is indicated.

Frank pancreatitis following a transcystic CBD exploration is rare.[21,27] Temporary hyperamylasemia without clinical pancreatitis is, however, fairly common. Intravenous glucagon administration during the transcystic CBD exploration and gentle handling of the instruments in the duct should minimize the likelihood of trauma to the distal duct and the sphincter of Oddi. If a clinical pancreatitis develops after a transcystic CBD exploration, it should be managed with standard supportive measures for pancreatitis.

Unsuspected retained stones should be rare if a completion cholangiography shows free contrast passage into the duodenum and no intraluminal filling defects. However, retained stones do occur and should be suspected if the patient develops epigastric pain along with rising liver function tests. Small fragments may pass spontaneously, but usually an ERC is indicated. It will document a clear duct if the stone has passed, but if a stone is present, a sphincterotomy and stone extraction to clear the duct can be done. The success rate of ductal clearance for postoperative ERC is 75% to 95%.[16,27]

Results

LCBDE have been performed for over a decade. As the technique has evolved and the instruments improved, LCBDE for CBD stones, has become a fairly standard procedure. The overall success rate for LCBDE (transcystic approach and choledochotomy) is well above 90%.[1,5,6,9,11,13,14,22,27–30] Several thousands of successful transcystic CBD explorations have been reported, but the transcystic approach can be applied in about 80% of patients with CBD stones. In most series, it is successful in clearing the duct in 70% to 95% of cases.[2,4,7,9,10,13,21,24]

The operative time for laparoscopic cholecystectomy and transcystic CBD exploration is at least an hour longer than that for the cholcystectomy alone. The reported mean operative time for LC and transcystic CBD exploration ranges from 95 to 228 min. The mean length of hospital stay for patients undergoing transcystic CBD exploration is 1.5 to 5.5 days.[7–9,13,14,21,24] Both the reported operative time and hospital stay are longer for laparoscopic choledochotomy than for the transcystic approach, or 175 to 225 min and 2 to 10 days, respectively.[6,9,14,24] In several nonrandomized trials, the morbidity and the mortality were significantly higher for laparoscopic choledochotomy than for laparoscopic transcystic CBD exploration.[6,7,8,14,27]

From our experience of doing an average of six (five to eight) LCBDE per year, for the past 5 years, we have noted how important practising routine intraoperative cholangiogram is for the whole team. For our total of 31 cases of LCBDE using a team approach, we have experienced no retained stones. Three transcystic–CBD explorations were converted to laparoscopic choledochotomy, and two were converted to an open procedure. One was converted to an open procedure because of an impacted stone (the right probes for the lithotripter were not available) and another because of retained stones on the completion cholangiogram in a patient who had previously undergone gastrectomy and Bilroth II anastomosis. Mean operative time overall was 215 min. Postoperatively, one patient developed mild pancreatitis, and three had a temporary hyperamylasemia without clinical panceatitis. One patient developed a bile leak after removal of a cystic duct drainage catheter, requiring an ERC and a stent placement for the leak to seal. These numbers are small; they do show, however, that a laparoscopic surgeon doing 50 to 70 laparoscopic cholecystectomies a year can offer their patients a single-stage approach for their choledocholithiasis with reasonable results.

Conclusion

LCBDE offers a minimally invasive approach for CBD stones in a single procedure. For approximately 80% of patients with CBD stones, the transcystic approach is appropriate and feasible. The success rate for clearing the duct using the transcystic approach is 75% to 95%, the morbidity and mortality rates are low, and the recovery is similar to that for laparoscopic cholecystectomy alone.[2,4,7,9,10,13,21,24] Performing LCBDE does require some additional skills of the surgeon and the team as well as additional equipment and instuments. Therefore, many surgeons performing laparoscopic cholecystectomy are reluctant and uncomfortable performing LCBDE and rely on pre- or postoperative endoscopic stone removal. However, clearing the CBD of stones with a single procedure and a single anaesthetic is clearly easier for the patient and has been shown to be cost-effective.[6,8,9,11,15]

References

1. Petelin JB. Laparoscopic approach to common duct pathology. Am J Surg 1993;165:487–491.
2. Hunter JG. Laparoscopic transcystic common bile duct exploration. Am J Surg 1992;163:53–58.
3. Philips EH, Rosenthal RJ, Carroll BJ, Fallas MJ. Laparoscopic trans-cystic common-bile-duct exploration. Surg Endosc 1994;8:1389–1394.
4. Petelin JB. Clinical results of common bile duct exploration. Endosc Surg 1993;1:125–129.
5. Berci G, Morgenstern L. Laparoscopic management of common bile duct stones. A multi-institutional SAGES study. Society of American Gastrointestinal Endosopic Surgeons. Surg Endosc 1994;8:1168–1174.
6. Rhodes M, Sussman L, Cohen L, Lewis MP. Randomised trial of laparoscopic exploration of common bile duct versus postoperative endoscopic retrograde cholangiography for common bile duct stones. Lancet 1998;351:159–161.
7. Martin I, Bailey I, Rhodes M, et al. Laparoscopic common bile duct exploration. Br J Surg 1998;85:412.
8. Memon MA, Hassaballa H, Memon MI. Laparoscopic common bile duct exploration: the past, the present, and the future. Am J Surg 2000;179:309–315.
9. Lauter D, Froines EJ. Laparoscopic common duct exploration in the management of choledocholithiasis. Am J Surg 2000;179:372–372.
10. Motson RW, Keeling N, Walsh CJ, Finch AC. Laparoscopic exploration of the common bile duct. Gut 1997;40:81A.
11. DePaula AL, Hashiba K, Bafutto M. Laparoscopic management of choledocholithiasis. Surg Endosc 1994;8:1399–1403.
12. Phillips EH, Liberman M, Caroll BJ, et al. Bile duct stones in the laparoscopic cholecystectomy era: is preoperative sphincterotomy necessary? Arch Surg 1995;130:880–886.
13. Berthou JC, Drouard F, Charbonneau P, Mousalier K. Evaluation of laparoscopic management of common bile duct stones in 220 patients. Surg Endosc 1998;12:16–22.
14. Cuschieri A, Lezoche E, Morino M, et al. E.A.E.S. multicenter prospective randomized trial comparing to-stage vs single-stage management of patients with gallstone disease and ductal calculi. Surg Endosc 1999;13(10):952–957.
15. Urbach DR, Khajanchee YS, Jobe BA, et al. Cost-effective management of common bile duct stones. Surg Endosc 2001;15:4–13.
16. Cotton PB. Endoscopic retrograde cholangiopancreatography and laparoscopic cholecystectomy. Am J Surg 1993;165:474–478.
17. Peppelenbosch AG, Naber AHJ, van Goor H. Recurrence rate of common bile duct stones is higher after endoscopic sphincterotomy than after common bile duct exploration in patients below 60 years of age: a longterm follow-up stay. Br J Surg 1998;85:54.
18. Freeman ML, Nelson DB Sherman S, et al. Complications of endoscopic biliary sphincterotomy. N Engl J Med 1996;335:909–963.
19. NIH Consensus Developmental Panel. Gallstones and laparoscopic cholecystectomy. JAMA 1993;269:1018–1024.
20. Koo KP, Traverso LW. Do preoperative indicators predict the presence of common bile duct stones during laparoscopic cholecystectomy. Am J Surg 1996;••:495–499.
21. Carroll BJ, Phillips EH, Rosenthal R, et al. Update on transcystic exploration of the bile duct. Surg Laparosc Endosc 1996;6:453–458.
22. Swanstrom LL, Marcus DR, Kenyon T. Laparoscopic treatment of known choledocholithiasis. Surg Endosc 1996;10:526–528.
23. Gompertz RHK, Rhodes M, Lennard TWJ. Laparoscopic cholangiography: an effective and inexpensive technique. Br J Surg 1992;79:233–234.
24. Hensman C, Crosthwaite G, Cuschieri A. Transcystic biliary decompression after direct laparoscopic exploration of the common bile duct. Surg Endosc 1997;11:1106–1110.
25. Meyer C, Vo Huu Le J, Rohr S, et al. Management of common bile duct stones in a single operation combining laparoscopic cholecystectomy and perioperative endoscopic sphincterotomy. Surg Endosc 1999;13:874–877.
26. Cox MR, Wilson TG, Toouli. Perioperative endoscopic sphincterotomy during laparoscopic cholecystectomy for choledocholithiasis. Br J Surg 1996;82:257–259.
27. Gigot JF, Navez B, Etienne J, et al. A stratified intraoperative surgical strategy is mandatory during laparoscopic common bile duct exploration for common bile duct stones. Surg Endosc 1997;11:772–728.
28. Giurgiu DI, Margulies DR, Carroll BJ, et al. Laparoscopic common bile duct exploration: long-term outcome. Arch Surg 1999;134(8):839–844.
29. Paganini AM, Lezoche E. Follow-up of 161 unselected consecutive patients treated laparoscopically for common bile duct stones. Surg Endosc 1998;12:23–29.
30. Arvidsson D, Berggren U, Haglund U. Laparoscopic common bile duct exploration. Eur J Surg 1998;164:369–375.

22
Laparoscopic Choledochotomy for Common Bile Duct Stones

Monty H. Cox and Thadeus L. Trus

Background and Historical Development

Operations for symptomatic gallbladder disease are among the most common abdominal operations in the United States, with approximately 650,000 cholecystectomies performed each year.[1] Since its introduction in 1987, laparoscopic cholecystectomy has gained widespread acceptance as the procedure of choice for the treatment of symptomatic gallbladder disease. The reported incidence of choledocholithiasis at the time of laparoscopic cholecystectomy is 4% to 15%.[2–6] It has been estimated that as many as 10% of these cases would become symptomatic if left untreated.[7] During the early acceptance phase of laparoscopic cholecystectomy at the end of the 1980s, the equipment and techniques for laparoscopic common bile duct exploration (LCBDE) simply did not exist. Because of this lack of appropriate equipment and, having no experience in performing laparoscopic common bile duct explorations, many surgeons turned to therapeutic endoscopic retrograde cholangiography (ERC) to clear the common bile duct (CBD) of stones either preoperatively or postoperatively. As a result, patients were often subjected to several (minimally) invasive procedures to treat their gallstone and common duct disease.

Intraoperative cholangiography allows surgeons to evaluate the common bile duct. Historically, techniques to remove stones from the bile duct relied on direct access to the common duct using mechanical skills borrowed from retrograde biliary endoscopy and endourology. Specialized equipment and new techniques have given the surgeon several different options for laparoscopic common bile duct exploration. These techniques include fluoroscopically guided transcystic duct exploration with basket retrieval of stones, transcystic choledochoscopy, and laparoscopic choledochotomy with choledochoscopy. This chapter describes the current technique, results, and potential pitfalls and complications of laparoscopic common bile duct exploration.

Cholangiography

Routine intraoperative cholangiography is advised for several reasons: it defines biliary anatomy and pathology, and it may decrease the occurrence or severity of common bile duct injury, and it allows common duct stones to be identified.[8] Also, by performing cholangiography routinely, the surgeon becomes proficient at bile duct access. Various catheters and specialized clamps are available. Regardless of the type of catheter used, one should use a digital C-arm unit with real-time fluoroscopy. "Spot" films do not allow the same visualization of the duct and impede any fluoroguided stone extractions.

Cholangiography may be performed using several techniques. One method is direct puncture of the gallbladder fundus and injection of contrast, filling the gallbladder and biliary tree (Fig. 22.1A). Alternatively, a specialized cholangiogram clamp (Nashville Surgical Instruments, Springfield, TN, USA) may be used to isolate the gallbladder infundibulum for cannulation and contrast injection, thus preventing retrograde filling of the gallbladder with contrast (Fig. 22.1B). The author's preferred method for cholangiography is direct cholangiogram catheter cannulation of the cystic duct (transcystic cholangiography; Fig. 22.1C). There are several reasons why this transcystic approach is favored over cholangiography performed via the gallbladder. (1) Stones in the gallbladder may be flushed into the common bile duct (CBD) during injection of contrast into the fundus. (2) Stones may be impacted in the neck of the gallbladder, preventing contrast flow into the CBD. (3) If CBD stones are found, laparoscopic techniques for stone retrieval involve exposure and cannulation of the cystic duct, which would have already been performed if one routinely used a transcystic approach.

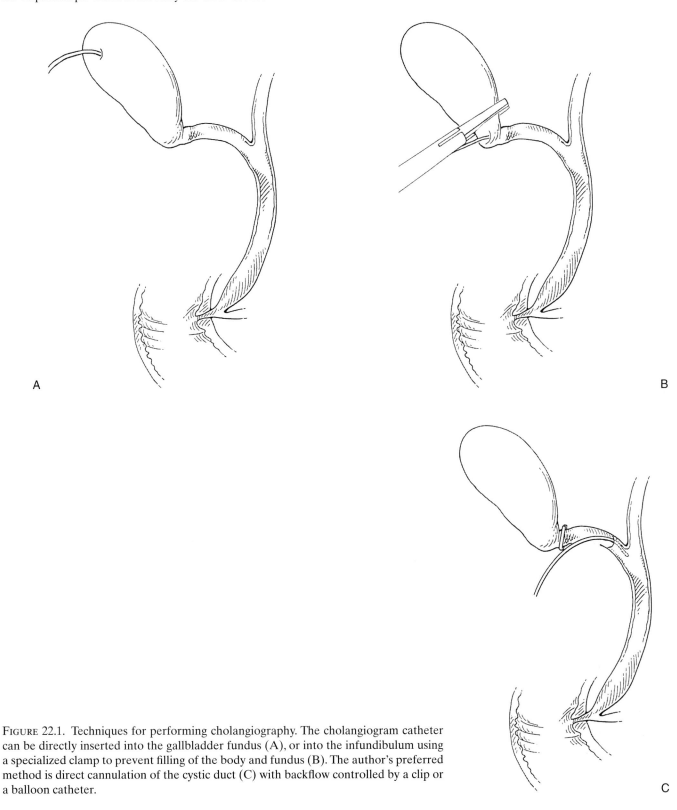

A

B

C

FIGURE 22.1. Techniques for performing cholangiography. The cholangiogram catheter can be directly inserted into the gallbladder fundus (A), or into the infundibulum using a specialized clamp to prevent filling of the body and fundus (B). The author's preferred method is direct cannulation of the cystic duct (C) with backflow controlled by a clip or a balloon catheter.

Laparoscopic cholecystectomy is initiated using standard trocar placement. The right upper quadrant port should be lateral to the anterior axillary line, just below the costal margin (Fig. 22.2). The cystic duct is skeletonized at the gallbladder–cystic duct junction. A hemoclip is applied proximally, and a small cystic duct ductotomy is made using microshears. The cholangiogram catheter (Cook Surgical, Bloomington, IN, USA) is

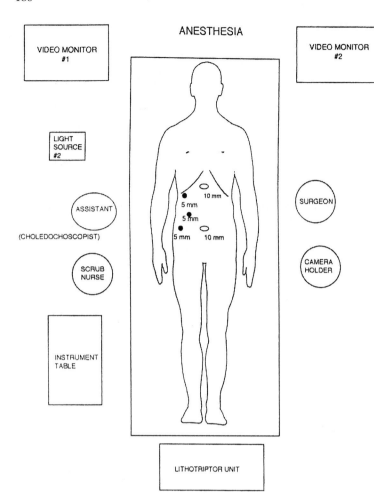

FIGURE 22.2. Recommended trocar placement and positioning of operating personnel and equipment for laparoscopic choledochotomy. Trocar placement is similar to standard laparoscopic cholecystectomy; an additional right epigastric site may be used for passage of a cholangiography catheter as well as the choledochoscope.

introduced into the abdomen percutaneously and fed into the cystic duct. Alternatively, it can be introduced through the right lateral trocar using a cholangiogram clamp (Karl Storz, Culver City, CA, USA).

Real-time imaging is performed while half-strength renograffin is introduced through the cholangiography catheter. False-positive cholangiograms may be a result of air bubbles in the duct or spasm of the sphincter of Oddi. Filling defects can be confirmed by obtaining views in different planes, where necessary.

When a filling defect is seen on cholangiogram, glucagon (1 mg, IV) should be administered immediately to relax the sphincter of Oddi before any instrument or basket is passed through this sphincter. The duct is then vigorously irrigated through the cholangiogram catheter with 10 ml normal saline to flush the CBD stone. The use of 1% lidocaine as an irrigant has also been described to further relax the sphincter. Fluoroscopy is used during irrigation to visualize stone movement and possible passage. Repeat cholangiography should then be performed to evaluate whether the stone has passed.

The necessary equipment for choledocotomy and choledochoscopy should be stored together on a separate

cart to minimize the amount of preparation time for CBD exploration. Ideal positioning of equipment and assistants is illustrated in Figure 22.2. It should be emphasized that the choledochoscope must be attached to a separate light source and camera. The image should be viewed on a viewed on a separate monitor or a split-screen monitor to allow simultaneous visualization of the laparoscopic and choledochoscope images. Although choledochoscopy can be performed by simply moving the camera from the laparoscope to the choledochoscope, this is not recommended. The laparoscope view should be fixed on the choledochoscope as it enters the cystic duct to avoid tearing of the cystic duct by excessive torque on the scope.

Choledochoscopy is performed by dissecting the cystic duct within 1 cm of the junction with the CBD. A cystic duct ductotomy is then performed. A guidewire is advanced into the cystic duct through a 3-mm reducer in the right subcostal trocar. Alternatively, if the cholangiogram catheter was placed percutaneously, the site can be dilated and a Berci cystic duct introducer (Cook Surgical) can be placed to pass the choledochoscope. The cystic duct is often too small to allow passage of the

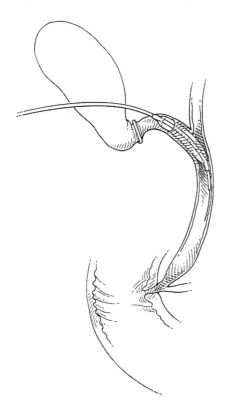

FIGURE 22.3. Balloon dilation of the cystic duct. The distal end of the balloon lies at the cystic duct–common bile duct junction, and approximately one-third of the length of the balloon protrudes from the cystic duct when the balloon is inflated.

choledochoscope and therefore must be dilated (in approximately 50% of cases). A deflated balloon catheter (5–8 mm in diameter; Cook Surgical) is advanced over the guidewire into the cystic duct until its distal end is at the cystic duct–common bile duct junction. Approximately one-third of the balloon will protrude from the cystic duct (Fig. 22.3). The balloon is then inflated to 3 to 10 atmospheres (depending on the size of the balloon) for 5 min. Direct visualization is maintained with the laparoscope to monitor for laceration of the cystic duct. If the cystic duct begins to tear during dilation, the balloon should be deflated and exchanged. Excessive traction on the gallbladder should also be avoided during balloon dilation to prevent cystic duct avulsion.

Maximum dilation of the duct should not exceed 8 mm; stones larger than 8 mm should be handled with lithotripsy, choledochotomy, or sphincterotomy. When the duct has been adequately dilated, the balloon is deflated and removed, leaving the guidewire in place. The choledochoscope can then be advanced over the guidewire into the dilated duct. Continuous saline irrigation through the choledochoscope under pressure no greater than 50 to 100 mmHg is used to facilitate visualization as the choledochoscope is advanced.

On visualizing a stone, the Segura stone basket is passed through the working channel of the choledochoscope. The basket is then opened so that the middle of the basket is aligned with the middle of the stone. Careful manipulation of the basket in an in-and-out manner aids in stone capture. When the stone is within the basket wires, the basket is closed around the stone, and the stone is pulled to the tip of the scope. Both the scope and basket are then withdrawn in unison (Fig. 22.4). If multiple stones are present, the process is repeated as necessary. The stones may be placed on the surface of the liver or in a plastic collection sac for retrieval at the completion of bile duct exploration. When the duct is cleared of stones, the scope should easily pass into the duodenum (additional glucagon may be used if more than 15 min has elapsed since the initial injection). Completion cholangiography is performed, and the cystic duct is closed with a pretied ligature.

Impacted stones can occasionally be dislodged with a Fogarty catheter if basket manipulation is unsuccessful. If use of the Fogarty catheter is unsuccessful, electrohydraulic lithotripsy or antegrade sphincterotomy may be performed. Hepatic duct visualization is usually unnecessary, because 90% of bile duct stones are found distal to the entry of the cystic duct. When a proximal bile duct stone is found, however, visualization can be difficult

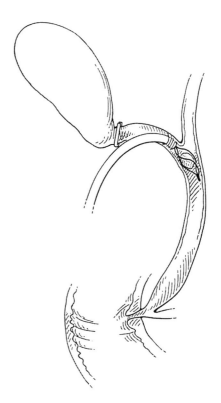

FIGURE 22.4. Transcystic choledochoscopy. The basket is closed around the stone, and the choledochoscope and basket are then withdrawn in unison.

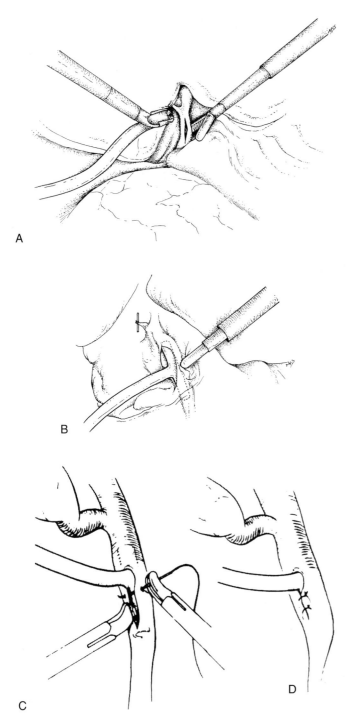

A

B

C

D

FIGURE 22.5. Repair of choledochotomy. A T-tube is placed in the common bile duct (A,B), and the choledochotomy is repaired using interrupted sutures (C,D).

because of the acute angle of the hepatic duct–cystic duct junction. Cannulation of the proximal bile duct system can sometimes be achieved by inferior traction on Hartmann's pouch to alter the angle of the cystic duct. Stones may also be encouraged to drop into the CBD by placing the patient in reverse Trendelenburg position or using

irrigation. If the stone is inaccessible, transcystic exploration should be abandoned for laparoscopic choledochotomy or postoperative ERC. To facilitate cannulation of the CBD during postoperative ERC, a guidewire may be left in the duct at operation, with the tip extending though the papilla into the duodenum.

Laparoscopic Choledochotomy

Up to 10% of CBD stones are not extractable through a transcystic approach. In general, if a stone is very large (8mm), the cystic duct is unfavorable (small or spiral), or a stone is in an inaccessible position in the proximal bile ducts, attempts at transcystic exploration should be abandoned and laparoscopic choledochotomy performed. One should not attempt choledochotomy on a normal-sized common bile duct. The additional equipment needed includes laparoscopic needle drivers (Olympus, Lake Success, NY, USA), fine suture such as 4-0 Vicryl (Ethicon, Cincinnati, OH, USA), and both a T-tube and closed suction drain.

With the gallbladder retracted cephalad, the dissection of the CBD is extended approximately 1 to 2cm distal to the junction of the cystic duct. Stay sutures, as used in open bile duct exploration, are usually not necessary with the laparoscopic technique. The choledochotomy is made in a vertical fashion with microscissors or an arthroscopy scalpel. The duct is then flushed wiht saline to remove any loose stones (a Fogarty catheter may also be used). The choledochoscope is passed directly into the CBD through the choledochotomy, and stones are removed with a basket retrieval technique similar to transcystic choledochoscopy. After clearing the duct of stones, a 12F or 14F T-tube is inserted into the choledochotomy and the ductal defect is closed with interrupted sutures (Fig. 22.5). Placing the camera in the epigastric port and suturing through the umbilical port may facilitate closure of the duct. The T-tube is brought out through the subcostal port, and a 7F closed-suction drain is brought out through the most lateral port.

Results of Laparoscopic Common Bile Duct Exploration

Laparoscopic common bile duct exploration is a safe and effective method of treating CBD stones in patients with symptomatic cholelithiasis. Several recently published series have reported that stones in the CBD can be successfully cleared laparoscopically in 80% to 96% of cases.[4,9–19] In most series the stones were cleared using a transcystic approach. Generally, open CBD clearance or postoperative ERCP was required in fewer than 5% of cases (Table 22.1). Complications were generally minor,

TABLE 22.1. Successful stone clearance rates, morbidity and mortality for laparoscopic and open common bile duct exploration.

Study	Total cases	Lap CBDE		Open CBDE		Morbidity		Mortality	
		No.	%	No.	%	No.	%	No.	%
Hunter (1992)[4]	20	17	85.0	3	15.0	1	5.0	0	0.0
DePaula (1994)[9]	114	108	94.7	3	2.6	7	6.1	1	0.9
Rhodes (1995)[10]	129	119	92.2	2	1.6	7	5.4	0	0.0
Phillips (1995)[11]	145	116	80.0	4	2.8	18	12.4	0	0.0
Lezoche (1996)[12]	100	96	96.0	4	4.0	7	7.0	1	1.0
Gigot (1997)[13]	92	77	83.7	11	12.0	14	15.2	2	2.2
Millat (1997)[14]	236	208	88.1	2	0.8	31	13.1	1	0.4
Drouard (1997)[15]	161	152	94.4	4	2.5	12	7.5	0	0.0
Rhodes (1998)[16]	40	30	75.0	1	2.5	7	17.5	0	0.0
Ferguson (1998)[17]	25	20	80.0	1	4.0	0	0.0	0	0.0
Berthou (1998)[18]	220	210	95.5	3	1.4	20	9.1	4	1.8
Snow (1999)[19]	136	114	83.8	11	8.1	13	9.6	2	1.5

Lap CBDE, laparoscopic common bile duct exploration; Open CBDE, open common bile duct exploration.

with transient hyperamylasemia being the most frequently encountered.

With the evolution of laparoscopic equipment and techniques, the approach to management of CBD stones has changed. In the past, many surgeons relied on preoperative or postoperative ERCP and endoscopic sphincterotomy. This trend was a result of unfamiliarity with the technique or unavailability of the necessary equipment for laparoscopic CBD exploration. However, endoscopic sphincterotomy is associated with a 1% mortality rate and an 8% complication rate, including bleeding, perforation, pancreatitis, and papillary stenosis.[20] Failure rates of up to 30% have been reported with endoscopic sphincterotomy. In addition, ERCP has been shown to be unnecessary in up to 85% of cases when performed for preoperative suspicion of CBD stones.[21] Therefore, the use of preoperative or postoperative ERCP can now be avoided in most cases. Preoperative ERCP should be

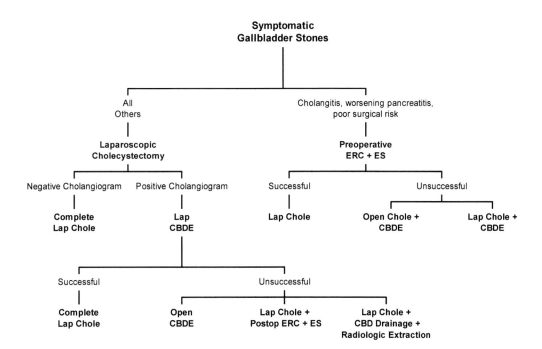

FIGURE 22.6. Recommended algorithm for the treatment of symptomatic gallbladder disease. Preoperative endoscopic retrograde cholangiography with endoscopic sphincterotomy (*ERC + ES*) is used selectively for patients with cholangitis, worsening pancreatitis, or poor surgical risk. If laparoscopic common bile duct exploration (*Lap CBDE*) is unsuccessful, alternatives include *Open CBDE*, postoperative ERC + ES, or common bile duct drainage with subsequent postoperative radiological extraction.

used selectively, such as in patients with cholangitis, or worsening pancreatitis, or those who are poor surgical risks. If the gallbladder is visualized at ERCP, only 10% to 15% of patients develop symptomatic cholelithiasis once the duct has been cleared of stones.[22] If the gallbladder does not fill with contrast at ERCP, the gallbladder should be removed, as most of these patients will have continued symptoms.

Several alternatives exist when laparoscopic techniques fail to clear the duct, including open CBD exploration, postoperative ERCP with endoscopic sphincterotomy, or laparoscopic bile duct drainage followed by radiographically guided stone extraction through the drainage catheter tract. The choice among these alternatives will be based on the skills and experience of the surgeon, the availability of necessary equipment, and the availability and reliability of nonsurgical alternatives. A suggested algorithm for management of common bile duct stones is presented in Figure 22.6.

Laparoscopic management of choledocholithiasis at the time of laparoscopic cholecystectomy is a safe and effective, single-stage treatment. Given the high success rate of laparoscopic common bile duct exploration, preoperative or postoperative ERCP and endoscopic sphincterotomy is not required in most cases.

References

1. Ellison EC, Carey LC. Cholecystostomy, cholecystectomy, and intraoperative evaluation of the biliary tree. In: Nyhus LM, Baker RJ, Fischer JF (eds) Mastery of Surgery, 3rd Ed. Boston: Little, Brown, 1997:1086–1093.
2. Stimpson REJ, Way LW. Common duct stones. In: Moody FG, Carey LC, Jones RC, et al. (eds) Surgical Treatment of Digestive Diseases. Chicago: Year Book Medical, 1986:306–322.
3. Hermann R. The spectrum of biliary stone disease. Am J Surg 1991;161:171–173.
4. Hunter JG. Laparoscopic transcystic common bile duct exploration. Am J Surg 1992;163:53–58.
5. Helms B, Czarnetski HD. Strategy and technique of laparoscopic common bile duct exploration. Endosc Surg 1993;1: 117–124.
6. Rosenthal RJ, Rossi RL, Martin RF. Options and strategies for the management of choledocholithiasis. World J Surg 1999; 22:1125–1132.
7. McEntee G, Grace PA, Bouchier-Hayes D. Laparoscopic cholecystectomy and the common bile duct. Br J Surg 1991;78:385–386.
8. Kullman E, Borch K, Lindstrom E, Svanvik J, Anderberg B. Value of routine intraoperative cholangiography in detecting aberrant bile ducts and bile duct injuries during laparoscopic cholecystectomy. Br J Surg 1996;83:171–175.
9. DePaula AL, Hashiba K, Bafutto M. Laparoscopic management of choledocholithiasis. Surg Endosc 1994;8(12): 1399–1403.
10. Rhodes M, Nathanson L, O'Rourke N, Fielding G. Laparoscopic exploration of the common bile duct: lessons learned from 129 consecutive patients. Br J Surg 1995;82(5):666–668.
11. Phillips EH, Liberman M, Carroll BJ, Fallas MJ, Rosenthal RJ, Hiatt JR. Bile duct stones in the laparoscopic era: is preoperative sphincterotomy necessary? Arch Surg 1995;130: 880–885.
12. Lezoche E, Pananini AM, Carlei F, Feliciotti F, Lomanto D, Buerrieri M. Laparoscopic treatment of gallbladder and common bile duct stones: a prospective study. World J Surg 1996;20:535–541.
13. Gigot JF, Navez B, Etienne J, et al. A stratified intraoperative surgical strategy is mandatory during laparoscopic common bile duct exploration for common bile duct stones: lessons and limits from an initial experience of 92 patients. Surg Endosc 1997;11(7):722–728.
14. Millat B, Atger J, Deleuze A, et al. Laparoscopic treatment for choledocholithiasis: a prospective evaluation in 247 consecutive unselected patients. Hepato-Gastroenterology 1997;44(13):28–34.
15. Drouard F, Passone-Szerzyna N, Berthou JC. Laparoscopic treatment of common bile duct stones. Hepato-Gastroenterology 1997;44(13):16–21.
16. Rhodes M, Sussman L, Cohen L, Lewis MP. Randomised trial of laparoscopic exploration of common bile duct versus postoperative endoscopic retrograde cholangiography for common bile duct stones. Lancet 1998;351:159–161.
17. Ferguson CM. Laparoscopic common bile duct exploration: practical application. Arch Surg 1998;133:448–451.
18. Berthou JC, Drouard F, Charbonneau P, Moussalier K. Evaluation of laparoscopic management of common bile duct stones in 220 patients. Surg Endosc 1998;12(1):16–22.
19. Snow LL, Weinstein LS, Hannon JK, Lane DR. Management of bile duct stones in 1572 patients undergoing laparoscopic cholecystectomy. Am Surg 1999;65:530–547.
20. Cotton PB, Lehman G, Vennes J, et al. Endoscopic sphincterotomy complications and their management: an attempt at consensus. Gastrointest Endosc 1991;37:383–393.
21. Southern Surgeons Club. A prospective analysis of 1,518 laparoscopic cholecystectomies. N Engl J Med 1991;324: 1073–1078.
22. Safrany L, Cotton PB. Endoscopic management of choledocholithiasis. Surg Clin N Am 1982;62:825–836.

23
Laparoscopic Management of Difficult Common Bile Duct Stones

Daniel M. Herron

During the first few years after the introduction of laparoscopic cholecystectomy, the cornerstone of management of common bile duct stones was avoidance. Surgeons relied heavily upon pre- and postoperative endoscopic retrograde cholangiopancreatography (ERCP) with papillotomy for the diagnosis and treatment of choledocholithiasis. As surgeons' technical skills evolved, the laparoscopic common duct exploration became an increasingly desirable alternative. At this time, laparoscopic transcystic common duct exploration and laparoscopic choledochotomy are recognized as safe and effective techniques that retain the benefits of minimal access while avoiding the need for a second procedure.

In the simplest scenario of laparoscopic common duct exploration, small stones near the cystic duct opening or choledochotomy site may be "milked out" using a laparoscopic grasper. Moderate-sized stones and those farther down the duct may often be flushed through the ampulla using an irrigating catheter. Larger stones, which may become impacted within the duct, are removed using balloon catheters and endoscopic baskets under fluoroscopic or choledochoscopic guidance.

Unfortunately, there remain difficult stones that elude these methods of retrieval. Such stones are difficult because of either their size or their location. Large stones, 1 cm or more in diameter, present several problems. First, because their diameter is greater than that of the cystic duct, a choledochotomy is mandatory. Second, these stones are more likely to become impacted within the common duct, potentially preventing the passage of balloon catheters or baskets past the stone. Even if these instruments can be appropriately positioned, the stone may be so firmly lodged within the inflamed and friable duct wall that it is unsafe to dislodge them with traction alone.

A nonimpacted stone may present difficulty if it lies in an inaccessible location. A stone may form proximal to a strictured common duct, beyond the reach of even small-diameter choledochoscopes. Or, a stone may be present in the hepatic duct after a choledochoenteric anastomosis, which may preclude endoscopic access.

In these situations it is helpful for the surgeon to have access to either intracorporeal or extracorporeal lithotripsy (from Greek, *lithos*—stone, and *tripsis*—to crush). Lithotriptors consist of an energy source and a means of transmitting the energy to the stone, causing fragmentation. Intracorporeal lithotriptors, which require placing a probe into the biliary tree, can be used in the operating room during the initial common duct exploration. Extracorporeal lithotripsy is useful postoperatively. After fragmentation, small stone particles frequently pass through the ampulla spontaneously. Fragments remaining within the common duct will be more amenable to traditional retrieval techniques because of their reduced size.

Intracorporeal Lithotripsy

Mechanical Lithotripsy

The simplest form of lithotripsy relies upon the direct application of mechanical force to the gallstones. A wire lithotripter, functionally similar to an endoscopic retrieval basket, may be inserted into the common duct under choledochoscopic or fluoroscopic guidance. The heavy wire noose is then maneuvered around the stone and tightened until the enclosed stone fractures. The resultant fragments can then be cleared from the common duct using standard stone retrieval techniques or copious irrigation.

The elegance of these catheters lies in their simplicity. No external power source is needed; the energy to crush the stones is provided by the surgeon's hand. Thus, this technique is significantly less expensive than other methods described here. Additionally, the procedure is effective: a 1997 series of 162 patients treated with endo-

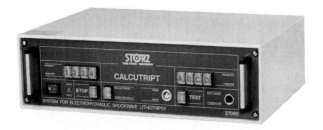

FIGURE 23.1. Electrohydraulic lithotriptor (EHL) unit. (Courtesy of Karl Storz Endoscopy-America Inc., Culver City, CA, USA.)

scopic mechanical lithotripsy reported an 84% stone clearance rate.[1]

Unfortunately, the technique presents several major problems. To transmit adequate force to the wire noose, the outer sheath must be able to resist the significant compressive force generated when the surgeon applies pressure to the handle. Accordingly, these catheters are quite heavy in their construction, making them bulkier and stiffer than the more commonly used retrieval baskets and thus suboptimal for a transcystic approach to the common duct. Also, even with their sturdy construction, the noose may jam while being tightened around the stone, creating the unfortunate situation in which the catheter is strongly affixed to an impacted stone that fails to fracture. A third disadvantage lies in the need to position the tip of the mechanical lithotripter *beyond* the stone; this is impossible in 14% of cases.[1] If the calculus is severely impacted, this maneuver may risk perforation of the duct wall.[2]

Electrohydraulic Lithotripsy

Electrohydraulic lithotripsy, or EHL, overcomes many of the disadvantages of the mechanical lithotriptor. The technology was initially developed in the Soviet Union for industrial use and was adapted for medical purposes in 1968 for the treatment of urinary bladder calculi. In 1975, the technique was applied to the biliary tree.[3] Dr. Arregui first reported its use laparoscopically in 1992.[4]

EHL causes fragmentation by creating a small explosion in immediate proximity to the stone. An electrical charge is built up in a capacitor within the power supply unit (Fig. 23.1). This energy is then discharged into a thin coaxial cable inserted through the irrigating port of the choledochoscope (Fig. 23.2). The resultant spark at the tip of the probe vaporizes a small amount of surrounding fluid and creates a high-amplitude shock wave. If the tip of the probe is located near the stone, the force of this shock may be sufficient to cause fragmentation. Because the energy transmitted by the shock waves dissipates with the square of the distance, structures further removed

from the spark discharge, namely the common duct wall, are relatively protected from injury.[5]

Certain guidelines must be followed if this technique is to be used safely. The tip of the EHL electrode must be kept continuously visualized during spark discharge to avoid injury to the common duct wall. It must remain approximately 6mm beyond the end of the choledochoscope to avoid damage to its optics. The tip of the electrode should be placed close to the stone, within 1 to 2mm, but not in direct contact, to ensure that enough fluid is present at the tip to create a shock wave upon vaporization. Because the destruction of stones creates clouds of suspended particles, frequent or continuous irrigation is essential for adequate visualization.

The violent discharge of energy from the EHL probe destroys the electrode after less than 1 min of continuous use. Thus, to maximize the life of the electrode and minimize the risk of common duct injury, the surgeon should activate the device in short bursts and use the lowest possible power setting. If the stone does not fragment adequately after several applications at a low power level, the power can be increased as needed. The goal of EHL is not to completely disintegrate the stone but to break it into fragments that are more easily managed by traditional common duct techniques such as basket retrieval. The essential caveat is that the tip of the probe must be kept away from the duct wall at all times. Brief contact may result in fibrosis of the wall, whereas more prolonged contact, particularly with the probe perpendicular to the wall, will result in perforation.[5]

The equipment required for EHL is relatively inexpensive when compared to lasers or extracorporeal

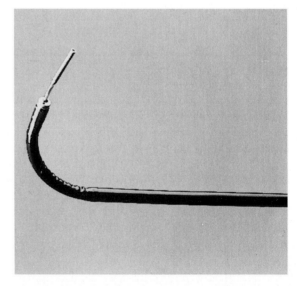

FIGURE 23.2. EHL probe emerging from working channel of choledochoscope. (Courtesy of Karl Storz Endoscopy-America Inc., Culver City, CA, USA.)

lithotriptors. The power unit costs approximately U.S. $10,000; the disposable probes present an additional expense. Because the electrodes are quite flexible and thin enough to be placed through the irrigation port of a choledochoscope, the technique is well suited to laparoscopic common duct exploration. If used correctly, EHL will fragment large or impacted stones quickly and safely.

Dr. Sheen-Chen reported a series of 10 patients in 1995 in which EHL was used to treat impacted distal common bile duct stones. All 10 patients experienced successful clearance of their ducts; the sole morbidity was mild hemobilia in 1 patient, which resolved spontaneously.[6] In another study, Dr. Arregui reviewed the treatment of 36 patients with suspected choledocholithiasis. Two patients had stones severely enough impacted to resist all attempts at removal via traditional techniques. EHL was successful in fracturing the stones endoscopically in both these cases.[4]

Laser Lithotripsy

In the early 1990s, a number of investigators evaluated the laser as an energy source for intracorporeal lithotripsy. Several different types of lasers have been described for this purpose. The coumarin green dye laser (wavelength, 504nm) is well absorbed by biliary calculi but poorly absorbed by hemoglobin and hemoglobin-containing tissues. A rhodamine-6G dye laser (wavelength, 594nm) creates an orange-red light; this has been used with a backscatter detector that automatically shuts off the laser if it is not pointed toward a stone.[7,8] These devices consist of a large housing for the laser hardware, which is connected by a series of mirrors to a flexible fiber optic that directs the beam intracorporeally (Fig. 23.3). Although the total energy contained in a single laser pulse is quite small, 60 to 100mJ, the peak power is as great as 100,000 watts.[9] The intense heat created when the laser beam is absorbed by the stone produces a plasma field and a resultant acoustic shock wave, which propagates through the stone with sufficient energy to cause fragmentation.

A holmium laser (wavelength, 2100nm) has also been described that functions in a different manner. The infrared energy produced by this device melts a hole in the stone; as fluid in the hole vaporizes, the internal pressure fractures the gallstone. This type of laser may have greater application with pure white cholesterol stones, which fail to absorb shorter wavelengths well.[10]

Proponents of the laser cite several advantages over EHL. The quartz fiber used to transmit the laser beam may be as small as a third of a millimeter in diameter and thus fits easily through the irrigation channel of the chole-dochoscope, while leaving adequate room for irrigant. The selective absorption of laser energy by different

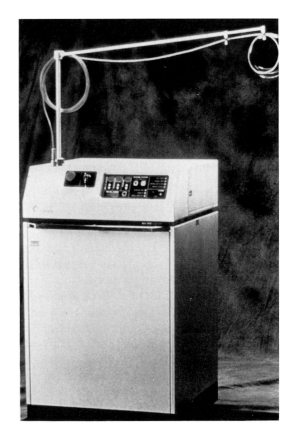

FIGURE 23.3. Laser lithotriptor unit. (Courtesy of Candela Corporation, Wayland, MA, USA.)

tissues is another theoretical benefit. A 1993 animal study demonstrated less mucosal injury after contact with the 504-nm laser than with the EHL probe.[11]

In 1992, Dr. Josephs treated eight patients with retained common bile duct stones using a 504-nm pulsed-dye laser inserted through a choledochoscope in a T-tube tract.[12] Using a pulse of 100 to 120mJ at a rate of 3 to 5 Hz, fragmentation was achieved in every patient. This series demonstrated a single morbidity: one patient manifested transient bacteremia after the procedure, which resolved with intravenous antibiotic therapy. In a 1995 study utilizing the rhodamine-6G dye laser, 16 patients with difficult bile duct stones were treated. Fragmentation was achieved in all 16 patients and complete bile duct clearance in 88%.[13]

Several precautions must be observed with the fine quartz fibers used to transmit the laser beam. The fibers are quite brittle and can break off within the common duct if forced against the duct wall, leaving a potentially lithogenic nidus behind. Additionally, because the fibers may perforate the side of the duct even without the laser activated, they must be kept under direct view at all times. The primary drawback to laser lithotripsy lies in its cost; the laser unit itself costs approximately U.S. $250,000. There is also a significant cost associated with the maintenance of this technically complex unit and its associated dye replacements. Additionally, special safety training is required for all personnel who will be exposed to laser radiation. Because the units are considerably larger than EHL devices, they are more difficult to position within the operating room and to store when not in use.

Extracorporeal Lithotripsy

EHL and laser lithotripsy both require access to the biliary tree. They are useless if such access is not available through the laparoscope or choledochoscope, as when stones form above a tight biliary stricture. In such situations extracorporeal shockwave lithotripsy (ESWL) may be of benefit. In ESWL, a shock wave is generated outside the patient's body using an electrostatic spark, an electromagnet, or a piezoelectric discharge. The high-amplitude wave is then focused, through one of a variety of mechanisms, onto the desired target. Early ESWL devices required the patient be immersed within a water bath to provide adequate acoustic coupling between the shockwave generator and the patient's abdomen. More recent machines allow the patient to lie flat on a table, with only a thin film of oil between the device and the patient's skin.

ESWL was first used in Germany in 1980 to destroy renal calculi with considerable success. Its use as a treatment for symptomatic cholelithiasis received considerable attention in the late 1980s before the widespread acceptance of laparoscopic cholecystectomy. A lead article in the *New England Journal of Medicine* in 1988 described the treatment of 175 patients with a combination of ESWL and oral litholytic therapy (chenodeoxycholic and ursodeoxycholic acid).[14] More than 90% of patients demonstrated disintegration of their gallstones after 12 to 18 months of therapy. Because of the significant length of time required for treatment for cholelithiasis, this technique fell out of favor following the general acceptance of laparoscopic cholecystectomy.

Although ESWL is no longer used for the treatment of cholelithiasis, it remains an important tool in the treatment of hard-to-reach common duct stones because it does not require direct access to the biliary tree. Current indications for its use include the treatment of stones above a common bile duct stricture and the nonoperative fragmentation of stones beyond the reach of the endoscope, such as in the patient with difficult Billroth II anatomy. It also provides a nonoperative alternative for the treatment of debilitated patients who cannot tolerate an invasive surgical procedure.

Unfortunately, ESWL is not as effective in treating biliary calculi as it is with renal calculi. A 1988 study of 50 patients evaluated ESWL in conjunction with oral dis-

solution therapy for the treatment of biliary calculi in the extra- and intrahepatic ducts.[15] After treatment, spontaneous passage of stone fragments occurred in only 10% of the subjects. However, ESWL fragmented impacted stones such that 86% could subsequently be removed endoscopically. A more recent study involved 27 patients with large common duct stones who had failed treatment with endoscopic sphincterotomy.[16] After treatment with piezoelectric-generated ESWL, stone clearance was achieved in 18 of the 27 patients (67%).

Alternative Techniques

Lithotripsy devices, whether intra- or extracorporeal, provide an effective means of treating the difficult impacted common duct stone when traditional techniques fail. Unfortunately, EHL, laser lithotripsy, and ESWL are unavailable in many hospital settings. Several simpler and less expensive techniques are more commonly available that may be useful adjuncts in treating the difficult impacted stone.

Pharmacological Relaxation of the Ampulla

The administration of intravenous glucagon (1 µg) will relax the ampulla of Vater. If this is followed by a brisk saline infusion through the duct, the duct may be cleared of stones up to 76% of the time.[17]

Transampullary Instrumentation

A flexible guidewire may be placed through the ampulla to facilitate successful ERCP and sphincterotomy postoperatively. The wire may be inserted through the cystic duct stump, and passed through the common duct and into the duodenum under fluoroscopic guidance. If an appropriate wire is not available, a cholangiogram catheter may be used. The cystic duct opening is then gently clipped or ligated around the wire, which is brought out of the abdomen through a lateral trocar site. Postoperatively, the endoscopist may use the wire as a guide over which to pass the ERCP catheter and sphincterotome. The ERCP may also be performed intraoperatively, but this is difficult with the patient in the supine position and may add 2h or more to the operation.[18]

A sphincterotomy may also be performed via an antegrade approach. First described by DePaula in 1993, laparoscopic antegrade sphincterotomy may be performed by threading an endoscopic sphincterotome through the cystic duct or choledochotomy.[19] After a side-viewing duodenoscope is used to confirm the positioning of the sphincterotome, the sphincter is divided with a cautery wire. Curet et al. reported the use of this technique in six patients in 1995.[20] Although transient asymptomatic hyperamylasemia occurred in half the patients, all had successful clearance of their common duct.

Several authors have advocated transcystic or transcholedochal dilatation of the sphincter of Oddi using a balloon catheter.[21,22] Proponents of this technique believe that it achieves adequate clearance of common duct stones while eliminating the risk of cautery to the ampulla. Although duct clearance rates of up to 85% have been described with this method, balloon-induced trauma to the ampulla results in hyperamylasemia or mild pancreatitis in 15% of patients.[21,23]

Postoperative Choledochal Access and Dissolution Therapy

A T-tube or drainage catheter may also be left in the common duct; this will permit both biliary drainage as well as postoperative access to the duct. If the cystic duct is of adequate size, a 14F red rubber catheter may be inserted through it. If a choledochotomy has been performed, a T-tube may be placed and the choledochotomy closed around it. Once a tract has formed, the stone may then be removed by an interventional radiologist under fluoroscopic guidance.

The presence of a catheter within the common duct also opens the possibility of chemical dissolution therapy. Although methyl-*tert*-butyl-ether (MTBE) has been demonstrated to provide excellent dissolution, it is difficult to use due to its volatility. Additionally, its use is associated with significant morbidity, including hemolysis, necrosis, and permanent dilatation of the bile duct in up to 79% of patients.[24] Mono-octanoin has been more widely used because of its greater safety, but it is successful in only 28% of cases.[25] Its efficacy may be improved by heating the chemical and providing high flow around the stone, but this adds complexity and expense to the therapy.[26]

Conclusion

Most common bile duct stones may be treated laparoscopically through a transcystic common bile duct exploration. If common duct stones are large in size or number, a laparoscopic choledochotomy may be more effective. In centers where the technology is available, intracorporeal and extracorporeal lithotripsy provide a valuable means of treating stones that are severely impacted or beyond the reach of the endoscope. If such devices are unavailable, pharmacological or mechanical dilatation of the ampulla or transampullary instrumentation may be helpful.

References

1. Cipolletta L, Costamagna G, Bianco MA, et al. Endoscopic mechanical lithotripsy of difficult common bile duct stones. Br J Surg 1997;84:1407–1409.
2. Cotton PB, Lehman G, Vennes JA. Endoscopic sphincterotomy complications and their management: an attempt at consensus. Gastrointest Endosc 1991;37:383–390.
3. Burhenne HJ. Electrohydraulic fragmentation of retained common duct stones. Radiology 1975;117:721–722.
4. Arregui ME, Davis CJ, Arkush AM, et al. Laparoscopic cholecystectomy combined with endoscopic sphincterotomy and stone extraction or laparoscopic choledochoscopy and electrohydraulic lithotripsy for management of cholelithiasis with choledocholithiasis. Surg Endosc 1992; 6:10–15.
5. Yucel O, Arregui ME. Electrohydraulic lithotripsy combined with laparoscopy and endoscopy for managing difficult biliary stones. Surg Laparosc Endosc 1993;3(5): 398–402.
6. Sheen-Chen S, Chou F. Intraoperative choledochoscopic electrohydraulic lithotripsy for difficultly retrieved impacted common bile duct stones. Arch Surg 1995;130: 430–432.
7. Neuhaus H, Hoffmann W, Gottlieb K, et al. Endoscopic lithotripsy of bile duct stones using a new laser with automatic stone recognition. Gastrointest Endosc 1994;40(6): 708–715.
8. Ell C, Hochberger J, May A, et al. Laser lithotripsy of difficult bile duct stones by means of a rhodamine-6G laser and an integrated automatic stone-tissue detection system. Gastrointest Endosc 1993;39(6):755–762.
9. Hunter JG, Soper NJ. Laparoscopic management of common bile duct stones. Surg Clin N Am 1992;72(5): 1077–1097.
10. Burdick JS, Magee DJ, Hernandez E, et al. Holmium laser for treatment of left hepatic duct stone. Gastrointest Endosc 1998;48(5):523–526.
11. Carroll B, Chandra M, Papaioannou T, et al. Biliary lithotripsy as an adjunct to laparoscopic common bile duct stone extraction. Surg Endosc 1993;7:356–359.
12. Josephs LG, Birkett DH. Laser lithotripsy for the management of retained stones. Arch Surg 1992;127:603–605.
13. Schreiber F, Gurakuqi GC, Trauner M. Endoscopic intracorporeal laser lithotripsy of difficult common bile duct stones with a stone-recognition pulsed dye laser system. Gastrointest Endosc 1995;42(5):416–419.
14. Sackmann M, Delius M, Sauerbruch T, et al. Shock-wave lithotripsy of gallbladder stones. N Engl J Med 1988;318(7): 393–397.
15. Greiner L, Wenzel H, Jakobeit C. Biliary lithotripsy of difficult bile duct stones. In: Burhenne HJ, Paumgartner G, Ferrucci JT (eds) Biliary Lithotripsy, vol II. Chicago: Year Book Medical, 1989:119–127.
16. Gilchrist AM, Ross B, Thomas WEG. Extracorporeal shock-wave lithotripsy for common bile duct stones. Br J Surg 1997;84:29–32.
17. Rhodes M, Nathanson L, O'Rourke N, et al. Laparoscopic exploration of the common bile duct; lessons learned from 129 consecutive cases. Br J Surg 1995;82(5):666–668.

18. Zucker KA, Bailet RW. Laparoscopic cholangiography and management of choledocholithiasis. In: Zucker KA (ed) Surgical Laparoscopy Update. St. Louis: Quality Medical, 1993:145–193.
19. DePaula AL, Hashiba K, Bafutto M, et al. Laparoscopic antegrade sphincterotomy. Surg Laparosc Endosc 1993; 3(3):157–160.
20. Curet MJ, Pitcher DE, Martin DT, et al. Laparoscopic antegrade sphincterotomy. A new technique for the management of complex choledocholithiasis. Ann Surg 1995; 221(2):149–155.
21. Carroll B, Phillips EH, Chandra M, et al. Laparoscopic transcystic duct balloon dilatation of the sphincter of Oddi. Surg Endosc 1993;7(6):514–517.
22. Fujisaki S, Nezu T, Miyake H, et al. Laparoscopic treatment for common bile duct stones by transcystic papilla balloon dilatation technique. Surg Endosc 1999;13(8):824–826.
23. Ido K, Tamada K, Kimura K, et al. The role of endoscopic balloon sphincteroplasty in patients with gallbladder and bile duct stones. J Laparoendosc Adv Surg Tech A 1997; 7(3):151–156.
24. Neoptolemos JP, Hall C, O'Connor HJ, et al. Methyl-tert-butyl-ether for treating common bile duct stones: the British experience. Br J Surg 1990;77(1):32–35.
25. Palmer KR, Hofmann AF. Intraductal mono-octanoin for the direct dissolution of bile duct stone: experience in 343 patients. Gut 1986;27(2):196–202.
26. Janssen D, Bommarito A, Lathrop J. A new technique for the rapid dissolution of retained ductal gallstones with monoctanoin in T-tube patients. Am Surg 1992;58(2):141–145.

24
Intraoperative Antegrade Common Duct Stone Treatments

Karl A. Zucker

Since its first description in Germany in 1985, laparoscopic cholecystectomy has become the procedure of choice in the management of nearly all individuals with symptomatic gallbladder disease.[1] Soon after the introduction of this innovative procedure, clinicians recognized that patients with concomitant choledocholithiasis might prove to be a particularly difficult challenge if they were also to be managed with laparoscopic techniques. For several years, most minimally invasive surgeons relied heavily on the efforts of the biliary endoscopist to identify and treat common bile duct stones before attempting laparoscopic cholecystectomy. If common bile duct stones were visualized in a patient undergoing an endoscopic retrograde cholangiography (ERC), an endoscopic sphincterotomy and stone extraction were performed, usually at the same setting.[2-5] However, even this approach to common bile duct disease did not eliminate all the potential problems that could face the laparoscopic surgeon. As many as 50% of patients with common bile duct stones are first discovered at the time of operative intervention, although this figure seems to be decreasing as the number of gastroenterologists trained in biliary endoscopy and therefore the number of ERCPs being performed have increased.[3-6] Surgeons are then faced with the choice of conversion to open laparotomy and a formal common bile duct exploration (losing the advantages of minimally invasive surgery) or completing the laparoscopic procedure followed by postoperative ERC and sphincterotomy. The latter option was troubling to many clinicians because of the dilemma faced if the endoscopist could not clear the common bile duct.

Progressive advances in minimally invasive techniques, equipment, and expertise have proven that laparoscopic common bile duct exploration is safe and successful in most patients with uncomplicated choledocholithiasis.[7-9] Current techniques of laparoscopic-guided transcystic common bile duct exploration or even direct attempts via a choledochotomy may be unsuccessful, however, in those patients with multiple bile duct stones or intrahepatic calculi or those with stones impacted at the ampulla. In the past, many of these patients would have undergone a drainage procedure to ensure adequate drainage of the biliary tree during the postoperative period. These options included prolonged T-tube drainage, a biliary enteric bypass, an open transduodenal sphincterotomy, or a perioperative endoscopic sphincterotomy.

In an attempt to extend the benefits of minimally invasive surgery to those difficult patients with complex biliary tract disease, an innovative physician from Brazil, Aureo Ludovicio DePaula, has described a technique known as laparoscopic antegrade biliary sphincterotomy.[10] This procedure combines the modalities of laparoscopic common bile duct exploration and flexible biliary endoscopy, thereby allowing the surgeon to provide definitive management to patients with complex choledocholithiasis at the time of laparoscopic surgery. It also allows the laparoscopic surgeon to perform a biliary drainage procedure so that any retained debris or small calculi may pass through the ampulla at a later time. Other antegrade techniques have also been adapted from the armenentarium of the flexible endoscopist for laparoscopic approaches, such as antegrade stent placement and lithotripsy.

Surgical Technique

Patients are screened for the possibility of choledocholithiasis before operative intervention by means of a detailed history and physical, an abdominal ultrasound, and blood studies to detect any pancreatic or hepatic enzyme abnormalities. If there is any suspicion of persistent choledocholithiasis, the patient is given the choice of undergoing a preoperative ERC or proceeding directly to laparoscopic surgery.

The standard four-puncture technique as described by Reddick is used to begin the laparoscopic cholecystectomy.[11] Routine intraoperative transcystic cholangiography is performed, preferably with a C-arm fluoroscopy unit. If choledocholithiasis is demonstrated on the cholangiogram, an attempt is first made at transcystic stone extraction. A common surgical practice is to first advance a balloon-tipped catheter catheter into the distal duct under fluoroscopic guidance. Radiographic contrast can be slowly infused while this catheter is being maneuvered past the stone(s). The balloon is next inflated while the catheter is slowly withdrawn. Often one or more stones can be extracted in this manner. If the stone(s) cannot be extracted with the balloon-tipped catheter, a three- or four-wire basket can be maneuvered into the main bile ducts using fluoroscopy. If this technique fails, one should proceed to transcystic choledochoscopy. In most cases an additional 5-mm port will be placed in the right upper quadrant for insertion of the choledochoscope. A small (outer diameter, 3.1 mm) flexible cholecochoscope (URF-P2 Choledochoscope; Olympus Corp., Japan) is then introduced through this additional cannula. In most cases, the choledochoscope can be inserted through the same cystic ductotomy made previously for the cholangiogram. If the choledochoscope cannot be maneuvered into the main bile duct, the opening in the cystic duct can be extended down onto the common bile duct; this almost always results in an opening large enough to allow the scope to pass easily into the distal and proximal common bile duct. After visualizing the stone(s), one should attempt to pass a four-wire basket through the working channel of the choledochoscope and position it around the calculus. The basket can then be closed under direct vision, and the choledochoscope, basket, and stone are then all withdrawn out of the common bile duct; this is necessary because the working channel of the scope is far too small (1–1.5 mm) to allow the stone to be removed via that route. The scope is reinserted to remove additional stone(s) or to ensure the duct is clear.

Indications for proceeding with antegrade sphincterotomy include multiple common bile duct stones, calculi impacted at the ampulla, or situations where it has proven impossible to remove all the stones within the bile ducts (i.e., intrahepatic stones). Another situation occasionally encountered is a stone(s) fractured while being retrieved with a wire basket, resulting in multiple smaller fragments that may prove difficult if not impossible to remove using the techniques just described. After deciding to proceed with an antegrade sphincterotomy, one should first remove the choledochoscope and then try to guide a standard endoscopic sphincterotome, as used for an ERCP, directly into the distal common bile duct. Again, the same opening in the cystic duct or common bile duct is used to introduce this instrument. The sphinctertome is then guided down the common bile duct, across the ampulla, and into the duodenum under direct vision.

Different types of endoscopic sphincterotomes are commercially available; they are the same devices used by the biliary endoscopist to perform an ERC with sphincterotomy. We typically use a 30-mm, short-nose sphincterotome (Microvasive Ultratome, Boston, MA, USA); DePaula in Brazil prefers a Classen-Demling or Billroth II type papillotome.[10] The sphincterotome is usually introduced through the fifth port using a "suture introducer" to minimize gas leakage. A grasping forceps is inserted through the subxiphoid sheath to help guide the sphincterotome into the lumen of the cystic duct or common bile duct. While the sphincterotome is being maneuvered into the biliary tree, another member of the team passes a side-viewing duodenoscope (Olympus TJF 100) or standard forward-viewing gastroscope (Olympus GIF) orally into the esophagus; this allows the surgeon to actually visualize the sphincterotome as it exits the ampulla. Ideally, a video endoscope is used so that it is easier for both the endoscopist and the surgeon to observe the duodenal lumen. Nasoorogastric tubes, esophageal stethoscopes, and temperature probes are first removed before passing the duodenoscope. It is frequently necessary to elevate the jaw while introducing the scope through the pharynx and proximal esophagus, which may require assistance from the anesthesia staff. This maneuver appears to be necessary because of the unusual patient positioning (supine) and the obstructing effect of the endotracheal tube. The scope is then guided through the remaining esophagus, stomach, antrum, and pylorus and finally into the duodenum. Glucagon is then administered (0.5–1.0 mg IV) to minimize duodenal peristalsis.

Sometimes it is difficult to adequately distend the duodenum with air because the muscle relaxation of the general anesthesia allows for free reflux of air back out the mouth. This can be diminished by *gentle* compression of the neck to seal the proximal esophagus around the duodenoscope. The duodenoscope is then positioned directly across from the ampulla. Using the view afforded by the side-viewing endoscope, the sphinctertome is guided by the surgeon so that the diathermic wire will extend toward the 12 o'clock position (Fig. 24.1).

It may prove difficult to pass the sphincterotome into the duodenum because of stones impacted at the ampulla. In these patients, one should try to pass a guidewire through the working channel of the choledochoscope and maneuver it through the ampulla under direct vision. The choledochoscope is then removed and the sphincterotome passed over the wire. A sphincterotomy is then performed using a blended electrical current and extended proximally to the first transverse fold of the ampulla (Fig. 24.2). In most cases the stones will then pass into the duodenum spontaneously or with gentle irrigation. Following successful sphincterotomy, repeat choledochoscopy is performed to ensure that all the stones

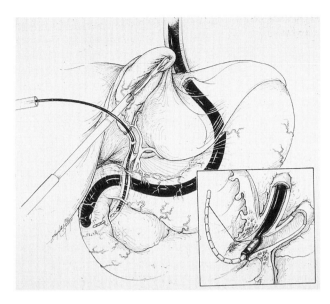

FIGURE 24.1. Schematic drawing of side-viewing endoscope positioned within the duodenum to visualize the sphincterotome.

have passed. The choledochoscope should pass easily all the way into the duodenum (Fig. 24.3).

There has been considerable discussion in the past few years regarding the need for mandatory T-tube catheter placement after laparoscopic common bile duct exploration. It is our opinion that, if common bile duct exploration and passage of the sphincterotome were done only via the cystic duct, the surgeon may choose to forgo insertion of a T-tube or similar ductal drainage catheter and simply secure the cystic duct with a pretied laparoscopic ligature, assuming adequate drainage at the ampulla. If the common bile duct is incised and directly instrumented, it is preferable to insert a 14 to 16 French T-tube with the other end of the catheter brought through the right lateral trocar site. Laparoscopic cholecystectomy is then completed. It is also wise to routinely place a closed-suction drain in the subhepatic space at the completion of the operative procedure to control any leakage from the operative sites. Occasionally, what initially appears to be a distal common duct stone is in fact an obstructing common duct or pancreatic cancer. In this case it is possible to place a transduodenal stent, either plastic (10–12 F) or expandable metal, transcystically or through the choledochotomy using the same deployment systems used in ERCP (Fig. 24.4).

Discussion

Emerging and evolving technology, instrumentation, and expertise have led surgeons to attempt common bile duct exploration laparoscopically. This technique has proven successful in most patients.[7–9,12] However, in some individuals the common bile duct cannot be cleared with current laparoscopic techniques, and it is these difficult patients who may benefit from antegrade sphincterotomy. Attempts have been made to perform intraoperative ERC and sphincterotomy; however, retrograde cannulation of the bile duct is extremely difficult to

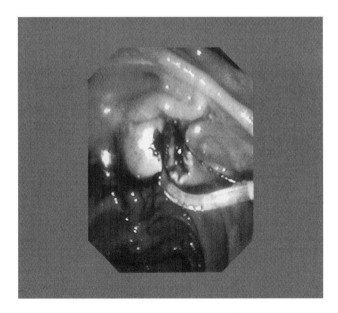

FIGURE 24.2. Duodenoscopic view of sphincterotomy after proper positioning of the diathermic wire.

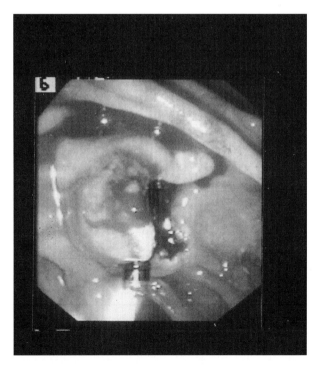

FIGURE 24.3. Following antegrade sphincterotomy, the choledochoscope easily traverses the ampulla.

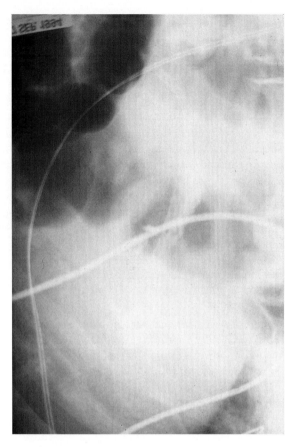

FIGURE 24.4. Intraoperative cholangiogram shows a 10 F biliary stent placed transcystically for a bile duct malignancy.

He stated that this procedure added only a mean of 18 min (range, 10–29 min) to perform this procedure[12] in addition to time spent attempting other methods of laparoscopic common bile duct exploration. DePaula reports his indications for this procedure include inability to clear the common bile duct of all stones or debris, patients with intrahepatic stones, and those individuals with suspected papillary stenosis. In our own experience, we were able to complete the sphincterotomy in just over 20 min, excluding time spent at attempted common bile duct exploration and waiting for the additional equipment to be brought into the operating suite.

Fortunately, to date, very few complications have been reported with this procedure. One reason is probably that most surgeons who have thus far attempted it have also been experienced endoscopists. Antegrade passage of the sphincterotome device also may be inherently a safer technique. A number of well-known problems are associated with retrograde biliary endoscopy (i.e., ERCP), including pancreatitis resulting from cannulation of the pancreatic duct, creation of false passages, and ductal and duodenal perforation.[14–16] These problems should be minimized with laparoscopic-guided antegrade sphincterotomy because it is much easier to pass the sphincterotome antegrade through the bile ducts, avoiding cannulation of the pancreatic duct or the creation of false passages. One patient in our series did have a duodenal mucosal injury from passage of the side-viewing endoscope into the duodenum. The large diameter of the duodenoscope was probably the major contributing factor for this injury as the individual was quite small in size (height, 53 in.). Use of a smaller standard gastroscope may obviate this problem but does not provide the same degree of visualization of the sphincterotomy process. In the same series, one patient developed clinical and laboratory signs of pancreatitis that delayed hospital discharge. In this patient, the total time to perform laparoscopic-guided antegrade sphincterotomy was significantly longer because of technical problems when the cystic duct was inadvertently transected. Three additional patients had asymptotic and transient hyperamylasemia postoperatively (mean, 252 IU/liter; nl < 114). In these cases, serum enzyme levels returned to normal within 3 days with no clinical manifestations of pancreatitis. Antegrade transduodenal stent placement can afford patients good palliation if they are found to have unsuspected malignant obstruction or if an obstructing stone cannot be dislodged.

One reason retrograde biliary endoscopy is so popular is that it can achieve duct clearance rates of 90% to 95%, although it must be remembered that authors reporting these results may have put the patient through two or even three endoscopic sessions to achieve successful stone clearance.[2,5,15,17] Laparoscopic common bile duct exploration alone has a reported duct clearance rate of

achieve in the operating room because the patient is not in the prone position typically used during biliary endoscopy. Another problem associated with intraoperative endoscopy is that the lumen of the small bowel can become massively distended with air from the insufflation port of the endoscope, which can dramatically hinder visualization of the operative field, rendering completion of the laparoscopic operation difficult if not impossible. Also, attempts at intraoperative ERC can markedly prolong anesthesia time and may be unsuccessful.

In contrast, laparoscopic-assisted antegrade procedures have proven to be a rapid and effective means of enhancing biliary drainage and clearing the bile ducts. Laparoscopic antegrade sphincterotomy has a number of advantages compared to conventional methods of endoscopic sphincterotomy. Although a side-viewing duodenoscope should be positioned in the proximal duodenum, it is only used to confirm proper positioning of the diathermic cutting wire. Passage of the sphincterotome antegrade through the ampulla is rapid compared to the retrograde cannulation required during ERC. DePaula has recently reported his updated series of 34 patients undergoing antegrade sphincterotomy.[13]

70% to 90%,[7,8,9,12] which should improve with the addition of antegrade sphincterotomy. In our current series, we were able to clear the common bile duct in all 12 patients with choledocholithiasis in which the antegrade sphincterotomy was successfully performed, despite the fact that these cases represented the most difficult to manage under laparoscopic guidance.[18] The one individual with the duodenal mucosal injury was opened to exclude a possible full-thickness perforation and thus underwent an open common bile duct exploration.

Another important aspect is patient expectation. Individuals prefer complete management of all their biliary tract problems at one setting (preferably with laparoscopic surgery) rather than multiple procedures before or after cholecystectomy or conversion to open laparotomy. The appeal of one minimally invasive procedure to completely handle cholelithiasis and choledocholithiasis cannot be overstated.

Antegrade sphincterotomy, however, is associated with a number of disadvantages. Operative and anesthesia times are prolonged, although with experience this should be less than 30 min, as mentioned previously. Surgeons who are already skilled at laparoscopic common bile duct exploration become adept at this technique very quickly. Antegrade sphincterotomy does require additional equipment in an already crowded operating room, and an experienced physician is required to operate the side-viewing endoscope, which is optimal for performing this procedure. This instrument is somewhat more difficult to maneuver than the standard forward-viewing endoscopes, and specialized training manipulating these devices and performing sphincterotomy is advised. Unfortunately, very few operating rooms are equipped with side-viewing endoscopes. These devices are therefore usually requested from the GI endoscopy unit. Preparation and transportation of the equipment may take some time. To avoid excessive delay, we were actually able to persuade one hospital to designate a portable antegrade sphincterotomy cart that could be transported to the operating room with only a few minutes notice.

Our experience and DePaula's report indicate that this procedure can be done safely and in a timely manner with excellent results. Patient selection criteria are still being developed. DePaula performs this procedure in patients with multiple common bile duct stones and proximal duct stones as well as for individuals with markedly dilated common bile ducts and suspected papillary stenosis.[10,13] In our series, laparoscopic-guided antegrade sphincterotomy was performed only if the common bile duct could not be cleared by more conventional laparoscopic techniques, usually because of multiple stones or one or more stones impacted at the ampulla. Clearly this experience is similar to that of Dr. DePaula's in that only a very small percentage of patients with choledocholithiasis should be considered candidates for this procedure.

The addition of laparoscopic antegrade sphincterotomy to the minimally invasive surgeon's armamentarium simply expands the options for treating those individuals with very complex choledocholithiasis. The appropriate option needs to be tailored to the individual patient, as well as the expertise of the surgeon. Biliary endoscopy (pre- and postoperative), open common bile duct exploration, or laparoscopic common bile duct exploration with or without antegrade sphincterotomy are all potential alternatives that should be given serious consideration.

References

1. NIH Consensus Conference Statement. Am J Surg 1993;165: 390–396.
2. Cotton PB. Endoscopic retrograde cholangiopancreatography and laparoscopic cholecystectomy. Am J Surg 1993;165: 474–478.
3. Flowers JL, Zucker KA, Graham SM, Scovill WA, Imbembo AL, Bailey RO. Laparoscopic cholangiography: results and indications. Ann Surg 1992;215:209–216.
4. Van Stiegmann G, Perlman NW, Goff JS, Sun JH, Norton LW. Endoscopic cholangiography and stone removal prior to cholecystectomy. Arch Surg 1989;124:787–790.
5. Traverso LW, Kozarek RA, Ball TJ, et al. Endoscopic retrograde cholangiopancreatography after laparoscopic cholecystectomy. Am J Surg 1993;165:581–586
6. Zucker KA, Bailey RW. Laparoscopic cholangiography and management of choledocholithiasis. In: Zucker KA(ed) Surgical Laparoscopy Update. St. Louis: Quality Medical, 1993:145–193.
7. Hunter JG. Laparoscopic transcystic common bile duct exploration. Am J Surg 1992;163:53–58.
8. Petelin JB. Laparoscopic approach to common duct pathology. Am J Surg 1993;165:487–491
9. Petelin JB. Laparoscopic approach to common duct pathology. Surg Laparosc Endosc 1991;1:33–41.
10. DePaula AL, Hashiba K, Bafutto M, Zago R, Machado MM. Laparoscopic antegrade sphincterotomy. Surg Laparosc Endosc 1993;3:157–160.
11. Reddick EF, Olsen DO. Laparoscopic laser cholecystectomy: a comparison with mini-laparotomy. Surg Endosc 1989;3:44–48.
12. Van Stiegmann G, Goff JS, Mansour A, Pearlman NW, Reveille RM, Norton L. Pre-cholecystectomy endoscopic cholangiography and stone removal is not superior to cholecystectomy, cholangiography and common duct exploration. Am J Surg 1992;163:227–230.
13. DePaula AL. Intraoperative endoscopic retrograde cholangiopancreaticography. In: Maurice E, Arregui ME (eds) Principles of Laparoscopic Surgery. Berlin: Springer, 1995: 185–210.
14. Cotton PB. Non-operative removal of bile duct stones by duodenoscopic antegrade sphincterotomy. Br J Surg 1980; 67:1–5.
15. Reiter JJ, Bayer HP, Menncken C, Manegold BC. Results of endoscopic papillotomy: a collective experience from

nine endoscopic centers in West Germany. World J Surg 1978;2:505–511.

16. Leese T, Neoptolemos JR, Carr-Locke DL. Successes, failures early complications and their management following endoscopic sphincterotomy: results in 394 consecu-tive patients from a single center. Br J Surg 1985;72:215–219.

17. Cotton PB, Lehman B, Vennes J, et al. Endoscopic sphincterotomy complications and their management: an attempt at consensus. Gastrointest Endosc 1991;37:383–393.

18. Curet MJ, Pitcher DE, Martin DT, Zucker KA. Laparoscopic antegrade sphincterotomy: a new technique for the management of complex choledocholithiasis. Ann Surg 1995;221:149–155.

25
Laparoscopic Choledochoenterostomies

Joseph Mamazza, Eric C. Poulin, Christopher M. Schlachta, Pieter A. Seshadri, and Margherita O. Cadeddu

Background and Historical Development

Endoscopic treatment of both benign and malignant causes of obstructive jaundice has enjoyed significant success with relatively low morbidity and mortality, with less overall cost.[1-3] Thus, surgical biliary drainage procedures have, in many instances, been replaced by endoscopic sphincterotomy with or without stent insertion. However, there still remains clinical conditions and situations where surgical intervention is required, particularly when endoscopic therapeutic measures have failed (Fig. 25.1). The surgical biliary drainage procedures most favored have been choledochoduodenostomy or Roux-en-Y choledochojejunostomy. Until recently, this required that patients undergo a formal laparotomy that could be quite debilitating, particularly in elderly patients or those with underlying malignancy. With new, minimally invasive surgical techniques, laparoscopic biliary enteric bypass surgery offers the patient a less invasive alternative than open laparotomy. Laparoscopy affords the patient all the advantages of minimally invasive surgery as well as a permanent and secure biliary drainage procedure.

It is important to emphasize that laparoscopic choledochoenterostomies are very difficult procedures, requiring advanced laparoscopic skills. To date, most of the reports on laparoscopic biliary bypass have focused on simpler procedures, such as laparoscopic cholecystojejunostomy and laparoscopic choledochoduodenostomy.[4-10] These reports have shown that these procedures not only are technically feasible but can be performed within reasonable operative times. More complex procedures, such as Roux-en-Y choledochojejunostomies, are extremely time consuming even in the most experienced of hands. Significant active research and innovation in the area of laparoscopic biliary enteric anastomoses may soon result in the emergence of a technically feasible and practical approach, most likely using some form of anastomotic device.[11,12]

Laparoscopic Side-to-Side Choledochoduodenostomy

Indications and Surgical Strategies

The indications for choledochoduodenostomy include common bile duct obstruction or stasis secondary to sludge, primary or recurrent stones, multiple common bile duct stones (when these cannot be cleared by endoscopic sphincterotomy and basket extraction), and distal common bile duct obstruction secondary to chronic pancreatitis or benign distal stricture. It is mandatory that the common bile duct be at least 1.5cm in diameter to ensure that a large anastomosis is created. A side-to-side choledochoduodenostomy should not be carried out in patients whose common bile duct is less than 1.5cm in diameter or if there is acute inflammation or excessive fibrosis of the duodenal wall or common bile duct wall. Likewise, patients with biliary obstruction secondary to carcinoma of the pancreatic head are not ideal candidates for a choledochoduodenostomy due to progressive encroachment of tumor on the anastomosis.

Several important technical considerations must be adhered to when creating a choledochoduodenostomy. Because a choledochoduodenostomy will permit the free passage of enteric content into the common bile duct, it is important that the anastomosis be large enough to permit food to pass back and forth freely. If the stoma is too small, the risk of recurrent cholangitis will increase. A 2.5-cm anastomosis should be created whenever possible. To minimize the risk of postoperative anastomotic leakage, the anastomosis must be created with no tension. Therefore, it is critical that the choledochotomy be created as far distal on the common bile duct as possible and that the tissues surrounding the duct wall are of

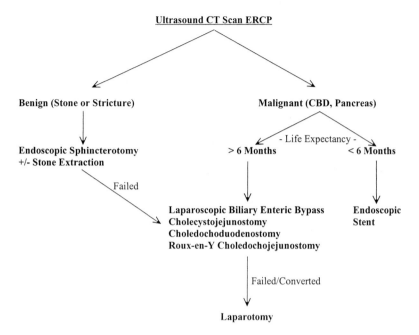

**COMMON BILE DUCT OBSTRUCTION
(JAUNDICE)**

FIGURE 25.1. Management of common bile duct obstruction.

satisfactory quality. Although it may not be required, kocherization of the duodenum is recommended to further reduce the tension on the anastomosis. A large, well-placed stoma will significantly reduce the risk of developing sump syndrome, which is essentially intermittent cholangitis resulting from the accumulation of food debris or calculi in the terminal portion of the common bile duct following choledochoduodenostomy.

Surgical Technique

After induction of satisfactory general anesthesia, the patient is placed in a supine position with the legs apart. The operator usually stands between the legs or to the left of the patient. The peritoneal cavity is entered by making a small incision at the umbilicus and introducing a 12-mm trocar under direct vision; this eliminates the risk of first trocar injuries. A pneumoperitoneum is created, and a 30° or 45° laparoscope is used because we believe this affords the best view of the duodenal and common bile duct anatomy. Under direct vision, a 12-mm trocar is introduced in the left upper quadrant in the subcostal region. Two 5-mm trocars are introduced, one in the right upper quadrant in the midclavicular line just above the umbilicus, and another more laterally at the level of the anterior axillary line (Fig. 25.2). If adhesions are present, these are lysed with sharp dissection, avoiding electrocautery wherever possible. The gallbladder, common bile duct, and duodenum are clearly identified. The fundus of the gallbladder is grasped with an atrau-

matic tissue grasper through the lateralmost trocar, and the gallbladder and liver are raised upward toward the right hemidiaphragm. This maneuver allows relatively easy access to, and good visualization, of the common bile duct. The peritoneum over the distal common bile duct is incised, exposing the common bile duct wall, and a

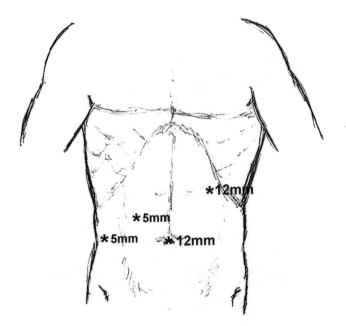

FIGURE 25.2. Laparoscopic choledochoduodenostomy: trocar positioning.

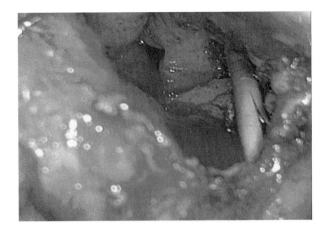

FIGURE 25.3. Common bile duct lumen with stent.

longitudinal incision along the anterior wall of the common bile duct is made for approximately 2.5 cm.

On opening the common bile duct wall, bile will flow out freely and a suction aspirator is used to minimize contamination. If a significant amount of stones and debris is seen within the common bile duct, these are either aspirated or collected and placed within a small sterile freezer bag to prevent contamination of the peritoneal cavity. In the case of common bile duct stones, a choledochoscope is introduced via one of the 5-mm trocar sites and passed proximally into the left and right hepatic ducts and distally along the length of the common bile duct (Fig. 25.3). Any residual stones may be cleared by either flushing the bile duct or basket extraction. A corresponding incision is then made along the longitudinal axis of the duodenum at a point close to the distal common duct (Fig. 25.4). Care must be taken not to make the duodenotomy too large because this will stretch to some degree during the procedure.

The anastomosis is then created by placing the first stitches at the midpoints of both the lateral and medial margins of the choledochotomy; these are correspondingly placed at the apex of the duodenotomy. These stitches are left long to act as stay sutures and to facilitate traction so that the orientation of the anastomosis can be maintained. The anastomosis is created with one layer of interrupted 3-0 PDS sutures on either a ski needle or straight needle. The posterior wall is approximated first, placing the first stitch at the inferior apex of the choledochotomy to the midpoint of the duodenotomy (Fig. 25.5). The back wall is further subdivided with full-thickness bites of the duodenum and common bile duct, completing the posterior half of the anastomosis (Fig. 25.6). The anterior wall of the anastomosis is completed by a row of full thickness interrupted stitches of 3-0 PDS sutures (Figs. 25.7, 25.8, 25.9). The anastomosis should be completed without tension.

A completion cholecystectomy is often done when the biliary bypass is performed for stone disease. Although not absolutely necessary, we routinely place a closed-suction drainage catheter in the vicinity of the anastomosis and bring this out through one of the lateral 5-mm trocar sites. To date, 17 cases of laparoscopic choledochoduodenostomies have been reported. All 17 cases achieved complete decompression of the biliary tree and resolution of jaundice. The operations were carried out with acceptable operative times with no significant postoperative complications. If a common bile duct exploration accompanied the procedure, operative times tended to be doubled.[7,8,9,13]

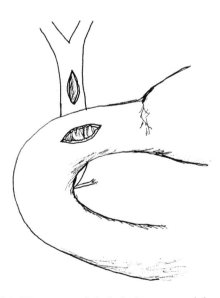

FIGURE 25.4. Placement of choledochotomy and duodenotomy.

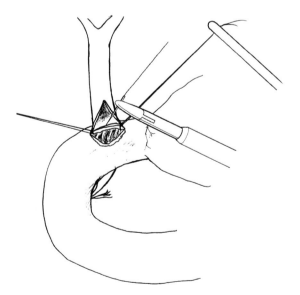

FIGURE 25.5. Posterior wall of choledochoduodenostomy. Stay sutures maintain traction.

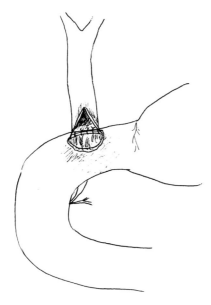

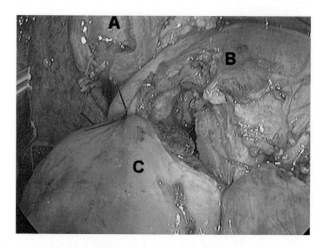

FIGURE 25.8. Partially completed choledochoduodenostomy. *A*, gallbladder; *B*, common bile duct; *C*, duodenum.

FIGURE 25.6. Choledochoduodenostomy. Posterior wall completed.

Laparoscopic Roux-en-Y Choledochojejunostomy

Indications and Surgical Strategies

When the common bile duct is less than 1.5 cm in diameter, a Roux-en-Y choledochojejunostomy should be performed to eliminate any undue tension on the anastomosis and, by diverting the food stream, prevent the occurrence of sump syndrome and recurrent cholangitis.

A choledochojejunostomy is recommended in those patients with common bile duct obstruction due to inoperable malignancy and greater than 6-month life expectancy.[14] This procedure reduces the risk of tumor encroachment and obstruction of the biliary–enteric anastomosis, which can occur if a choledochoduodenostomy is used. It is the preferred biliary bypass in patients with Caroli's cholangiohepatitis, hepatic duct stones, or benign common bile duct stricture. It should also be performed where there is significant duodenal inflammation or fibrosis of the duodenum or common bile duct.

When a Roux-en-Y segment of jejunum is anastomosed to the common bile duct, the risk of postoperative anastomotic failure approaches 0. There are fewer long-term complications, and mortality rate is also quite low.[15] It is clearly the safest of the biliary intestinal anastomoses. It is important that the choledochojejunostomy be constructed with a Roux-en-Y segment that is at least 50

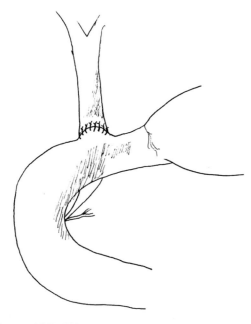

FIGURE 25.7. Side-to-side choledochoduodenostomy.

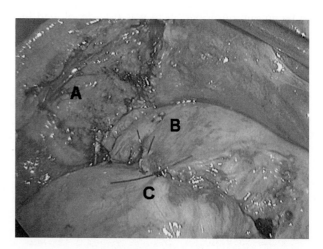

FIGURE 25.9. Completed side-to-side choledochoduodenostomy. *A*, gallbladderl; *B*, common bile duct; *C*, duodenum.

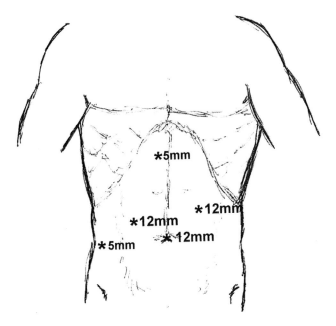

FIGURE 25.10. Laparoscopic choledochojejunostomy: trocar positioning.

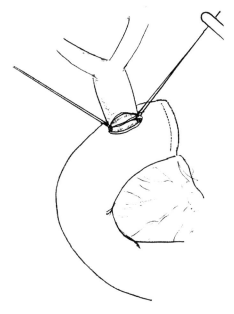

FIGURE 25.11. End-to-side choledochojejunostomy. Stay sutures maintain traction.

to 60 cm long to prevent any possibility of food regurgitating into the bile ducts. Care must be taken when constructing the Roux-en-Y limb so that there is sufficient length to reach the common bile duct. In most cases, this can be accomplished by dividing the marginal artery just distal to the second arcade vessels. Then, by dividing the third or fourth arcade vessels beyond this, sufficient length can usually be achieved.

Surgical Technique

Laparoscopic Roux-en-Y choledochojejunostomy is technically a very demanding and time-consuming procedure. It requires a high level of laparoscopic skill that presently precludes it from widespread adoption. The technique described here was first developed in an animal model in our laboratory and demonstrates that this operation is technically feasible.[13] The patient positioning and operating room setup are the same as previously described for laparoscopic choledochoduodenostomy. Trocar positioning is similar, except that we use three 12-mm trocars and two 5-mm trocars (Fig. 25.10). The extra 12-mm trocar allows us to use an endoscopic linear stapling device to perform the enteric anastomosis as well as transect the distal common duct.

Once the 30° laparoscope is inserted, a thorough examination of the portal triad and duodenal area is carried out to see if a surgical bypass can be performed. We prefer to create the Roux-en-Y jejunal limb first. The transverse colon is raised, exposing the ligament of Treitz and the proximal jejunum. The mesentery is divided just distal to the second arcade of vessels and extended down to the

third or fourth arcade, depending on the length required. Once the mesentery has been divided, an endoscopic linear stapling device is used to transect the jejunum.

The peritoneum over the distal common bile duct is then incised and the bile duct is carefully dissected free from the other portal triad structures. A right-angle dissector is often helpful in this dissection. When adequate mobilization of the distal common duct has been achieved, a 30-mm linear stapler is used to divide the distal common bile duct. The staple line on the proximal common bile duct is then excised, and an end-to-side single-layer handsewn anastomosis is created to the prepared jejunal limb (Figs. 25.11, 25.12, 25.13). A 2-0

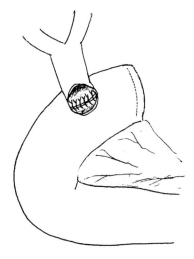

FIGURE 25.12. Choledochojejunostomy. Posterior wall completed.

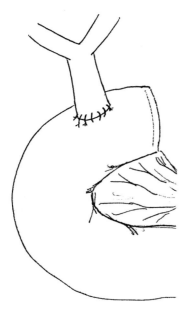

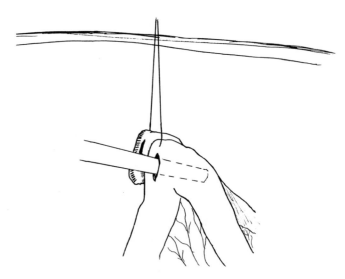

FIGURE 25.15. Side-to-side stapled enteroenterostomy.

FIGURE 25.13. Completed end-to-side choledochojejunostomy.

prolene suture on a straight needle is then passed through the abdominal wall, and seromuscular bites are taken through the proximal jejunal limb and the distal jejunum at an appropriate distance (50–60 cm) from the biliary–enteric anastomosis. This suture acts to stabilize the two jejunal limbs as well as to maintain orientation (Fig. 25.14). An enterotomy is made in both jejunal limbs that is large enough to fit the jaws of the stapling device (Fig. 25.15). Care must be taken to avoid twisting of the bowel, which would result in tangential stapling. A side-

to-side anastomosis is created using a 45-mm endoscopic linear stapler. The enterotomy sites are then closed with either an additional application of the stapler or a hand-sewn closure.

To date, there have been few reports of choledochojejunostomies, except for experimental animal models. There have been no reported cases of Roux-en-Y choledochojejunostomy in humans, and it is too early to tell whether laparoscopic choledochojejunostomy can be carried out quickly and safely enough to usurp present treatment options, including open surgery. However, because of new developments in anastomotic devices and animal models using fibrin glue, these clinical reports will probably soon emerge.[11,12,16] Ultimately, the final deciding factor in making this procedure useful in humans will be the surgeon who develops the expertise in intracorporeal suturing required to perform laparoscopic choledochojejunostomy in a safe, effective, and timely fashion.

References

1. Safrany L. Endoscopic treatment of biliary tract diseases (an international study). Lancet 1978;2:983–985.
2. Anderson JR, Sorensen SM, Kruse A. Randomized trial of endoscopic endoprosthesis versus operative bypass in malignant obstructive jaundice. Gut 1989;30:1132–1135.
3. Brandabuc JJ, Kozarek RA, Ball TJ, et al. Nonoperative versus operative treatment of obstructive jaundice in pancreatic cancer: cost and survival analysis. Am J Gastroenterol 1988;83:1132–1139.
4. Rhodes M, Nathanson L, Fielding G. Laparoscopic biliary and gastric bypass: a useful adjunct in the treatment of carcinoma of the pancreas. Gut 1995;36:778–780.
5. Shimi S, Banting S, Cuschieri A. Laparoscopy in the management of pancreatic cancer: Endoscopic cholecystoje-

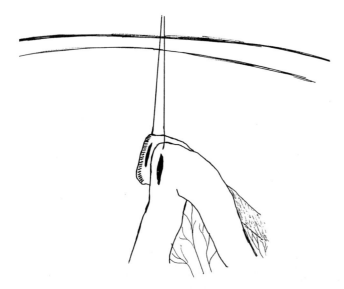

FIGURE 25.14. Stay suture maintains orientation of jejunal limbs.

junostomy for advanced disease. Br J Surg 1992;79:317–319.

6. Fletcher DR, Jones RM. Laparoscopic cholecystojejunostomy as palliation for obstructive jaundice in inoperative carcinoma of the pancreas. Surg Endosc 1992;6:147–149.

7. Farello GA, Cerofolini A, Bergamaschi G, et al. L'astomose cholédoco-duodénale par voie laparoscopique. J Chir Paris 1993;130:226–230.

8. Gurbuz AT, Watson D, Fenoglio ME. Laparoscopic choledochoduodenostomy. Am Surgeon 1999;65:212–214.

9. Rhodes M, Nathanson L. Laparoscopic choledochoduodenostomy. Surg Laparosc Endosc 1996;6:318–321.

10. Chekan EG, Clark L, Wu J, et al. Laparoscopic biliary and enteric bypass. Semin Surg Oncol 1999;16:313–320.

11. Schöb OM, Schmid RA, Schlump FR, et al. New anastomosis technique for (laparoscopic) instrumental small-diameter anastomosis. Surg Endosc 1995;9:444–449.

12. Schöb OM, Schmid RA, Morimoto AK, et al. Laparoscopic Roux-en-Y choledochojejunostomy. Am J Surg 1997;173:312–319.

13. Mamazza J, Seshadri PA, Schlachta CM, et al. Laparoscopic choledochoduodenostomy. Video submission to SAGES 1999.

14. van den Bosch RP, van der Schelling GP, Klinkenbijl JHG, et al. Guidelines for the application of surgery and endoprosthesis in the palliation of obstructive jaundice in advanced cancer of the pancreas. Ann Surg 1994;14:21918–21924.

15. Bismuth H, Franco D, Corlette MB, et al. Long term results of Roux-en-Y hepaticojejunostomy. Surg Gynecol Obstet 1978;146:161–167.

16. Jones DB, Brewer JD, Meininger TA, et al. Sutured or fibrin-glued laparoscopic choledochojejunostomy. Surg Endosc 1995;9:1020–1027.

Section IV
Laparoscopic Adrenalectomy and Splenectomy

Nathaniel J. Soper, MD
Section Editor

26
Laparoscopic Adrenalectomy

L. Michael Brunt

The surgical approach to the adrenal glands has changed dramatically in the past decade because of the development of laparoscopic techniques for performing adrenalectomy. Laparoscopic adrenalectomy has become the preferred method for removing most types of adrenal tumors, most of which are small and have a low risk of malignancy. Open adrenalectomy requires making a large incision to remove a small tumor because of the location of the adrenals deep in the retroperitoneum. The advantages of laparoscopic adrenalectomy, therefore, include reduced postoperative pain, a shortened hospitalization, and a faster recovery. In addition, the morbidity of performing adrenalectomy should also be reduced. This chapter reviews the current state of the various laparoscopic approaches to adrenalectomy and provides a framework for proper recognition of these tumors and selection of patients for operation.

Background and Historical Development

Historically, a variety of different open operative approaches for adrenalectomy have been used: these include the transabdominal approach, the flank approach, the retroperitoneal approach, and the thoracoabdominal approach.[1] The transabdominal approach is carried out via either a midline or bilateral subcostal incision. It has the advantage of allowing full exploration of the abdominal cavity and examination or removal of both adrenal glands via one incision. Before laparoscopic adrenalectomy, this approach was used primarily for patients with pheochromocytomas, large adrenal tumors, or suspected adrenal malignancies. The principal indications for open transabdominal adrenalectomy today are large tumors that are not amenable to laparoscopic excision as well as the suspicion of a large primary adrenal malignancy. The postero-lateral or flank approach is also

a transabdominal approach that is performed via a lengthy flank incision and usually involves resection of the 11th rib. It creates a wide surgical field and direct access to the adrenal, but has not been widely utilized in recent years because the incision is painful and does not allow access to the contralateral gland.

Open posterior adrenalectomy is an extraperitoneal, extrapleural approach that is carried out with the patient in a prone position. A hockey stick-shaped incision is made in the lower back, and the 11th or 12th rib is resected. The advantages of this approach are that it provides direct access to the adrenals and avoids entry into the peritoneal cavity. This approach has been associated with decreased morbidity compared to the open transabdominal approach.[2,3] The surgical exposure is somewhat limited, however, which restricts this procedure to patients with small adenomas or hyperplastic glands. Another disadvantage of this approach is that it has been associated with prolonged postoperative incisional pain.[4] Consequently, the posterior approach has been almost totally supplanted by laparoscopic adrenalectomy. The thoracoabdominal approach, which is rarely performed today, is reserved for patients with extremely large malignant lesions with probable vascular invasion who require en bloc resection of the tumor and adjacent viscera.

Laparoscopic adrenalectomy was first performed by Petelin[5] in 1992. Gagner et al.[6] subsequently reported three patients who underwent laparoscopic adrenalectomy via a transperitoneal lateral approach. This innovative approach was popularized by Gagner[7] and was rapidly adopted throughout North America and worldwide. Techniques for performing endoscopic adrenalectomy via a retroperitoneal approach were developed experimentally in 1993,[8] and the first clinical series of retroperitoneal endoscopic adrenalectomy was reported by Mercan and colleagues in 1995.[9] Several groups have since reported a high degree of success with the transabdominal and retroperitoneal approaches and, in most centers, laparoscopic adrenalectomy has replaced open adrenalectomy as the procedure of choice for patients with benign adrenal neoplasms.

Adrenal Anatomy

The adrenal glands lie in the retroperitoneum along the superomedial aspect of each kidney. They are composed of a cortex and medulla, each of which has distinct endocrine functions and separate embryological origins. The adrenal cortex is derived from the coelomic mesoderm and is the site for synthesis and secretion of cortisol, aldosterone, and adrenal androgens. The medulla arises from cells of the neural crest and is the site for synthesis of the catecholamines. The dimensions of the normal adrenal are approximately 4 to 5 cm × 2 to 3 cm × 0.5 to 1 cm, and the gland weighs 4 to 6 g. The right adrenal is somewhat pyramidal in shape, whereas the left gland is more flattened or crescentic and more closely applied to the kidney than the right. The high lipid content of the adrenals gives them a golden-orange color that is helpful in distinguishing them from the retroperitoneal fat in which they are embedded. Although the gland has a fibrous capsule, it is friable and can be easily disrupted and fragmented with surgical manipulation.

A thorough understanding of the surgical anatomy of the adrenals and their relationship to adjacent structures is essential to successful adrenalectomy, regardless of the technique employed. As shown in Figure 26.1, the right adrenal gland is adjacent to the diaphragm posteriorly and laterally, the liver and right triangular ligament anteriorly, the inferior vena cava anterior and medially, and the kidney inferiorly. A portion of the anteromedial

border of the adrenal may lie posterior to the inferior vena cava. The relationships of the left adrenal gland are as follows: posteriorly, the diaphragm; medially, the spleen; laterally, the kidney; and inferiorly, the kidney, renal vessels, pancreas, and splenic vein.

The adrenal is highly vascularized and derives its blood supply from branches of the inferior phrenic artery, aorta, and renal arteries (Fig. 26.2). These small arterial branches enter the gland from the superior, medial, and inferior aspects. On the right, the medial arterial branches course posterior to the inferior vena cava before entering the gland. Each gland is drained by a single adrenal vein. The right adrenal vein is short (about 1 cm long) and enters the inferior vena cava directly. In some cases, an accessory right adrenal vein may enter the inferior vena cava or hepatic veins more superiorly. The left adrenal vein is longer and, after exiting the infero-medial border of the gland, runs obliquely toward its junction with the left renal vein. The left adrenal vein is usually joined by the inferior phrenic vein within 1.5 cm of its entry into the renal vein. Surgical control of the adrenal veins is probably the most critical aspect of laparoscopic adrenalectomy. The right adrenal vein is especially vulnerable to tearing or avulsion from the inferior vena cava because of its short course.

Adrenal Physiology

Adrenal Cortex

The adrenal cortex is the site for synthesis and secretion of three types of hormones: cortisol, androgens, and aldosterone. Cholesterol is the precursor from which all

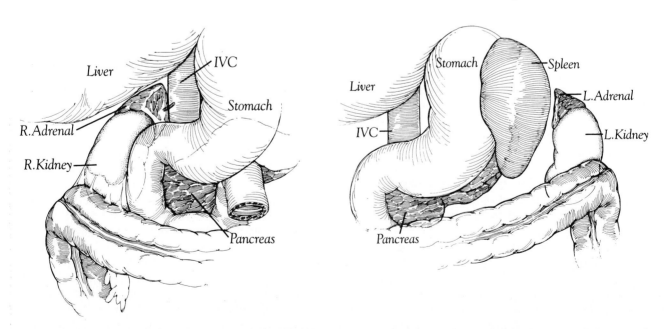

FIGURE 26.1. Anatomic relationships of the adrenal glands to surrounding structures. *IVC*, inferior vena cava.

FIGURE 26.2. Adrenal blood supply. (Reprinted with permission from Brunt LM. Laparoscopic adrenalectomy. In: Eubanks S, et al. (eds) Mastery of Endoscopic and Laparoscopic Surgery. Philadelphia: Lippincott, 2000:321.)

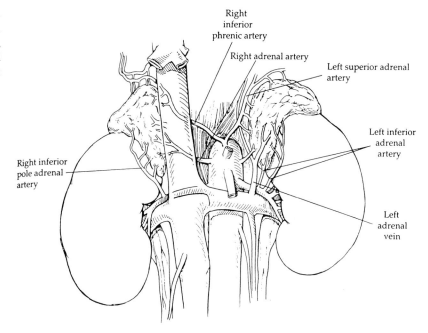

adrenal steroids are synthesized, and conversion of cholesterol to pregnenelone is the rate-limiting step in hormone synthesis and the major site of action of adreno-corticotrophic hormone (ACTH). Aldosterone is synthesized exclusively in the zona glomerulosa, which lacks the 17-α hydroxylase enzyme necessary for synthesis of cortisol and androgens. The zona fasciculata and zona reticularis, which synthesize cortisol and androgens, lack the required enzymes for synthesis of aldosterone.

Glucocorticoids

Approximately 10 to 30 mg of cortisol is secreted daily, and as much as 200 mg of cortisol may be produced each day during periods of maximal stress. Secretion of cortisol is regulated by the hypothalamus and the pituitary, which secrete corticotropin-releasing factor (CRF) and ACTH, respectively, under a classic negative feedback loop. Secretion follows a diurnal rhythm with peak cortisol levels occurring between 4 and 8 A.M. and the nadir between 8 P.M. and midnight. Increased secretion occurs in response to physical and emotional stress including surgery, trauma, pain, hemorrhage, exercise, and acute anxiety.

The glucocorticoids exert a broad range of metabolic effects on a variety of cells and tissues. They act to spare carbohydrates by increasing hepatic gluconeogenesis, increasing glycogen storage in the liver, and promoting conversion of amino acids to carbohydrates. They inhibit peripheral glucose uptake, resulting in a compensatory hyperinsulinism. Cortisol inhibits protein synthesis and increases protein catabolism, which leads to muscle weakness in patients with cortisol excess. Glucocorticoids also stimulate lipolysis of fat and cause redistribution of fat into truncal areas. Other effects include inhibition of intestinal calcium absorption and induction of negative calcium balance, leading to osteoporosis. Steroids also impair collagen synthesis and inhibit fibroblast activity, which adversely affects postoperative wound healing. Steroids exert a variety of anti-inflammatory effects as well, including decreasing cytokine production and inhibiting function of neutrophils and other inflammatory cells. Finally, glucocorticoids enhance cardiovascular stability, as evidenced by the cardiovascular collapse that may occur in patients with acute adrenal insufficiency. Chronic excess circulating glucocorticoids cause atrophy of the normal adrenal cortex and inability to increase cortisol secretion in response to stress.

Adrenal Androgens

The principal adrenal androgens are dehydroepiandrosterone (DHEA), its sulfated derivative DHEA sulfate, and androstenedione. The androgens have little direct biological activity until converted peripherally to testosterone and dihydrotestosterone. Secretion is regulated and stimulated by ACTH. In normal males, adrenal androgens count for less than 5% of total testosterone production. States of increased production include Cushing's syndrome, adrenal carcinoma, and congenital adrenal hyperplasia. Because of the low contribution of the adrenals to overall testosterone production in normal adult males, the clinical effects of increased adrenal androgen production in male patients are often minimal. In prepubertal boys, however, excessive adrenal androgens may cause early development of secondary sexual characteristics. In women, excess androgen states are associated with the development of acne, hirsutism, virilization, and menstrual irregularities.

Aldosterone

Aldosterone is produced exclusively by cells of the zona glomerulosa. Aldosterone acts to regulate sodium and potassium balance and maintain extracellular fluid volume. Secretion is regulated by the renin–angiotensin–aldosterone axis. The juxtaglomerular cells of the kidney secrete renin in response to decreased perfusion pressure in the renal afferent arterioles. Renin stimulates conversion of angiotensin to angiotensin I, which is in turn converted to angiotensin II by a converting enzyme in the lung. Angiotensin II is a potent vasoconstrictor that stimulates secretion of aldosterone by the adrenal. Aldosterone, in turn, stimulates renal tubular reabsorption of sodium in exchange for potassium, resulting in fluid reabsorption and volume expansion.

Adrenal Medulla

The biologically active catecholamines dopamine, norepinephrine, and epinephrine are synthesized in the adrenal medulla and select central nervous system neurons. Tyrosine, derived from dietary sources and from phenylalanine, serves as the substrate for catecholamine synthesis. Conversion of norepinephrine to epinephrine is catalyzed by the enzyme phenylethanolamine-N-methyl transferase (PNMT), which is found only in the adrenal medulla and organ of Zuckerkandl. The high local concentrations of cortisol found in the adrenal medulla are necessary for induction of PNMT activity. Catecholamines are secreted in response to various stimuli including exercise, hemorrhage, surgery, trauma, myocardial ischemia, hypoglycemia, and anoxia. Peripherally, the actions of the catecholamines are mediated via interactions with α- and β-adrenergic receptors. Stimulation of α-adrenergic receptors results in vasoconstriction; β_1 receptors mediate increased heart rate and contractility whereas activation of β_2 receptors results in vasodilatation and bronchial dilatation.

Adrenal Tumors and Associated Clinical Syndromes

Aldosteronoma

The syndrome of primary hyperaldosteronism (Conn's syndrome) is characterized by autonomous increased production of aldosterone from the zona glomerulosa. Because of negative feedback on the juxtaglomerular cells due to expansion of the extracellular fluid volume,

renin production is suppressed. Prevalence rates for primary hyperaldosteronism have been estimated at 0.7% of the hypertensive population,[10] although a much higher incidence of this disorder has been observed recently in some centers.[11,12] The most common cause of primary hyperaldosteronism is an aldosterone-producing adenoma, which accounts for approximately 70% to 80% of cases; between 20% and 30% of cases are caused by idiopathic hyperaldosteronism from bilateral cortical hyperplasia.[13] Aldosterone-producing carcinomas are extremely rare lesions, accounting for less than 1% of surgically treated cases.

The signs and symptoms of hyperaldosteronism are nonspecific but may include muscle weakness, fatigue, and polyuria, all of which are due to hypokalemia. The diagnosis should be suspected in any patient who presents with hypertension and spontaneous hypokalemia. Demonstration of elevated plasma or urine aldosterone levels in conjunction with suppressed plasma renin activity (plasma aldosterone:plasma renin activity ratio, >20–30) in a patient with hypokalemia establishes the diagnosis biochemically.[13–15] Twenty-four-hour urine potassium losses should exceed 30 mEq/day.

Once the diagnosis of primary hyperaldosteronism has been established biochemically, the next step is to determine the etiology. It is important to distinguish an aldosterone-producing adenoma from idiopathic hyperaldosteronism because the latter should be managed medically with spironolactone and not by adrenalectomy. Radiographic imaging should be carried out, preferably with a computed tomographic (CT) scan, which is more sensitive for detecting small adenomas than magnetic resonance imaging (MRI). If a discrete adenoma (>1 cm) is present and the contralateral adrenal appears normal by CT, then the patient should undergo unilateral adrenalectomy. If the nodule is smaller than 1 cm (microadenoma) or if there are bilateral nodules, then bilateral adrenal vein sampling for aldosterone and cortisol should be undertaken to determine if a unilateral gradient of increased aldosterone production exists.[16] If increased aldosterone production lateralizes to one gland, then the patient should undergo adrenalectomy. Aldosterone-producing adenomas are ideal cases for laparoscopic excision because most of these lesions are small and benign.

Cushing's Syndrome

Cushing's syndrome is the clinical state that results from chronic excessive production of cortisol by the adrenal cortex. Obesity is the most constant feature of Cushing's syndrome and has a characteristic truncal distribution including the development of moon facies, a buffalo hump over the upper back, and increased supraclavicular fat deposition. Other common features include facial plethora, hirsutism, hypertension, muscle weakness, skin striae, and easy bruisability. The most common cause of Cushing's syndrome is excessive ACTH secretion by a pituitary adenoma, which accounts for about 60% to 70% of all cases.[17] Primary adrenal tumors are much less common and comprise only 15% to 20% of cases. Occasionally, a patient may have Cushing's syndrome caused by primary adrenal hyperplasia, also known as pigmented micronodular adrenal hyperplasia or macronodular adrenal hyperplasia.[18] Ectopic production of ACTH by nonadrenal tumors accounts for about 15% of cases.

The diagnostic evaluation of a patient with suspected Cushing's syndrome involves two steps: (1) establishing the presence of excessive cortisol secretion and (2) determining the cause of the excess cortisol production.[17,19] The diagnosis is best established by demonstration of elevated 24-h urine free cortisol levels or by failure to suppress morning plasma cortisol levels to less than 5 μg/dl after administration of 1 mg dexamethasone the night before. Once the presence of hypercortisolism is confirmed, further diagnostic testing is indicated to determine the etiology. Patients with elevated plasma ACTH levels should have further testing to distinguish pituitary from ectopic ACTH sources. If the plasma ACTH level is low, an adrenal source should be suspected, and the patient should then undergo adrenal imaging with either a CT scan or MRI. Cortisol-producing adenomas are best treated by unilateral adrenalectomy. Bilateral adrenalectomy is indicated for the occasional patient with persistent Cushing's syndrome caused by failed treatment of pituitary tumors or ectopic ACTH syndrome or the rare patient who has Cushing's syndrome from primary adrenal hyperplasia.

Adrenocortical Carcinoma

Adrenocortical carcinoma is a rare lesion with an incidence of approximately 1 per 2 million population.[20,21] The lesion occurs somewhat more commonly in females than males, with a peak incidence between the ages of 30 and 50 years. Adrenocortical carcinoma may also present in children, in whom it occurs at a frequency greater than that of benign lesions. Most patients with adrenocortical carcinoma have a large mass at the time of diagnosis that may be palpable in some patients. In two large series of adrenocortical carcinoma, the mean tumor size was 12 and 15 cm, respectively.[22,23] Approximately one-half of adrenocortical carcinomas are biologically active and secrete cortisol, androgens, and other metabolites. The most common clinical features are those of Cushing's syndrome; about 10% of patients have virilizing features and 12% have evidence of feminization. In addition to measurement of urine cortisol levels, diagnostic evaluation should include assessment of urinary 17-ketosteroids and plasma DHEA sulfate levels. Small adrenocortical carcinomas (<5 cm in size) are rare but have been reported.[24–28]

Complete resection of all tumor at the initial surgery offers the only chance for cure of adrenocortical carcinoma. Because of the large size of these lesions and because of the increased risk of fracture with the laparoscopic approach, they should be removed surgically via an open transabdominal incision. Occasionally, a thoracoabdominal approach is needed for extremely large tumors with contiguous organ involvement that may require en bloc resection. On the right, the tumor may involve the inferior vena cava and even extend into the right atrium, which may require cardiopulmonary bypass for removal. Overall 5-year survival rates are approximately 35%,[20,23,29] approaching 50% with complete resection.[20,23] Surgical debulking may be indicated for hormonally active tumors that cannot be completely resected to alleviate hormonal symptoms. Partial responses to chemotherapy with mitotane have been observed in some patients. Adjuvant chemotherapy following surgical resection appears to be of no benefit.

The diagnosis of adrenocortical carcinoma can be difficult histologically. Because tumor size (>6 cm diameter) and weight (>100 g) are two of the best predictors of malignancy,[30,31] one should probably not attempt laparoscopic removal of large, primary adrenocortical tumors that meet these criteria. Other histological features associated with malignancy include evidence of vascular or capsular invasion, increased mitotic activity, and tumor necrosis and hemorrhage. Locally these tumors spread to lymph nodes, adjacent structures, and distant metastatic sites including the lung, liver, and bone. Harrison and associates[22] found that increased tumor size more than 12 cm, high mitotic activity (up to 6 mitoses/10 higher-power fields), and intratumor hemorrhage were all adverse prognostic signs.

Pheochromocytoma

Pheochromocytomas are catecholamine-secreting tumors that arise in the adrenal medulla and sympathetic ganglia. These tumors account for about 0.1% of cases of diastolic hypertension and are characterized by a 10% frequency of distribution: 10% to 15% extraadrenal, 10% familial, 10% malignant, 10% bilateral, and 10% in children. Extraadrenal tumors can occur anywhere along the sympathetic chain where chromaffin cells reside, but the most common extraadrenal site is in the organ of Zuckerkandl located to the left of the aorta between the inferior mesenteric artery and aortic bifurcation. Extraadrenal tumors have a higher risk of malignancy than adrenal pheochromocytomas. Familial pheochromocytomas can occur in a variety of settings including multiple endocrine neoplasia types 2A and 2B and von Hippel–Lindau syndrome. Pheochromocytomas in these

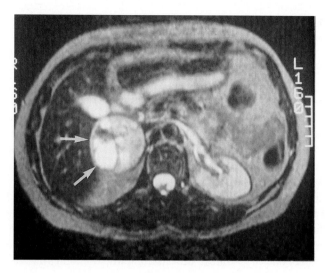

FIGURE 26.3. T$_2$-weighted MRI in a patient with a right adrenal pheochromocytoma.

patients often present at a younger age and have a high incidence of bilaterality.

The classic presentation of a pheochromocytoma is one of hypertension associated with spells consisting of palpitations, tachycardia, headache, and anxiety. Patients may also experience sweating and pallor from peripheral vasoconstriction. Some patients may present in a hypertensive crisis with profound elevation of the blood pressure and complications of congestive heart failure, myocardial infarction, and stroke. Hypertension is sustained in about 50% of patients.[32]

The diagnosis of pheochromocytoma is established by demonstrating elevated levels of catecholamines (norepinephrine and epinephrine) and metabolites (metanephrines) in a 24-h urine collection. Documentation of elevation of plasma catecholamines during a hypertensive episode can also be diagnostic but is mainly reserved for patients with normal or marginal urinary levels. The use of provocative tests is rarely indicated and is potentially dangerous. Once the diagnosis is established, imaging should be carried out with either CT or MRI. Pheochromocytomas typically have a bright appearance on T$_2$-weighted MRI sequences[33] (Fig. 26.3). Pheochromocytomas can also be imaged with the radionuclide agent ^{131}I-meta-iodylbenzylguanidine (^{131}I-MIBG), which detects pheochromocytomas but not normal adrenal tissue.[34] The main indications for scanning with ^{131}I-MIBG are (1) to search for an occult tumor in a patient with clinical and biochemical evidence of a pheochromocytoma in whom the CT and MRI scans are negative, (2) to evaluate patients with extraadrenal tumors, and (3) to follow patients with malignant pheochromocytomas.

Once a diagnosis of pheochromocytoma has been established, the patient should be prepared for adrenalectomy. A laparoscopic approach is appropriate for most patients, although large, obviously malignant pheochromocytomas with evidence of local tissue invasion should be managed in an open fashion. It is critical that all patients with pheochromocytomas be prepared pharmacologically for surgery to avoid a hypertensive crisis from catecholamine release during the stress of surgery and tumor manipulation. Alpha-adrenergic receptor blockade with phenoxybenzamine should be carried out for several days before the operation. The goal of therapy is to control hypertension and tachycardia as well as symptoms. Fluids should be given liberally to achieve adequate volume expansion preoperatively. β-Receptor blockade should be used only for patients with tachyarrhythmias or predominantly epinephrine-secreting tumors. Failure to adequately prepare the patient pharmacologically can result in a severe hypertensive crisis intraoperatively with potentially fatal consequences.

Incidental Adrenal Mass

Adrenal masses are detected in approximately 0.4% to 4.4% of all abdominal CT scans.[35–38] Consequently, the incidentally discovered adrenal mass is the most common adrenal lesion seen by surgeons today. Once an incidental mass is discovered, one should determine (1) whether the lesion is hormonally active and (2) whether it is potentially malignant. The evaluation should begin with a careful history and physical examination with particular attention to the presence of hypertension and other stigmata of the various hormone syndromes described here. All patients should have measurement of urinary catecholamines and metabolites to exclude a pheochromocytoma. Subclinical hypercortisolism due to partially autonomous cortisol secretion has been observed in 2% to 15% of patients with adrenal incidentalomas.[39–41] Screening for hypercortisolism should be carried out with the low-dose overnight dexamethasone test.[41,42] Biochemical evaluation for hyperaldosteronism is reserved for patients who have hypertension or spontaneous hypokalemia. Patients with larger tumors (≥4cm) or potentially malignant lesions should have measurement of plasma DHEA sulfate levels, which are more likely to be elevated in patients with malignant lesions. Adrenalectomy is indicated for all hyperfunctioning lesions.

Size is an important factor in determining whether an adrenal incidentaloma should be removed. Most adrenal adenomas are less than 4cm in diameter, whereas the incidence of carcinoma in tumors greater than 6cm ranges from 35% to 98%.[30,31,43] The imaging characteristics of the lesion may also be useful in determining the risk of malignancy. Cortical adenomas are usually well-circumscribed, low-attenuation lesions on noncontrast CT imaging (<10 Hounsfield units).[44,45] Malignant lesions, in contrast, typically are inhomogeneous with irregular borders and associated evidence of local invasion, and on

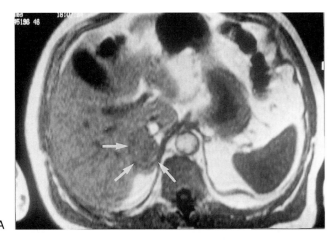

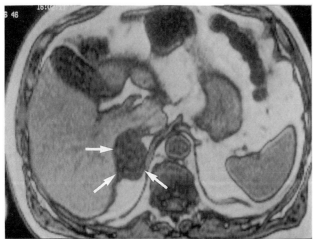

FIGURE 26.4. Chemical shift MRI sequences in a patient with an adrenal adenoma. A. In-phase images. B. Opposed-phase images show a loss of signal intensity compared to in-phase sequences.

according to the radiographic tumor appearance, patient preference, and other factors. Laparoscopic adrenalectomy may be appropriate for selected patients with nonfunctioning adrenal tumors, but the ability to perform this procedure should not lead to a more liberal policy of adrenalectomy. Patients who do not undergo adrenalectomy should have follow-up imaging with CT or MRI in 3 and 12 months to evaluate for possible growth of the mass.

Adrenal Metastasis

Per unit weight, the adrenal is one of the most common sites for metastasis. Primary tumors with a high incidence of adrenal metastases include lung carcinoma and renal cell carcinoma, but other cancers including colorectal,

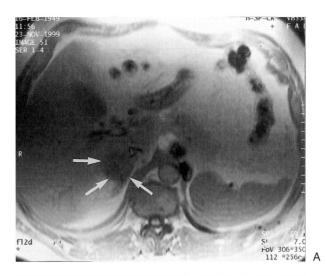

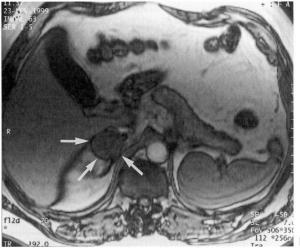

FIGURE 26.5. Chemical shift MRI sequences in a patient with a right adrenal metastasis from renal cell carcinoma. A. In-phase images. B. Opposed-phase images show no loss of signal intensity compared to in-phase sequences.

noncontrast scans they usually have high attenuation values (>18 Hounsfeld units). MRI can also be useful in evaluating these tumors. Benign lesions typically exhibit a loss in signal intensity on opposed-phase MRI sequences[46,47] (Figs. 26.4, 26.5), whereas malignant lesions should show no loss of signal. Fine-needle aspiration (FNA) cytology is not usually indicated for the evaluation of patients with primary adrenal masses and should never be carried out unless a pheochromocytoma has first been excluded biochemically. The primary role of FNA is in the patient with a known extraadrenal malignancy who has a unilateral adrenal mass.

The precise size cutoff for which adrenalectomy should be performed is controversial. Most endocrine surgeons recommend observation of lesions less than 4 cm and removal of those 6 cm or larger. Whether adrenalectomy should be performed in patients with intermediate-size lesions (4–6 cm) is a decision that must be individualized

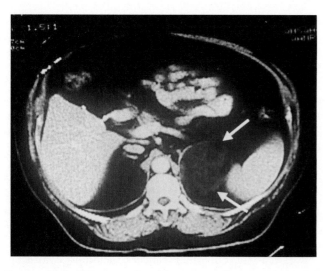

FIGURE 26.6. CT scan of a 10-cm myelolipoma of the left adrenal. (Reprinted with permission from Brunt LM, Moley JF. World J Surg 2001; 25(7):905–915.)

breast, lymphoma, and melanoma may also spread to the adrenal. In most cases, adrenal metastases occur in the setting of systemic metastatic disease, although an occasional patient will be appropriate for resection. In patients with a known extraadrenal primary tumor who also have metastatic disease in other sites, the incidence of metastasis to the adrenal has ranged from 13% to 26%.[42,48,49] Candel et al.[50] found that the risk of metastasis in a patient with a known extraadrenal primary increased with increasing size of the lesion. In their series, adrenal masses less than 3 cm in size were benign in 87% of cases whereas more than 95% of lesions greater than 3 cm were malignant. Fine-needle aspiration biopsy may be warranted in the patient with an adrenal mass and a history of an extraadrenal malignancy. Biopsy should not be performed, however, until biochemical studies have excluded the presence of a pheochromocytoma. Prolonged survival has been reported in a small percentage of cases after resection of unilateral adrenal metastasis.[51–53] In a review of Veterans hospital admissions, the 5-year survival rate after resection was 13%.[54] Laparoscopic resection of adrenal metastases has been reported[55,56] but is controversial. Laparoscopic adrenalectomy should not be attempted in this setting unless the surgeon is highly experienced and the lesion is well circumscribed and can be completely resected with negative margins.

Other Adrenal Tumors

A variety of other less common adrenal tumors can be seen. Myelolipomas are benign lesions composed of fat and bone marrow elements; they are usually discovered incidentally during CT imaging and can become quite large. Most are asymptomatic, but symptoms may occur with very large tumors or those in which there has been recent hemorrhage. These lesions are recognized radiographically by the characteristic CT (Fig. 26.6) or MRI appearance and high lipid content.

Adrenal cysts are usually discovered incidentally during CT or MRI scanning. Most are pseudocysts or lymphangiectatic cysts. The size is variable, and they are typically unilateral. Acute symptoms may result from hemorrhage into the cyst. Surgical resection is not indicated unless the patient has hemorrhaged into the cyst or the diagnosis is uncertain.

Ganglioneuromas are benign tumors comprised of mature ganglion cells with associated Schwann cells and neurofibrils in a collagen fibrous tissue matrix; they are typically asymptomatic and most often occur in older children and adults. About 30% arise from the adrenal medulla, but they can arise anywhere along the sympathetic chain,[57] and they may occasionally secrete vasoactive substances. These lesions can become large and may adhere to adjacent structures, which makes excision difficult. A variety of other tumors that may also occur less commonly in the adrenal include lymphoma, hemangioma, sarcoma, and other neuroblastic tumors including neuroblastoma.

Laparoscopic Adrenalectomy

Indications and Contraindications

Adrenalectomy is indicated for any patient with a hormonally active or functional tumor or suspected primary adrenal malignancy. Most hormonally active tumors are benign lesions less than 6 cm in size and are, therefore, appropriate for laparoscopic excision (Table 26.1).

TABLE 26.1. Indications and contraindications for laparoscopic adrenalectomy.

Indications
  Aldosteronoma
  Cushing's syndrome
    Cortisol-producing adenoma
    Primary adrenal hyperplasia
    Failed treatment of ACTH-dependent Cushing's
Pheochromocytoma (sporadic or familial)
Nonfunctioning cortical adenoma (>5 cm or atypical radiographic
   appearance)
Adrenal metastasis
Miscellaneous tumors (myelolipoma, adrenal cyst, ganglioneuroma)
Contraindications
  Large adrenocortical carcinoma (>5–6 cm)
  Malignant pheochromocytoma
  Large adrenal mass >8–10 cm diameter
  Existing contraindication to laparoscopic surgery

Laparoscopic adrenalectomy is also a valid approach for removal of hyperplastic glands in patients with ACTH-dependent Cushing's syndrome who have failed treatment of the pituitary or ectopic ACTH source and for Cushing's syndrome due to nodular adrenal hyperplasia. Laparoscopic adrenalectomy has also been used for the treatment of congenital adrenal hyperplasia.[58]

The role of laparoscopic adrenalectomy in the management of patients with primary adrenal malignancies has not yet been established. However, for several reasons most endocrine surgeons recommend an open approach to the patient with a large adrenal mass that appears malignant.[59] First, large tumors are more difficult to manipulate laparoscopically, which could increase the risk of tumor spillage. Second, adrenal malignancies may invade contiguous organs, soft tissue, or lymph nodes that require resection. The lack of tactile feedback and reduced ability to manipulate the adrenal also become more dominant factors as the lesion enlarges. Isolated case reports of tumor recurrence after laparoscopic adrenalectomy have recently appeared (see Complications, following).[60–63] These reports raise concerns that patients with malignant adrenal lesions could be at increased risk for inadequate resection and tumor spillage, as has been observed for patients undergoing laparoscopic procedures in the setting of gallbladder cancer[64,65] and colon cancer.[66,67] For these reasons, the practice in our institution has been to approach primary adrenal malignancies more than 6 cm in diameter by open adrenalectomy.

The precise size cutoff for which laparoscopic adrenalectomy is appropriate in nonmalignant-appearing adrenal masses is unclear. However, laparoscopic resection of adrenal masses greater than 8 cm in diameter has been reported by several groups,[60,68–73] and it has been technically possible to remove lesions up to 13–14 cm in diameter.[68,69,74] Because of the increased technical difficulty associated with laparoscopic removal of larger tumors, an appropriate size cutoff might be 8 to 10 cm for noncortical tumors such as pheochromocytomas or myelolipomas and 6 cm for adrenal cortical tumors. Only the most skilled and experienced laparoscopic endocrine surgeons should attempt to remove adrenal masses in this size range.

Several groups have used laparoscopic adrenalectomy to remove nonfunctioning adrenal masses. As discussed here, it is important that the indications for removal of these lesions not be liberalized because of the availability of the laparoscopic approach.

Patient Preparation

Patients with hormonally active tumors must be properly prepared preoperatively to minimize the risks of surgery and anesthesia. Hypertension should be under control, and electrolyte abnormalities should be corrected. Patients with aldosteronomas may benefit from treatment with spironolactone as well as oral potassium supplementation. Patients with Cushing's syndrome have atrophy of the contralateral adrenal and, therefore, require administration of stress steroids perioperatively.

Patients with pheochromocytomas should have stable pharmacologic blockade with an α-adrenergic receptor blocking agent. The goal is to control hypertension and tachycardia and eliminate spells or paroxysms. Our practice has been to start patients on phenoxybenzamine at a dose of 10 mg twice daily and titrate the dose upward until the above goals have been met. Most patients experience mild orthostatic hypotension with adequate blockade, which often requires 1 week of therapy to accomplish. Patients should take oral fluids liberally as the blockade progresses and are usually given intravenous fluids the night before surgery.

Perioperative monitoring consists of an electrocardiogram, pulse oximetry, and urinary catheter in all patients. Patients who have labile hypertension and all patients with pheochromocytomas should have an arterial line intraoperatively. A central venous pressure line is reserved for patients with large tumors or active pheochromocytomas. Occasionally, a patient with significant underlying cardiac disease requires placement of a pulmonary artery catheter intraoperatively. Patients with pheochromocytomas must be given adequate fluids intraoperatively and, if they become hypotensive, should be treated with aggressive fluid resuscitation rather than vasopressors. Hypertensive exacerbations intraoperatively are treated with intravenous nitroprusside (Nitropress). Hypertensive exacerbations and tachycardia are most likely to occur during anesthetic induction, insufflation of CO_2 pneumoperitoneum, and with direct tumor manipulation.

Equipment

The minimum equipment requirements for performing laparoscopic adrenalectomy include a video laparoscopy cart with a high-quality imaging system, an angled laparoscope, and basic laparoscopic instruments. The cost of disposable supplies can be minimized by the use of reusable trocars, clip appliers, and suction-irrigation devices. A right-angle clamp is useful for isolating the adrenal vein, and a retractor is necessary for elevating the liver during right adrenalectomy. An ultrasonic coagulator can be useful for performing the dissection if the tumor is large or if there is much retroperitoneal fat, especially for left-sided lesions. Laparoscopic ultrasound may also be beneficial in selected cases, as discussed next. An impermeable entrapment bag is used for specimen removal.

Surgical Technique

A variety of laparoscopic approaches to adrenalectomy have been described that closely mimic their open counterparts: the transabdominal flank approach, the retroperitoneal approach and the anterior transabdominal approach. The transabdominal lateral flank approach is the most widely utilized of these procedures. The advantages of this approach are that it provides the surgeon with a large working space and allows excellent access to the superior retroperitoneum. Although the patient is in a lateral decubitus position, anatomic landmarks to help maintain orientation of the dissection are readily apparent. Retraction of adjacent viscera is facilitated by gravity as a result of the patient's position. One can also examine other intraabdominal organs and perform concomitant procedures such as cholecystectomy or liver biopsy. Excellent results have also been reported with this technique in several different centers.[69,71–73,75–77] The disadvantages of this approach are that some retraction of adjacent viscera is required and, on the left side, the colon must be partially mobilized, which can result in a transient period of postoperative ileus. One is also unable to approach the contralateral adrenal because of the lateral decubitus position. Therefore, for bilateral adrenalectomy, the patient must be repositioned between sides. The risk of injury to other intraperitoneal organs should be minimal with this technique, but it is more difficult if the patient has had extensive previous upper abdominal surgery.

The retroperitoneal approach avoids entry into the peritoneal cavity altogether and involves minimal retraction of adjacent organs. The disadvantages of this technique are that the working space is small and it can be more difficult to establish one's orientation anatomically, especially if the patient has a large amount of retroperitoneal fat (e.g., Cushing's syndrome). It is also more difficult to manage larger tumors (≥5 cm) with this approach, and if a peritoneal tear occurs during the operation the working space may be further compromised. A potential advantage of this technique is that patients may have less postoperative ileus because the peritoneal cavity is usually not violated. The retroperitoneal approach has also been used to perform bilateral adrenalectomy without the need for repositioning the patient.

The anterior transabdominal approach is carried out with the patient supine. The principal advantages of this approach are that it provides a conventional view of intraabdominal anatomy and allows access to both the right and left adrenal glands. The operative exposure can be more difficult, however, because of the extra effort required to retract other abdominal organs and the need for placement of additional trocars.

Transabdominal Lateral Flank Approach

The operating room setup is shown in Figure 26.7. Video monitors are positioned at the head of the table on either side. The patient is placed in a lateral decubitus position with the affected side up and is secured in this position with a gel-padded beanbag mattress. The hips and legs are secured to the table with tape and a safety strap, and compression stockings are placed on the legs. All pressure points including the hips, legs, and axilla are amply padded to prevent nerve compression injuries. The operating room table should be flexed to open up the flank for better port access. The table is then tilted into reverse Trendelenburg to facilitate exposure in the retroperitoneum.

The surgeon should stand in a position that is comfortable for working with a two-handed technique. In most cases, standing on the right side is preferable for a right-hand-dominant surgeon and the left side for a left-handed individual. The camera operator should stand opposite the side being operated on, and the assistant is across from the surgeon.

Initial access to the peritoneal cavity is usually obtained with a Veress needle inserted just medial to the anterior axillary line about two fingerbreadths below the costal margin. Alternatively, initial access can be obtained at the umbilicus using an open technique with a Hasson cannula. In larger individuals, however, the umbilical port may not provide adequate access to the superior retroperitoneum. Once initial access has been obtained, three additional ports are inserted in the subcostal and flank region (Fig. 26.8). Our preference is to use one 10- to 12-mm port for insertion of the 10-mm clip applier and for specimen extraction; the remaining ports can be 5 mm

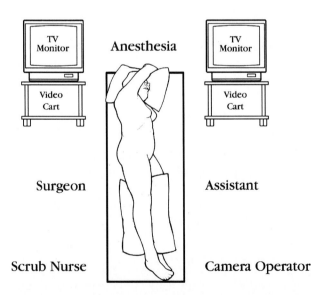

FIGURE 26.7. Operating room setup for laparoscopic right adrenalectomy with the transabdominal lateral approach.

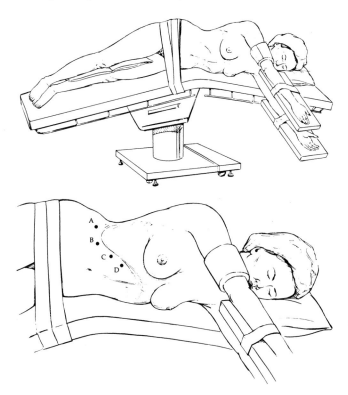

so that the liver can be rotated and retracted medially, thereby exposing the right retroperitoneum, adrenal gland, and inferior vena cava. It is rarely necessary to mobilize either the hepatic flexure of the colon or the duodenum using this approach. The inferior vena cava should be identified early in the procedure, and one must be aware of its location at all times during the dissection. Beginning along the medial border of the gland, the peritoneum between the adrenal and the inferior vena cava is incised. A combination of blunt dissection and the hook cautery is used for much of the dissection. The medial border of the adrenal should be cleanly defined and dissected away from the inferior vena cava until the right adrenal vein is identified. Hemostasis should be meticulous because even minor bleeding will stain the tissues and tissue planes and make the dissection difficult and dangerous.

The adrenal gland and tumor should be retracted by gently pushing or elevating it with a blunt instrument. The gland may also be retracted by grasping the periadrenal fat, but one should avoid grasping the gland or

FIGURE 26.8. Patient position and port site placement for laparoscopic right adrenalectomy using the transabdominal lateral approach. Initial access to the peritoneal cavity is usually accomplished at sites *C* or *D*. Port sizes are as follows: *A*, 5mm; *B*, 11mm; *C*, 5mm; *D*, 5mm. Further details regarding positioning and port placement are given in the text. (Reprinted with permission from Brunt LM. Laparoscopic adrenalectomy. In: Eubanks S, et al. (eds) Mastery of Endoscopic and Laparoscopic Surgery. Philadelphia: Lippincott, 2000:324.)

or even needlescopic depending on the individual case and the patient's body habitus. Left adrenalectomy can be carried out using only three ports total in selected cases. All ports should be spaced 5cm or more apart to allow freedom of movement externally.

The keys to success for laparoscopic adrenalectomy, regardless of the surgical approach chosen, include adequate exposure of the adrenal gland in the retroperitoneum, meticulous hemostasis to keep a clear surgical field, and extracapsular dissection of the adrenal to avoid bleeding or tumor spillage. The initial exposure is enhanced by adequate mobilization of adjacent organs and by allowing gravity to aid in retraction of those organs.

Right Adrenalectomy

The first step in laparoscopic right adrenalectomy using the lateral approach is to divide the right triangular ligament of the liver (Fig. 26.9). The L-hook electrocautery works well for this purpose. This ligament should be divided from the inferior vena cava up to the diaphragm

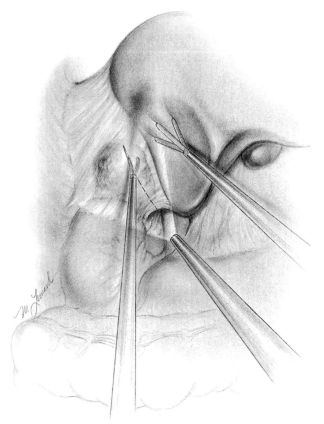

FIGURE 26.9. Technique for medial retraction of the liver and division of the right triangular ligament during laparoscopic right adrenalectomy. (Reprinted with permission from Brunt LM. Laparoscopic adrenalectomy. In: Eubanks S, et al. (eds) Mastery of Endoscopic and Laparoscopic Surgery. Philadelphia: Lippincott, 2000:325.)

Regardless of the method employed, one must exert tremendous caution during this portion of the dissection because the vein can be easily torn up into the vena cava. Once the vein has been divided, the medial, superior, and inferior borders of the adrenal are further dissected. Arterial branches are ligated with either clips or the ultrasonic coagulator. Smaller vessels can be divided with electrocautery. As these edges are mobilized, the gland is bluntly elevated and dissection is continued along the posterior border, where it is mobilized off the diaphragm. Finally, the lateral areolar attachments to the gland are divided. The adrenal is then placed in impermeable entrapment sack for removal. The retroperitoneum should be irrigated and inspected for hemostasis, but drains are not routinely inserted. The fascia at all 10-mm port sites is closed with absorbable 0-suture, and the skin is closed with a subcuticular layer.

Left Adrenalectomy

For left adrenalectomy, the splenic flexure of the colon must be mobilized from the left paracolic gutter to the inferior pole of the spleen. It is usually necessary to complete this maneuver before the most dorsal fourth port can be inserted. One must take care not to dissect posterior to the left kidney as this will cause the kidney to fall medially over the adrenal. The splenorenal ligament should then be divided from the inferior splenic pole to the diaphragm to allow the spleen and tail of the pancreas to rotate medially, exposing the left retroperitoneum (Fig. 26.11). Often the stomach and short gastric vessels are visible as the most cephalad portion of the splenorenal ligament is divided. The adrenal gland should at this point be identifiable between the spleen and superior pole of the kidney. It may be difficult at first to recognize the adrenal gland on the left side, especially if the patient has a large amount of retroperitoneal fat or if the gland harbors a small tumor or is hyperplastic. Laparoscopic ultrasound may be helpful in this setting to localize the gland and define its relationship to adjacent structures (see following). The tail of the pancreas should be visualized during splenic mobilization and should not be mistaken for the adrenal. Gentle retraction should be used around the pancreas to avoid bleeding or parenchymal injury.

Once the left adrenal gland has been located, its borders should be clearly defined. If the inferomedial border of the gland is visible, dissection may proceed directly in this area to expose and ligate the left adrenal vein (Fig. 26.12). However, exposure in this area is often difficult, and in most cases the superior, medial, and lateral borders of the adrenal are dissected first. It is important that the dissection stay close to the adrenal to avoid injury or ligation of renal arterial vessels. The inferior phrenic vein frequently joins the adrenal vein just

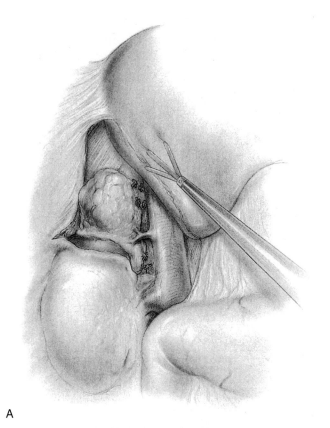

A

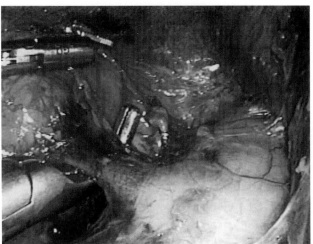

B

FIGURE 26.10. A. Dissection of the right adrenal gland with exposure of the right adrenal vein. B. Operative view of isolated right adrenal vein. The tumor is to the left and the inferior vena cava to the right.

tumor itself because the gland is friable and may bleed or the tumor may be violated. A right-angle dissector is useful in isolating the adrenal vein, which is usually ligated with two endoclips proximally on the vena cava side and one distally (Fig. 26.10). Alternatively, one can ligate the vein with sutures or an endovascular stapler.

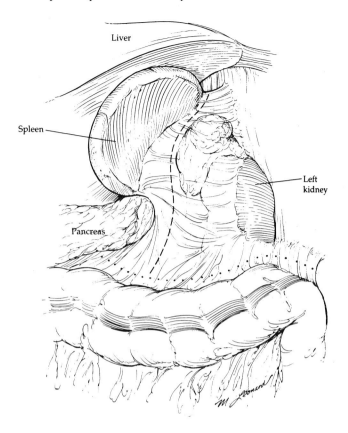

FIGURE 26.11. Exposure of the left adrenal gland during laparoscopic left adrenalectomy. The splenic flexure of the colon is divided first (*dotted line*) followed by division of the splenorenal ligament (*dashed line*). (Reprinted with permission from Brunt LM. Laparoscopic adrenalectomy. In: Eubanks S, et al. (eds) Mastery of Endoscopic and Laparoscopic Surgery. Philadelphia: Lippincott, 2000:326.)

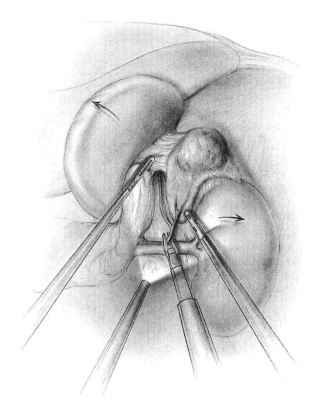

FIGURE 26.12. Laparoscopic view of the exposed left adrenal gland, spleen, tail of pancreas, kidney, adrenal vein, and left renal vein.

above its junction with the left renal vein and must also be looked for. Once the vein has been divided, the remaining attachments posterior to the gland are divided. The ultrasonic coagulator can be very helpful during dissection of the left side because of the surrounding retroperitoneal fat, especially in patients with Cushing's syndrome or in obese individuals. In dissecting larger tumors, one must also be aware medially of the proximity of the aorta to the adrenal and laterally of the renal capsule. Other structures that are at risk for injury during left adrenalectomy include the colon, spleen, tail of the pancreas, diaphragm, and renal vessels. A drain should be placed in the retroperitoneum if there is any suspicion of pancreatic injury.

Specimen Extraction

The adrenal gland and tumor are placed in an impermeable entrapment sack for removal (Fig. 26.13). For tumors 4 cm or less in diameter, the specimen can usually be removed via the 12-mm port side by enlarging the inci-

sion to 2 to 3 cm. For larger tumors, one should consider removal at the umbilicus or in the suprapubic region, especially in muscular males. Morcellation of the specimen has been advocated by some surgeons, but our preference has been to remove the specimen intact to allow thorough pathological evaluation. It is important that the

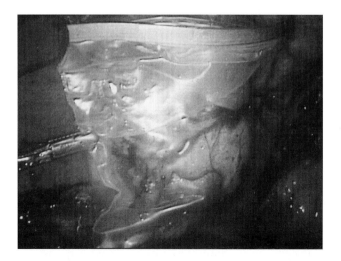

FIGURE 26.13. Extraction of a left adrenal adenoma via an entrapment bag.

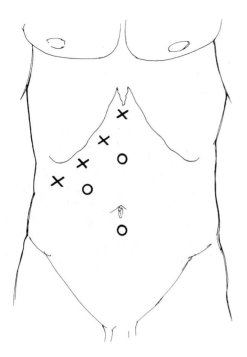

approach, the patient is put in a prone or semi-jackknife position with the hips flexed. The first port is usually inserted just lateral or inferior to the tip of the 12th rib (Fig. 26.15). A 12-mm incision is made, and sharp and blunt dissection is used to dissect through subcutaneous tissue and muscle to allow digital entry into the retroperitoneal space. The retroperitoneal space is then expanded with a balloon dissector or spacemaker device. The initial port is then inserted and the retroperitoneum insufflated to 12 to 20 mmHg^{2+} CO_2 pressure. Further expansion of the space is accomplished bluntly all the way to the diaphragm. Once the space has been adequately developed, two or three additional ports are inserted in the configuration shown in Figure 26.15B. In many cases, the adrenal gland can be difficult to visualize initially because of surrounding retroperitoneal fat. It may be helpful to define the upper pole of the kidney or use laparoscopic ultrasound to identify both the adrenal and kidney. One can also begin the dissection along the less vascular lateral border of the adrenal. On the right side, the

FIGURE 26.14. Port site placement for the anterior transabdominal approach: *x*, location of the primary ports; *o*, sites for accessory ports as needed. Initial access may be achieved at the umbilicus.

entrapment bag be impermeable as one may otherwise risk spilling cells if the tumor ruptures during manipulation and extraction through the incision.

Anterior Transabdominal Approach

The anterior transabdominal approach is carried out with the patient in a supine or hemilateral position. A total of four to six ports may be required (Fig. 26.14).[78,79] Initial peritoneal access is usually achieved at the umbilicus. For right adrenalectomy, the liver must be elevated superiorly as well as retracted medially. In addition, the transverse colon and hepatic flexure are mobilized and retracted inferiorly, and one may also have to Kocherize the second duodenum. The dissection is then carried out in a sequence similar to that for the transabdominal flank approach. For left adrenalectomy, the splenic flexure of the colon is first mobilized. The splenorenal ligament is then divided and the spleen and tail of the pancreas are retracted medially. Gerota's fascia is incised to expose the superior pole of the left kidney and the adrenal. The dissection then proceeds as described for the lateral approach.

Retroperitoneal Approach

Retroperitoneal endoscopic adrenalectomy may be performed using either a posterior lumbar/dorsal approach or a lateral approach. For the posterior lumbar or dorsal

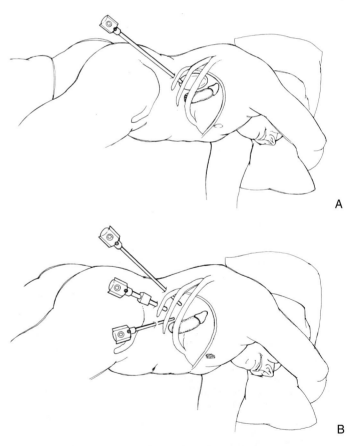

FIGURE 26.15. Port site placement for retroperitoneal endoscopic adrenalectomy (posterior lumbar or dorsal approach). A. The initial port is inserted just lateral or inferior to the tip of the 12th rib. A balloon device is then used to establish the retroperitoneal working space. B. Location of laparoscopic ports for the dorsal approach.

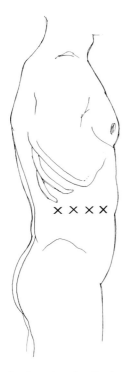

FIGURE 26.16. Port site location for the lateral retroperitoneal approach to laparoscopic adrenalectomy.

adrenal vein is at the posteromedial aspect of the gland and on the left it is at the medioinferior aspect. The dissection technique should be the same as described for the lateral approach.

Retroperitoneal adrenalectomy can also be carried out with the patient in a lateral position. Initial access is achieved via an incision placed in the midaxillary line about 3 cm above the iliac crest between the latissimus dorsi and external oblique muscles. The retroperitoneum is entered bluntly as for the posterior approach, and the space is also expanded with a balloon device. The additional ports are placed as shown in Figure 26.16. An addi-

TABLE 26.2. Potential applications of laparoscopic ultrasound during laparoscopic adrenalectomy.

Adrenal gland and tumor localization
    Learning curve phase
    Left adrenalectomy in obese patients
    Obese patients with small tumors or hyperplastic glands
    Retroperitoneal endoscopic approach to adrenalectomy
Guide to the dissection
    Identify relationship of adrenal to adjacent structures in difficult
      cases
Evaluation of pathology in other organs
Evaluation of laparoscopic resectability
    Large tumors >4 cm diameter
    Tumors with "suspicious" preoperative imaging characteristics on
      CT or MRI
Partial adrenalectomy

tional fifth port may be needed in some cases to retract the liver or if the peritoneum has been lacerated.[80] An advantage of the lateral retroperitoneal approach is that it can be converted to a transperitoneal approach if there is difficulty with the dissection.

Laparoscopic Adrenal Ultrasound

Laparoscopic ultrasound has been shown to be useful in selected patients undergoing laparoscopic adrenalectomy (Table 26.2).[81,82] In some patients, the adrenal gland and tumor may be difficult to localize surgically because of inexperience, the patient's anatomy, or increased retroperitoneal fat. In obese patients with small tumors, the left adrenal gland can be especially difficult to locate, and laparoscopic ultrasound has been helpful in this setting.[81–83] In our experience, however, it has not been necessary to use ultrasound to localize the right adrenal. Laparoscopic ultrasound also allows one to define the relationship of the adrenal gland and tumor to adjacent structures, including the renal artery and vein (Fig. 26.17) and the inferior vena cava. The adrenal vein is difficult to visualize, however, because of its small size and compressibility.[82] Laparoscopic ultrasound has also been used to demonstrate encapsulation of large or potentially malignant tumors so that one can safely proceed with laparoscopic resection (Fig. 26.18). Other potential applications of laparoscopic ultrasound during adrenalectomy include the evaluation of pathology in other organs and a guide to performing partial adrenalectomy.

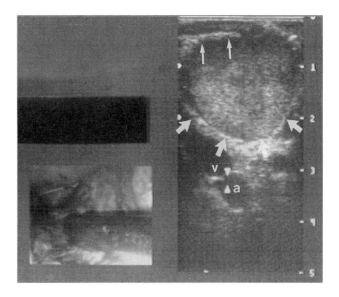

FIGURE 26.17. Laparoscopic ultrasound shows a left adrenal pheochromocytoma (*thick arrows*) with a contiguous normal adrenal limb (*thin arrows*). The renal artery (*a*) and vein (*v*) are seen just inferior to the tumor. (Reprinted with permission from Brunt LM, et al. Am J Surg. 1999;178(6):491.)

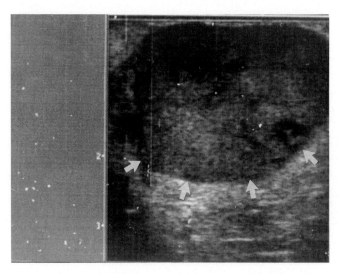

FIGURE 26.18. Laparoscopic ultrasound of metastatic renal cell carcinoma to the left adrenal. Intraoperative ultrasound showed that the lesion was well circumscribed and could be safely resected laparoscopically.

Results

The results of the various operative approaches to laparoscopic adrenalectomy have been reported in several large series. The greatest experience has been with the transperitoneal lateral approach (Table 26.3).[60,69,71–73,75–77,84–86] Conversion rates have ranged from 0% to 18%, with the most conversions occurring early during the surgeon's "learning curve" for the procedure. The most common reasons for conversion have been inexperience, bleeding (often from the adrenal vein), and difficulty in resecting larger tumors. Operative times have ranged from 2 to 3h in most cases, and blood loss has been minimal, with only the rare patient requiring transfusion. Most tumors in these series have been small (<6cm), but removal of tumors ranging in size from 8 to 14cm has been reported by several groups.[68,69,71–73]

The results of the less commonly utilized anterior transabdominal approach are summarized in Table 26.4.[70,87–89] Earlier reports of this procedure were associated with prolonged operative times and increased blood loss compared to the lateral transperitoneal approach. However, Filipponi and colleagues[70] recently achieved results comparable to the lateral approach in a large series of adrenalectomies. With their technique, only four trocars were used and operative times averaged less than 2h. Therefore, this approach does appear feasible in experienced hands and may be especially applicable to the patient who requires bilateral adrenalectomy.

The results of retroperitoneal endoscopic adrenalectomy from several series are shown in Table 26.5.[9,68,90–92] Operative times and conversion rates have been comparable to the transperitoneal lateral approach. The principal reasons for conversion to open operation have been bleeding, dissection and exposure difficulties, and loss of retropneumoperitoneum, probably from peritoneal tears. As with the other approaches, the conversion rates have decreased with increasing experience. A potential advantage of the lateral retroperitoneal approach is that it can be converted to a conventional transperitoneal approach if a peritoneal tear or other difficulty with the dissection develops. In the series reported by Takeda et al.,[93] three of six patients with Cushing's syndrome approached retroperitoneally required conversion to the transperitoneal approach.

Transperitoneal Versus Retroperitoneal Approaches

Several groups have compared outcomes from the transperitoneal lateral and retroperitoneal approaches in nonrandomized studies (Table 26.6).[68,80,92–94] In most of these reports, operative times, conversion rates, blood loss, hospital length of stay, and pain medication requirements have been similar for the two techniques. Baba et al.[94] noted significantly longer operative times and a

TABLE 26.3. Results: transperitoneal flank approach.

Series	Year	No. of cases (patients)	Conversions	Operative time (min)	Postoperative length of hospital stay (days)	Tumor size (cm) mean (range)
Miccoli et al.[72]	1995	25 (24)	0	109	3	3.1 (1–9)
Staren et al.[73]	1996	21 (21)	2 (9.5%)	206	2.2	3.2 (1–8)
Rutherford et al.[76]	1996	67 (67)	0	124	5.1	—
Marescaux et al.[71]	1996	27 (27)	5 (18%)	140	4.6	2.0 (0.5–8)
Gagner et al.[69]	1997	97 (88)	3 (3.4%)	123	2.7	4.6 (0.7–14)
de Canniere et al.[60]	1997	54 (52)	2 (4%)	80	4	4 (1.5–12)
Thompson et al.[84]	1997	50 (50)	7 (14%)	167	3.1	2.9
Terachi et al.[77]	1997	100 (100)	3 (3%)	240	—	—
Brunt et al.[82]	1999	45 (43)	0	175	2.8	3.1 (0.7–10)
Pujol et al.[86]	1999	30 (27)	2 (7%)	156	3	3.1 (1–5.7)
Imai et al.[85]	1999	41 (41)	1 (2.4%)	180	12	2.8

Table 26.4. Results: anterior transabdominal approach.

Series	Year	No. of cases (patients)	Conversions	Operative time (min)	Postoperative length of hospital stay (days)	Tumor size (cm) mean (range)
Suzuki et al.[87]	1993	12	0	278	—	2.3 (1.2–4.3)
Takeda et al.[89]	1994	17	1 (5.9%)	240	11.6	—
Stuart et al.[88]	1995	14 (14)	1 (7.1%)	157	3	—
Filliponi et al.[70]	1998	51 (50)	0	112	2.5	(1.5–8.5)

higher blood loss for the transperitoneal approach; however, the hemilateral position used for the transperitoneal operation may have accounted for these differences. In a study by Bonjer et al.,[80] the outcomes appeared to favor the retroperitoneal approach; however, inclusion of the converted patients (2/9 transperitoneal, 1/10 retroperitoneal) in the analysis may have skewed the results, given the small numbers in each group.

Fernandez-Cruz and colleagues[92] measured various physiological parameters in patients undergoing laparoscopic adrenalectomy and found that both approaches were associated with elevated pH, elevated CO_2, higher end tidal CO_2 pressures, increased base deficit, and decreased pH. Somewhat higher pCO_2 values and higher mean arterial pressure readings were recorded for the transperitoneal group. The clinical significance of these differences is unclear. However, these data suggest that either the transperitoneal or retroperitoneal approach is satisfactory for the non-obese patient with a small tumor. Patients who are obese or who have tumors ≥5 cm diameter are probably best approached transperitoneally. If the patient has had extensive upper abdominal surgery on the affected side, then a retroperitoneal approach is preferred.

Laparoscopic Versus Open Adrenalectomy

No prospective randomized trials comparing laparoscopic to open adrenalectomy have been carried out because the benefits of the laparoscopic approach became readily apparent with the introduction of this procedure. However, several groups have retrospectively compared the results of laparoscopic with open adrena-

lectomy. The largest of these series are shown in Table 26.7.[75,84,85,95–103] Operative times have been longer for laparoscopic adrenalectomy in almost every series; however, each of these studies has included the learning curve phase for the laparoscopic procedures in the results, and operative times have been shown to decrease with increasing surgical experience. Laparoscopic adrenalectomy has consistently been associated with decreased blood loss, reduced postoperative pain, a faster return to normal diet, and reduced hospital length of stay compared to open adrenalectomy performed either transabdominally or retroperitoneally. Although the magnitude of some of these differences may have been influenced by the noncontemporary nature of these retrospective comparisons as well as changing practice patterns over time, the conclusions from these various studies are probably valid. Fewer serious complications have also been reported with the laparoscopic approach, including a lower rate of blood transfusions.[75] The best data supporting the advantages of laparoscopic adrenalectomy come from two case-controlled studies. Thompson and associates[84] compared the results of 50 laparoscopic adrenalectomies with a demographically matched group of 50 patients treated by open posterior adrenalectomy. Operative times averaged 40 min longer in the laparoscopic group, but the other parameters all favored laparoscopic adrenalectomy. Similar results were achieved in a case-controlled study from Imai et al.,[85] who compared laparoscopic adrenalectomy to the open lateral approach.

No detailed cost analysis of the impact of laparoscopic adrenalectomy has been carried out. From the limited data that have been reported, it would appear that total hospital charges for this procedure are less than for open

Table 26.5. Results: retroperitoneal approach.

Series	Year	No. of cases (patients)	Conversions	Operative time (min)	Postoperative length of hospital stay (days)	Tumor size (cm) mean (range)
Mercan et al.[9]	1995	11 (8)	0	150	3	3.6 (1.5–8)
Heintz et al.[90]	1996	20 (18)	3 (15%)	180	5	—
Walz et al.[91]	1996	30 (27)	4 (13%)	124	—	(1–7)
Duh et al.[68]	1996	14	0	202	1.5	2.6 (1–6)
Fernandez-Cruz et al.[92]	1999	20 (17)	2 (10%)	105	2.8	—

TABLE 26.6. Comparative trials of laparoscopic transperitoneal versus retroperitoneal endoscopic adrenalectomy.

Series	Year	Approach	No. of cases	Conversions	Mean operative time (min)	Mean blood loss (ml)	Prostoperative hospital days
Duh et al.[68]	1996	Transperitoneal	23	0	226	—	2.2
		Retroperitoneal	14	0	202	—	1.5
Baba et al.[94]	1997	Transperitoneal	33	3 (9%)	252	101	6.1
		Retroperitoneal/posterior	13	1 (7.7%)	142	32	5.6
		Retroperitoneal/lateral	5	0	194	22	5.6
Bonjer et al.[80]	1997	Transperitoneal	9	2 (22%)	150	150	6
		Retroperitoneal	10	1 (10%)	75	20	4
Takeda et al.[93]	1997	Transperitoneal	27	—	232	155	—
		Retroperitoneal	11	1	248	151	—
Fernandez-Cruz et al.[92]	1999	Transperitoneal	22 (19)	2 (10.5%)	89	160	3
		Retroperitoneal	20 (17)	2 (10%)	105	180	2.8

transabdominal adrenalectomy and approximately the same as for the open posterior approach. Because operating room costs account for a significant percentage of the overall costs of laparoscopic adrenalectomy, limiting the use of disposable laparoscopic instrumentation and reducing operative time should make this a more cost-effective procedure.

Functional Results

Few studies have evaluated the functional outcomes of laparoscopic adrenalectomy. Filliponi and colleagues[70]

reported normalization of all biochemical data in 29 patients with hormonally active tumors, including 13 patients with hypercortisolism, 13 patients with aldosteronomas, and 3 patients with pheochromocytomas. Follow-up was short, however, at 8.5 months or less after surgery. Shen and associates[104] compared the impact of laparoscopic versus open adrenalectomy on clinical outcomes in patients with primary hyperaldosteronism. Forty-two patients underwent laparoscopic adrenalectomy, and 38 had open adrenalectomy; patients in the open group had more severe hypertension and hypokalemia preoperatively. At a follow-up interval

TABLE 26.7. Comparative series of laparoscopic versus open adrenalectomy.

Series	Year	Approach	No. of cases (patients)	Operative time (min)	Blood loss (ml)	Length of hospital stay (days)	Return to work (days)	Costs (US$)
Guazzoni et al.[99]	1995	Laparoscopic	20	170	100	3.4	9.7	—
		Open	20	145	450	9	16	—
Prinz et al.[38]	1995	Laparoscopic	10	212	228	2.1	—	—
		Open posterior	13	139	288	5.5	—	—
		Open anterior	11	174	391	6.4	—	—
Brunt et al.[75]	1996	Laparoscopic	24	183	104	3.2	10.7	13,184
		Open posterior	17	136	366	6.2	—	12,267
		Open anterior	25	142	408	8.7	—	16,972
MacGillivary et al.[96]	1996	Laparoscopic	17 (14)	289	198	3	8.9	—
		Open	12 (9)	201	500	7.9	14.6	—
Jacobs et al.[98]	1997	Laparoscopic	19 (19)	164	109	2.3	—	10,929
		Open	19 (19)	151	263	5.1	—	13,720
Thompson et al.[84]	1997	Laparoscopic	50	167	—	3.1	26	7,000
		Open posterior	50	127	—	5.7	49	6,000
Linos et al.[97]	1997	Laparoscopic	18	116	—	2.3	—	2,920
		Open posterior	61	109	—	4.5	—	2,724
		Open anterior	86	155	—	8	—	—
Vargas et al.[100]	1997	Laparoscopic	20	193	245	3.1	21	—
		Open	20	178	283	7.2	49	—
Winfield et al.[101]	1998	Laparoscopic	21	219	183	2.7	22	—
		Open	17	140	266	6.2	45	—
Imai et al.[114]	1999	Laparoscopic	41	180	40	12	—	7,000
		Open	40	127	162	18	—	8,000
Schell et al.[102]	1999	Laparoscopic	22	280	—	1.7	—	8,698
		Open	17	260	—	7.8	—	12,610
Dudley et al.[103]	1999	Laparoscopic	36	158	—	3.5	—	—
		Open	23	85	—	8.5	—	—

ranging from 4 months to 6 years after surgery, the two groups had similar outcomes as determined by measurement of blood pressure and serum potassium levels. Blood pressure normalized in 81% of the open group compared to 88% of the laparoscopically treated patients. Also, fewer postoperative complications were observed in the laparoscopic group. Clearly, further studies are needed to validate the functional outcomes of laparoscopic adrenalectomy for biochemically active adrenal tumors.

Specific Problems in Laparoscopic Adrenal Surgery

Pheochromocytomas

Pheochromocytomas can be challenging tumors to remove laparoscopically because of their size, vascularity, and potential for inducing hemodynamic instability intraoperatively. Patients must be pharmacologically prepared for surgery, as already discussed. Because of the potential hemodynamic consequences of increased catecholamine release from tumor manipulation, an effort should be made to ligate the adrenal vein as early as possible in the procedure. The malignant potential of pheochromocytomas should also be considered when dealing with large tumors. The liver should be examined carefully laparoscopically, both as a potential site for metastasis from the pheochromocytoma and, in patients with multiple endocrine neoplasia type 2, for metastatic medullary thyroid carcinoma. In one series,[105] 4 of 17 patients undergoing laparoscopic adrenalectomy for pheochromocytoma were found unexpectedly to have liver metastases from their pheochromocytomas.

Some surgeons have reported increased operative times, a longer hospital length of stay, and a higher complication rate in patients undergoing laparoscopic adrenalectomy for pheochromocytoma than for other indications.[105] However, Fernandez-Cruz and associates[106] found that outcomes following laparoscopic adrenalectomy were similar in patients with pheochromocytomas as opposed to other adrenal neoplasms. When compared to patients with pheochromocytomas who underwent open adrenalectomy, the results in the laparoscopic group were superior by all parameters measured, including less pronounced intraoperative hemodynamic changes (including lower mean arterial pressure, pulmonary wedge pressure, and systemic vascular resistance) and a lesser degree of elevation of plasma catecholamines. The author has observed that hemodynamic changes during laparoscopic adrenalectomy occur primarily during CO_2 insufflation and with tumor manipulation.[106] Long-term follow-up studies have not been carried out in patients undergoing laparoscopic

adrenalectomy for pheochromocytoma, except for one study of eight patients evaluated 2 to 20 months postoperatively.[107] Urinary catecholamines were normal in all except one patient who developed a recurrent pheochromocytoma on the contralateral side at the site of a prior open adrenalectomy.

Bilateral Laparoscopic Adrenalectomy

Bilateral adrenalectomy is occasionally indicated for the treatment of patients with Cushing's syndrome (see Table 26.1) or familial bilateral pheochromocytomas. Each of the various operative approaches has been used for performing laparoscopic bilateral adrenalectomy, and all except the prone retroperitoneal approach and the supine transabdominal approach require repositioning the patient between sides. Consequently, laparoscopic bilateral adrenalectomy is a lengthy and sometimes difficult procedure, especially in obese patients with Cushing's syndrome who typically have large amounts of fragile retroperitoneal fat. Operative times have averaged 4.5 to 5.5h in most series,[108–111] but postoperative pain and hospital length of stay have been shorter than for open adrenalectomy.[109] The frequency of postoperative wound complications also appears low in the small number of cases reported.

Compared to unilateral adrenalectomy, laparoscopic bilateral adrenalectomy has been associated with a somewhat slower recovery, including a longer hospital stay and a slower return to full activity. Some of this delay may be explained by the need for hormone replacement postoperatively in the total adrenalectomy group. Clinical recurrence of Cushing's syndrome after laparoscopic bilateral adrenalectomy has not been reported. However, evidence of stimulated cortisol production in response to exogenously administered ACTH has been observed in four patients from different series.[74,108,109] In one of these cases, the adrenal gland was ruptured intraoperatively due to technical difficulties.[109] Long-term follow-up data are needed to demonstrate that the functional results of bilateral laparoscopic adrenalectomy for Cushing's syndrome are equivalent to those from the era of open adrenal surgery.[112]

Partial Adrenalectomy

Laparoscopic techniques have been used to perform partial adrenalectom in selected patients.[113–115] Walz and colleagues[113] carried out subtotal resections in 22 patients with various adrenal tumors, including 11 aldosteronomas, 4 pheochromocytomas, 4 Cushing's adenomas, and 3 nonfunctioning adenomas. The tumors were excised with a 0.5- to 1.0-cm margin of normal adrenal without bleeding complications. Preservation of the adrenal vein was possible in 11 cases. All patients were clinically and biochemically cured at 1 to 31 months follow-up.

Despite the apparent success of this technique, total adrenalectomy should remain the procedure of choice for patients with a unilateral tumor. The risk of developing a tumor in the contralateral gland in such patients is low, whereas the potential for spilling tumor cells and developing a recurrence of even benign lesions is probably increased by partial resection. At this time, laparoscopic partial adrenalectomy should be reserved for carefully selected patients with small, peripherally located tumors who either have bilateral lesions or have undergone prior adrenalectomy on the contralateral side.

Complications

Complications reported with laparoscopic adrenalectomy are listed in Table 26.8. A lower incidence of major complications has been consistently observed with laparoscopic adrenalectomy when compared to the open procedures.[75,85,97–99,101–103] The most frequent major complication of laparoscopic adrenalectomy has been bleeding, which has also been the primary reason for conversion to open adrenalectomy. The transfusion rate for this procedure, however, has been low. The adrenal

TABLE 26.8. Complications of laparoscopic adrenalectomy.

Hemorrhage
Intraperitoneal Organ Injury
   Liver, spleen, pancreas, kidney, colon, diaphragm
Pancreatitis/pancreatic fistula
Wound
   Infection
   Trocar site hernias
Neurological
   Nerve compression
   Compartment syndrome
Other
   Acute adrenal insufficiency
   Lymphocele
   Renovascular hypertension
   Tumor recurrence
GI
   Ileus
Urinary tract
   UTI
Pulmonary
   Pneumonia
   Atelectasis
   Pneumothorax
Thromboembolic
   Deep venous thrombosis
   Pulmonary embolus
Cardiovascular
   Arrhythmias

vein can be a major source of hemorrhage, especially on the right side if a clip is dislodged or if the vein is torn at the vena cava. Other potential sites of bleeding during laparoscopic adrenalectomy include the adrenal gland itself, retroperitoneal vessels, the liver (which can be lacerated by retractors or dissection), the pancreas, spleen, and short gastric vessels. One must be especially cautious on the left side where bleeding from the tail of the pancreas can be triggered by retraction or dissection and can be difficult to control with cautery or clips. Meticulous dissection of the adrenal with extracapsular dissection of the gland, avoiding direct grasping of the adrenal, and a thorough knowledge of the anatomy are the keys to preventing this complication. As with other laparoscopic procedures, the risk of significant intraoperative hemorrhage and conversion to open adrenalectomy appears to diminish with increased experience.

Several other technical complications have been reported with laparoscopic adrenalectomy, including injury to the tail of the pancreas, leading to a pancreatic leak or pancreatitis, injury to the diaphragm, and pneumothorax. With the patient in a lateral position, the liver, kidney, spleen, and colon are also at risk for injury from puncture by either the Veress needle or a trocar. Wound complications including infection and trocar site hernias have occasionally occurred but have been much less common than with open adrenalectomy. Cardiopulmonary complications such as atelectasis and pneumonia have been rare. Deep venous thrombosis has been reported in 0.8% of patients and pulmonary embolus in 0.5%, and there have been no perioperative myocardial infarctions. Only two perioperative deaths have been reported, both in patients with severe end-stage Cushing's syndrome.[68,103] In neither case was the death thought to be directly related to the laparoscopic procedure.

Renovascular hypertension is an uncommon complication of adrenalectomy; however, three cases have been observed following laparoscopic adrenalectomy. In one series, two patients developed renovascular hypertension[69,74]: one patient had atherosclerotic renal artery stenosis that was probably unrelated to the laparoscopic procedure, and the second patient developed stenosis of a polar renal artery branch with a segmental perfusion defect on the side of the adrenalectomy. Fibromuscular dysplasia was present on the opposite side. In another report,[116] a patient developed severe renovascular hypertension after laparoscopic adrenalectomy for Cushing's syndrome due to a left adrenal adenoma. The patient was subsequently found to have complete occlusion of the left renal artery. The mechanism of the occlusion was unclear, but it was postulated that it could have been caused by an intimal tear from trauma or retraction during the dissection. These cases, although rare, illustrate the importance of clarity in the dissection to avoid injury to the renal vessels; this is especially critical on the left side where the adrenal is in close apposition to the superior pole of the kidney and the renal hilar vessels.

Isolated cases of tumor recurrence after laparoscopic adrenalectomy have recently been reported. de Canniere and colleagues[60] reported a patient who underwent laparoscopic left adrenalectomy for an adrenal metastasis. Four months later, the patient required a left nephrectomy for tumor recurrence in the hilum of the left kidney. Ushiyama and associates[61] noted the development of multiple metastases at the adrenalectomy site 14 months after en bloc laparoscopic excision of a 5-cm left adrenal adenoma in a patient with Cushing's syndrome. Foxius and colleagues[62] removed a 2.7-cm "atypical unencapsulated" right adrenal aldosteronoma from a patient who developed recurrent hyperaldosteronism from extensive carcinomatosis 11 months postoperatively. At laparotomy, tumor was found in the greater omentum, left paracolic gutter, and behind the spleen, but there was no evidence of locoregional recurrence. The patient expired 20 months after the original operation. The pattern of tumor recurrence in this latter case suggested a possible role for dissemination of tumor cells by the pneumoperitoneum, as has been observed for colorectal and gallbladder cancers.[64–67] Iacconi et al.[63] removed a 7-cm right adrenal mass laparoscopically that showed no evidence of extraadrenal invasion in a patient with preclinical Cushing's syndrome. The mass was completely excised laparoscopically, and the patient was given mitotane postoperatively for a pathological diagnosis of adrenocortical carcinoma. Twenty-six months later, the patient was reoperated on for locoregional recurrence of the tumor as well as multiple port site metastases.

The extent to which the laparoscopic procedure contributed to tumor recurrence or dissemination in these cases is unclear, because tumor progression resulting from unrecognized micrometastases at the time of the initial surgery can also occur with open adrenalectomy. To some extent, therefore, these cases may simply reflect the natural history and biological behavior of the tumors being resected. However, the cases of Foxius[62] and Iacconi[63] do point to a probable contributory role for the laparoscopic procedure based on the pattern of tumor recurrence. Consequently, until further follow-up data are available, caution and restraint should be exercised in attempting to remove any potentially malignant adrenal lesion, including large tumors with benign imaging characteristics. Such lesions are probably best managed by highly skilled, experienced laparoscopic adrenal surgeons or by open adrenalectomy. In no case, regardless of one's experience, should established oncologic principles of complete resection with negative margins be compromised as a result of overzealous application of laparoscopic techniques.

Postoperative Care

Most patients can be cared for on a regular nursing unit following laparoscopic adrenalectomy. Patients who have had significant hemodynamic disturbances, especially with resection of pheochromocytomas, or who have severe underlying cardiopulmonary disease may require overnight observation in the intensive care unit. Liquids are usually begun the morning after surgery, and the diet is advanced to regular food as tolerated. Pain medications are administered as needed, but parenteral narcotics are usually unnecessary beyond the first 24 h. A complete blood count should be checked the morning after surgery, and electrolytes are monitored as clinically indicated. Discharge from the hospital is usually within 24 to 48 h of operation. Patients who require steroid replacement after bilateral adrenalectomy are often observed for 72 to 96 h. Patients can be discharged home without physical activity limitations and should return to work and full activity within 2 weeks of surgery. An initial follow-up visit is scheduled for 2 to 3 weeks postoperatively.

Patients with Cushing's syndrome and those who undergo bilateral adrenalectomy require perioperative administration of stress doses of steroids. Oral hydrocortisone is then administered at a maintenance dose of 12 to 15 mg/m^2 per day. In the patient with Cushing's syndrome caused by an adrenal cortical adenoma, substitution therapy should be continued until recovery of the hypothalamic–pituitary–adrenal axis has been demonstrated with ACTH stimulation testing. Eighteen to 24 months may be required for the contralateral adrenal gland to completely recover.[117] Patients who have undergone bilateral adrenalectomy also require lifelong mineralocorticoid replacement with fludrocortisone (100 µg/day). One must be alert to the possible development of acute adrenal insufficiency in patients with Cushing's syndrome or after bilateral adrenalectomy. The presenting manifestations can include cardiovascular collapse with hypotension and shock as well as abdominal pain, weakness, fever, nausea, vomiting, and leukocytosis. Treatment is prompt administration of intravenous hydrocortisone, as this condition can be fatal if not promptly recognized and treated.

Following resection of a pheochromocytoma, patients can become hypotensive and may require large amounts of intravenous fluids because of loss of α-receptor-mediated sympathetic tone and expansion of intravascular capacity. Hypoglycemia is also a potential risk due to rebound hyperinsulinism from the loss of inhibition of insulin secretion by circulating catecholamines. These patients should, therefore, undergo bedside glucose monitoring periodically for the first 24 to 36 h after resection. Urinary catecholamines should be measured within the first several weeks after surgery and on an annual basis thereafter.

References

1. Scott HW Jr. Anatomy of the adrenal glands and bilateral adrenalectomy. In: Nyhus LM, Baker RJ, Sabiston DC (eds) Mastery of Surgery, 2nd Ed. Boston: Little, Brown, 1992:1373–1378.

2. Russell CF, Hamberger B, van Heerden JA, Ilstrup DM. Adrenalectomy: anterior or posterior approach? Am J Surg 1982;144:322–324.

3. Proye CAG, Huart JY, Cuvillier XD, Assez NML, Gambardella B, Carnaille BML. Safety of the posterior approach in adrenal surgery: experience in 105 cases. Surgery (St. Louis) 1993;114:1126–1131.

4. Buell JF, Alexander HR, Norton JA, Yu KC, Fraker DL. Bilateral adrenalectomy for Cushing's syndrome: anterior versus posterior surgical approach. Ann Surg 1997;225:63–68.

5. Petelin JB. Laparoscopic adrenalectomy. In: Proceedings, Third World Congress Endoscopic Surgery, Bordeaux, France, September 1992.

6. Gagner M, Lacroix A, Bolte E. Laparoscopic adrenalectomy in Cushing's syndrome and pheochromocytoma. N Engl J Med 1992;327:1033.

7. Gagner M, Lacroix A, Bolte E, Pomp A. Laparoscopic adrenalectomy: the importance of a flank approach in the lateral decubitus position. Surg Endosc 1994;8:135–138.

8. Brunt LM, Molmenti EP, Kerbl K, Soper NJ, Stone AM, Clayman RV. Retroperitoneal endoscopic adrenalectomy: an experimental study. Surg Laparosc Endosc 1993;4:300–306.

9. Mercan S, Seven R, Ozarmagan S, Tezelaman S. Endoscopic retroperitoneal adrenalectomy. Surgery (St. Louis) 1995;118:1071–1076.

10. Melby JC. Diagnosis and treatment of primary aldosteronism and isolated hypoaldosteronism. Clin Endocrinol Metab 1985;14:977–995.

11. Young WF. Primary hyperaldosteronism: a common and curable form of hypertension. Cardiol Rev 1999;7:207–214.

12. Gordon RD, Stowasser M, Tunny TJ, Klemm SA, Rutherford JC. High incidence of primary aldosteronism in 199 patients referred with hypertension. Clin Exp Pharmacol Physiol 1994;21:315–318.

13. Ganguly A. Primary aldosteronism. N Engl J Med 1998;339:1828–1834.

14. Young WF, Hogan MJ, Klee GG, Grant CS, van Heerden JA. Primary aldosteronism: diagnosis and treatment. Mayo Clin Proc 1990;65:96–110.

15. Blumenfeld JD, Sealey JE, Schlussel Y, et al. Diagnosis and treatment of primary hyperaldosteronism. Ann Intern Med 1994;121:877–885.

16. Young WF, Stanson AW, Grant CS, Thompson GB, van Heerden JA. Primary aldosteronism: adrenal venous sampling. Surgery (St. Louis) 1996;120:913–920.

17. Newell-Price J, Trainer P, Besser M, Grossman A. The diagnosis and differential diagnosis of Cushing's syndrome and pseudo-Cushing's states. Endocr Rev 1988;19:647–672.

18. Zeiger MA, Nieman LK, Cutler GB, et al. Primary bilateral adrenal causes of Cushing's syndrome. Surgery (St. Louis) 1991;110:1106–1115.

19. Orth DN. Cushing's syndrome. New Engl J Med 1995;332:791–803.

20. Pommier RF, Brennan MF. An eleven-year experience with adrenocortical carcinoma. Surgery (St. Louis) 1992;112:963–971.

21. Copeland P. The incidentally discovered adrenal mass. Ann Intern Med 1983;98:940–945.

22. Harrison LE, Gaudin PB, Brennan MF. Pathologic features of prognostic significance for adrenocortical carcinoma after curative resection. Arch Surg 1999;134:181–185.

23. Icard P, Chapuis Y, Andreassian B, Bernard A, Proye C. Adrenocortical carcinoma in surgically treated patients: a retrospective study on 156 cases by the French Association of Endocrine Surgery. Surgery (St. Louis) 1992;112:972–980.

24. Herrera MMF, Grant CS, van Heerden JA, Sheedy PF, Ilstrup DM. Incidentally discovered adrenal tumors: an institutional perspective. Surgery (St. Louis) 1991;110:1014–1021.

25. Fishman EK, Deutch BM, Hartman DS, Goldman SM, Zerhouni EA, Siegelman SS. Primary adrenocortical carcinoma: CT evaluation with clinical correlation. AJR 1987;148:531–535.

26. Hofle G, Gasser RW, Lhotta K, Janetschek G, Kreczy A, Finkenstedt G. Adrenocortical carcinoma evolving after diagnosis of preclinical Cushing's syndrome in an adrenal incidentaloma. Horm Res 1998;50:237–242.

27. Gross MD, Shapiro B, Francis IR, et al. Incidentally discovered bilateral adrenal masses. Eur J Nucl Med 1995;22:315–321.

28. Van Erkel AR, van Gils AP, Lequin M, Kruitwagen C, Bloem JL, Falke TH. CT and MR distinction of adenomas and nonadenomas of the adrenal gland. J Comp Assist Tomogr 1994;18:432–438.

29. Crucitti F, Belantone R, Ferrante A, Boscherina M, Crucitti P. The Italian registry for adrenal cortical carcinoma: analysis of a multinational series of 129 patients. Surgery (St. Louis) 1996;119:161–170.

30. Page DL, DeLellis RA, Hough AJ. Tumors of the adrenal. Washington, DC: AFIP, 1986.

31. Ross NS, Aron DC. Hormonal evaluation of the patient with an incidentally discovered adrenal mass. N Engl J Med 1990;323:1401–1405.

32. Bravo EL. Evolving concepts in the pathophysiology, diagnosis, and treatment of pheochromocytoma. Endocr Rev 1994;15:356–368.

33. Shady KL, Brown JJ. MR imaging of the adrenal glands. MRI Clin N Am 1995;3:73–85.

34. Thompson NW, Allo MD, Shapiro B, Sisson JC, Beierwaltes W. Extra-adrenal and metastatic pheochromocytoma: the role of ^{131}I meta-iodylbenzylguanidine (^{131}I MIBG) in localization and management. World J Surg 1984;8:605–611.

35. Glazer HS, Weyman PJ, Sagel SS, McLennan BL. Nonfunctioning adrenal masses: incidental discovery on computed tomography. AJR 1982;139:81–85.

36. Belledgrun A, Hussain S, Seltzer SE, Loughlin KR, Gittes RF, Richie JP. Incidentally discovered mass of the adrenal gland. Surg Gynecol Obstet 1986;163:203–208.

37. Kley HK, Wagner H, Jaresh S, et al. Endokrin inaktiv nebennierentumoren. In: Allolio B, Schulte HM (eds) Moderne diagnostik und therapeutische strategien bei nebennierentumoren. New York: Schattauer, 1990:189–197.

38. Prinz RA, Brooks MH, Churchill R, et al. Incidental asymptomatic adrenal masses detected by computed tomographic scanning: is operation required? JAMA 1982;248:701–704.

39. Osella G, Terzolo M, Borreta G, et al. Endocrine evaluation of incidentally discovered adrenal masses (incidentalomas). J Clin Endocrinol Metab 1994;79:1532–1539.

40. Mantero F, Masini AM, Opocher G, Giovagnetti M, Arnaldi G. Adrenal incidentaloma: an overview of hormonal data from the National Italian Study Group. Horm Res (Basel) 1997;47:284–289.

41. Reincke M, Nieke J, Krestin GP, Saeger W, Allolio B, Winkelmann W. Preclinical Cushing's syndrome in adrenal "incidentalomas": comparison with adrenal Cushing's syndrome. J Clin Endocrinol Metab 1992;75:826–832.

42. Kloos RT, Gross MD, Francis IR, Korobkin M, Shapiro B. Incidentally discovered adrenal masses. Endocr Rev 1995;16:460–484.

43. Peplinski GR, Norton JA. In: Zinner MJ, Schwartz SI, Ellis H (eds) The adrenal glands, 10th Ed. Stamford, CT: Appleton & Lange, 1997:723–760.

44. Paivansalo M, Lahde S, Merikanto J, Kallionen M. Computed tomography in primary and secondary adrenal tumours. Acta Radiol 1988;29:519–522.

45. Lee MJ, Hahn PF, Papanicolaou N, et al. Benign and malignant adrenal masses: CT distinction with attenuation coefficients, size, and observer analysis. Radiology 1991;179:415–418.

46. Korobkin M, Lombardi TJ, Aisen AM, et al. Characterization of adrenal masses with chemical shift and gadolinium-enhanced MR imaging. Radiology 1995;197:411–418.

47. Mayo-Smith WW, Lee MJ, McNicholas MM, Hahn PF, Boland GW, Saini S. Characterization of adrenal masses <5 cm by use of chemical shift MR imaging: observer performance versus quantitative measures. AJR 1995;165:91–95.

48. Siekavizza JL, Bernardino ME, Samaan NA. Suprarenal mass and its differential diagnosis. Urology 1981;18:625–632.

49. Hussain S, Belledgrun A, Seltzer SE, Richie JP, Gittes RF, Abrams HL. Differentiation of malignant from benign adrenal masses: predictive indices on computed tomography. AJR 1985;144:61–65.

50. Candel A, Gattuso P, Reyes CV, Prinz RA, Castelli MJ. Fine-needle aspiration biopsy of adrenal masses in patients with extraadrenal malignancy. Surgery (St. Louis) 1993;114:1132–1137.

51. Lo CY, van Heerden JA, Soreide JA, et al. Adrenalectomy for metastatic disease to the adrenal gland. Br J Surg 1995;83:528–531.

52. Ayabe H, Tsuji H, Hara S, et al. Surgical management of adrenal metastasis from bronchogenic carcinoma. J Surg Oncol 1995;58:149–154.

53. Ettingshausen SE, Burt ME. Prospective evaluation of unilateral adrenal masses in patients with operable non-small-cell lung cancer. J Clin Oncol 1991;9:1462–1466.

54. Wade TP, Longo WE, Virgo KS, Johnson FE. A comparison of adrenalectomy with other resections for metastatic cancers. Am J Surg 1998;175:183–186.

55. Elashry OM, Clayman RV, Soble JJ, McDougall EM. Laparoscopic adrenalectomy for solitary metachronous contralateral adrenal metastasis from renal cell carcinoma. J Urol 1997;157:1217–1222.

56. Heniford BT, Arca MJ, Walsh RM, Gill IS. Laparoscopic adrenalectomy for cancer. Semin Surg Oncol 1999;16:293–306.

57. Stowens D. Neuroblastoma and related tumors. Arch Pathol 1957;63:451–459.

58. Nasir J, Royston C, Walton C, White MC. 11B-hydroxylase deficiency: management of a difficult case by laparoscopic bilateral adrenalectomy. Clin Endocrinol 1996;45:225–228.

59. Wells SA Jr, Merke DP, Cutler GB Jr, Norton JA, Lacroix A. Therapeutic controversy: the role of laparoscopic surgery in adrenal disease. J Clin Endocrinol Metab 1998;83:3041–3042.

60. de Canniere L, Michel L, Hamoir E, et al. Multicentric experience of the Belgian Group for Endoscopic Surgery (BGES) with endoscopic adrenalectomy. Surg Endosc 1997;11:1065–1067.

61. Ushiyama T, Suzuki K, Kageyama S, Fujita K, Oki Y, Yoshimi T. A case of Cushing's syndrome due to adrenocortical carcinoma with recurrence 19 months after laparoscopic adrenalectomy. J Urol 1997;157:2239.

62. Foxius A, Ramboux A, Lefebvre Y, Broze B, Hamels J, Squifflet J-P. Hazards of laparoscopic adrenalectomy for Conn's adenoma: when enthusiasm turns to tragedy. Surg Endosc 1999;13:715–717.

63. Iacconi P, Bendinelli C, Miccoli P, Bernini GP. Re: A case of Cushing's syndrome due to adrenocortical carcinoma with recurrence 19 months after laparoscopic adrenalectomy. J Urol 1999;161:1580–1586.

64. Clair DG, Lautz DB, Brooks DC. Rapid development of umbilical metastases after laparoscopic cholecystectomy for unsuspected gallbladder carcinoma. Surgery (St. Louis) 1993;113:355–358.

65. Z'graggen K, Birrer S, Maurer CA, Klaiber C, Baer HU. Incidence of port site recurrence after laparoscopic cholecystectomy for preoperatively unsuspected gallbladder carcinoma. Surgery (St. Louis) 1998;124:31–38.

66. Fusco MA, Paluzzi MW. Abdominal wall recurrence after laparoscopic colectomy for adenocarcinoma of the colon: a case report. Dis Colon Rectum 1993;36:858–861.

67. Ramos JM, Gupta S, Anthine GJ, Ortega AE, Simons AJ, Beart RW Jr. Laparoscopy and colon cancer—is the port site at risk? A preliminary report. Arch Surg 1994;129:897–899.

68. Duh Q-Y, Siperstein AE, Clark OH, et al. Laparoscopic adrenalectomy: comparison of the lateral and posterior approaches. Arch Surg 1996;131:870–876.

69. Gagner M, Pomp A, Heniford BT, Pharand D, Lacroix A. Laparoscopic adrenalectomy: lessons learned from 100 consecutive procedures. Ann Surg 1997;226:238–247.

70. Filliponi S, Guerrieri M, Arnaldi GGM, Masini AM, Lezoche E, Mantero F. Laparoscopic adrenalectomy: a report on 50 operations. Eur J Endocrinol 1998;138:548–553.

71. Marescaux J, Mutter D, Wheeler MH. Laparoscopic right and left adrenalectomies: surgical procedures. Surg Endosc 1996;10:912–915.

72. Miccoli P, Iacconi P, Conte M, Goletti O, Buccianti P. Laparoscopic adrenalectomy. J Laparoendosc Surg 1995;5:221–226.

73. Staren ED, Prinz RA. Adrenalectomy in the era of laparoscopy. Surgery (St. Louis) 1996;120:706–711.

74. Lacroix A. Therapeutic controversy: five-year experience with laparoscopic adrenalectomy at Hotel-Dieu in Montreal: endocrinologist's perspective. J Clin Endocrinol Metab 1998;83:3043–3046.

75. Brunt LM, Doherty GM, Norton JA, Soper NJ, Quasebarth MA, Moley JF. Laparoscopic compared to open adrenalectomy for benign adrenal neoplasms. J Am Coll Surg 1996;183:1–10.

76. Rutherford JC, Stowasser M, Tunny TJ, Klemm SA, Gordon RD. Laparoscopic adrenalectomy. World J Surg 1996;20:758–761.

77. Terachi T, Matsuda T, Terai A, et al. Transperitoneal laparoscopic adrenalectomy: experience in 100 cases. J Endourol 1997;11:361–365.

78. Fernandez-Cruz L, Saenz A, Benarroch G, Torres E, Astudillo E. Technical aspects of adrenalectomy via operative laparoscopy. Surg Endosc 1994;8:1348–1351.

79. Guerrieri M, Paganini A, Feliciotti F, Zenobi P, Mantero F, Lezoche E. Laparoscopic adrenalectomy: report of 70 cases. Surg Endosc 1998;12:611.

80. Bonjer HJ, Lange JF, Kazemier G, De Herder WW, Steyerberg EW, Bruining HA. Comparison of three techniques for laparoscopic adrenalectomy. Br J Surg 1997;84:679–682.

81. Heniford BT, Ianniti DA, Hale J, Gagner M. The role of intraoperative ultrasonography during laparoscopic adrenalectomy. Surgery (St. Louis) 1997;122:1068–1074.

82. Brunt LM, Bennett HF, Teefey SA, Moley JF, Middleton WD. Laparoscopic ultrasound imaging of adrenal tumors during laparoscopic adrenalectomy. Am J Surg 1999;178:490–495.

83. Prinz RA. Editorial: Laparoscopic adrenalectomy. J Am Coll Surg 1996;183:71–73.

84. Thompson GB, Grant CS, van Heerden JA, et al. Laparoscopic versus open posterior adrenalectomy: a case-control study of 100 patients. Surgery (St. Louis) 1997;122:1132–1136.

85. Imai T, Kikumori T, Ohiwa M, Mase T, Funahashi H. A case-controlled study of laparoscopic compared with open lateral adrenalectomy. Am J Surg 1999;178:50–54.

86. Pujol J, Viladrich M, Rafecas A, et al. Laparoscopic adrenalectomy: a review of initial 30 cases. Surg Endosc 1999;13:488–492.

87. Suzuki K, Kageyama S, Ueda D, et al. Laparoscopic adrenalectomy: clinical experience with 12 cases. J Urol 1993;150:1099–1102.

88. Stuart RC, Chung SCS, Lau JYW, et al. Laparoscopic adrenalectomy. Br J Surg 1995;82:1498–1499.

89. Takeda M, Go H, Imai T, Nishiyama T, Morishita H. Laparoscopic adrenalectomy for primary aldosteronism: report of initial ten cases. Surgery (St. Louis) 1994;115:621–625.

90. Heintz A, Walgenbach S, Junginger T. Results of endoscopic retroperitoneal adrenalectomy. Surg Endosc 1996;10:633–635.

91. Walz MK, Peitgen K, Hoermann R, Giebler RM, Mann K, Eigler FW. Posterior retroperitoneoscopy as a new minimally invasive approach for adrenalectomy: results of 30 adrenalectomies in 27 patients. World J Surg 1996;20:769–774.

92. Fernandez-Cruz L, Saenz A, Taura P, Benarroch G, Astudillo E, Sabater L. Retroperitoneal approach in laparoscopic adrenalectomy? Is it advantageous? Surg Endosc 1999;13:86–90.

93. Takeda M, Go H, Watanabe R, et al. Retroperitoneal laparoscopic adrenalectomy for functioning adrenal tumors: comparison with conventional transperitoneal laparoscopic adrenalectomy. J Urol 1997;157:19–23.

94. Baba S, Miyajima A, Uchida A, Asanuma H, Miyakawa A, Murai M. A posterior lumbar approach for retroperitoneoscopic adrenalectomy: assessment of surgical efficacy. Urology 1997;50:19–24.

95. Huber DF, Martin EW Jr, Cooperman M. Cholecystectomy in elderly patients. Am J Surg 1983;146:719–722.

96. MacGillivray DC, Shichman SJ, Ferrer FA, Malchoff CD. A comparison of laparoscopic vs open adrenalectomy. Surg Endosc 1996;10:987–990.

97. Linos DA, Stylopoulos N, Boukis M, Souvatzoglou A, Raptis S, Papadimitriou J. Anterior, posterior, or laparoscopic approach for the management of adrenal diseases? Am J Surg 1997;173:120–125.

98. Jacobs JK, Goldstein RE, Geer RJ. Laparoscopic adrenalectomy: a new standard of care. Ann Surg 1997;225:495–502.

99. Guazzoni G, Montorsi F, Bocciardi A, et al. Transperitoneal laparoscopic versus open adrenalectomy for benign hyperfunctioning adrenal tumors: A comparative study. J Urol 1995;153:1597–1600.

100. Vargas HI, Kavoussi LR, Bartlett DL, et al. Laparoscopic adrenalectomy: a new standard of care. Urology 1997;49:673–678.

101. Winfield HN, Hamilton BD, Bravo EL, Novick AC. Laparoscopic adrenalectomy: the preferred choice? A comparison to open adrenalectomy. J Urol 1998;160:325–329.

102. Schell SR, Talamini MA, Udelsman R. Laparoscopic adrenalectomy for nonmalignant disease: improved safety, morbidity, and cost effectiveness. Surg Endosc 1999;13:30–34.

103. Dudley NE, Harrison BJ. Comparison of open posterior versus transperitoneal laparoscopic adrenalectomy. Br J Surg 1999;86:656–660.

104. Shen WT, Lim RC, Siperstein AE, et al. Laparoscopic vs open adrenalectomy for the treatment of primary hyperaldosteronism. Arch Surg 1999;134:628–632.

105. Gagner M, Breton G, Pjarand D, Pomp A. Is laparoscopic adrenalectomy indicated for pheochromocytomas? Surgery (St. Louis) 1996;120:1076–1080.

106. Fernandez-Cruz L, Taura P, Saenz A, Benarroch G, Sabater L. Laparoscopic approach to pheochromocytoma: hemodynamic changes and catecholamine secretion. World J Surg 1996;20:762–768.

107. Col V, de Canniere L, Colard E, Michel L, Donckier J. Laparoscopic adrenalectomy for phaeochromocytoma: endocrinological and surgical aspects of a new therapeutic approach. Clin Endocrinol 1999;50:121–125.

108. Bax TW, Marcus DR, Galloway GQ, Swanstrom LL, Sheppard BC. Laparoscopic bilateral adrenalectomy following failed hypophysectomy. Surg Endosc 1996;10:1150–1153.

109. Chapuis Y, Chastanet S, Dousset B, Luton J-P. Bilateral laparoscopic adrenalectomy for Cushing's disease. Br J Surg 1997;84:1009.

110. Fernandez-Cruz L, Saenz A, Benarroch G, Sabater L, Taura P. Total bilateral laparoscopic adrenalectomy in patients with Cushing's syndrome and multiple endocrine neoplasia (IIa). Surg Endosc 1997;11:103–107.

111. Lanzi R, Montorsi F, Losa M, et al. Laparoscopic bilateral adrenalectomy for persistent Cushing's disease after transsphenoidal surgery. Surgery (St. Louis) 1998;123:144–150.

112. Kemink L, Hermus A, Pieters G, Benraad T, Smals A, Kloppenborg P. Residual adrenocortical function after bilateral adrenalectomy for pituitary-dependent Cushing's syndrome. J Clin Endocrinol Metab 1992;75:1211–1214.

113. Walz MK, Peitgen K, Saller B, et al. Subtotal adrenalectomy by the posterior retroperitoneoscopic approach. World J Surg 1998;22:621–627.

114. Imai T, Tanaka Y, Kikumori T, et al. Laparoscopic partial adrenalectomy. Surg Endosc 1999;13:343–345.

115. Mugiya S, Suzuki K, Saisu K, Fujita K. Unilateral laparoscopic adrenalectomy followed by contralateral retroperitoneoscopic partial adrenalectomy in a patient with multiple endocrine neoplasia type 2a syndrome. J Endourol 1999;13:99–104.

116. Wu T-H, Tsai S-H, Tsai C-Y, Huang T-P. Renovascular hypertension after laparoscopic adrenalectomy in a patient with adrenal adenoma. Nephron 1996;74:464–465.

117. Doherty GM, Nieman LK, Cutler GB Jr, Chrousos GP, Norton JA. Time to recovery of the hypothalamic-pituitary-adrenal axis after curative resection of adrenal tumors in patients with Cushing's syndrome. Surgery (St. Louis) 1990;108:1085–1090.

27
Laparoscopic Splenectomy

Eric D. Whitman and L. Michael Brunt

The spleen is one of the most common solid organs removed by laparoscopic techniques. Laparoscopic splenectomy (LS) was first performed by Delaitre in 1992[1] and is one of the most challenging laparoscopic procedures because of the bulk and vascularity of the spleen and the wide range of pathological conditions that affect it. Although conversion rates for laparoscopic splenectomy have been higher than those reported for most other advanced laparoscopic procedures, laparoscopic splenectomy has become the preferred method of splenectomy in patients with normal or near normal sized spleens. Laparoscopic techniques have also been used to carry out splenectomy successfully in selected patients with splenomegaly.

The purpose of this chapter is to describe the development of laparoscopic splenectomy as a viable surgical procedure, culminating in a discussion of the various techniques possible and the specific technical recommendations of the authors. The indications, results, and complications of laparoscopic splenectomy are presented along with an analysis of the cost-effectiveness of this procedure in comparison to the historical standard of open splenectomy (OS).

Anatomy and Physiology

The spleen is located in the left upper quadrant of the abdomen, just dorsal and lateral to the stomach. The normal spleen weighs between 75 and 100 g and usually undergoes a slight decrease in size with age.[2] Protected by the rib cage anteriorly, laterally, and posteriorly, the spleen is suspended in position by ligaments attaching it to the diaphragm, stomach, kidney, and splenic flexure of the colon. These ligaments attach to the splenic capsule, fixing the spleen to the retroperitoneum (Fig. 27.1).

The spleen receives arterial blood from two principal sources, the splenic artery and the short gastric arteries.

The splenic artery, a branch of the celiac axis, approaches the spleen along the superior and posterior aspects of the pancreas, entering the central portion of the spleen, or hilum, just lateral to the tail of the pancreas. Two patterns of vascular distribution of the arterial blood supply to the spleen have been described.[3,4] In the distributed mode, which is the most common pattern, multiple arterial branches arise from the main splenic artery 2 to 3 cm from the hilum. This pattern can often be recognized by notching of the anterior border of the spleen. In contrast, in the magistral mode, the main splenic artery enters the splenic hilum as a compact structure without branching. The short gastric vessels lie within the gastrosplenic ligament, generally entering the upper portion of the spleen superomedial to the hilum and splenic artery. The short gastric vessels are variable in length and number but, in general, three or four vessels, each about 3 cm long, enter the spleen. The principal venous drainage of the spleen is through the splenic vein, which runs parallel to the splenic artery along the posterior aspect of the pancreas before converging with the superior mesenteric vein to form the portal vein. Minor venous drainage may occur through the other suspensory ligaments already listed, which may be more numerous and enlarged in patients with portal hypertension.

The spleen has two principal physiological functions. First, it is a hematopoietic filter and a primary component of the body's reticuloendothelial system. It eliminates antigenic and nonantigenic particulate matter (i.e., damaged, modified, or senescent circulating blood cells, encapsulated microorganisms, immune complex products, and hemoglobin or iron breakdown products) from the circulation. Filtered particles are subsequently phagocytized by splenic macrophages and reticular cells. Second, the spleen serves as a secondary component of the body's immune system, producing opsonins that promote complement activation and bacterial phagocytosis, and antibodies, especially IgM. The spleen may be particularly important in protecting against infection

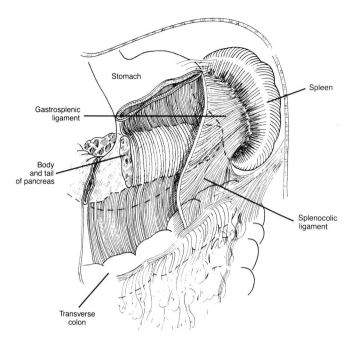

FIGURE 27.1. Peritoneal attachments of the spleen. Not shown is the splenorenal ligament that attaches to the spleen posteriorly. (From Dierks MM, et al. Splenectomy. In: Jones DB, Wu JS, Soper NJ (eds) Laparoscopic Surgery: Principles and Procedures. St. Louis: Quality Medical Publishing, 1997:294, with permission.)

with encapsulated organisms, which are most effectively removed from the circulation by the spleen.

Splenic Pathology

Splenic pathology can be related to either a derangement in normal splenic physiology or damaging, yet physiological, responses of the spleen to congenital or acquired hematopoietic dysfunction. Although not usually treated with laparoscopic techniques, probably the most common form of splenic pathology is traumatic injury to the spleen. Although the spleen may be injured from penetrating trauma, most splenic injuries occur as a result of blunt abdominal trauma in which the thin capsule and splenic parenchyma may be ruptured by a sudden impact from an external object or sudden acceleration/deceleration forces. The high blood flow (averaging 300 ml/min) and filtration function of the spleen make traumatic injuries potentially life-threatening, unless rapidly diagnosed and treated. The current inherent limitations of laparoscopic abdominal surgery minimize the role of laparoscopy in the treatment of splenic trauma except for diagnostic purposes (see following). However, the use of a hand-port device to assist in laparoscopic removal of the spleen may allow application of this technique to selected cases of splenic injury.

Surgical disorders of the spleen may be classified broadly as hemolytic anemias, thrombocytopenias, lymphomas/leukemias, myeloproliferative disorders, and various miscellaneous conditions. The hemolytic anemias constitute a variety of disorders that result from increased destruction of red blood cells due to either an intrinsic or acquired abnormality. The most common hemolytic anemias are hereditary spherocytosis and idiopathic autoimmune hemolytic anemia. Hereditary spherocytosis is an autosomal dominant condition associated with a defective red blood cell (RBC) membrane. These defective RBCs, also known as spherocytes because of their morphological appearance, exhibit increased fragility and are unable to pass easily through the splenic pulp where they are sequestered and destroyed, leading to anemia, splenomegaly, and, in some cases, jaundice. Pigmented gallstones are present in up to 30% to 60% of cases, and splenectomy is the only effective treatment. Other congenital hemolytic anemias for which splenectomy may occasionally be indicated include hereditary elliptocytosis, hemolytic anemia due to enzyme deficiency, thalassemia, and sickle cell disease. Autoimmune hemolytic anemia is an acquired condition caused by the formation of autoantibodies to red blood cells that leads to their increased destruction. This disorder is seen primarily in adults over the age of 50 years. About 50% of patients have palpable splenomegaly and 25% have gallstones. Splenectomy is indicated for patients who fail to respond to corticosteroid therapy.

Idiopathic or immune thrombocytopenia purpura (ITP) is an autoimmune disorder in which IgG autoantibodies to platelet glycoprotein result in increased platelet sequestration and destruction. The spleen itself is a major source of antibody production in this disorder as well as the principal site of sequestration and removal of antibody-coated platelets. Bone marrow analysis usually demonstrates normal or increased numbers of megakaryocytes. ITP occurs in two forms. In the childhood variety, 80% of patients recover completely without any specific therapy.[5] In contrast, adult patients with ITP do not usually undergo spontaneous remission and are treated initially with corticosteroids. Patients who fail or do not tolerate steroid therapy, or who relapse after steroids are discontinued, should undergo splenectomy. Patients who remain thrombocytopenic after corticosteroid treatment may respond to infusion of intravenous IgG to boost the platelet count preoperatively. Approximately 70% to 80% of patients with ITP undergo a complete remission after splenectomy.[6–8] An additional 15% exhibit improved although not normal platelet levels, and approximately 5% have no response to splenectomy. In addition to the idiopathic form, ITP may also occur in association with systemic lupus erythematosis (SLE) or human immunodeficiency virus (HIV) infection.[9] The response rate to splenectomy in these groups is similar to that for other patients with ITP.

Thrombotic thrombocytopenia purpura (TTP) is a disorder of unknown pathogenesis in which there is vascular occlusion of the microcirculation by platelet aggregates. Clinical features consist of a consumptive thrombocytopenia, hemolytic anemia, fever, central nervous system dysfunction, and renal insufficiency. TTP has a high mortality rate, and the primary therapy is plasmapheresis. Splenectomy may be indicated for patients who relapse or fail to respond initially to plasmapheresis.

Other pathological conditions of the spleen include primary or secondary neoplastic transformation. Primary lymphoid neoplasms include various lymphomas and leukemias, which frequently present with splenic enlargement. Splenectomy is occasionally indicated in these patients, either for diagnostic reasons or because of associated cytopenias, but less commonly for staging purposes.

The myeloproliferative disorders of the spleen include myelofibrosis or myeloid metaplasia, polycythemia vera, and idiopathic thrombocytosis.[10] The etiology of these various disorders is unclear. Common features include splenomegaly which is often massive and symptomatic, hypersplenism, and variable hemostatic disturbances including anemia, thrombocytopenia or thrombocytosis, and leukocytosis. Myelofibrosis is a panproliferative process involving the bone marrow, liver, spleen, and lymph nodes. It tends to occur in middle-aged and older adults and is frequently accompanied by extramedullary hematopoiesis. Clinical features often include anemia, purpura, symptomatic splenomegaly, hepatomegaly, and hyperuricemia. Diagnosis is established on a peripheral red blood cell smear that shows fragmentation, immature forms, and poikilocytosis; bone marrow analysis typically shows varying degrees of fibrosis. Patients with myelofibrosis may require splenectomy because of symptoms of pain or compression from the markedly enlarged spleen or to facilitate control of anemia and thrombocytopenia. The spleen is often massively enlarged in these patients and typically not amenable to laparoscopic removal. The morbidity and mortality rates for patients undergoing splenectomy for myelofibrosis are higher than for any other splenic pathology, and these patients are especially at increased risk for postoperative thrombotic complications, including splenic or portal vein thrombosis.[11]

Indications and Results

The primary therapy for most nontraumatic splenic disorders is medical and not surgical. Surgical intervention for nontraumatic splenic pathology is generally warranted only after the failure of medical therapy, as a palliative adjunct to medical therapy in situations where the spleen itself causes significant symptomatology, or for the diagnosis and staging of malignancy. The current indications for splenectomy, either by laparoscopic or open techniques, are listed in Table 27.1. Laparoscopic splenectomy is appropriate for almost all patients with normal or near normal sized spleens. The most common indication for laparoscopic splenectomy is ITP, which accounts for 40% to 100% of cases in some published series (Table 27.2).[3,6,12-23] The spleen is usually normal in size in ITP, and there appears to be no greater risk of bleeding with the laparoscopic approach compared to open splenectomy. The platelet count should be optimized preoperatively in patients with ITP by administration of corticosteroids or, in some cases, infusion of intravenous IgG. Although ideally the platelet count should be $40,000/mm^3$ or higher before splenectomy, laparoscopic splenectomy has been safely performed in patients with platelet counts of 5,000 to $10,000/mm^3$.[3,12,16]

The role of laparoscopic splenectomy in the management of patients with hematological malignancies has been somewhat controversial. Advances in noninvasive radiographic staging of Hodgkin's lymphoma have reduced the need for surgical staging in this group. Splenectomy for Hodgkin's lymphoma is currently indicated only when there are equivocal radiologic findings or when splenic tissue is required to clarify the disease status after therapy. Splenectomy may occasionally be indicated for patients with non-Hodgkin's lymphoma or leukemia for diagnosis or for treatment of associated hypersplenism and cytopenias. Laparoscopic staging of

TABLE 27.1. Indications for splenectomy.

Hemolytic anemias
  Acquired autoimmune anemias
  Congenital hemolytic anemias
  Congenital hemoglobinopathies
Thrombocytopenias
  Idiopathic thrombocytopenic purpura (ITP)
  Thrombotic thrombocytopenic purpura (TTP)
  Felty's syndrome
Myeloproliferative and lymphoproliferative disorders
Hematologic malignancies
  Leukemia and non-Hodgkin's lymphoma
  Hairy cell leukemia
  Hodgkin's lymphoma
Hypersplenism from other causes
  Storage disease
  Gaucher's disease
Splenic vein occlusion/thrombosis
Splenic cyst/pseudocyst
Splenic abscess
Vascular anomalies
Splenic artery aneurysm
Traumatic injury

TABLE 27.2. Institutional series of laparoscopic splenectomy.

Year	Authors[a]	n	Operative time (min)	Length of stay (days)	Conversions	Accessory (spleens)	ITP	Complications
1995	Emmermann et al. [12]	27	170	4.4	5 (19%)	0%	74%	11%
1995	Gigot et al.[13]	50	203	5.4	5 (10%)	14%	62%	34%
1996	Bove et al.[14]	21	158	4.4	2 (10%)	0%	33%	16%
1996	Flowers et al.[15]	43	144	2.7	8 (19%)	0%	51%	16%
1998	Szold et al.[17]	43	79	2.3	0 (0%)	19%	84%	7%
1998	Katkhouda et al.[3]	103	161	2.5	4 (4%)	17%	65%	6%
1998	Decker et al.[18]	35	221	5.0	3 (9%)	17%	34%	23%
1999	Harold et al.[6]	27	—	1.5	1 (4%)	11%	100%	4%
1999	Walsh and Heniford[19]	57	185	2.4	0 (0%)	0%	0%	2%
1999	Brody et al.[20]	27	190	2.6	5 (19%)	4%	100%	9%
1999	Stanton[21]	30	150	2.3	2 (7%)	21%	100%	13%
1999	Gossot et al.[22]	20	127	4.3	0 (0%)	25%	70%	5%
2000	Trias et al.[23]	111	153	4.0	9 (8%)	14%	50%	17%
2000	Park et al.[27]	203	146	2.7	6 (3%)	15%	64%	6%
	Total/mean	797	153	3.2	50 (6.3%)	12%	61%	11%

[a] Minimum 20 cases, ordered chronologically by publication year.

lymphoma may also be performed in conjunction with splenectomy when clinically indicated.[24] Patients with hematological malignancies often have enlarged spleens that can be difficult to manage laparoscopically. In a recent retrospective examination of LS cases for hematological malignancies, the conversion rate to open splenectomy was 41% versus a conversion rate of 3% in patients with benign hematological disorders (p = 0.001).[25]

Contraindications to laparoscopic splenectomy include massive splenomegaly, the presence of bulky splenic hilar adenopathy, portal hypertension, and a diagnosis of a myeloproliferative disorder. Obesity increases the difficulty of laparoscopic splenectomy but does not absolutely contraindicate a laparoscopic approach. Portal hypertension should be a contraindication to laparoscopic splenectomy because of the increased risk of major hemorrhage from engorged vessels within the splenic hilum and splenic accessory ligaments. Proliferative disorders such as myelofibrosis are associated with massive splenomegaly and are probably best approached by open splenectomy, because of both the massive spleen size and the increased risk of splenectomy in this particular population. Traumatic splenic rupture is at this time a relative contraindication to attempted laparoscopic splenectomy because of the difficulty in controlling active major splenic hemorrhage. Laparoscopy may play a role, however, in the diagnosis of splenic trauma and has been used to manage mild splenic injuries.[26]

Laparoscopic splenectomy is a more challenging procedure in patients with significant splenomegaly. With experience, most patients with moderately enlarged spleens (15–20cm in longitudinal dimension or <1000g in weight) can usually be resected laparoscopically.[27,28] However, the presence of massive splenomegaly poses an increased challenge for this approach because of the difficulty in manipulating the enlarged spleen and exposing the relevant ligaments and vessels and an increased risk of hemorrhage. The precise size limit for attempting laparoscopic splenectomy is still under evaluation, but it would appear that spleens 28 to 30cm or greater in longitudinal dimension and 3000g or more in weight are best approached in open fashion because of the low success rate with the laparoscopic approach.[27–29] The use of a hand-assisted technique for performing laparoscopic splenectomy may allow wider application of minimally invasive surgery to patients with moderate or marked splenomegaly, as discussed next. Considerable experience should be developed with laparoscopic splenectomy in nonenlarged spleens before attempting this procedure in patients with marked splenomegaly.

The data presented in Table 27.2 describe the larger published series of LS (focusing on adults), and Table 27.3 shows the results of laparoscopic versus open splenectomy series in which a minimum of 20 laparoscopic cases were performed. The results can be summarized as follows.

1. LS is technically feasible in a growing variety of clinical situations. It should be considered the favored surgical approach for patients with ITP who fail medical management.[16,17,30–33]

2. Operative times for LS have been longer than those for OS in almost all studies; this is partially a reflection of a "learning curve" as multiple studies have cited a progressive decrease in operative times with increasing LS experience.[3,20,21,30,34–36]

3. Hospital length of stay (LOS) for LS patients is significantly shorter than case-control matched OS patients. Patients also routinely have a shorter duration

TABLE 27.3. Comparative series of laparoscopic versus open splenectomy.[a]

Series	No. of cases		Conversions	Op Time (min)		LOS (days)		Accessory Spleen		ITP		Complications	
	LS	OS		LS	OS	LS	OS	LS	OS	LS	OS	LS	OS
Rhodes et al.[36]	24	11	2 (8%)	120	75	3	7	—	—	—	—	12.5%	27%
Brunt et al.[37]	26	20	0	202	134	2.5	5.8	12%	5%	65%	20%	23%	30%
Glasgow et al.[35]	52	28	6 (11%)	196	156	4.8	6.7	16%	21%	44%	57%	10%	14%
Friedman et al.[40]	63	74	5 (7%)	153	121	3.5	6.7	17%	14%	50%	25%	14%	34%
Rescorla et al.[44]	50	32	0	115	83	1.4	2.5	18%	25%	16%	19%	6%	3%
Lozano-Salazar et al.[48]	22	27	2 (9%)	270	162	4	6	9%	11%	100%	100%	27%	37%
Park et al.[45]	147	63	4 (3%)	145	77	2.4	9.2	15%	5%	65%	60%	10%	35%
Targarona et al.[28][b]	66	43	3 (4%)	143	43	3.7	8	—	—	68%	79%	11%	28%
Donini et al.[41]	44	56	1 (2%)	130	133	5.1	7.2	9%	9%	55%	14%	7%	23%
Berman et al.[25]	22	77	9 (41%)	203	120	4	6	—	—	0	0	32%	36%
Tanoue et al.[8]	35	41	0	204	100	9.6	20	11%	12%	100%	100%	11%	46%
Total/mean	551	472	32 (5.8%)	159	99	3.6	7.9	14%	12%	59%	50%	12%	28%

LS, laparoscopic splenectomy; OS, open splenectomy; LOS, length of postoperative hospital stay.
[a] Minimum 20 cases of LS required for inclusion.
[b] Excludes reported patients with spleens >400 g.

of postoperative ileus and are able to tolerate a regular diet sooner.[25,30,35–38]

4. Conversion rates from LS to OS are generally decreasing in frequency and are believed to be related to experience and patient selection.[35] From a technical perspective, creation of a larger incision to facilitate removal of a laparoscopically detached spleen is still considered a laparoscopic splenectomy.[15,22,25,34] Almost all cases requiring conversion to OS are due to either intraoperative hemorrhage[15] or splenomegaly beyond the capability of current instrumentation.[28]

5. The complication rate of LS is relatively low and is equivalent to or better than reported complication rates from OS procedures.[8,27,28,36,37,39–42] Perioperative mortality is often from underlying medical problems unrelated to the LS surgery itself, particularly in patients with hematological malignancies.[15,25,35,36]

6. As with any new procedure, initial cost analysis of LS suggests a higher per case cost than OS[39,43]; however, subsequent studies have shown either similar or lower costs of LS compared to OS,[30,35,44,45] as discussed further here.

7. Results in all patients seem equivalent to OS,[19,21,25,46–48] with some concern over early relapse in ITP.[3,13] Long-term follow-up is not available at this point for a procedure introduced less than 10 years ago.

In summary, the indications for laparoscopic splenectomy are evolving based on clinical advances and cumulative surgical experience. For surgeons with minimal LS experience, the procedure should be reserved for patients with small or normal-sized spleens, with reasonable medical response to anticoagulopathy treatments, and with otherwise acceptable medical risks for operation. In more experienced hands, only patients with massive

splenomegaly (≥28 cm or ≥3000 g), portal hypertension, or splenic fracture from trauma are at present excluded from an attempt at LS. Future advances in laparoscopic technology and techniques may enable LS even in some of those cases.

Operative Treatment

Preoperative Preparation

The decision to perform splenectomy should be made by both the surgeon and hematologist/oncologist. The surgeon should review all diagnostic studies, including abdominal imaging studies and bone marrow aspirate results. Routine imaging studies are not necessary in patients with benign hematological disorders (e.g., ITP) but should be carried out in all patients with hematological malignancies or palpable splenomegaly. Preoperative consultation and evaluation includes a complete history and physical examination, with attention to any abdominal surgical scars and general medical disorders that may increase the overall risk to the patient from the surgery itself. Patients considered appropriate candidates for LS are advised of the risks and benefits of this procedure, including the potential for conversion to an open procedure.

Standard preoperative laboratory studies and other tests are obtained, including a type and screen or cross-match for blood products. Initially, we cross-matched two units of packed red blood cells preoperatively on all patients. However, in some centers, including our own, patients with normal-sized spleens who are at low risk for intraoperative hemorrhage may be typed and screened only. Any patient with splenomegaly or anemia should have a minimum of two units of blood cross-matched and readily available. Patients with autoimmune hematological disorders and ITP are likely to have difficulty being cross-matched by the blood bank because of multiple serum antibodies, and therefore the patient should be screened for antibodies 1 day before the scheduled surgery. Although some surgeons advocate preoperative platelet transfusion to obtain counts above 50,000/mm³, this has not been necessary in our experience and for others.[49] Platelets should be available for intraoperative transfusion, however, in patients with severe thrombocytopenia. Preoperative vaccination with polyvalent pneumococcal vaccine (Pneumovax) and *Hemophilus influenzae* type B vaccine is performed, ideally several weeks before surgery. Children should also be vaccinated against *Neisseria meningitidis*. Corticosteroids may be given preoperatively to patients with ITP to boost the platelet count before surgery. Patients who have recently been treated with steroids should receive perioperative "stress-dose" corticosteroids. Preoperative embolization of the splenic artery is not recommended because it may actually increase the difficulty of the procedure by inducing an inflammatory reaction around the spleen; also, it is costly and painful to the patient.

Laparoscopic splenectomy is generally performed as a same-day surgery unless the patient is already hospitalized because of the underlying disease process. At least one large-bore peripheral intravenous line should be placed (preferably two in patients with splenomegaly). Perioperative antibiotic coverage in the form of a single dose of a first-generation cephalosporin is given routinely. Some surgeons have administered cathartics to cleanse the colon, but this is unnecessary in most patients.

Operating Room and Patient Setup

A range of surgical techniques, patient positions, and operative instrumentation have been used for laparoscopic splenectomy. The following sections note, where possible, the various alternatives but emphasize the authors' preferences.

Laparoscopic splenectomy is carried out under general endotracheal anesthesia. Nitrous oxide is to be avoided because it can lead to distension of the colon, which can interfere with the laparoscopic view. Sequential compression stockings should be placed on the patient's legs to prevent deep venous thrombosis, and a urinary catheter should be inserted. Patient positioning, if not controversial, is at least a source of disagreement among surgeons with extensive LS experience. Our preference is a flexed right lateral or semilateral decubitus position[50–52] on a beanbag device[53] (Fig. 27.2), which is a modification of the "hanged spleen" approach described in 1995 by Delaitre.[54] Other options include supine/lithotomy[25] and supine with table tilting.[55] Once the patient is

in the semilateral decubitus position, the beanbag is molded around the torso. The table is then elevated, flexed, and put in slight reverse Trendelenburg. Padding supports the chest wall to protect the brachial plexus, and the lower extremities are well padded also. The combination of these maneuvers exposes the left upper quadrant to the surgical team, with the space between the left costal margin and the iliac crest maximized by flexion and elevation of the head of the table, which causes the patient's abdominal viscera to gently fall toward the feet. The table may be rotated from side to side during the procedure to improve exposure to the abdomen or lateral/posterior flank as needed.[56,57] The prepped area should extend from the nipple line superiorly to the pubis inferiorly and table to table on the sides. The umbilicus should be exposed in the sterile field as a reference point and as a potential site for access.

Equipment

A recommended list of equipment for performing laparoscopic splenectomy is shown in Table 27.4. The video imaging system should be of high quality, and our preference is to use a 5-mm, 30° laparoscope to eliminate one of the larger ports. The initial access port (5mm) is usually disposable as is the primary working port (12mm), but the other ports can be nondisposable. A 5-mm flexible arm retractor (Genzyme, Cambridge, MA, USA) or fan-type retractor can be useful for retracting and elevating the spleen, and a 10-mm, 90° dissector is helpful in isolating large vessels. Much of the dissection of the fatty splenic ligaments is carried out with an ultrasonic coagulator, especially division of the short gastric

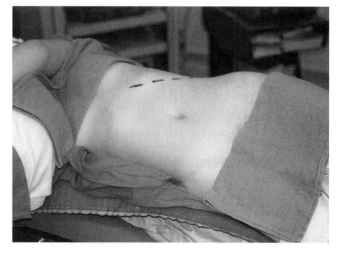

FIGURE 27.2. Patient position for laparoscopic splenectomy. The patient is in a semilateral position on a gel-padded beanbag mattress. The left costal margin is marked with a *dashed line*.

TABLE 27.4. Equipment for laparoscopic splenectomy.

Basic laparoscopic instrument set
5-mm retractor
Trocars:
    12mm (1)
    5mm (3)
5- or 10-mm 30° laparoscope
Endoscopic linear cutting stapler (vascular cartridge)
Ultrasonic coagulation device
Clip applier
Specimen extraction bag
18-mm trocar

vessels. An endoscopic linear cutter stapler with vascular load staple cartridges should be available for dividing the splenic hilar vessels. A large impermeable entrapment bag is necessary for specimen removal, and an 18-mm disposable laparoscopic port is usually needed to insert this device. Use of a hand-assisted device may be warranted in selected patients with splenomegaly, as discussed next.

Operative Procedure

Step 1: Port Placement

Laparoscopic splenectomy can be performed using either three or four ports, depending on the size of the spleen, anticipated difficulty of the dissection, and teaching considerations. The precise location of the ports also varies depending upon the patient's size, body habitus, and the size of the spleen. In patients with a small body habitus and in those with splenomegaly, initial access is usually established at the umbilicus with an open Hasson cannula insertion technique. The other ports are placed in the subcostal region so as to form a triangle in relationship to the umbilical port (Fig. 27.3A). For most patients, however, the optimal port of configuration is in an arc that parallels the costal margin (Fig. 27.3B). Initial access for this approach is usually obtained with a Veress needle puncture about 2cm inferior to the left costal margin at or just medial to the anterior axillary line. A 5-mm disposable trocar with safety shield is then inserted at the Veress needle site, and the remaining ports are inserted under direct laparoscopic vision. Alternatively, one can use an optical trocar for initial access to observe progression through the abdominal wall layers into the peritoneal cavity. This latter method requires a straight-viewing (0°) laparoscope. The second port (5mm) is placed near the midline, and the third port (12mm) is inserted about 5cm lateral to the first port. After the initial ports have been placed, preliminary search for accessory spleens is performed, although a more complete exam is not possible until some of the splenic ligaments have been divided (see following).[58]

Step 2: Inferolateral Dissection

The first step in the dissection is to divide any adhesions between the spleen, colon at the splenic flexure, and the lateral abdominal wall (Fig. 27.4A). The patient's lateral decubitus position often exaggerates the appearance of these adhesions and facilitates their retraction and division. The splenic flexure is then taken down, using either the ultrasonic coagulator or electrocautery (Fig. 27.4B). Our preference is to use the ultrasonic device because there is less risk of thermal injury and it provides excellent hemostasis.[59,60] Division of the splenic flexure attachments is continued from medially to laterally from the inferior pole of the spleen until the colon has fallen away

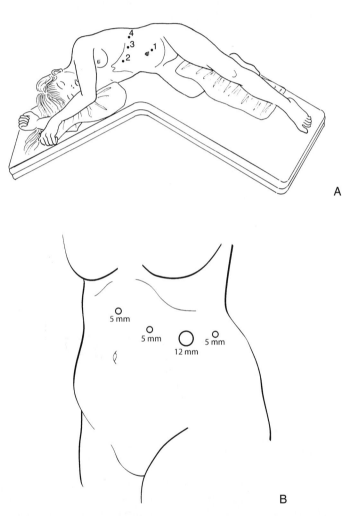

FIGURE 27.3. Port site placement for laparoscopic splenectomy. A. Port placement (1–4) in patient with a small body habitus. Initial access is at the umbilicus. (From Dierks MM, et al. Splenectomy. In: Jones DB, Wu JS, Soper NJ (eds) Laparoscopic Surgery: Principles and Procedures. St. Louis: Quality Medical, 1997:296, with permission.) B. Subcostal port placement. This port alignment works best for most adult patients with normal or near normal size spleens.

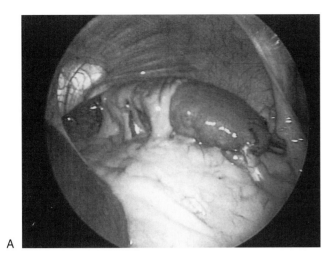

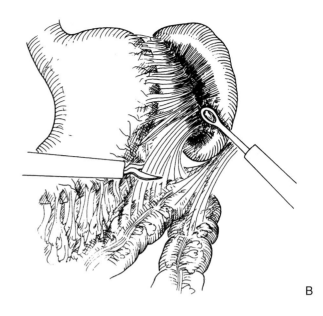

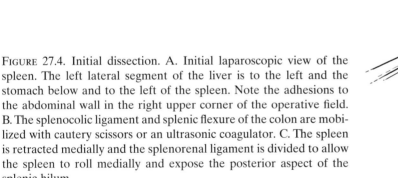

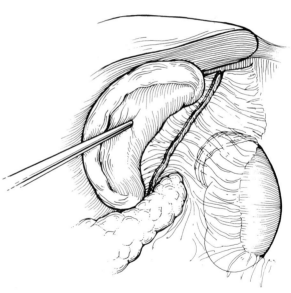

FIGURE 27.4. Initial dissection. A. Initial laparoscopic view of the spleen. The left lateral segment of the liver is to the left and the stomach below and to the left of the spleen. Note the adhesions to the abdominal wall in the right upper corner of the operative field. B. The splenocolic ligament and splenic flexure of the colon are mobilized with cautery scissors or an ultrasonic coagulator. C. The spleen is retracted medially and the splenorenal ligament is divided to allow the spleen to roll medially and expose the posterior aspect of the splenic hilum.

from the operative field. At this time, a fourth (5-mm) port may safely be placed under direct vision at about the posterior axillary line, 2 cm below the left costal margin. The next step is to divide the splenorenal ligament from the inferior border of the spleen to the diaphragm (Fig. 27.4C). This dissection is also done with an ultrasonic coagulator, and care must be taken at this juncture to avoid dissecting in the splenic hilum or along the tail of the pancreas. The splenorenal ligament should be completely divided so that the spleen can be easily rolled medially, providing posterior access to the hilum. Alternatively, one may perform the medial dissection (step 3, below) before dividing the splenorenal ligament.

Special Note: Splenic Retraction

The spleen, because of its bulk, vascularity, and fragility can be difficult to maneuver laparoscopically. One should never try to grasp the spleen directly, regardless of the relatively atraumatic nature of the instrument. Also, grasping, pulling, or retracting soft tissue next to the spleen must be done carefully as this may tear the splenic capsule and lead to bleeding that obscures the operative field and makes continued laparoscopic dissection difficult or impossible.

One option is to use a fan retractor (10 mm) for splenic retraction,[61] but this requires placement of a second

10-mm port. Initially, it is used unopened to push the spleen superiorly or medially while dissection is performed on the inferior or lateral splenic attachments. Once the inferior and lateral attachments are divided, it is generally possible to "open" the fan retractor and elevate the spleen, with the spokes of the fan encompassing the splenic hilum to facilitate completion of the laparoscopic splenectomy. Alternatively, one can use a 5-mm dissecting instrument or a flexible snake-type retractor to retract or elevate the spleen. The shaft of a grasper or dissecting instrument can also be used to roll the spleen back and forth to view the medial and lateroposterior aspects as the dissection progresses.

Step 3: Medial Dissection

The spleen is rolled back laterally so that the medial aspect is visualized. The gastrosplenic ligament is then divided with the ultrasonic scalpel, and one may also divide the short gastric vessels at this point if the exposure is adequate. A careful search for accessory spleens should also be made during this part of the dissection. When the gastrosplenic ligament has been divided, it should be possible to visualize the main splenic artery trunk as it courses along the superior border of the pancreas. In some cases, it may be advisable to isolate the splenic artery proximal to the splenic hilum and then ligate it with a single clip or suture (Fig. 27.5). It is our practice to do this in cases in which the dissection is difficult, such as in obese individuals, when the spleen is enlarged, or if the patient is markedly thrombocytopenic.

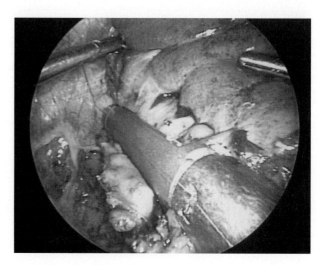

FIGURE 27.6. Division of the splenic hilum. The spleen is elevated, and the hilar vessels are divided with one or more applications of an endoscopic vascular load linear cutter stapler.

Step 4: Splenic Hilum

When the gastrosplenic and splenorenal ligaments and short gastric vessels have been divided, the splenic hilum can be approached. It may be necessary to dissect some areolar tissue away from the hilum to allow more precise visualization of the relationship of the splenic vessels and tail of the pancreas. Dissection of the hilum is facilitated by elevating the spleen with retractors or dissecting instruments. The most commonly employed method for ligation and division of the splenic hilar vessels involves application of an endoscopic linear cutting stapler using a vascular load cartridge (Fig. 27.6). This method is fast, efficient, and provides excellent hemostasis, although occasionally bleeding from the stapled edge of a vessel may require application of a clip or suture. One or more firings of the stapler may be necessary to secure the entire hilum. One should also know the exact location of the tail of the pancreas before firing the stapler to avoid injury to this structure. Although it is possible to dissect and individually isolate and clip the splenic artery and vein, this technique is time consuming and is more likely to result in significant hemorrhage. Furthermore, the use of clips may interfere with subsequent application of the endoscopic stapler if bleeding does occur.

Step 5: Final Dissection and Specimen Removal

Depending on the extent of dissection performed laterally and on the short gastric vessels, the spleen is generally attached superiorly by only a small amount of tissue following division of the hilum. The spleen is elevated and rotated back and forth to maximize visualization of any remaining medial and superior attachments, which are divided by the ultrasonic coagulator with attention to

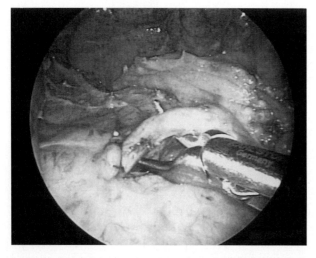

FIGURE 27.5. Ligation of the main splenic artery. The main splenic artery trunk can be ligated along the superior border of the pancreas before dissection of the splenic hilum. A right-angle dissector is used to isolate the vessel, which is then occluded with a single clip.

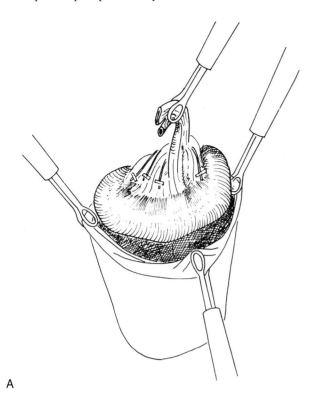

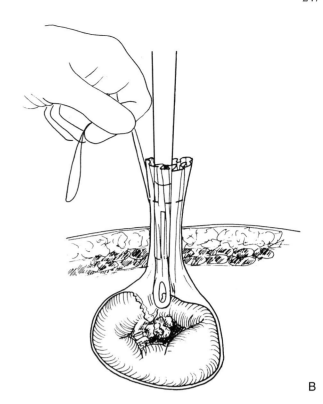

A   B

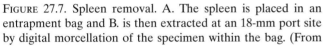

FIGURE 27.7. Spleen removal. A. The spleen is placed in an entrapment bag and B. is then extracted at an 18-mm port site by digital morcellation of the specimen within the bag. (From Dierks MM. Splenectomy. In: Jones DB, Wu JS, Soper NJ (eds) Laparoscopic Surgery: Principles and Procedures. St. Louis: Quality Medical Publishing, 1997:301, with permission.)

avoiding the wall of the stomach. Once the spleen has been completely detached from the patient, the dissection site should be inspected for hemostasis. The spleen is then removed via the 12-mm port site, which is first exchanged under direct vision for an 18-mm port. It is the authors' preference to use a bag preattached to an expandable ring (EndoCatch II; US Surgical, Norwalk, CT, USA) to entrap and remove the spleen. The EndoCatch device is placed into the abdomen through the 18-mm port and deployed with the spleen behind it. The back rim of the EndoCatch is next rotated under the back edge of the spleen and, with a sudden pronation of the first assistant's wrist, the spleen is scooped into the bag (Fig. 27.7). The EndoCatch rim is then leveled and elevated to the anterior abdominal wall, simultaneously shaking the instrument to open the bag and allow the spleen to fall further into the bag itself. The bag is then closed by pulling the pursestring suture, and the device is removed along with the port, so that the end of the pursestring suture is protruding out of the abdominal wall. The suture is pulled out of the port site, bringing the opening of the entrapment sack outside of the abdomen. It is usually necessary at this point to extend the skin and fascial incision by a few millimeters to facilitate extraction of the specimen. Sponges are placed around the inci-

sion to prevent spillage of any blood or splenic tissue into the wound. The spleen is then removed piecemeal with a digital fracture technique. A ring forceps is helpful in extracting the splenic fragments from the bag until the remaining specimen is small enough to allow the entire bag to be removed from the patient (Fig. 27.7). Suction should be used to evacuate blood from the bag as the spleen is fractured. If a mechanical morcellator is used, the bag must be strong enough so that it does not tear. Obviously, care must be taken to avoid puncturing the bag and to prevent leakage of splenic tissue back into the abdominal cavity from the skin surface. After specimen removal, the surgeon changes gloves, and all sponges and instruments that have touched splenic tissue are taken away from the operative field.

Step 6: Inspection and Closure

The 18-mm port is replaced into the lateral site. It may be necessary to partially close the fascia or to secure the skin around the port with towel clips to allow reconstitution of pneumoperitoneum. The left upper quadrant is irrigated and inspected. Particular attention is paid to the area of the splenic hilum, the vascular staple lines, and at the site of division of the short gastric vessels along the greater curvature of the stomach. A drain is not routinely placed unless there is concern that the pancreatic parenchyma may have been injured.

The abdomen is then evacuated of CO_2 and the ports are removed. The fascia at all 10-mm or larger port sites should be closed with interrupted #0 or #1 absorbable sutures. The skin is closed with absorbable 4–0 sutures or with steri-strips. The dressings are placed, and the patient is awakened, rolled supine, and extubated.

Approach to Patients with Splenomegaly and Hematological Malignancies

Choice of Technique

Historically, the presence of splenomegaly has been one of the most important predictors of surgical difficulty and outcome in patients undergoing open splenectomy.[62,63] Laparoscopic splenectomy is especially challenging in these patients, both for technical reasons and because of the underlying disease process. Many patients with splenomegaly have associated hematological malignancies and are older, thus potentially complicating operative management. The surgical approach to these patients and consequent outcomes, therefore, deserve special consideration.

Compared to patients with normal-sized spleens, laparoscopic splenectomy in patients with splenomegaly and hematological malignancies has been associated with increased operative times,[25,28,29,64,65] increased transfusion requirements, and an increased rate of conversion to open splenectomy. In some series of patients with splenomegaly, conversion rates to open splenectomy as high as 21% to 40% have been reported.[25,28,29] Complication rates have also been somewhat higher than in patients with normal-sized spleens. Despite these observations, however, laparoscopic splenectomy appears to still be advantageous when compared to open splenectomy for splenomegaly; proven benefits include a shorter postoperative hospitalization, reduced morbidity, and a lower transfusion rate despite longer operative times. In one series of laparoscopic splenectomy, complications and conversion rates were highest in patients whose spleens weighed 1000 g or more compared to patients with smaller spleens.[28]

The precise size limit for attempting laparoscopic splenectomy has been the subject of much debate. In most series, patients whose spleens are 28 to 30 cm or more in longitudinal dimension or that weigh 3000 g or more have almost uniformly been converted to an open procedure.[27–29] Park and colleagues[27] have suggested that the relationship between spleen size and the patient's size and body habitus is a better predictor of success of the laparoscopic approach than the absolute spleen weight. Spleen weight can be difficult to judge preoperatively, and our approach is to obtain radiographic imaging (ultrasound or CT) in any patient who has palpable splenomegaly or a diagnosis of hematological malignancy. In addition to defining the size and bulk of the spleen, imaging can also be useful in identifying patients with bulky splenic hilar adenopathy that might preclude a laparoscopic approach. The spleen that is just palpable below the costal margin may weigh as much as 750 to 1000 g.[66] The massively enlarged spleen that is palpable at the midline or down to the iliac crest will usually weigh 3000 g or more and should be approached with an open incision. As discussed next, the use of a hand-assisted technique for performing laparoscopic splenectomy has the potential to expand the current limitations on spleen size and to enhance the success rate of a laparoscopic approach in patients with spleens 20 to 30 cm long or that weigh 1000 to 3000 g.

Several modifications in technique should be considered in approaching the patient with splenomegaly. Trocar placement may need to be modified by avoiding the left upper quadrant and instead using the midline and lower abdomen. An open insertion technique at the umbilicus or upper midline should be used for initial access to reduce the risk of splenic puncture. Additional trocars may be necessary for insertion of extra retractors to facilitate manipulation of the spleen, although placement of a hand-assist device usually obviates the need for this. Preligation of the splenic artery proximal to the hilum in the lesser sac along the superior border of the pancreas early in the dissection is highly recommended to reduce the bleeding risk, decrease splenic engorgement, and provide some degree of autotransfusion for the patient.

The use of a hand-assisted technique for performing laparoscopic splenectomy in patients with marked splenomegaly has been reported to improve the success rate of the procedure, reduce the bleeding risk, and expand indications.[67–70] In addition, the hand-assisted technique may reduce operative time, and it also facilitates extraction of specimens that are too large to place into a retrieval bag.

The hand-assist device may be placed at a variety of locations depending upon the patient's size and body habitus, the spleen size, and the preferred operating position of the surgeon (Fig. 27.8). The incision should be positioned such that the surgeon can insert the non-dominant hand within the peritoneal cavity and operate using laparoscopic instruments in the dominant hand. The incision for the hand device is usually made after initial laparoscopic access and inspection of the peritoneal cavity. The incision length should match the width of the surgeon's hand and should be placed such that one can reach the limits of the spleen superiorly. The hand

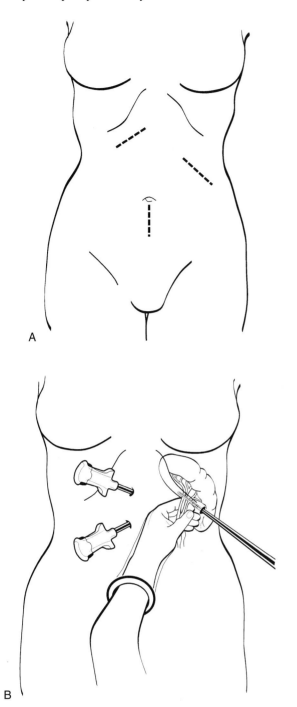

FIGURE 27.8. Hand-assisted technique for laparoscopic splenectomy. A. Possible incision options for placement of the hand-assist device. B. Operating technique with the hand access port in place.

can then be used to facilitate exposure, retraction, and manipulation of the spleen and to tamponade bleeding vessels. Matthews and associates[69] have recommended starting the procedure with the hand device if the spleen is 23 cm or more in cranial–caudad dimension or 19 cm or more in width. In other cases, the procedure may be

started using an entirely laparoscopic approach, and the hand device is held in reserve only to be used if difficulty is encountered. The principles of dissection should be the same as already described. Even with the hand device incision, extraction of the specimen can be challenging for very large spleens. If the spleen cannot be removed intact through this incision, it may be possible to manipulate the spleen into a large retrieval bag intraabdominally using the hand and then morcellating the specimen within the bag at the hand incision site. Intraperitoneal fragmentation of the specimen should be avoided because of the risk of splenic implants and recurrent disease.

Postoperative Care

Following laparoscopic splenectomy, the majority of patients can be discharged on the first postoperative day. The urinary catheter is removed on the evening of surgery, and the diet is advanced as tolerated. Postoperative laboratory testing consists of a complete blood count in the recovery room and again on the first postoperative day. Patients able to tolerate a regular diet, who are voiding without difficulty, and who have a stable hemoglobin/hematocrit are discharged by early afternoon the day after surgery. They are given complete discharge instructions for showers to begin the next day and activity as tolerated. Contact sports should be avoided for the first 7 to 14 days after surgery. Most patients report returning to normal activity levels somewhere between the 7th and the 10th postoperative day, with a wide range of responses.[37]

Complications of Laparoscopic Splenectomy

Intraoperative

Table 27.5 lists the reported intraoperative complications of laparoscopic splenectomy, taken from the series listed in Tables 27.2 and 27.3 and other references. The overall incidence of complications from LS has varied considerably among different reports but is probably in the 5% to 15% range overall. Predictors of complications from LS include surgeon experience, patient age, spleen weight, and malignant disease process.[71] Reported complications include injury to the spleen and adjacent organs, as a result of either technical difficulties or failure to recognize important anatomic structures during surgery. The most important and common complication of laparoscopic splenectomy is hemorrhage, which accounts for most conversions to open splenectomy (see following).[72] Hemorrhage can occur from the spleen itself, either from laceration of the splenic capsule[14] or

TABLE 27.5. Potential complications of laparoscopic
splenectomy.

Abdominal/gastrointestinal
  Port site hernia (incarcerated, obstructed)
  Gastrotomy
  Colonic perforation
  Pancreatitis
  Pancreatitis fistula
  Small bowel obstruction
Cardiovascular
  Myocardial infarction
  Deep venous thrombosis
  Pulmonary embolism
  Arrhythmias
Hematological
  Missed accessory spleens(s)
  Splenosis/splenic implants
Hemorrhagic
  Intraabdominal hemorrhage
  Port site hemorrhage
Infectious (nonpulmonary)
  Wound infection
  Cellulitis
  Fever
  Subphrenic abscess
Pulmonary/thoracic
  Atelectasis
  Pneumothorax
  Pleural effusion
  Pneumonia
  Diaphragmatic perforation
Other
  Urinary retention
  Paresthesias

inadequate ligature or control of the splenic vessels.[14,61] In the authors' experience, long-term steroid use may make the splenic capsule more prone to rupture. Other sources of hemorrhage during LS include the short gastric vessels, variable arterial supply to the lower pole of the spleen, the left gastroepiploic artery, and bleeding from small vessels in the retroperitoneal attachments of the spleen and from vessels along the tail of the pancreas.[20] Interestingly, despite the high incidence of thrombocytopenia in LS patients, the frequency of intraoperative hemorrhagic complications related to laparoscopic port sites is extremely low, in both the published literature[16,17,30–33] and the authors' experience, perhaps because the circulating platelets in such patients are functionally normal.

Injury to adjacent organs such as the colon, pancreas, and stomach may occur rarely during laparoscopic splenectomy. The splenic flexure of the colon is initially in the operative field in most patients, and one of the first steps in LS is to mobilize the splenic flexure. During this part of the procedure, cautery injury or direct trauma from the ultrasonic dissector is possible. The colon may also be injured with the Veress needle or trocar during the initial access phase. The most important issue concerning intraoperative colonic injury is to recognize the problem and repair it at the time of the laparoscopic procedure. Primary repair of small colonic injuries may be possible laparoscopically. However, through-and-through colon injuries may require conversion to an open procedure. If the injury is not noted intraoperatively, the patient may present later with peritoneal sepsis that requires emergency laparotomy and possible colostomy. Pancreatic injury is most likely to occur if the tail of the pancreas is close to the splenic hilum. It should be possible at the time of surgery to identify the pancreatic tail and dissect it away from the spleen enough to allow ligation of the hilar vessels without pancreatic disruption.[49] If the pancreatic parenchyma has been violated at the time of LS, a closed-suction drain should be placed. Unrecognized pancreatic injury may present with a left upper quadrant abscess, fluid collection, or clinical evidence of pancreatitis,[3,6,16,22] fistula,[13] or, in severe cases, sepsis. Pancreatic injury should rarely be serious enough that conversion to open operation is necessary. Gastric injury may occur when dissecting the short gastric vessels away from the spleen.[25] The ultrasonic dissector can injure the stomach wall directly if applied incorrectly, but thermal injuries should be rare. Gastric perforation or gastric serosal injuries during LS should be treated with laparoscopic suture repair.

Other reported causes of conversion to open splenectomy include splenomegaly (especially early in an institution's experience),[18,25,34] obesity,[30] extensive adhesions,[15] pulmonary insufficiency from chronic obstructive pulmonary disease restricting pneumoperitoneum,[20] and various other technical considerations.[12,25]

A final intraoperative complication of LS is failure to identify and remove accessory spleens.[58] The reported incidence of accessory spleens varies widely, ranging up to 30% in autopsy studies.[13] Failure to remove accessory spleen(s) may lead to disappointing long-term therapeutic results from the splenectomy itself. Experience is undoubtedly an important factor in locating accessory spleens,[13,58] but in most cases, they should be readily identifiable with standard laparoscopic techniques. The splenic hilum, gastrosplenic omentum, gastrocolic ligament, and region along the tail of the pancreas should be inspected carefully for the presence of accessory splenic tissue (Fig. 27.9). This compulsive visual exploration should take place at the beginning of the operation rather than at its conclusion. Preoperative imaging does not appear to be of sufficient sensitivity to justify its use on the basis of localizing accessory splenic tissue alone. The removal of accessory spleens laparoscopically is usually straightforward, dissecting the accessory organ with cautery or an ultrasonic coagulator and removing it with an impermeable entrapment bag. One option is to leave the accessory spleen in situ until the splenic dissection has been completed so that it can be placed in the same specimen bag as the spleen for removal. Patients with persistent or recurrent ITP after LS should undergo radionuclide imaging to identify any residual accessory splenic tissue.[65] Patients with a positive scan may be candidates for laparoscopic accessory splenectomy.[73] Residual splenic function may also occur because of splenosis from implantation of splenic tissue at the time of splenectomy.[65,72] This complication emphasizes the importance of avoiding disruption of the splenic capsule during and after the dissection.

Postoperative

Postoperative complications of LS are thus far infrequently reported. The most common problem is the same as that for OS: failure of the splenectomy to reverse the underlying clinical syndrome. In most cases, this is related to the underlying disease process and is not due to missed accessory splenic tissue. Nonetheless, consideration should be given to the latter possibility in patients with primary failure of the splenectomy, and a radiographic search for accessory spleens may be warranted, as already noted. Late presentation of intraabdominal organ injury to the colon, pancreas, or stomach may also occur. Any patient with an atypical course after laparoscopic splenectomy who has increased abdominal pain, fever, or an elevated white blood cell count should be aggressively

evaluated, beginning with an abdominal CT scan. Thrombosis of the splenic vein or portal vein is also a recognized complication after splenectomy,[11] primarily occurring in patients with markedly enlarged spleens and underlying coagulopathies. These patients usually present with abdominal pain and fever, and the diagnosis can often be made on a contrast enhanced CT scan. Splenectomized patients may also be at increased risk for overwhelming sepsis from encapsulated microorganisms.[74] The groups at highest risk for this complication are pediatric patients with underlying hematological disorders. To date, no cases of overwhelming postsplenectomy sepsis have been reported following laparoscopic splenectomy.

Wound-related problems such as infection are uncommon after laparoscopic splenectomy. Incisional hernias may develop at any port site that is 10mm or larger in diameter.[13,37,48] Port site hernias should be surgically repaired to eliminate the risk of intestinal obstruction or strangulation.[47] This complication should be avoidable in most cases by compulsive operative closure of the fascia at all port sites of 10mm or larger. Other potential complications of LS include wound infection,[12,15,20,34,36] atelectasis,[19,34] pneumonia,[3,37,71] pleural effusions,[13–15,50] diaphragmatic perforation,[28,34] pneumothorax,[27] deep venous thrombosis,[13,18,27] pulmonary embolism,[18,27] cardiac arrhythmias,[15] myocardial infarction,[20,27,36] and miscellaneous others listed in Table 27.5. It would appear that these complications occur less frequently than after open splenectomy. Patients have also developed "late" bleeding requiring reoperation.[12,25,34,48] Perioperative mortality, often related to underlying medical problems or hematological disorders, has also been reported.[15,25,35,36,48]

Conversion to Open Splenectomy

As with any laparoscopic procedure, intraoperative conversion to an "open" procedure is a judgment-based decision of the operating surgeon. The most common reason to convert from a laparoscopic to open splenectomy is bleeding. This decision to convert should be based on the surgeon's experience and comfort with LS procedures, as many instances of bleeding encountered early in one's learning curve are more easily handled laparoscopically with continued operative experience. For example, when ligating the splenic hilum, initial bleeding from vessels, if not severe enough to immediately obscure the laparoscopic view, may often be controlled with an additional application of the endoscopic GIA vascular load stapler; the same is true of bleeding from the short gastric vessels, which often can be controlled with either the ultrasonic scalpel or clips. Oozing from the spleen itself may occur during sequential ligature and division of the splenic vessels. This dark venous blood can often obscure the operative field temporarily, but again this can be con-

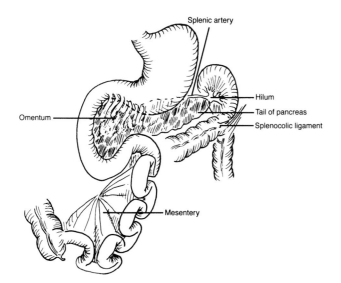

FIGURE 27.9. Sites of accessory spleens in decreasing order of frequency: splenic hilum, tail of the pancreas, greater omentum, along the course of the splenic artery, and within the splenocolic ligament. Less common sites include the small bowel mesentery and along the course of the gonadal vessels. (From Dierks MM, et al. Splenectomy. In: Jones DB, Wu JS, Soper NJ (eds) Laparoscopic Surgery: Principles and Procedures. St. Louis: Quality Medical, 1997:296, with permission.)

TABLE 27.6. Cost comparison of laparoscopy versus open splenectomy.

Year	Authors	Cost LS	Cost OS	p value	Comment
1996	Smith et al.[43]	$17,071	$13,196	NS	Adults, charges
1996	Friedman et al.[30]	$8,271	$10,890	NS	Adults, costs
1997	Diaz et al.[39]	$18,015	$14,524	0.04	Adults, costs
1997	Glasgow et al.[35]	$8,939	$14,022	0.03	Adults, costs
1998	Rescorla et al.[44]	$5,713	$6,564	NS	Children, charges

LS, Laparoscopic splenectomy; OS, open splenectomy.

trolled with completion of the splenic hilum division. Another cause of splenic bleeding is retractor injury to the splenic capsule, something that occurs very commonly but should not, with experience, necessarily lead to conversion. Another option in the patient with troublesome but not brisk bleeding is to insert a hand port device to allow improved exposure and tamponade of the bleeding site until control can be attained.

Conversion to open splenectomy may occur through multiple incisions, including midline, left subcostal, or transverse. The optimal incision for conversion depends on the patient's position and size of the spleen. Our preference, in most cases, is to convert to a left subcostal incision, connecting the posterior flank port site to the main operative port site in the left upper quadrant of the abdomen. In patients with splenomegaly, it may be preferable to convert via a midline incision. With ongoing hemorrhage, the emphasis at the time of conversion of the case is to enter the abdomen as quickly and safely as possible. The oblique muscles in the left subcostal area may be rapidly divided and the abdomen entered within seconds if necessary. This incision may be extended anteriorly as needed, but often the splenectomy may be completed through a 10- to 15-cm incision in this area. Patients can usually be discharged from the hospital on the third or fourth postoperative day after this open procedure.

Outcomes and Costs

Although health care payors in the United States increasingly seek cost data, it remains difficult for physicians and hospitals to consistently identify the exact cost of caring for an individual patient. Often, hospital charge data are presented, yet the relationship between insurance charges (even Medicare), reimbursements, and costs are inconsistent. Charge data also cannot account for the indirect costs and benefits to society from procedures that minimize patients' postoperative disability and hasten their return to work.

As such, it is extremely difficult with new procedures to validate cost differences between the old procedure, OS, and the new one, LS. Multiple publications have taken a preliminary approach to examining this problem. As noted in Tables 27.2 and 27.3, the outcome from LS

cases appears relatively good. The increased costs of these procedures are related primarily to resource utilization (operative time, inpatient days, personnel, capital, and disposable equipment). LS appears to consistently require more lengthy operative times (with attendant increased personnel and material costs) but has shorter inpatient hospitalizations. The relative cost of these two opposing factors is difficult to calculate as it necessarily varies by hospital and geographic region. With experience, the extended operative times for LS should be reduced to that of OS, while still maintaining an advantage in inpatient hospitalization days, reflected in a lower nonoperating cost for LS.[30] The costs of personnel and equipment are much harder to estimate and are not addressed well by current publications. LS utilizes more disposable equipment than OS, and reported costs from the operating room are consistently greater in LS than OS cases.[43] The indirect savings of smaller incisions, faster discharge, and more rapid return to full activity are very difficult to estimate, but it is likely that LS results in "societal" cost savings over OS. Table 27.6 lists several estimates of the differential hospital costs between LS and OS, excluding professional fees. There are no clear trends in these numbers, other than the overall suggestion that the total hospital costs of the two procedures are probably equivalent. Overall, the cost-effectiveness of LS relative to OS should increase with time, as surgeons become more experienced (leading to shorter operative times and less hospital/personnel resource utilization) and disposable equipment usage is minimized or replaced by nondisposable, depreciable, capital equipment.

Conclusion

Laparoscopic splenectomy should be considered the standard of care for patients who require splenectomy for ITP, hemolytic anemia, and other hematological disorders with primary splenic manifestations. Relative to open splenectomy, laparoscopic splenectomy appears to have equivalent clinical outcomes in terms of cure of the underlying disorder. However, LS results in less patient disability, shorter hospitalization, and probably less perioperative morbidity, although there are no prospective, randomized comparisons of the open and laparoscopic procedures. The cost of laparoscopic splenectomy to the health care institution may initially be higher, but medical cost differences will likely evolve in favor of the laparoscopic over the open procedure with increasing surgical experience. The indirect savings to society from reduced disability are significant but difficult to calculate.

Indications for LS are expanding based on the accrued experience of laparoscopic surgeons and the excellent outcomes to date. With continued advances in techniques and instrumentation, even patients with splenic trauma or massive splenomegaly may some day be managed laparoscopically.

References

1. Delaitre B, Maignien B, Icard P. Laparoscopic splenectomy. Br J Surg 1992;79:1334.
2. Schwartz SI. Spleen. In: Schwartz SI, Shires GT, Spencer FC (eds) Spleen, 5th Ed. St. Louis: McGraw-Hill, 1989:1441–1457.
3. Katkhouda N, Hurwitz MB, Rivera RT, et al. Laparoscopic splenectomy: outcome and efficacy in 103 consecutive patients. Ann Surg 1998;228:568–578.
4. Michels N. The variational anatomy of the spleen and splenic artery. Am J Anat 1942;70:21–72.
5. George J, El-Harake M, Raskob G. Chronic idiopathic thrombocytopenic purpura. N Engl J Med 1994;331:1207–1211.
6. Harold KL, Schlinkert RT, Mann DK, et al. Long-term results of laparoscopic splenectomy for immune thrombocytopenic purpura. Mayo Clin Proc 1999;74:37–39.
7. Meyer G, Wichmann MW, Rau HG, Hiller E, Schildberg FW. Laparoscopic splenectomy for idiopathic thrombocytopenic purpura. Surg Endosc 1998;12:1348–1352.
8. Tanoue K, Hashizume M, Morita M, et al. Results of laparoscopic splenectomy for immune thrombocytopenia purpura. Am J Surg 1999;177:222–226.
9. Lord R, Coleman M, Milliken S. Splenectomy for HIV-related immune thrombocytopenia. Arch Surg 1998;133:205–210.
10. Tefferi A. Myelofibrosis with myeloid metaplasia. N Engl J Med 2000;342:1255–1265.
11. Rattner D, Ellman L, Warshaw A. Portal vein thrombosis after elective splenectomy. Arch Surg 1993;128:565–570.
12. Emmermann A, Sornig C, Peiper M, Weh JH, Broelsch CE. Laparoscopic splenectomy: technique and results in a series of 27 cases. Surg Endosc 1995;9:924–927.
13. Gigot JF, Legrand M, Cadiere GB. Is laparoscopic splenectomy a justified approach in hematologic disorders? Int Surg 1995;80:299–303.
14. Bove T, Delvaux G, Van Eijkelenburg P, De Backer A, Willems G. Laparoscopic assisted surgery of the spleen: clinical experience in expanding indications. J Laparoendosc Surg 1996;6:213–217.
15. Flowers JL, Lefor AT, Steers J, Heyman M, Graham SM, Imbembo A. Laparoscopic splenectomy in patients with hematologic diseases. Ann Surg 1996;224:19–28.
16. Tsiotos G, Schlinkert RT. Laparoscopic splenectomy for immune thrombocytopenic purpura. Arch Surg 1997;132:642–646.
17. Szold A, Sagi B, Merhav H, Klausner MM. Optimizing laparoscopic splenectomy: technical details and experience in 59 patients. Surg Endsoc 1998;12:1078–1081.
18. Decker G, Millat B, Guillon F, Atger J, Linon M. Laparoscopic splenectomy for benign and malignant diseases: 35 consecutive cases. World J Surg 1998;22:62–68.
19. Walsh R, Heniford B. Laparoscopic splenectomy for non-Hodgkin's lymphoma. J Surg Oncol 1999;70:116–121.
20. Brody FJ, Chekan EG, Pappas TN. Conversion factors for laparoscopic splenectomy for immune thrombocytopenic purpura. Surg Endosc 1999;13:789–791.
21. Stanton C. Laparoscopic splenectomy for idiopathic thrombocytopenic purpura. Surg Endosc 1999;13:1083–1086.
22. Gossot D, Fritsch S, Celerier M. Laparoscopic splenectomy: optimal vascular control using the lateral approach and ultrasonic dissection. Surg Endosc 1999;13:21–25.
23. Trias M, Targarona E, Espert J, et al. Impact of hematological diagnosis on early and late outcome after laparoscopic splenectomy. Surg Endosc 2000;14:556–560.
24. Baccarani U, Carroll BJ, Hiatt JR, et al. Comparison of laparoscopic and open staging in Hodgkin disease. Arch Surg 1998;133:517–522.
25. Berman RS, Yahanda AM, Mansfield PF, et al. Laparoscopic splenectomy in patients with hematologic malignancies. Am J Surg 1999;178:530–536.
26. Targarona E, Trias M. Laparoscopic treatment of splenic injuries. Semin Laparosc Surg 1996;3:44–49.
27. Park AE, Birgisson G, Mastrangelo MJ, Marcaccio MM, Witzke DB. Laparoscopic splenectomy: outcomes and lessons learned from over 200 cases. Surgery (St. Louis) 2000;128:660–667.
28. Targarona EM, Espert JJ, Cerdain G. Effect of spleen size on splenectomy outcome: a comparison of open and laparoscopic surgery. Surg Endosc 1999;13:559–562.
29. Schlachta CM, Poulin EC, Mamazza J. Laparoscopic splenectomy for hematologic malignancies. Ann Surg 1998;228:35–39.
30. Friedman RL, Fallas MJ, Carroll BJ, Hiatt JR, Phillips EH. Laparoscopic splenectomy for ITP: the gold standard. Surg Endosc 1996;10:991–995.
31. Watson DI, Coventry BJ, Chin T, Gil PG, Malycha P. Laparoscopic versus open splenectomy for immune thrombocytopenic purpura. Surgery (St. Louis) 1997;121:18–22.
32. Marassi A, Vignali A, Zuliani W, Biguzi E, Bergamo CGL, Di Carlo V. Splenectomy for idiopathic thrombocytopenic purpura. Surg Endosc 1999;13:17–20.
33. Shimomatsuya T, Horiuchi T. Laparoscopic splenectomy for treatment of patients with idiopathic thrombocytopenic purpura. Comparison with open splenectomy. Surg Endosc 1999;13:563–566.
34. Trias M, Targarona EM, Espert JJ, Balague C. Laparoscopic surgery for splenic disorders. Surg Endosc 1998;12:66–72.
35. Glasgow RE, Yee LF, Mulvihill SJ. Laparoscopic splenectomy: the emerging standard. Surg Endosc 1997;11:108–112.
36. Rhodes M, Rudd M, O'Rourke N, Nathanson L, Fielding G. Laparoscopic splenectomy in patients with hematologic disorders. Ann Surg 1995;222:43–46.

37. Brunt LM, Quasebarth MA, Whitman ED. Comparative analysis of laparoscopic versus open splenectomy. Am J Surg 1996;172:596–601.
38. Yee LF, Carvajal SH, de Lorimier AA, Mulvihill SJ. Laparoscopic splenectomy. The initial experience at University of California, San Francisco. Arch Surg 1995;130:874–879.
39. Diaz J, Eisenstat M, Chung R. A case-controlled study of laparoscopic splenectomy. Am J Surg 1997;173:348–350.
40. Friedman R, Hiatt J, Korman JFK, Cymerman J, Phillips E. Laparoscopic or open splenectomy for hematologic disease: which approach is superior? J Am Coll Surg 1997;185:49–54.
41. Donini A, Baccarani U, Terrosu G, et al. Laparoscopic vs open splenectomy in the management of hematologic diseases. Surg Endosc 1999;13:1220–1225.
42. Janu PG, Rogers DA, Love TE. A comparison of laparoscopic and traditional open splenectomy in childhood. J Pediatr Surg 1996;31:109–114.
43. Smith CD, Meyer TA, Goretsky MJ, Hyamus D, Michetle FA, Fegelman EJ. Laparoscopic splenectomy by the lateral approach: a safe and effective alternative approach to open splenectomy for hematologic diseases. Surgery (St. Louis) 1996;120:789–794.
44. Rescorla FJ, Breitfeld PP, West KW, Williams D, Engum SA, Grosfeld JL. A case controlled comparison of open and laparoscopic splenectomy in children. Surgery (St. Louis) 1998;124:670–676.
45. Park A, Marcaccio M, Sternbach M, Witzke D, Fitzgerald P. Laparoscopic vs open splenectomy. Arch Surg 1999;134:1263–1269.
46. Zamir O, Szold A, Matzner Y, et al. Laparoscopic splenectomy for immune thrombocytopenic purpura. J Laparoendosc Surg 1996;6:301–304.
47. Katkhouda N, Waldrep DJ, Feinstein D, Soliman H, Stain SC, Artega AE. Unresolved issues in laparoscopic splenectomy. Am J Surg 1996;172:585–590.
48. Lozano-Salazar R.R., Herrera MF, Vargas-Vorachkova F, Lopez-Karpovitch X. Laparoscopic versus open splenectomy for immune thrombocytopenic purpura. Am J Surg 1998;176:366–369.
49. Schlinkert RT, Teotia SS. Laparoscopic splenectomy. Arch Surg 1999;134:99–103.
50. Park A, Gagner M, Pomp A. The lateral approach to laparoscopic splenectomy. Am J Surg 1997;173:126–130.
51. Hashizume M, Sugimachi K, Kitano S, et al. Laparoscopic splenectomy. Am J Surg 1994;167:611–614.
52. Trias M, Targarona EM, Balague C. Laparoscopic splenectomy: an evolving technique. A comparison between anterior and lateral approaches. Surg Endosc 1996;10:389–392.
53. Saldinger PF, Matthews JB, Mowschenson PM, Hodin RA. Stapled laparoscopic splenectomy: initial experience. J Am Coll Surg 1996;182:459–461.
54. Delaitre B. Laparoscopic splenectomy: the "hanged spleen" technique. Surg Endosc 1995;9:528–529.
55. Lefor AT, Melvin WS, Bailey RW, Flowers JL. Laparoscopic splenectomy in the managment of immune thrombocytopenia purpura. Surgery (St. Louis) 1993;114:613–618.
56. Richardson WS, Smith CD, Branum GD, Hunter JG. Leaning spleen: a new approach to laparoscopic splenectomy. J Am Coll Surg 1997;185:412–415.
57. Dexter SPL, Martin IG, Alao D, Norfolk DR, McMahon MJ. Laparoscopic splenectomy: the suspended pedicle technique. Surg Endosc 1996;10:393–396.
58. Gigot JF, Jamar F, Ferrant A, et al. Inadequate detection of accessory spleens and splenosis with laparoscopic splenectomy. Surg Endosc 1998;12:101–103.
59. Laycock WS, Hunter JG. New technology for the division of short gastric vessels during laparoscopic Nissen fundoplication: a prospective randomized trial. Surg Endosc 1996;10:71–73.
60. Rothenberg SS. Laparoscopic splenectomy using the harmonic scalpel. J Laparendosc Surg 1996;6S:61–63.
61. Miles WFA, Greig JD, Wilson RG, Nixon SJ. Technique of laparoscopic splenectomy with a powered vascular linear stapler. Br J Surg 1996;83:1212–1214.
62. Horowitz J, Smith JL, Wever TK, Rodriguez-Bigas MA, Petrelli NJ. Postoperative complications after splenectomy for hematologic malignancies. Ann Surg 1996;223:290–296.
63. Nelson EW, Mone MC. Splenectomy in high-risk patients with splenomegaly. Am J Surg 1999;178:581–586.
64. Terrosu G, Donini A, Baccarani U, et al. Laparoscopic versus open splenectomy in the management of splenomegaly: our preliminary experience. Surgery (St. Louis) 1998;124:839–843.
65. Targarona E, Espert J, Balague C, et al. Residual splenic function after laparoscopic splenectomy. Arch Surg 1998;133:56–60.
66. Morgenstern L, Skandalakis JE. Anatomy and embryology of the spleen. In: Hiatt JR, Phillips EH, Morgenstern L (eds) Surgical Diseases of the Spleen. Berlin: Springer, 1997:15–24.
67. Southern Surgeons' Club Study Group. Handoscopic surgery: a prospective multicenter trial of a minimally invasive technique for complex abdominal surgery. Arch Surg 1999;134:477–485.
68. Pratt C, Anderson T, Demeure MJ. Hand-assisted laparoscopic splenectomy: retained benefits of laparoscopic splenectomy over open splenectomy. Presented at the SAGES 2000 meeting in Atlanta, GA.
69. Matthews BD, Backus CL, Walsh RM, Pratt BL, Greene FL, Heniford BT. Laparoscopic versus hand-assisted splenectomy in patients with massive splenomegaly. Presented at the SAGES 2000 meeting, Atlanta, GA.
70. Yood SM, Kelly J, Sandor A, Roll S, Cohen R, Litwin DEM. Hand-assisted laparoscopic splenectomy for splenomegaly. Presented at the SAGES 2000 meeting, Atlanta, GA.
71. Targarona E, Espert J, Bombuy E, et al. Complications of laparoscopic splenectomy. Arch Surg 2000;135:1137–1140.
72. Navarro R, Korman J, Phillips E. Complications of laparoscopic splenectomy. Semin Laparosc Surg 1997;4:182–189.
73. Szold A, Kamat M, Nadu A. Laparoscopic accessory splenectomy for recurrent idiopathic thrombocytopenic purpura and hemolytic anemia. Surg Endosc 2000;14:761–763.
74. Schilling RF. Estimating the risk of sepsis after splenectomy for hereditary spherocytosis. Ann Intern Med 1995;122:187–188.

Section V
Laparoscopic Hernia Repair

Maurice E. Arregui, MD
Section Editor

Part I
Laparoscopic Inguinal Hernia Repair

28
History of the Preperitoneal Approach for Inguinal Hernia: Rationale and Various Approaches

Lloyd M. Nyhus

The early approaches to groin hernia repair were via the abdominen intraperitoneal. The term repair is used advisedly, because identification of the hernia sac and ligation of same in most instances completed the operation. Here again, the word "completed" needs clarification. Marcy[1] of Boston brought to our attention (English translation) a description of a hernia operative procedure detailed by Demetrius de Cantemir,[2] Prince of Moldavia, and translated (from the French) by M. De Joncquieres in 1743. Cantemir related that "the inhabitants of Albania and Epirus, otherwise called by the Turks Arnaut, excelled in the cure of ruptures; and after he (Cantemir) has spoken of their skill in many respects, he related a process which he observed himself."

> As to the cure of ruptures (says he) they undertake it upon all sorts of people and at all ages: their method is coarse, but yet successful. When I was at Constantinople I had the operation performed upon my secretary, who was an elderly man, in my own palace. Having agreed as to the expense, they tied the patient down upon a broad plank, and secured him from his breast to his feet with proper bandages: then the operator made an incision in the inferior part of the abdomen with a kind of razor or bistoury. The peritoneum being opened, he pulled out about the bulk of a hand of the internal substance, under the skin, and drew up the intestine, which was fallen into the scrotum, into its proper place. Afterward he sew'd up the peritoneum with strong thread, and a knot at the end of it to hinder it from slipping; and the lips which hung over were cut off with the same razor. Then the wound was rubbed with hog's lard, and cauterized with a red-hot iron. Before the dressing was applied, they lifted up a little of the legs of the patient, who was almost dead, and pour'd the whites of nine new-laid eggs into the wound; and if that liquour fermented and bubbled within the space of an hour or two, it was certain sign of a cure; on the contrary, if there was no appearance of that kind in three hours, they made no favorable prognostic. They attribute ill success to the age or weakness of the patient, which obstructs the cure, for they never doubt of the efficacy of their method: and indeed there seldom die two out of an hundred of those whom they under-take. Convalescence was prolonged, as it lasted from 20 to 40 days, this being the time needed for the separation of the thread.

It is clear why it is important to separate the concept of approach and that of type of repair. Today, the intraabdominal and preperitoneal (posterior) approaches have strong advocates, but we must all agree the techniques of repair are legion in their variety. The posterior approach has waxed and waned in its popularity. It has not been since the past several decades that a clear understanding of the detailed anatomy of the posterior inguinal wall has evolved. Following the use of a prosthetic mesh buttress complemented by intraabdominal pressure, that is, Pascal's law, a satisfactory result has regularly been obtained. Pascal (1623–1662) a French scientist, mathematician, and religious writer, proposed the principle that "gas or liquid at rest in a closed container will transmit pressure change without loss to every portion of the gas or fluid and to the walls of the container." As is discussed here, it was Rives[3] and Stoppa et al.[4] who recognized that this principle would apply to the pressures within the peritoneal and extraperitoneal spaces as a salutary mechanism in the use of prosthetic mesh in preperitoneal hernia repair.

Intraperitoneal Approach

Meade[5] and Read[6] have summarized the many attempts to repair groin hernias from within the peritoneal cavity. Although surgeons in the late nineteenth century claimed a relatively good "cure" rate for the era, the lack of prolonged enthusiasm for this approach suggests a less than stellar outcome. Here again, we must separate the approach from the repair; the peritoneal cavity was readily entered, but concepts of anatomic repair were lacking.

Some confusion exists concerning the position of LaRoque[7] in the historical sequence under consideration.

This surgeon suggested that the peritoneal cavity be entered at the outset through an opening slightly above the standard hernia incision. He then removed the hernial sac and performed a high ligation of the neck of the sac. LaRoque made no attempt to repair the posterior inguinal wall but performed a standard anterior Bassini repair.

More recent exploration of intraabdominal techniques may be found in studies of Jacobson,[8] Mansfield,[9] Phetteplace,[10] and Williams.[11] The intra-abdominal approach and repair (IPOM) via the laparoscopic methodology is reviewed next.

The Preperitoneal (Posterior) Approach and Repair

The term preperitoneal has caused some confusion, yet as I coined the term as connoting before—"pre"—the peritoneum to indicate the anatomic plane of dissection, there is an obvious wish on my part for its use to continue. Condon[12] clarified the subject by the following observation: "Preperitoneal is a hybrid from the Latin (pre) and Greek (peritoneum). Some object to it as etymologically illegitimate and recommended the form properitoneal. Those who raise such an objection, however, do not object to retroperitoneal, which also is an etymologic hybrid (retro, Latin; peritoneal, Greek). I prefer preperitoneal because it clearly conveys the intended meaning and has wide clinical acceptance. Further, preperitoneal is accepted by the O.E.D., which should satisfy even the most abstemious etymologist."

The evolution of the posterior approach from that of intraperitoneal visualization of groin hernia defects to the current careful and precise dissection and repair of the posterior inguinal wall in the preperitoneal space has encompassed a century of "trial and error and success." Table 28.1[13–41] reviews the highlights of the saga beginning in 1876 with the presentation of Annandale.[13] He did not perform a fascial repair. Lawson Tait of Birmingham, England, in 1891 reported the advantages of the treatment of hernia by "median abdominal section."[15] He also recognized that, for "radical cure" to occur, "elements of the tendinous aperture must be agglutinated in order that the aperture may be effectively closed." Thus, the concept of repair of the posterior inguinal wall was presented in association with the preperitoneal approach. There were many similar suggestions in the literature at this time. The September 26, 1891, issue of the *British Medical Journal* is particularly interesting because it contains many allusions to the posterior approach, as presented to the Annual Meeting of the British Medical Association in Bournemouth, England, July 1891.

Bates[16] of Seattle should be credited with further advancing this concept. Bates repaired the defect from the posterior approach using transversalis fascia. The historical impact of the Bates contribution is significant. Although McEvedy[17] usually is credited with exposure of the preperitoneal space lateral to the rectus abdominis muscle (in contrast to the vertical linea alba incision of Cheatle[18,19] and of Henry[20]), the words of Bates suggest that in 1913 he pioneered this lateral transverse incision. Therefore, the first paragraph of Bates' paper is quoted:

"This operation consists in making an incision, about two inches long, parallel with Poupart's ligament. The end of the incision should be about one inch above the usual location of the internal ring. The fascia of the external oblique muscle is divided in line of its fibers. The arching fibers of internal oblique are separated and retracted. The fascia of the transversalis together with the peritoneum is opened. If adhesions are encountered they can be broken up by traction and blunt dissection with the finger within the sac."

The preperitoneal approach concept was slow to gain adherents; however, during subsequent decades, a number of advocates presented views on the subject (see Table 28.1).[21–41]

Cheatle and later Henry suggested that the approach might facilitate the technical handling of inguinal and femoral hernias. However, with few exceptions, the approach was used primarily for femoral hernias. There was little use of the approach for direct hernias.

The historical flow of posterior repair methods is clearly shown in Table 28.1. Note the early reference to the iliopubic tract in terms of anatomic hernia repair in our presentation of 1960.[28] The clear separation of the inguinal ligament from its "shelving edge," that is, the iliopubic tract of the posterior inguinal wall by Condon,[12] was a major step in advancing our understanding of groin anatomy as seen posteriorly.

Iliopubic Tract

The iliopubic tract was first described by Alexander Thomson[42,43] (frequently misspelled Thompson) in 1836. Thomson recognized this important thickening in the posterior inguinal wall as an entity distinctly separate from the inguinal ligament. He wrote: "There is not one single fiber coming from the external oblique muscle . . . We always find behind the tendinous portion of the external oblique, which forms Poupart's ligament, a strong aponeurotic bandelette, which has been, but wrongly, confused with the tendon itself."

Eugene Polya[44] also was a strong proponent of the individuality of the iliopubic tract. Polya made several interesting comments concerning this structure: "The opinions are not unanimous whether the ligament is part of the transversalis fascia, Poupart's ligament, femoral sheath or the psoas fascia. As far as I am concerned, and most of

TABLE 28.1. Methods of anatomic repair of a defect with a preperitoneal approach to hernioplasty.

Author	Type of hernia	Method of repair
Annandale (1876)[13]	Indirect	Ligation of hernial sac: no repair
	Direct	Ligation of hernial sac: no repair
	Femoral	Obscure
Maunsell (1877)[14]	Femoral	Suture of pectineus fascia and pectineal line to Poupart ligament
Tait (1891)[15]	Indirect	Suture of fascial defect, "external column of ring to inner column"
	Femoral	Obscure
Bates (1913)[16]	Indirect	Suture of transversalis fascia of internal ring; transverse incision lateral to rectus
McEvedy (1950)[17]	Femoral	Suture of conjoined tendon to Cooper ligament; vertical incision lateral to rectus
Cheatle (1920)[18]	Indirect	Occlusion of internal ring by suture
	Femoral	Flap periosteum of pubis to Poupart ligament
Cheatle (1921)[19]	Indirect	High ligation of sac only
	Femoral	Flap periosteum of pubis to Poupart ligament
Henry (1936)[20]	Indirect	Plastic to internal ring: transversalis fascia to fascia deep surface internal oblique muscle
	Femoral	Flap of pectineus fascia to Poupart ligament
		Cheatle and Henry incisions; lower abdomen vertical midline
Jennings et al. (1942)[21]	Indirect	Plastic closure of internal ring: suture of transversalis fascial sling lateral to the cord
Musgrove and McCready (1949)[22]	Femoral	Suture of Poupart ligament to Cooper ligament
Riba and Mehn (1952)[23]	Indirect	Plastic closure of internal ring: suture of transversalis fascial sling, combined with prostatectomy
	Direct	Suture of transversalis fascia to Cooper ligament
Hull and Ganey (1953)[24]	Femoral	Suture of Poupart ligament to Cooper ligament or pectineus fascia flap technique of Henry
Mikkelsen and Berne (1954)[25]	Femoral	Suture of transversalis fascia and transversus aponeurosis to Cooper ligament
	Small indirect	Plastic repair of internal ring: transversalis fascia
	Large indirect	Similar to femoral closure
Mouzas and Diggory (1956)[26]	Femoral	Suture of conjoined tendon to Cooper ligament
Nyhus et al. (1959)[27]	Indirect	Suture of transversalis fascial sling medial to the cord
	Direct	Suture of transversalis fascia to Cooper ligament
	Femoral	Suture of transversalis fascia to Cooper ligament
		Use of synthetic (Ivalon) to buttress posterior wall repair
Nyhus et al. (1960)[28]	Indirect	Suture of transversalis fascial sling medial or lateral to the cord or both
	Direct	Suture of transversalis fascia, arch of transversus abdominis aponeurosis, or both to iliopubic tract
	Femoral	Suture of iliopubic tract to Cooper ligament
Estrin et al. (1963)[29]	Femoral	Suture of transversalis fascia to Cooper ligament
	Indirect	Suture of transversalis fascia to inguinal ligament
	Direct	Suture of transversalis fascia to Cooper ligament
Stoppa et al. (1972)[30]	Indirect, direct	Preperitoneal insertion of large Dacron prosthesis without fascial repair (GPRVS)
Stoppa et al. (1984)[31]	Femoral, recurrent	Same
Ger (1982)[32]	Indirect	(L) Laparoscopic closure neck of sac: no repair
Gazayerli (1992)[33]	Indirect or direct	(L) Suture of transversalis fascia to iliopubic tract
Filipi et al. (1992)[34]	All types	(L) Intraperitoneal onlay mesh (IPOM)
Arregui et al. (1992)[35]	Indirect or direct	(L) Transabdominal preperitoneal patch repair (TAPP)
Dion (1993)[36]	All types	(L) Adapted from Nyhus (see below)
McKernan and Laws (1992)[37]	Indirect	(L) Total extraperitoneal mesh (TEP)
McKernan and Laws (1993)[38]	Direct	(L) (TEP)
Phillips et al. (1993)[39]	Indirect, direct	(L) (TEP)
Patino (1998)[40]	All types	As under Nyhus (see below)
Greenburg (1999)[41]	All types	Similar to Nyhus (see below)
Nyhus (2003) (current)[a]	Type I: internal ring not dilated	High ligation of sac only
	Type II: Small indirect	Suture of transversalis fascial sling medial or lateral to the cord
	Type IIIA: direct	Suture of transversalis fascia and transversus abdominis aponeurosis to iliopubic tract; buttress with Marlex mesh
	Type IIIB: large indirect	Suture of transversalis fascia and transversus abdominis apouneurosis to iliopubic tract medial to cord; occasionally, one or two sutures placed between transversalis fascial sling and iliopubic tract lateral to cord to ensure adequate closure of internal ring; cord at level of femoral vessels; if massive, use components of direct repair as well; buttress with Marlex mesh
	Type IIIC: femoral	Suture of iliopubic tract to Cooper ligament, no mesh
	Type IV: recurrent	Repair defect and buttress with Marlex mesh

[a] All indirect and femoral hernia sacs ligated; direct sac usually inverted, not opened.

the other authors agree, this ligament constitutes a part of the transversalis fascia."

In his anatomic dissections, Condon[12] transected or excised the inguinal ligament to visualize the iliopubic tract. Polya in 1912[44] recognized the importance of this technique to adequately demonstrate this structure. It was Polya who suggested that the bandelette iliopubienne be named the ligamentum iliopubicum Thomsonii. Fruchaud[45,46] described the iliopubic tract in great detail both in script and pictorially.

Classification of Hernia

It has been the habit of surgeons to find one operative technique for hernial repair and to use the same for all types of hernias. I term this the "haberdashery" approach or "one size fits all." Zollinger[47] has summarized the current status of attempts to develop a helpful hernia classification. Because hernia types and methods of repair are alluded to in my historical review, a brief outline is given of our classification for reference. Our guide allows objective evaluation of treatment and verification of results.[48]

Classifying hernias and matching the types of hernia with specific operations serves as a technical guide to hernia repair. For example, prosthetic mesh is not necessary for all hernia repairs. Mesh is useful in patients with large direct or combined direct–indirect hernias but is rarely necessary for femoral hernia repair.

Type I hernias are indirect inguinal hernia in which the internal abdominal ring is of normal size, configuration, and structure. They usually occur in infants, children, or young adults. The boundaries are well delineated, and the Hesselbach triangle is normal. An indirect hernial sac extends variably from just distal to the internal abdominal ring to the middle of the inguinal canal.

Type II hernias are indirect inguinal hernias in which the internal ring is enlarged and distorted without impinging on the floor of the inguinal canal. The Hesselbach triangle (floor of the canal) is normal when palpated through the opened peritoneal sac. The hernial sac is not in the scrotum, but it may occupy the entire inguinal canal.

Type III hernias are of three subtypes: direct, indirect, and femoral.

Type IIIA are direct inguinal hernias in which the protrusion does not herniate through the internal abdominal (inguinal) ring. The weakened transversalis fascia (posterior inguinal wall medial to the inferior epigastric vessels) bulges outward in front of the hernial mass. All direct hernias, small or large, are type IIIA.

Type IIIB hernias are indirect inguinal hernias with a large dilated ring that has expanded medially and encroaches on the posterior inguinal wall (floor) to a greater or lesser degree. The hernial sac frequently is in the scrotum. Occasionally, the cecum on the right or the sigmoid colon on the left makes up a portion of the wall of the sac. These sliding hernias always destroy a portion of the inguinal floor. (The internal abdominal ring may be dilated without displacement of the inferior epigastric vessels. Direct and indirect components of the hernial sac may straddle those vessels to form a pantaloon hernia.)

Type IIIC hernias are femoral hernias, a specialized form of posterior wall defect.

Type IV hernias are recurrent hernias. They can be direct (type IVA), indirect (type IVB), femoral (type IVC), or a combination of these types (type IVD). They cause intricate management problems and carry a higher morbidity than do other hernias.

The Role of Prosthetic Mesh in Posterior Repair

Usher[49] is credited with the wave of interest in prosthetic meshes. Through his diligent and pioneering work, polypropylene mesh was perfected and used successfully for large direct and indirect defects repaired by either the anterior Bassini or the Halsted technique. Although we reported the use of synthetic material (Ivalon) as a buttress for hernial repair from the preperitoneal approach in 1959,[27] it is clear that Stoppa et al.[31] deserve credit for bringing to our attention the value of prosthetic meshes in buttressing the posterior inguinal wall. Note that the word "repair" was not used because Stoppa's technique relied entirely upon the hydrostatic principle of Pascal to maintain the mesh (Merseline-Dacron) in the appropriate position to cover the defects of concern. This procedure has been named the giant prosthetic reinforcement of the visceral sac, or GPRVS. Earlier proponents of mesh placement unilaterally within the preperitoneal space included Estrin,[29] Rives,[3] Read,[50] and Mahorner and Goss.[51] An anterior transinguinal approach to the posterior wall was used by several of these authors. It was our practice from the mid-1950s to perform transversalis fascia suture closure of groin defects without the routine use of mesh buttress. However, after our comparative study published in 1988[52] in which we demonstrated a clear advantage of recurrent hernia repair with Marlex mesh buttress (1.7% rerecurrent hernia rate) versus suture repair only (5% recurrence), we converted to repair plus buttress as our standard operation. This position does not apply to femoral hernia repair, wherein the use of mesh is usually unnecessary. Although the use of prosthetic material to plug hernial defects has had some advocates during the past decade, this therapeutic modality has not found a significant role as used from the posterior approach.

Laparoscopic Hernioplasty

The first laparoscopic approach to the problem of groin hernia is credited to Ger,[32] who intraabdominally stapled the neck of a hernial sac. Interestingly, Ger was one of the few surgeons who took his ideas to the animal laboratory for study (15 beagle dogs). A flurry of new concepts, that is, techniques, appeared in the early 1990s, which included Gazayerli[33] (a classic posterior suture repair), Filipi et al.,[34] Arregui et al.,[35] Dion,[36] Schultz,[53] and Corbitt[54] (insertion of rolls of prosthetic material into hernia defects). This "plug" method later was discarded because of an unacceptable recurrence rate.

Laparoscopic Intraperitoneal Onlay Mesh (IPOM)

Colleagues from Omaha[34] also entered the research laboratory (using pigs) and reviewed the concept of the placement of onlay prosthetic mesh over peritoneal defects in the lower abdominal wall. Moving to the human patient population, they reported good results. However, other surgeons reported difficulty with intraabdominal trocar placement with injury to bowel and major blood vessels, especially during the learning curve.

Transabdominal Preperitoneal Mesh (TAPP)

Arregui and colleagues[35] transabdominally opened into the preperitoneal space and covered the target posterior inguinal wall with prosthetic mesh. This laparoscopic approach probably is the most popular in use today, particularly for bilateral inguinal hernias. The method has found a niche as well in our approach to the ever-present recurrent hernia.

Total Extraperitoneal Mesh (TEP)

Because all prior laparoscopic approaches traversed the peritoneal cavity, each had potential morbidity and even mortality because of the aforementioned complications. McKernan and Laws[37,38] and Phillips and colleagues[39] devised the total extraperitoneal technique for placement of mesh into the preperitoneal space. McKernan demonstrated that very few posterior wall staples or sutures into the mesh were necessary (using the Pascal–Stoppa phenomenon), obviating the injury to intramural nerves. TEP is continuing to find adherents throughout the surgical world.

The New Millennium

We have reviewed the historical background of the posterior approach to groin hernia problems from the Middle Ages (Ottoman Empire), through open preperitoneal techniques, the addition of prosthetic mesh buttresses, and finally the various laparoscopic methods in which prosthetic mesh has played a key role. It does appear that we enter the next 1000 years confident that most complex groin hernias can be cured with minimal morbidity if approached posteriorly. The preoperative and operative classification of hernia types will allow our surgical progeny to select the most appropriate technique for repair of a given type of hernia. I know that there will be continuing controversy. Troidl[55] stated, "Despite numerous interventions and investment by industry, the role of endoscopic surgery for hernia is still open to debate."

We look forward to the continuing dialogue of the pros and cons of all hernia operative approaches and repairs. In the interest of providing the best care for our patients, we will keep aware of new developments.

References

1. Marcy HO. The anatomy and surgical treatment of hernia. New York: Appleton, 1892:263.
2. de Cantemir D. Histoire d'agrandissement de l'empire Ottoman (trans M. De Joncquieres). 1743;2:397–461.
3. Rives J. Surgical treatment of the inguinal hernia with Dacron patch: principles, indications, technic and results. Int Surg 1967;47:360–361.
4. Stoppa RE, Rives JL, Warlaumont CR, et al. The use of Dacron in the repair of hernias of the groin. Surg Clin N Am 1984;64:269–285.
5. Meade RH. The history of the abdominal approach to hernia repair. Surgery (St. Louis) 1965;57:908–914.
6. Read RC. Properitoneal herniorrhaphy: a historical review. World J Surg 1989;13:532–540.
7. LaRoque GP. The permanent cure of inguinal and femoral hernia: a modification of the standard operative procedures. Surg Gynecol Obstet 1919;29:507–510.
8. Jacobson P. Inguinal herniorrhaphy from the intraabdominal perspective. Am J Surg 1946;71:797–808.
9. Mansfield RD. A new approach to the treatment of hernia of the groin. Am J Surg 1960;100:462–464.
10. Phetteplace CH. The intraabdominal (LaRoque) approach to hernioplasty. West J Surg 1955;63:490–496.
11. Williams C. The advantages of the abdominal approach to inguinal hernia. Ann Surg 1938;107:917–922.
12. Condon RE. The anatomy of the inguinal region and its relation to groin hernia. In: Nyhus LM, Condon RE (eds) Hernia, 4th Ed. Philadelphia: Lippincott, 1995:16–72.
13. Annandale T. Case in which a reducible oblique and direct inguinal and femoral hernia existed on the same side and were successfully treated by operation. Edinb Med J 1876; 21:1087–1091.

14. Maunsell HW. Advantages of suprapubic laparotomy in strangulated femoral hernia. N Z Med J 1887;1:23–25.

15. Tait L. Treatment of hernia by median abdominal section. Br Med J 1891;2:685–691.

16. Bates UC. New operation for the cure of indirect inguinal hernia. JAMA 1913;60:2032–2033.

17. McEvedy PG. Femoral hernia. Ann R Coll Surg Engl 1950; 7:484–496.

18. Cheatle GL. An operation for the radical cure of inguinal and femoral hernia. Br Med J 1920;2:68–69.

19. Cheatle GL. An operation for inguinal hernia. Br Med J 1921;2:1025–1026.

20. Henry AK. Operation for femoral hernia by a midline extraperitoneal approach. Lancet 1936;1:531–533.

21. Jennings WK, Anson BJ, Wright RR. A new method of repair for indirect inguinal hernia considered in reference to parietal anatomy. Surg Gynecol Obstet 1942;74:697–707.

22. Musgrove JE, McCready FJ. The Henry approach to femoral hernia. Surgery (St. Louis) 1949;26:608–611.

23. Riba LW, Mehn WH. Retropubic prostatectomy and inguinal hernia repair. J Urol 1952;67:106–116.

24. Hull HC, Ganey JB. The Henry approach to femoral hernia. Ann Surg 1953;137:57–60.

25. Mikkelsen WP, Berne CJ. Femoral hernioplasty: suprapubic extraperitoneal (Cheatle–Henry) approach. Surgery (St. Louis) 1954;35:743–748.

26. Mouzas GL, Diggory PLC. A modification of the McEvedy repair of femoral hernia. Lancet 1956;2:1073–1074.

27. Nyhus LM, Stevenson JK, Listerud MB, et al. Preperitoneal herniorrhaphy: a preliminary report in fifty patients. West J Surg 1959;67:48–54.

28. Nyhus LM, Condon RE, Harkins HN. Clinical experiences with preperitoneal hernial repair for all types of hernia of the groin. Am J Surg 1960;100:234–242.

29. Estrin J, Lipton S, Block IR. The posterior approach to inguinal and femoral hernias. Surg Gynecol Obstet 1963; 116:547–550.

30. Stoppa R, Petit J, Henry X, et al. Plastie des hernies de l'aine par voie médiane sous-péritonéale. In: Actualités Chirurgicales, 74th Congres Français de Chirurgie, Association Française de Chirurgie. Paris: Masson, 1972: 448–453.

31. Stoppa RE, Rives JL, Warlaumont, et al. The use of Dacron in the repair of hernias of the groin. Surg Clin N Am 1984; 64:269–285.

32. Ger R. The management of certain abdominal herniae by intraabdominal closure of the neck of the sac. Ann R Coll Surg Engl 1982;64:342–344.

33. Gazayerli MM. Anatomical laparoscopic hernia repair of direct and indirect inguinal hernias using the transversalis fascia and iliopubic tract. Surg Laparosc Endosc 1992;2:49–52.

34. Filipi CJ, Fitzgibbons RF Jr, Salerno GM, et al. Laparoscopic herniorrhaphy. Surg Clin N Am 1992;72:1109–1124.

35. Arregui ME, Davis CJ, Yucel O, et al. Laparoscopic mesh repair of inguinal hernia using a preperitoneal approach: a preliminary report. Surg Laparosc Endosc 1992;2:53–58.

36. Dion YM. Laparoscopic inguinal herniorrhaphy: an individualized approach. Surg Laparosc Endosc 1993;3:451–455.

37. McKernan JB, Laws H. Laparoscopic preperitoneal prosthetic repair of inguinal hernias. Surg Rounds 1992;15:597–608.

38. McKernan JB, Laws H. Laparoscopic repair of inguinal hernias using a totally extraperitoneal prosthetic approach. Surg Endosc 1993;7:26–28.

39. Phillips EH, Carroll B, Fallas M. Laparoscopic preperitoneal inguinal hernia repair without peritoneal incision: technique and early clinical results. Surg Endosc 1993;7: 159–162.

40. Patino JF, Garcia-Herreros LG, Zundel N. Inguinal hernia repair: the Nyhus posterior preperitoneal operation. Surg Clin N Am 1998;78:1063–1074.

41. Greenburg G. Personal communication, September 1999.

42. Thomson A. Cause anatomique de la hernia inguinal externe. J Conn Med Prat 1836;4:137.

43. Rheault MJ, Oppenheimer GJ, Nyhus LM. Portrait of the anatomist Alexander Thomson. Surg Gynecol Obstet 1965; 121:601–606.

44. Polya J. Anatomical forms of hernial relapses. Orvosihetif (Budapest) 1912;56:449.

45. Fruchaud H. Anatomie chirurgicale des hernies de l'aine. Paris: Doin, 1956.

46. Fruchaud H. Le traitement chirurgical des hernies de l'aine chez l'adulte. Paris: Doin, 1956.

47. Zollinger RM Jr. Establishing a registry for hernia management. Presented to second Annual Meeting of the American Hernia Society, Las Vegas, NV, February 24, 1999.

48. Nyhus LM. Individualization of hernia repair: a new era. Surgery (St. Louis) 1993;114:1–2.

49. Usher FC, Ochsner J, Tuttle LL Jr. Use of Marlex mesh in the repair of incisional hernias. Am Surg 1958;24:969–974.

50. Read RC. Preperitoneal prosthetic inguinal herniorrhaphy without a relaxing incision. Am J Surg 1976;132:749–752.

51. Mahorner H, Goss CM. Herniation following destruction of Poupart's and Cooper's ligaments: a method of repair. Ann Surg 1962;155:741–748.

52. Nyhus LM, Pollak R, Bombeck CT, et al. The preperitoneal approach and prosthetic mesh buttress repair for recurrent hernia: the evolution of a technique. Ann Surg 1988;208: 733–737.

53. Schultz LS, Graber J, Pietrafitta J, et al. Laser laparoscopic herniorrhaphy: a clinical trial preliminary results. Surg Laparosc Endosc 1991;1:41–45.

54. Corbitt JD Jr. Laparoscopic herniorrhaphy. Surg Laparosc Endosc 1991;1:23–25.

55. Troidl H. Endoscopic surgery: innovation versus evaluation: introduction. World J Surg 1999;23:743–744.

29
Musculoskeletal and Neurovascular Anatomy of the Inguinal Preperitoneal Space

Mary E. Schultheis, Robert J. Fitzgibbons, and Thomas H. Quinn

The widespread use of laparoscopic herniorrhaphy necessitates an understanding of the inguinal region to prevent iatrogenic neurovascular damage. The anatomy of this region is complex and is conventionally taught beginning with the superficial structures and proceeding to the deeper structures; each tissue layer is reviewed in the sequence that it would be encountered during a laparotomy.[1] However, the view seen through a laparoscope is reversed, and this could prove to be disorienting to surgeons accustomed to the traditional presentation. The goal of this chapter therefore is to reorient the laparoscopic surgeon and to present the anatomy of the inguinal preperitoneal region as it would be encountered in laparoscopic herniorrhaphy.

Characteristics of the Interior Aspect of the Anterior Abdominal Wall

Peritoneal Folds and Fossae

Inspection of the interior aspect of the anterior abdominal wall with a laparoscope reveals five peritoneal folds or ligaments that flare out inferior to the umbilicus (Fig. 29.1).[2] The midline or *median umbilical ligament* is a peritoneal fold over the urachus, the fibrous remnant of the fetal allantois. It courses superiorly from the fundus of the bladder to the umbilicus. On either side of the median umbilical fold are the *medial umbilical ligaments*; these are the peritoneal folds covering the obliterated portions of the umbilical arteries. These vessels originate from the internal iliac arteries and course superomedially toward the umbilicus, giving off the superior vesical branches from the proximal patent portion of the arteries. On either lateral side of these folds are the *lateral umbilical ligaments*. These ligaments are folds of peritoneum that contain the inferior epigastric vessels.

The medial and lateral umbilical ligaments as well as the fundus of the bladder delineate three depressions, or fossae, within the peritoneum.[3] The *lateral fossa* is situated laterally on either side of the lateral umbilical ligaments. It contains the internal (deep) inguinal ring and is therefore the site of indirect hernias that traverse the deep inguinal ring. The *medial fossa* is bordered by the medial umbilical ligament and the lateral umbilical ligament. It is the site of Hesselbach's triangle and both direct and femoral hernias. The *supravesical fossa* is situated between the medial and median umbilical ligaments. Hernias in this fossa occur rarely because the fossa is reinforced by the rectus abdominis muscle and the rectus sheath.[4]

Contents of the Preperitoneal Space

On dissection of the peritoneum away from the transversalis fascia, *the extraperitoneal space is opened.* Although this space is continuous throughout the entire abdomen and retroperitoneum, the anterior portion of the space, called the *preperitoneal space*, is of primary importance during laparoscopic herniorrhaphy.[5] It is entered during both the transabdominal preperitoneal (TAPP) and the totally extraperitoneal approach (TEPA) herniorrhaphies.[6] The space contains adipose tissue, blood vessels, lymphatic channels, and nerves and therefore is a site for potential iatrogenic injury during laparoscopic herniorrhaphy. The preperitoneal space can be further subdivided into several different clinically significant spaces.

The Musculopectineal Orifice of Fruchaud and Its Contents

The *musculopectineal orifice of Fruchaud* (Fig. 29.2) is a space within the anterior abdomen with the following boundaries: the inferior borders of the transversus abdominis and internal oblique muscles superiorly, the rectus abdominis muscle medially, the iliopsoas muscle

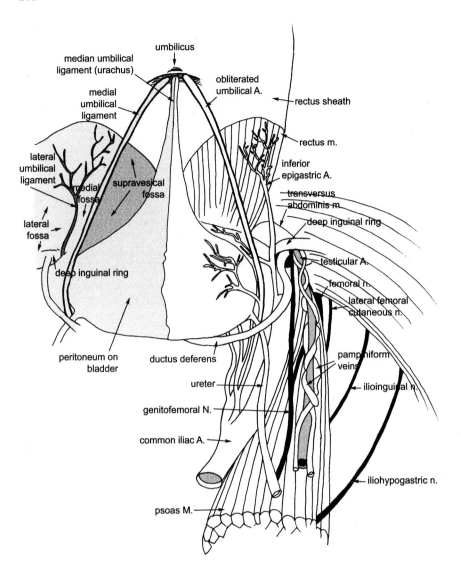

FIGURE 29.1. The anterior abdominal wall and the deep inguinal region. The *shaded area* to the left of the midline represents the peritoneum, ligaments formed by it, and the umbilical fossae. The area to the right of the midline shows the structures underlying the peritoneum.

laterally, and the pecten of the pubis inferiorly.[7] The space is of great clinical significance because it is considered a "hole in the muscle" and therefore a weak site in the abdomen where hernias may occur. It houses the inguinal triangle and important sites for abdominal herniation: the deep inguinal ring that opens into the inguinal canal and the femoral ring that opens into the femoral canal.

The Inguinal (Hesselbach's) Triangle

The inguinal triangle (Fig. 29.2), located within the medial fossa, was originally described by Hesselbach as the area of the abdominal wall bounded by the inferior epigastric vessels superiolaterally, the lateral border of the rectus sheath medially, and Cooper's ligament inferiorly.[8] These borders were modified by surgeons performing conventional herniorrhaphy to substitute the inguinal ligament for the inferior border of the triangle in place of Cooper's ligament because the inguinal ligament was visible during conventional herniorrhaphy.[1] However,

with the advent of laparoscopic herniorrhaphy, Cooper's ligament can be viewed quite well, and Hesselbach's original definition of the triangle is more suitable for this procedure.[7–9]

Inguinal Canal

The inguinal canal (Fig. 29.3) is a 4-cm-long inferomedially directed passage through which pass the spermatic cord, or the round ligament in females, the ilioinguinal nerve, the genital branch of the genitofemoral nerve, and the blood and lymphatic vessels.[3] It has an interior opening into the abdomen (the deep inguinal ring), a passageway formed by the various components of the abdominal wall at that level, and a superficial opening, the superficial inguinal ring. The deep inguinal ring is visible by laparoscope on the interior aspect of the anterior abdominal wall as a fingertip-sized indentation just lateral to the lateral umbilical ligament. Dissecting away the peritoneum reveals the deep inguinal ring as a con-

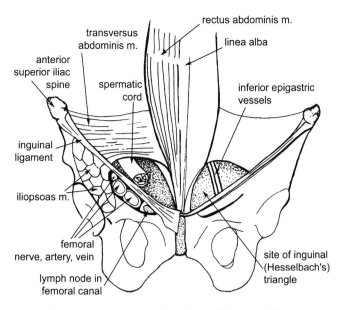

FIGURE 29.2. The myopectineal orifice of Fruchaud. Its superior component consists of the area inferior to the aponeurotic arch of the transversus abdominis, including the inguinal (Hesselbach's) triangle. The lower part of the orifice is inferior to the inguinal ligament and contains the femoral canal, femoral sheath and its contents, and the iliopsoas muscle. The inguinal ligament divides the two portions.

cord originates at the deep inguinal ring and courses through the inguinal canal and superficial inguinal ring to end in the scrotum on the posterior surface of the testes. The cord consists of several fascial layers that it accumulates as it passes through the inguinal canal, each layer being superimposed on the one before it.[9,10] As the contents of the spermatic cord enter the deep inguinal ring, they are surrounded by a layer of transversalis fascia called the *internal spermatic fascia*. As the cord courses inferomedially through the canal, it is enveloped by a layer of the internal oblique fascia named the *cremasteric fascia*. As it exits the canal through the superficial inguinal ring, the most superficial layer of the cord is acquired, the *external spermatic fascia*, derived from the external oblique aponeurosis.

Femoral Sheath

The femoral sheath (Fig. 29.5) has been described as a funnel-shaped tube composed of transversalis fascia that envelops the femoral artery, femoral vein, and the femoral canal.[7] It creates a passageway for these structures as they pass under the inguinal ligament from the pelvis into the femoral triangle of the lower extremity. The femoral sheath is subdivided by two vertical fascial septa into three compartments.[7,9] The lateral compart-

densation of the transversalis fascia known as the transversalis fascia sling.[9,10] The ring is just lateral to the weak area of Hesselbach's triangle; it is separated from it by the lateral umbilical ligament.

The inguinal canal itself has an anterior and posterior wall, a roof, and a floor (Fig. 29.3).[10] When thinking of these boundaries, it is helpful to remember the oblique path of the canal and the contents of the anterior abdominal wall at that level. The boundaries of the canal include an anterior wall composed of the aponeurosis of the external oblique muscle; a posterior wall formed by the transversalis fascia laterally and the conjoined tendon (when present as such) medially; and a floor formed by a reflected portion of the inguinal ligament, the lacunar ligament.[4] The iliopubic tract (another condensation of the transversalis fascia described below) provides a landmark for the inferior edge of the deep inguinal ring.[1] The superficial opening into the scrotum, the superficial inguinal ring, is composed of fibers from the aponeurosis of the external oblique muscle and is located lateral to the pubic tubercle.

The spermatic cord (Figs. 29.3, 29.4) is the conduit for many structures that travel to or from the testes. Its contents include the ductus deferens and its vascular supply, the testicular artery and the pampiniform plexus, the cremasteric artery, sympathetic nerve fibers, the genital branch of the genitofemoral nerve, and lymphatics. The

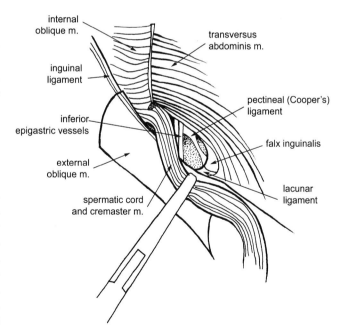

FIGURE 29.3. The femoral canal with the spermatic cord retracted. The external oblique aponeurosis is divided and retracted, thereby removing the fibers of the external inguinal ring. Note that the cremaster muscle fibers arise from the internal abdominal oblique muscle. The falx inguinalis is formed by the aponeurotic insertion of the transversus abdominis muscle.

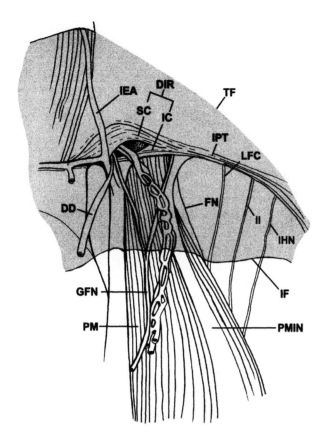

FIGURE 29.4. The anterior abdominal wall and the deep inguinal region. The *shaded portion* represents the area that is covered by peritoneum and transversalis fascia. Clockwise from the left: *IEA*, inferior epigastric artery; *DIR*, deep inguinal ring; *SC*, *IC*, superior and inferior crus of the diaphragm, respectively; *TF*, transversalis fascia; *IPT*, iliopubic tract; *LFC*, lateral femoral cutaneous nerve; *II*, ilioinguinal nerve; *IHN*, iliohypogastric; *IF*, iliac fascia; *PMIN*, psoas minor; *FN*, femoral nerve; *GFN*, genitofemoral nerve; *PM*, psoas major; *DD*, ductus deferens.

ment contains the femoral artery. The femoral nerve courses lateral to this compartment and is separated from it by the iliopubic tract. The middle compartment contains the femoral vein. The medialmost compartment contains the femoral canal.

Femoral Canal

The femoral canal (Figs. 29.2, 29.5) is a 1- to 2-cm-long canal that contains adipose tissue and lymphatics.[7] The canal can be thought of as a cone oriented so that the apex courses into the thigh while the base remains in the abdomen. When viewing the interior aspect of the anterior abdominal wall during laparoscopy, the canal is not usually visible, but its location can be approximated by observing other visible landmarks on the interior surface of the anterior abdominal wall. The abdominal opening

to this canal, the *femoral ring*, is inferomedial to the deep inguinal ring and directly inferior to the weak area within Hesselbach's triangle. The ring is composed of fibers from the iliopubic tract anteriorly, the superior ramus of the pubis, the pectineus muscle and Cooper's (pectineal) ligament posteriorly, the femoral vein laterally, and the lacunar ligament medially.[9] Although the ring is usually closed by a layer of connective tissue, the *septum femorale*, bowel can herniate through this opening and into the canal, causing a femoral hernia.[7]

Vessels Within the Musculopectineal Orifice of Fruchaud

Several important vessels pass through this preperitoneal space on their way to the inguinal area and the femoral region (Figs. 29.1, 29.2, 29.4). The main source of these vessels is the external iliac artery and vein. These vessels are formed by a bifurcation of the common iliac vessels and course parallel to the pelvic brim on top of the psoas muscle. Proximal to the iliopubic tract and the inguinal ligament, the external iliac vessels give off the inferior epigastric vessels medially and the deep circumflex iliac vessels laterally. The inferior epigastric vessels course superiorly, giving off the artery to the cremasteric muscle and entering the space of Bogros.[1,11] The cremasteric artery then courses inferolaterally to enter the medial portion of the inguinal ring on its way through the inguinal canal. The deep circumflex iliac artery originates from the external iliac artery laterally just before its

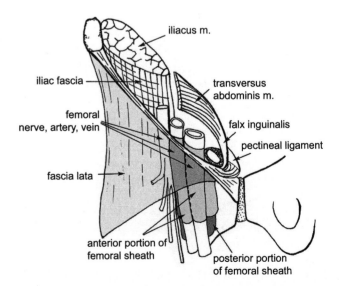

FIGURE 29.5. The femoral sheath and the femoral canal. The anterior femoral sheath is formed by the transversalis fascia and blends inferiorly with the adventitia of the femoral vessels. The posterior sheath is continuous with the iliac fascia, itself merely a named portion of the transversalis fascia.

entrance into the femoral sheath. It travels laterally between the iliopubic tract and the iliopectineal arch to its final destination between the transversus abdominis muscle and the internal oblique muscle where it anastomoses with the iliolumbar artery.[1] The testicular artery is a paired branch of the abdominal aorta. It travels inferiorly in the retroperitoneum along the medial border of the psoas muscle. It crosses the common iliac artery proximal to its bifurcation and travels with these vessels until it reaches the femoral ring where it courses superiorly to enter the inguinal canal.[1]

Nerves Coursing Through the Musculopectineal Orifice of Fruchaud

In addition, several sensory nerves arising from the lumbar plexus (Figs. 29.1, 29.4) course through the preperitoneal space on their way to the upper extremities or into the genital area. Therefore, they are of great importance during laparoscopic herniorrhaphy in the prevention of postoperative pain or anesthesia within the groin and upper thigh.[5,9] The ilioinguinal nerve arises posterior to the lateral border of the psoas muscle and descends inferolaterally along the quadratus lumborum muscle. It then travels laterally along the iliac crest to dive deep to the transversus abdominis muscle into the internal oblique to travel between the external and internal oblique muscles. It travels medially sandwiched between these two muscles and then enters the deep inguinal ring and travels through the inguinal canal on the surface of the spermatic cord. After exiting the canal, the nerve supplies sensation to the skin of the scrotum, the base of the penis, and the medial thigh.

The iliohypogastric nerve (Fig. 29.4) also arises from the lateral border of the psoas muscle and courses inferolaterally on the ventral surface of the quadratus lumborum to reach the transversus abdominus muscle. It penetrates this muscle and travels medially to pierce both the internal oblique and the external oblique muscles 2 to 4 cm above the superficial inguinal ring where it supplies sensation to the skin in this region.[1,7,9]

The genitofemoral nerve (Fig. 29.4) arises from L1 and L2. It travels inferiorly, passing through the psoas muscle, and then divides into a medial genital branch (external spermatic nerve) and a lateral femoral branch (lumboinguinal nerve). The genital branch continues inferiorly parallel to the course of the external iliac artery. At the origin of the inferior epigastric artery, the genital branch courses superomedially to enter the inguinal canal within the spermatic cord on its dorsal aspect.[1,7,10] The femoral branch also courses along the pathway of the external iliac artery to enter the femoral sheath lateral to the artery.[4,10] It then pierces the fascia lata of the thigh and supplies the sensory innervation to the anterior portion of the thigh.

The femoral nerve (Figs. 29.1, 29.4) is derived from the second, third, and fourth ventral divisions of the lumbar nerves. It emerges from the inferolateral portion of the psoas muscle and courses inferiorly along its lateral border on the surface of the iliacus muscle. The nerve then dives inferior to the iliopectineal arch and continues its inferior course just lateral to the femoral vessels.[4] It then passes beneath the inguinal ligament on the surface of the iliopsoas muscle just lateral to the femoral vessels but is separated from them by the iliopectineal arch.[4,10]

The lateral femoral cutaneous nerve (see Fig. 29.4) contains the ventral primary divisions of the second and third lumbar nerves. It can be seen arising near the middle portion of the psoas muscle and running in an inferolateral direction across the iliacus muscle toward the anterior iliac spine.[4,7,8,10] It comes within 1 cm of the anterior superior iliac spine when it dives beneath the inguinal ligament lateral to the iliopsoas muscle and medial to the sartorius muscle.[4] It supplies sensory innervation to the lateral aspect of the thigh.

The Prevesical Space of Retzius

A triangular portion of the preperitoneal space underlying the supravesical fossa (Fig. 29.1) and the medial fossa constitutes the *prevesical space of Retzius*.[3,7] The space of Retzius contains connective and adipose tissue and vessels. The boundaries of this space include: the symphysis pubis and the rectus abdominis muscle anteriorly; the umbilicus superiorly, the lateral umbilical ligaments laterally; the umbilicovesical fascia covering the bladder posteriorly; the lateral surface of the bladder medially; and the fusion of the umbilicovesical fascia with the transversalis fascia superiorly.[11] The umbilicovesical fascia is a layer of connective tissue that originates at the umbilicus and fans out inferiorly to envelop the urachus, the obliterated umbilical arteries, and the inferior epigastric vessels and then covers the anterior portion of the bladder to terminate at the bladder neck.[4,11]

Within the space of Retzius, aberrant obturator arteries occur in 25% to 40% of individuals in the United States.[7] An aberrant obturator artery arising from the inferior epigastric artery tends to course inferolateral and cross over the pectineal ligament before entering the obturator canal and anastomosing with a normal obturator artery arising from the internal iliac artery.[4,7] This arrangement creates what has become known as the *corona mortis* or crown of death because of the significant intraoperative hemorrhage that can be caused by accidental incision of this anastomosis.[11] Aberrant obturator veins are actually more common and if incised can cause severe postoperative bleeding.[7,12]

Bogros' Space

A lateral extension of the space of Retzius within the preperitoneal space was described by a French anatomist named Bogros in 1823. Bogros' space is important in herniorrhaphy during reconstruction of the inguinal canal floor.[3,7,11] The space is entered by incising transversalis fascia from the medial border of the deep inguinal ring to the pubic crest.[11,12] Its boundaries include the iliac fascia laterally, the transversalis fascia anteriorly and the peritoneum medially.[11]

Just posterior to the iliopubic tract and the inguinal ligament, the external iliac vessels (see Fig. 29.1) give off the inferior epigastric vessels medially and the deep circumflex iliac vessels laterally. The inferior epigastric artery courses medially within the walls of the space of Bogros and then superiorly to pierce the transversalis fascia and enter the rectus abdominis sheath.[4] On entering the rectus space, the artery travels superiorly and anastomoses with the superior epigastric artery. There are also small anastomoses between the inferior epigastric artery and the obturator artery through pubic branches.[4]

The venous circulation within the preperitoneal space of Bogros has recently been elucidated. A venous anastomosis between the iliopubic vein and the rectusial vein exists in the space of Bogros in various forms.[12] The iliopubic vein passes deep but parallel to the iliopubic tract; the rectusial vein courses along the lateral border of the rectus abdominis muscle.[5,12] Knowledge of this venous circulation will help to prevent hemorrhage and hematoma formation during and after surgery.

Transversalis Fascia and Its Derivatives

Transversalis Fascia

The fascial layer immediately external to the peritoneum is the transversalis fascia (Fig. 29.6). This layer is also known as the endoabdominal fascia because it invests the entire internal surface of the abdomen. The term transversalis fascia was coined by Sir Astley Cooper to refer to the structure that covered the internal surface of the transversus abdominis muscle.[1,7,9] There is considerable debate as to the number of layers contained within the transversalis fascia.[1,10] The original description by Cooper was a bilaminar structure containing an anterior layer and a posterior layer. The anterior layer closely enveloped the transversus abdominis muscle and its aponeurosis and has an inferior insertion onto Cooper's ligament and a medial insertion to the rectus sheath.[4,8] The posterior layer joins superiorly with the linea semicircularis, medially with the linea alba, and inferiorly inserts on the superior ramus of the pubis.[4,5]

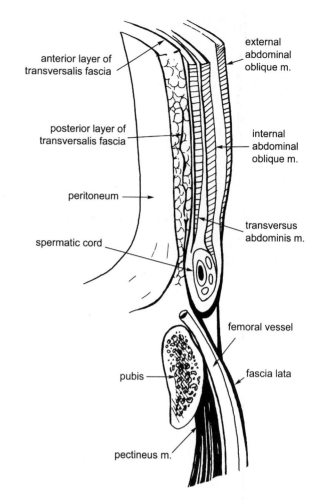

FIGURE 29.6. Longitudinal section of the anterior abdominal wall and inguinal region. Note the posterior layer of the transversalis fascia. Although not universally accepted as a lamina of the transversalis fascia, most agree that a thickened layer of fascia is encountered in this area in most individuals.

This posterior layer is also known as the preperitoneal fascia. The space between the posterior and anterior layers of the transversalis fascia contains the umbilical arteries medially and the inferior epigastric vessels laterally. If this space is mistakenly entered during a TAPP herniorrhaphy, damage to these vessels may result in bleeding. The bladder also lies within this plane and can be damaged by medial dissection.

Derivatives of the Transversalis Fascia

Many structures derive from thickenings or condensations of the fascia itself.[1] They serve as important landmarks for the laparoscopic surgeon during laparoscopic herniorrhaphy. In some cases, they can serve as anchors for staples. The internal (deep) inguinal ring, already dis-

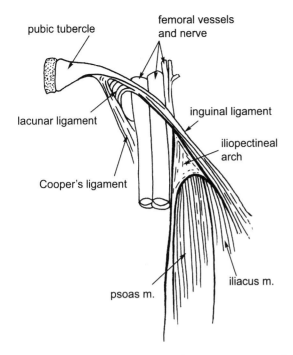

FIGURE 29.7. The muscular and vascular compartments of the deep inguinal region are divided by the iliopectineal arch. It is a continuation of the psoas minor tendon when this muscle is present. The lacunar ligament covers the area between the medial part of the inguinal ligament and the pectineal (Cooper's) ligament. Cooper's ligament is actually a thickened periosteal layer on the pecten pubis. Only the superior surface of the the pubic symphysis and pubic tubercle are seen.

cussed briefly, is formed when the testicle migrates from the abdomen to the scrotum and pulls with it a layer of transversalis fascia. The direction of the migration is slightly more oblique than the orientation of the transversalis fascia, and this results in a redundancy of the medial portion of the deep inguinal ring called the transversalis fascia sling (Figs. 29.1, 29.4). The sling itself has superior and inferior portions that serve to close off the ring like a sphincter during times of straining; this helps to prevent indirect herniation.

The iliopubic tract (see Fig. 29.4) is a transversalis fascia condensation that is attached laterally to the inner lip of the iliac crest, on the anterior superior iliac spine and on the iliopectineal arch. It courses anteriorly in a plane deep but parallel to the inguinal ligament. It bridges the external iliac vessels as they enter the femoral canal and attaches to (or fuses with) the medial portion of Cooper's ligament. During its course, the iliopubic tract also forms the inferior border of the deep inguinal ring as well as the posterior wall of the inguinal canal. Although identification of the tract itself is not always feasible during a TAPP herniorrhaphy, its approximate location should always be sought for staple placement. Staples should always be placed above the iliopubic tract

to avoid damage to the testicular artery, the pampiniform plexus, and branches of the lumbar plexus.

Cooper's ligament (Figs. 29.3, 29.7) is easily identified during laparoscopic herniorrhaphy as the white glistening structure covering the superior pubic ramus. Some anatomists consider it a fusion of the iliopubic tract, the transversalis fascia, and the periosteum whereas others consider it a lateral extension of the lacunar ligament. It originates on the superior aspect of the pubic ramus and reaches laterally to the pubic tubercle. Its strength makes Cooper's ligament an important substrate for staples or sutures.

The iliopectineal arch (Fig. 29.7) is a condensation of the transversalis fascia that attaches laterally to the superior anterior iliac spine and travels medially to insert on the iliopectineal eminence. During its course, it provides fibers for the iliopubic tract, the external and internal oblique muscles, and the transversus abdominis muscles of the abdominal wall. The arch divides the structures that pass through the abdomen into the upper extremity into a medial compartment containing the femoral canal and the femoral vessels and a lateral muscular compartment containing the iliopsoas muscle and the femoral nerve.

References

1. Quinn TH, Annibali R, Dalley AF II, Fitzgibbons RJ Jr. Dissection of the anterior abdominal wall and the deep inguinal region from a laparoscopic perspective. Clin Anat 1995;8:245–251.
2. Quinn TH. Anatomy of the groin: a view from the anatomist. In: Fitzgibbons RJ, Greenburg AG (eds) Nyhus and Condon's Hernia, 5th Ed. Philadelphia: Lippincott/Williams & Wilkins, 2001:55–70.
3. Annibali R, Camps J, Nagan RF, et al. In: Arregui ME, et al. (ed) Principles of Laparoscopic Surgery: Basic and Advanced Techniques. New York: Springer-Verlag, 1995:409–425.
4. Moore KL, Dalley AF II. Clinically Oriented Anatomy, 4th Ed. Baltimore: Lippincott/Williams & Wilkins, 1999.
5. Colborn GL, Skandalakis JE. Laparoscopic inguinal anatomy. Hernia 1998;2:179–191.
6. Eubanks S. Hernias. In: Sabiston DC, Lyerly HK (eds) Sabiston's Textbook of Surgery: The Biological Basis of Modern Surgical Practice, 15th Ed. Philadelphia: Saunders, 1997:1216–1219.
7. Richards AT, Quinn TH, Fitzgibbons RJ Jr. Abdominal wall hernias. In: Greenfield LJ, Mulholland MW, Oldham KT, Zellenock GB, Lillemoe KD (eds) Surgery: Scientific Principles and Practice. Philadelphia: Lippincott/Williams & Wilkins, 2001:1185–1223.
8. Ponka J. Hernias of the Abdominal Wall. Philadelphia: Saunders, 1980:18–39.
9. Quinn TH, Ryberg A, Annibali R, Fitzgibbons R. Anatomy of the anterior abdominal wall and deep inguinal region

from the laparoscopic surgeon's perspective. In: Lanzafame RJ (ed) Prevention and Management of Complications in Minimally Invasive Surgery. New York: Igaku-Shoin, 1996: 107–117.

10. Clemente CD (ed) Gray's Anatomy, American Edition. Philadelphia: Lea & Febiger, 1985.

11. Read RC. Anatomy of abdominal herniation. The parietoperitoneal spaces. In: Nyhus LM, Baker RJ, Fisher JE (eds) Mastery of Surgery, 3rd Ed, vol II. Boston: Little Brown, 1997:1795–1806.

12. Bendavid R. The space of Bogros and the deep inguinal venous circulation. Surg Gynecol Obstet 1992;174:355–358.

30
Laparoscopic Hernia Repair: Indications and Contraindications

David L. Crawford and Edward H. Phillips

Initial enthusiasm for laparoscopic herniorrhaphy was driven by dissatisfaction with the pain, disability, and recurrence following traditional anterior hernia repairs. It was hoped that the minimally invasive approach would eliminate the chronic pain and disability that affect the occasional patient following anterior herniorrhaphy. Laparoscopic herniorrhaphy allows identification of contralateral hernias while offering a safer repair of recurrent hernias by avoiding the cord structures and regional nerves in the prior operative site.

Over the past decade, laparoscopic hernia repair has changed from an operation in evolution to several well-defined techniques of transperitoneal or totally extraperitoneal approaches. The complex technical descriptions and names of the procedures can sometimes obscure the fact that they all accomplish a posterior reinforcement with prosthetic material of the myopectineal orifice of Fruchaud.[1]

When physicians are presented with a new technology or a new operation, they must consider several questions. The physician must decide by their own experience, the recommendations of others, or the published results which patients, if any, would be best served by the new technology or operation. Is the added expense of the new technology worth the potential benefits to their patient? Is the operation safe? Do the benefits outweigh the risks? Is it practical to train surgeons in practice? Do practicing surgeons have the time or skills to overcome the learning curve associated with learning the operation? These are the difficult questions that have been repeatedly asked about laparoscopic herniorrhaphy.

This chapter discusses the indications for laparoscopic hernia repair as well as some reasons for choosing one technique over another. We then discuss the most common contraindications to laparoscopic herniorrhaphy.

Indications

Recurrent Hernia

Recurrence of groin hernias after a seemingly adequate repair is a part of every surgeon's practice. The mechanism for recurrences after conventional inguinal herniorrhaphy include suture pullthrough; tension repairs leading to tissue breakdown and the creation of new defects; missed hernia; and intrinsically weak tissue caused by a disorder of collagen metabolism. Repairs such as that of Bassini, McVay, Maloney, and even the Shouldice repair all involve some degree of tension. This tension results in tissue breakdown and subsequent repair failure. Recurrence has been reported as high as 30% for the Bassini repair to less than 1% for the Shouldice repair. Recurrence rates improved with the introduction of the Shouldice technique and the increased use of mesh, popularized by the preperitoneal repairs of Nyhus and Stoppa, and the anterior tension-free mesh repair popularized by Lichtenstein. Recurrence rates with these repairs have been reported as low as 1% to 5% at 10 years.[2-5]

It would not be unrealistic to estimate the recurrence rate after anterior herniorrhaphy in the general community to be 5% to 10% at 10 years using the various anterior repair techniques (Fig. 30.1). Thus, every surgeon is forced to formulate a plan of action to handle recurrent hernias. Anterior repair of a recurrent hernia is a technically demanding operation and is associated with a much higher risk of regional nerve injury and testicular ischemia.

Table 30.1 displays the results following open repair techniques when applied to recurrent hernias. Nyhus et al.,[6] using his preperitoneal approach, added a piece of prosthetic mesh when repairing recurrent defects and reported a 1.7% rerecurrence rate in 115 hernias over a 10-year period. Greenburg[7] used the same approach but used a prosthetic patch in only a small percentage of

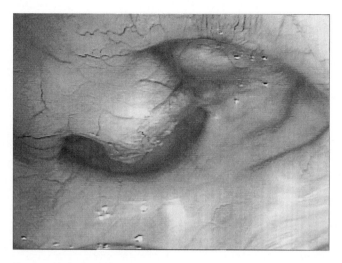

FIGURE 30.1. Intraoperative photo of a recurrent direct hernia after a "plug and patch" type repair.

laparoscopic technique uses a large prosthetic mesh to cover the entire myopectineal orifice, thus covering all three potential sites of recurrence (direct, indirect, femoral). Laparoscopy also allows visualization of the entire pelvis to avoid missing any unexpected hernias or potential sites of recurrence. Table 30.2 shows the results of several laparoscopic series that address the repair of recurrent inguinal hernias.[11–15] The transabdominal preperitoneal repair (TAPP) technique is more prevalent in these series, presumably because the totally extraperitoneal (TEP) repair was developed after the TAPP and more surgeons perform the TAPP technique. The results of these series of laparoscopic herniorrhaphy are impressive considering that laparoscopic hernia surgery is only 10 years old.

his patients, experiencing a 4.3% rerecurrence rate as a result. Glassow,[8] reporting the Shouldice clinic experience, had a 3.3% rerecurrence rate. Lichtenstein et al.[9] used a relatively tension-free anterior plug technique and reported a 1.6% rerecurrence. Stoppa[5] reported a series of 529 repairs using a giant posterior prosthetic reinforcement of the abdominal wall. In this large personal series, his patients experienced a rerecurrence rate of only 1.1%. The results (see Table 30.1) show that a posterior repair utilizing prosthetic mesh provides excellent outcomes.

As mentioned earlier, hernias recur because excess tension results in tissue failure, a direct hernia or an indirect hernia sac is missed, the entire posterior inguinal wall is weak, or the initial repair was inadequately performed. Felix et al.[10] repaired 90 recurrent hernias laparoscopically and found 42% were due to recurrent direct defects and 29% to persistent indirect sacs; 25% showed a pantaloon hernia, and 9% were femoral defects that were missed initially or created by anterior tension from the original repair. The laparoscopic approach addresses all these areas. Laparoscopic herniorrhaphy also provides a posterior approach so that the previously dissected tissue is avoided, thereby reducing the chance of regional nerve injury and vascular compromise of the testicle. The

Bilateral Hernias

Bilateral inguinal hernias are an ideal indication for laparoscopic repair. The reasons are multiple, including the ability to detect any unexpected unilateral or contralateral hernias at the same time, the ability to repair unilateral or bilateral hernias through the same three small incisions, and the reduced pain and disability associated with the laparoscopic bilateral repair.

When the diagnosis of a contralateral hernia is not certain, laparoscopy is clearly indicated and allows repair of subclinical hernias at the same time as the symptomatic hernia. The pediatric surgical literature has shown the effectiveness of laparoscopy in detecting the presence of contralateral inguinal hernias.[16–18] In 1998, the authors reported a series of 253 patients who underwent laparoscopic hernia repair. Fifty of the 73 patients believed to have unilateral hernias preoperatively had their diagnosis changed by diagnostic laparoscopy. Operative findings in this group were bilateral hernias in 37, different unilateral inguinal hernias in 7, and 6 additional femoral hernias. Unexpected contralateral hernias were found in 42 (57%) patients. In patients preoperatively diagnosed with bilateral inguinal hernia, 91 of the 180 had their diagnosis changed by laparoscopy. The findings included 63 different inguinal hernias on either side, 21 additional femoral hernias, and 7 hernias that were only unilateral. Unexpected hernias found at laparoscopic exploration

TABLE 30.1. Open repair of recurrent inguinal hernias.

Author	Year	No. of hernias	Technique	Rerecurrence rate (%)	Follow-up (months)
Glassow[8]	1986	1874	Shouldice	3.3	48–360
Greenburg[7]	1987	413	Preperitoneal (no mesh)	4.3	48–60
Nyhus[6]	1988	201	Preperitoneal (mesh)	1.7	6–120
Lichtenstein[9]	1993	1500	Lichtenstein (plug)	1.6	26–240
Stoppa[5]	1995	529	GPRVS	1.1	12–120

GPRVS, giant prosthetic reinforcement of the visceral sac.

TABLE 30.2. Laparoscopic repair of recurrent inguinal hernias.

Author	Year	No. of hernias	Technique	Rerecurrence rate (%)	Follow-up (months)
Leibel[11]	1996	210	TAPP	0.9	6–36
Sandbichler[12]	1996	200	TAPP	0.5	9–31
Birth[13]	1996	117	TAPP	0	3–36
Felix[14]	1998	173	TAPP/TEP	0.8	24
Ferzli[15]	1999	75	TEP	0	6–72

TAPP, transabdominal preperitoneal repair; TEP, totally extraperitoneal repair; IPOM, intraperitoneal onlay mesh repair.

before or during repair changed the preoperative diagnosis in 141 patients (56%).[19] Elsewhere in the adult literature, the reported incidence of unsuspected contralateral hernias is 10% to 25%.[20–21]

When one considers that a unilateral laparoscopic hernia repair can be performed with a minimum of 2 cm of total incision (10-mm trocar, ×1; 5-mm trocar, ×2) and a maximum 3-cm total incision (10-mm trocar, ×3), the patient already has an advantage in incisional pain and disability compared to anterior repairs. If you extrapolate this to a patient requiring bilateral repairs, the benefits are clear. The ability to avoid bilateral inguinal incisions, dissection, and postoperative disability is a significant advantage that should not be minimized. Most of the discomfort that patients experience in the postoperative period is associated with the incisions for the working ports in the TEP technique and, additionally, the dissection of the peritoneum from the underside of the abdominal wall in the TEP technique, not the internal inguinal dissection. The indurated groin wound and the manipulation of the spermatic cord of the anterior repair are avoided.

Pain and Disability

Numerous prospective randomized studies have compared laparoscopic and open (anterior) hernia repair techniques (Tables 30.3, 30.4).[22–50] Postoperative pain has been assessed using various pain measurement scales including quantification of consumption of analgesics. Measuring when a patient returns to normal activity is difficult; this is affected not only by the patient's ability to do so but also by the patient's desire (or lack thereof) to return to work/activity. The best way to measure the patient's ability to be active is with exercise testing. Unfortunately, this is difficult and expensive, so most studies use a patient questionnaire that asks when patients returned to "normal activity."

Kozol et al.[36] performed a prospective, randomized, blinded comparison of both repairs with regard to postoperative pain, using two standardized pain scales and the cumulative dosages of analgesics during the first 48 h. In these 62 patients, all of whom had general anesthetics, postoperative pain was significantly less in those having laparoscopic repairs. No difference in complications was found between the two groups.

TABLE 30.3. Open versus laparoscopic hernia repair: prospective randomized series 1994–1996.

Reference	Year	Technique	No. of patients (O/L)	Postoperative pain	Return to activity (days) (O/L)	Follow-up (months)
Stoker[22]	1994	D/TAPP	75/75	<Lap*	28/14*	7†
Payne[23]	1994	L/TAPP	52/48	NR	17/9*	10‡
Champault[24]	1994	S/TEP	89/92	<Lap*	24/12*	12†
Maddern[25]	1994	D/TAPP	44/42	ND	30/17*	8‡
Vogt[26]	1995	B/V/IPOM	31/30	<Lap	18/7	8†
Barkun[27]	1995	SC/TAPP	49/43	ND	11/9	14‡
Lawrence[28]	1995	D/TAPP	66/58	<Lap*	28/22	1.5
Leibl[29]	1995	S/TAPP	48/54	<Lap*	38/21*	16†
Schrenk[30]	1996	S/TAPP/TEP	34/28/24	<Lap*	ND	3†
Bessell[31]	1996	S/TEP/TAPP	72/29/3	<Lap*	32/30	7‡
Filipi[32]	1996	L/TAPP	29/24	ND	ND	11†
Tschudi[33]	1996	S/TAPP	43/44	<Lap*	48/25*	7‡
Wright[34]	1996	SC/TAPP	64/67	<Lap*	NR	NR
Hauters[35]	1996	S/TAPP	35/35	<Lap	10/6	30

Lap, laparoscopic; O, open; TAPP, transabdominal preperitoneal repair; TEP, totally extraperitoneal; IPOM, intraperitoneal onlay mesh; S, Shouldice; D, darn; L, Lichtenstein; B, Bassini; V, McVay; SC, surgeon's choice of repair; P, plug and patch; ST, Stoppa; PPO, preperitoneal open; ND, no difference; NR, not reported; *p < 0.05 open vs. lap; †, values are means; ‡, values are medians.

TABLE 30.4. Open versus laparoscopic hernia repair: prospective randomized series 1997–1999.

Reference	Year	Technique	No. of patients (O/L)	Postoperative pain	Return to activity (days) (O/L)	Follow-up (months)
Kozol[36]	1997	SC/TAPP	32/30	<Lap*	NR	1.5†
Liem[37]	1997	SC/TEP	507/487	<Lap*	10/6*	20‡
Heikkinen[38]	1997	L/TAPP	18/20	<Lap*	19/14*	2
Liem[39]	1997	SC/TEP	48/57	NR	10/6*	1.5
Tanphiphat[40]	1997	B/TAPP	60/60	<Lap*	14/8*	32†
Kald[41]	1997	S/TAPP	100/100	NR	23/14*	12
Champault[42]	1997	SC/TEP	49/51	<Lap*	35/17*	36†
Zieren[43]	1998	S/P/TAPP	80/80/80	<Lap & P*	26/18/16*	25†
Wellwood[44]	1998	L/TAPP	200/200	<Lap*	21/17*	3†
Heikkinen[45]	1998	L/TAPP	20/20	ND	21/14*	17‡
Paganini[46]	1998	L/TAPP	56/52	ND	ND	28‡
Aitola[47]	1998	PPO/TAPP	25/24	<Lap*	5/7	18‡
Dirksen[48]	1998	B/TAPP	87/88	<Lap*	27/17*	24†
Khoury[49]	1998	P/TEP	142/150	<Lap*	15/8*	17‡
Juul[50]	1999	S/TAPP	130/138	<Lap*	18/13*	12‡
Total: Tables 30.2, 30.3.			2365/2233			

Lap, laparoscopic; O, open; TAPP, transabdominal preperitoneal repair; TEP, totally extraperitoneal; IPOM, intraperitoneal onlay mesh; S, Shouldice; D, darn; L, Lichtenstein; B, Bassini; V, McVay; SC, surgeon's choice of repair; P, plug and patch; ST, Stoppa; PPO, preperitoneal open; ND, no difference; NR, not reported; *$p < 0.05$ open vs. lap; †, values are means; ‡, values are medians.

In another study (by Liem et al.[39]), 105 patients were prospectively randomized (48 open, 57 TEP) to accurately determine patient ability to return to normal activity by measuring their muscular performance with exercise testing. These results were then compared to questionnaires assessing activities of daily living (ADL) and return to normal activity. The results of the exercise tests and ADL questionnaires after operation in patients who had laparoscopic herniorrhaphy were significantly better than those with anterior repairs. Patients who had laparoscopic herniorrhaphy returned to normal activities sooner (6 versus 10 days; $p = 0.0003$). At 1 week postoperatively, the laparoscopic herniorrhaphy patients were able to perform more repetitions of situps and straight leg raises ($p < 0.0001$), and their ADL scores were significantly better ($p = 0.0001$) than those patients undergoing open repairs. The authors concluded that laparoscopic herniorrhaphy results in a quicker recovery.

Another study by Khoury[49] compared plug and patch repairs ($n = 142$) to TEP ($n = 150$) with an 89% follow-up at 17 months (median) postoperatively. Initially, laparoscopic repair was slower than open but became 10 min faster after 75 repairs. Patients undergoing TEP repair consumed fewer narcotic analgesics and returned to their normal activities 1 week earlier than their open counterparts ($p < 0.01$). Hospital stay did not differ between the two groups. Postoperative complications occurred in 23% of open patients and 13% of TEP patients ($p < 0.01$). Recurrence rates at follow-up were 3% for plug and patch and 2.5% for TEP. The author concluded that patients with inguinal hernias who undergo extraperitoneal laparoscopic repair have the same hospi-

tal stay and recurrence rates but recover faster, use less pain medication, and have fewer minor complications than those who undergo plug and patch repair.

Wellwood et al.[44] reported a large experience in which 400 patients were prospectively randomized to undergo either TAPP or Lichtenstein repairs. Patients with both unilateral and bilateral hernias were included. Follow-up in 86% of patients at 3 months revealed the following data. More patients in the open group (96%) than in the laparoscopic group (89%) were discharged on the same day as the operation ($p = 0.01$). Although pain scores were lower in the open group while the local anesthetic effect persisted, scores after open repair were significantly higher for each day of the first week, on day 7, and during the second week ($p < 0.01$). At 1 month, there was a greater improvement in mean SF-36 scores (measurement of well-being) over baseline in the laparoscopic group compared with the open group on seven of eight parameters, reaching significance on five ($p = 0.01$). For every activity considered, the median time until return to normal was significantly shorter for the laparoscopic group.

Other randomized studies support these outcomes in showing reduced postoperative pain,[22,24,26,28,29,31,33,35,40,42,43,47,48,50] reduced analgesic requirements,[26,31,33,40,43,48,49] and earlier return to work[22,23,26,29,33,40–45,48–50] when compared to anterior approaches. These same studies in many cases have shown laparoscopic herniorrhaphy to demonstrate no significant difference in convalescence[26–28,30–32,35,46,47] or postoperative pain.[25,27,33,45,46] As the number and quality of the prospective randomized studies increase, evidence favoring the laparoscopic

TABLE 30.5. Collected series of TAPP versus TEP.

Author (year)	Hernias (no.)	Repair type	Complications (%)	Recurrence (%)
Felix (1995)[51]	733	TAPP	1.2	0.2
	382	TEP	0	0.2
Ramshaw (1996)[52]	300	TAPP	4.3	2
	600	TEP	0.8	0.3
Dellemagne (1996)[53]	254	TAPP	NR	1.5
	371	TEP	NR	0
Fielding (1996)[54]	386	TAPP	0.5	1
	218	TEP	0	0.9
Kald (1997)[55]	339	TAPP	11	2
	87	TEP	8	0
Cocks (1998)[56]	148	TAPP	27	2
	313	TEP	12	0.3
Felix (1999)[57]	472	TAPP	5.6	NR
	678	TEP	1.0	NR

NR, not reported.

approach is accumulating. It is clear (see Tables 30.3, 30.4) that the majority of studies that examine the parameters of pain and return to activity favor the laparoscopic groups.

Technique-Specific (TAPP Versus TEP): Indications and Contraindications

Once the decision to perform laparoscopic herniorrhaphy has been made, the choice of laparoscopic repair technique, TAPP or TEP, may also influence the outcome significantly. Recently there has been an increase in the performance of the TEP technique and a trend away from TAPP. It is important that surgeons understand both techniques, however, because some TEP repairs need to be converted to TAPP to be completed safely and successfully and others should be started as TAPP.

If a laparoscopic approach has been chosen over open and the patient has a simple unilateral, bilateral, or recurrent hernia, then the TEP technique should be chosen. Several nonrandomized studies have looked at the question of TAPP versus TEP, and TEP is shown to have fewer complications and equivalent if not superior recurrence rates (Table 30.5).[51–57] TEP has several advantages over TAPP in the majority of cases. If the Phillips technique[58] is used, then the peritoneal cavity can be inspected before repair to rule out unexpected defects and after repair to ensure no peritoneal tears occurred. The surgeon can make sure that the hernia was not reduced "en masse," and that the mesh is in correct position. TEP avoids the large peritoneal incisions of TAPP that can result in either adhesive or incarcerated small bowel obstructions. TEP also allows better visual control in the medial part of the operative field where it is important to see that the mesh crosses the midline. In patients with previous midline pelvic incisions, TEP is preferable because the preperitoneal space can be entered posterior to the rectus muscle and followed inferiorly to the pubis. Transverse incisions prevent this, and these patients are better treated with the TAPP approach.

If concomitant diagnostic laparoscopy is required, then TAPP is the best approach to use; this allows the operating surgeon to have two graspers available intraperitoneally to move the viscera about and thoroughly examine all surfaces. TEP (with peritoneoscopy) can be used if the pelvic floor or surface of the liver needs to be inspected, but without graspers available intraperitoneally the inspection can be limited.

Although TEP is indicated for the treatment of the majority of hernias, TAPP can help the surgeon approach large scrotal, incarcerated, and complex recurrent hernias with a higher margin of safety and ease (Table 30.6). The indirect sac of a large scrotal hernia can be difficult or

TABLE 30.6. Indications for repair techniques (TAPP, TEP, OPEN).

	TEP	TAPP	OPEN (tension free)
Hernia type			
Unilateral	✓		✓
Bilateral	✓		✓
Recurrent	✓		✓
Large scrotal		✓	✓
Incarcerated		✓	✓
Failed laparoscopic repair			✓
Diagnostic		✓	
Previous pelvic incision			
Transverse		✓	✓
Midline	✓		✓
S/P prostatectomy			✓
H/O pelvic radiation			✓
H/O severe pelvic infections			✓
Cardiopulmonary insufficiency			✓

impossible to encircle from the extraperitoneal space. With such a large orifice to the indirect sac, it is simpler to approach the defect from the peritoneal cavity where the surgeon can check both sides of the peritoneum while reducing the sac far enough to amputate and close the defect. The TAPP approach also allows the surgeon the luxury of not worrying about a peritoneal tear, which might otherwise compromise visibility during a difficult dissection. If the scrotal hernia is too large, a "scrotal tunic" must be placed preoperatively so that the scrotum will not preferentially inflate and adequate intraperitoneal CO_2 pressure can be maintained. In fact, intraabdominal distension cannot be obtained in patients who have lost the right of domain from a longstanding giant scrotal hernia.

Incarcerated hernias are another indication for the TAPP approach. The intraperitoneal instruments and visualization assist the surgeon during reduction of the incarcerated viscera. The surgeon can then closely inspect the viscera for viability during and after the repair process. If, on initial inspection, immediate conversion to open technique for extensive resection is indicated, then valuable operating time is not lost. If at the end of the repair, a small segment is in question, then it can be exteriorized through a small incision and resection performed.

Although simple recurrent hernias can be well managed using TEP, surgeon preference and experience with other transperitoneal posterior approaches to complex groin hernias may encourage them to use TAPP for complex recurrent hernias. If the previous repairs were open/anterior, then either repair technique works well because the tissue has not been previously dissected; this is not true with preperitoneal plug repairs, Rives' repair, or other preperitoneal mesh repairs performed via anterior access. However, if mesh has been placed posteriorly by either open or laparoscopic techniques, the repair is much more complicated. Dissecting the peritoneum off mesh is difficult and frequently results in breaches in the peritoneum, making visualization from the preperitoneal space suboptimal. If there is posterior mesh and there has been no previous anterior dissection, then the surgeon should consider an anterior repair as well.

Contraindications

Cardiopulmonary Insufficiency

The adverse physiological effects resulting from pneumoperitoneum are related to both hypercarbia and the mechanical effects of patient positioning and increased intraabdominal pressure. The physiological effects of carbon dioxide pneumoperitoneum are important to understand, especially when operating on elderly patients with significant comorbid conditions.

Hypercarbia is partially related to transperitoneal absorption of CO_2 and results in elevated pCO_2 and end-tidal CO_2 ($ETCO_2$). Too rapid insufflation causing peritoneal stretching may cause a vagal response, resulting in bradycardia and potentially cardiovascular collapse. Intraabdominal hypertension increases venous resistance, decreases venous return, and increases mean systemic pressure and afterload. The increased afterload results from mechanical compression of the splanchnic circulation and neurohormonal response to hypotension. Increased venous resistance is a result of inferior vena cava (IVC) compression and decreasing venous return. On the other hand, the increase in mean systemic pressure from compression of the capacitance vessels acts as a pump to increase venous return and plays a role in preload. In those patients who are euvolemic or hypovolemic, the influence of the increased venous resistance predominates and venous return is decreased with pneumoperitoneum. In hypervolemic patients, the influence of increased systemic pressure predominates with minimal compression of the IVC, resulting in increased venous return.[59,60]

In patients undergoing laparoscopic surgery with a 15mmHg pneumoperitoneum, McLaughlin et al.[61] demonstrated increases in systolic blood pressure (11.3%), diastolic blood pressure (19.7%), mean arterial pressure (MAP) (15.9%), and central venous pressure (CVP) (30%). In addition, decreased stroke volume (29.5%) and cardiac index (29.5%) were reported. In another human study with a 15mmHg pneumoperitoneum, Westerband et al.[62] reported a decrease in cardiac output (30%), increased MAP (15%), and total peripheral vascular resistance (79%). The increased afterload may increase the myocardial oxygen consumption and the possibility of myocardial infarction in susceptible patients. As a result, patients at risk should undergo careful perioperative evaluation and monitoring to reduce the possibility of cardiac morbidity or perhaps forgo the laparoscopic approach altogether.

Changes in pulmonary function are primarily caused by the mechanical effects of pneumoperitoneum. The increase in intraabdominal pressure and volume results in decreased diaphragmatic excursion with an increase in intrathoracic and peak airway pressure and a decrease in pulmonary compliance and vital capacity. Most pulmonary effects related to pneumoperitoneum are limited and easily compensated for with an increase in tidal volume or respiratory rate.[63]

It is important that surgeons performing laparoscopic procedures understand the physiological consequences of pneumoperitoneum. However, the larger risk to the fragile patient being considered for laparoscopic herniorrhaphy is not the pneumoperitoneum but the general anesthetic. All inhalational anesthetics are myocardial depressants to varying degrees. Unfortunately, even a deep intravenous sedation in a fragile cardiac patient can have myocardial repercussions. There are small series where hernias have been successfully treated laparoscopically using regional anesthetics (epidural and local). However, the most commonly performed laparoscopic hernia repair, TAPP, is not well suited to regional anesthetics because of the necessity of intraperitoneal CO_2 and its accompanying peritoneal irritation. Therefore, if a patient is not a candidate for general anesthesia for reasons of cardiac or pulmonary disease, the hernia should not be repaired laparoscopically.

The Hostile Abdomen

Many different events in a patient's past medical or surgical history can predispose to extra or intraperitoneal scarring that can make laparoscopic herniorrhaphy difficult and dangerous. These events, in most cases, can be discovered during a thorough history and physical.

A patient who has a history of extensive intraabdominal pelvic infections such as ruptured diverticulitis or appendicitis, pelvic inflammatory disease, or complicated Crohn's disease more than likely has adhesions of the bowel to the underside of the abdominal wall. These adhesions, often dense, make TAPP impossible and TEP inadvisable. Even if the extraperitoneal space has been spared from the disease prosess and a TEP repair is initiated, the adherent viscera make the peritoneum more difficult to dissect off the abdominal wall, and if tears occur they are more dangerous to repair. For these reasons, history of extensive intraabdominal infections should cause the prudent surgeon to perform an open repair.

A history of pelvic radiation such as that used for treatment of rectal, prostate, or gynecological carcinoma is a contraindication to laparoscopic herniorrhaphy. The radiation causes tissue damage that results in dense scarring and therefore obliteration of the extraperitoneal space. With dense scar tissue occupying this usually easily entered sapce, dissection of the peritoneum off the abdominal wall, a prerequisite for both TAPP and TEP, is impossible.

Surgical procedures that are performed extraperitoneally, such as prostatectomy or bladder neck operations for the treatment of incontinence, result in the scarring of this space. Thus, the peritoneum is difficult to dissect off the abdominal wall, making laparoscopic repair inadvisable. This problem brings up the controversial question of whether a recurrent hernia, initially treated laparoscopically, is a contraindication to laparoscopic rerepair. Reports concerning laparoscopic repair of recurrent inguinal hernias have already been published that include laparoscopic reoperative cases.[64,65] Just as recurrences following anterior repairs can be performed through an anterior approach, laparoscopic recurrence following TEP or TAPP repairs can be performed laparoscopically. In such cases, however, the patient should be aware conversion to an anterior approach may be needed. These cases are difficult due to the adhesions of the peritoneum to the mesh and require careful dissection. Proceeding laparoscopically in such a situation would not be for the novice laparoscopist and, in most situations, should be treated via an anterior tension-free repair.

Conclusion

Laparoscopic herniorrhaphy is being performed by an increasing number of surgeons. Although there is a considerable learning curve, the short-term recurrence and complication rates are low. These results have made laparoscopic hernia repair the preferred treatment option for patients with bilateral and recurrent hernias.

TEP is preferable to TAPP because of its lower complication and recurrence rates. TAPP should be reserved for patients with large scrotal hernias, incarcerated hernias, prior transverse lower abdominal wall incisions, and patients requiring diagnostic laparoscopy.

The inability to tolerate general anesthesia for any reason and a hostile abdomen are clear contraindications to laparoscopic hernia repair. Surgeons must carefully evaluate their patients to ensure that laparoscopic technology is properly applied, especially because anterior repair techniques are safe and provide good results. Laparoscopic herniorrhaphy is an excellent technique, but it is not minimally invasive. It may be too stressful an operation for the young patient with a unilateral hernia or an older patient who is better served with a less invasive operation performed under local anesthesia.

References

1. Stoppa RE, Warlaumont CR. The preperitoneal approach and prosthetic repair of groin hernia. In: Nyhus LM, Condon RE (eds) Hernia, 3rd Ed. Philadelphia: Lippincott, 1989:154–177.
2. Glassow F. Inguinal hernia repair using local anesthesia. Ann R Coll Surg Engl 1984;66:382–387.
3. Nyhus LM. The recurrent groin hernia: therapeutic solutions. World J Surg 1989;13:541–544.
4. Lichtenstein IL, Shulman AL, Amid PK, et al. The tension-free hernioplasty. Am J Surg 1989;157:188–193.
5. Stoppa RE. The preperitoneal approach and prosthetic repair of groin hernia. In: Nyhus LM, Condon RE (eds) Hernia, 4th Ed. Philadelphia: Lippincott, 1995:188–206.
6. Nyhus LM, Pollak R, Bombeck C, et al. The preperitoneal approach and prosthetic buttress repair for recurrent hernia: the evolution of a technique. Ann Surg 1988;208:733–737.
7. Greenberg AG. Revisiting the recurrent groin hernia. Am J Surg 1987;154:35–40.

8. Glassow F. The Shouldice Hospital technique. Int Surg 1986;71:148–153.

9. Lichtenstein IL, Shulman AG, Amid PK. The cause, prevention and treatment of recurrent groin hernias. Surg Clin N Am 1993;73(3):529–543.

10. Felix EL, Michas C, McKnight RL. Laparoscopic repair of recurrent groin hernia. Surg Laparosc Endosc 1994;4:200–204.

11. Leibel B, et al. Endoscopic hernia surgery (TAPP)—gold standard in the management of recurrent hernias? Chirurg 1996;67(12):1226–1230.

12. Sandbichler, et al. Laparoscopic repair of recurrent inguinal hernias. Am J Surg 1996;171(3):366–368.

13. Birth M, et al. Laparoscopic transabdominal preperitoneal hernioplasty: results of 1000 consecutive cases. J Laparosc Surg 1996;6(5):293–300.

14. Felix EL, et al. Laparoscopic repair of recurrent hernia. Am J Surg 1996;172:580–584.

15. Sayad P, Ferzli G. Laparoscopic preperitoneal repair of recurrent inguinal hernias. J Laparoendosc Adv Surg Tech 1999;9(2):127–130.

16. Pellegrin K, Bensard DD, Karrer FM, et al. Laparoscopic evaluation of contralateral patent processus vaginalis in children. Am J Surg 1996;72:602–606.

17. Holcomb GW, Morgan WM, Brock JW. Laparoscopic evaluation for contralateral patent processus vaginalis: Part II. J Pediatr Surg 1996;31(8):1170–1173.

18. Wulkan ML, Wiener ES, VanBalen N, et al. Laparoscopy through the open ipsilateral sac to evaluate presence of contralateral hernia. J Pediatr Surg 1996;31(8):1174–1177.

19. Crawford DL, Hiatt JR, Phillips EH. Laparoscopy identifies unexpected groin hernias. Am Surg 1998;64(10):976–978.

20. Panton ONM, Panton RJ. Laparoscopic hernia repair. Am J Surg 1994;167:535–537.

21. Quilici PJ, Greaney EM, Quilici J, et al. Transabdominal preperitoneal laparoscopic inguinal herniorrhaphy: results of 509 repairs. Am Surg 1996;62(10):849–852.

22. Stocker DL, Spiegelhalter DJ, Singh R, et al. Laparoscopic versus open inguinal hernia repair: randomized prospective trial. Lancet 1994;343:1243–1244.

23. Payne JH Jr, Grininger LM, Izawa MT, et al. Laparoscopic or open inguinal herniorrhaphy? A randomized prospective trial. Arch Surg 1994;129:979–981.

24. Champault G, Benoit J, Lauroy J, Rizk P. Hernies de l'aine de l'adulte. Chirurgie laparoscopique vs opération de Shouldice. Étude randomisée contrôlée: 181 patients. Résultats préliminaires. Ann Chir 1994;48:1003.

25. Maddern GJ, Rudkin G, Bessell JR, et al. A comparison of laparoscopic and open hernia repair as a day surgical procedure. Surg Endosc 1994;8:1404–1408.

26. Vogt DM, Curet MJ, Pitcher DE, et al. Preliminary results of a prospective randomized trial of laparoscopic onlay versus conventional inguinal herniorrhaphy. Am J Surg 1995;169:84–90.

27. Barkun JS, Wexler MJ, Hinchley EJ, et al. Laparoscopic versus open inguinal herniorrhaphy: preliminary results of a randomized controlled trial. Surgery (St. Louis) 1995;118:703–710.

28. Lawrence K, McWhinnie D, Goodwin A, et al. Randomized controlled trial of laparoscopic versus open repair of inguinal hernia: early results. BMJ 1995;311:981–985.

29. Leibl B, Däubler P, Schwarz J, et al. Standardisierte laparoskopische Hernioplastik vs. Shouldice-Reparation. Chirurg 1995;66:895–898.

30. Schrenk P, Woisetschläger R, Rieger R, et al. Prospective randomized trial comparing postoperative pain and return to physical activity after transabdominal preperitoneal, total preperitoneal or Shouldice technique for inguinal hernia repair. Br J Surg 1996;83:1563–1566.

31. Bessell JR, Baxter P, Riddell P, Watkin S, Maddern GJ. A randomized controlled trial of laparoscopic extraperitoneal hernia repair as a day surgical procedure. Surg Endosc 1996;10:495–500.

32. Filipi CJ, Gaston-Johnson F, McBride PJ, et al. An assessment of pain and return to normal activity. Laparoscopic herniorrhaphy vs. open tension-free repair. Surg Endosc 1996;10(10):983–986.

33. Tschudi J, Wagner M, Klaiber C, et al. Controlled multicenter trial of laparoscopic transabdominal preperitoneal hernioplasty vs. Shouldice herniorrhaphy. Early results. Surg Endosc 1996;10(8):845–847.

34. Wright DM, Kennedy A, Baxter JN, et al. Early outcome after open versus extraperitoneal endoscopic tension-free hernioplasty: a randomized clinical trial. Surgery (St. Louis) 1996;119(5):552–557.

35. Hauters P, Meunier D, Urgayan S, et al. Prospective controlled study comparing laparoscopy and the Shouldice technique in the treatment of unilateral inguinal hernia. Ann Chir 1996;50(9):776–781.

36. Kozol R, Lange PM, Kosir M, et al. A prospective, randomized study of open vs. laparoscopic inguinal hernia repair: an assessment of postoperative pain. Arch Surg 1997;132:292–295.

37. Liem MSL, Van Der Graaf Y, Van Steensel CJ, et al. Comparison of conventional anterior surgery and laparoscopic surgery for inguinal hernia repair. N Engl J Med 1997;336(22):1541–1547.

38. Heikkinen T, Haukipuro K, Leppälä J, et al. Total costs of laparoscopic and Lichtenstein inguinal hernia repairs: a randomized prospective study. Surg Laparosc Endosc 1997;7(1):1–5.

39. Liem MSL, Van Der Graaf Y, Zwart RC, et al. A randomized comparison of physical performance following laparoscopic and open inguinal hernia repair. Br J Surg 1997;84:64–67.

40. Tanphiphat C, Tanprayoon T, Sansubhan C, et al. Laparoscopic versus open inguinal hernia repair: a randomized, controlled trial. Surg Endosc 1998;12:846–851.

41. Kald A, Anderberg B, Carlsson P, et al. Surgical outcome and cost-minimization analyses of laparoscopic and open hernia repair: a randomized prospective trial with one year follow-up. Eur J Surg 1997;163:505–510.

42. Champault GG, Rizk N, Catheline JM, et al. Totally preperitoneal laparoscopic approach versus Stoppa operation: randomized trial of 100 cases. Surg Laparosc Endosc 1997;7(6):445–450.

43. Zieren J, Zieren HU, Jacobi CA, et al. Prospective randomized study comparing laparoscopic and open tension-

free inguinal hernia repair with Shouldice's operation. Am J Surg 1998;175:330–333.

44. Wellwood J, Sculpher MJ, Stoker D, et al. Randomized controlled trial of laparoscopic versus open mesh repair for inguinal hernia: outcome and cost. BMJ 1998;317:103–110.

45. Heikkinen TJ, Haukipuro K, Hulkko A. A cost and outcome comparison between laparoscopic and Lichtenstein hernia operations in a day-case unit. Surg Endosc 1998;12:1199–1203.

46. Paganini AM, Lezoche E, Carle F, et al. A randomized, controlled, clinical study of laparoscopic versus open tension-free inguinal hernia repair. Surg Endosc 1998;12:979–986.

47. Aitola P, Airo I, Matikainen M. Laparoscopic versus open preperitoneal inguinal hernia repair: a prospective randomized trial. Ann Chir Gynaecol 1998;87:22–25.

48. Dirksen CD, Beets GL, Go PMNYH, et al. Bassini repair compared with laparoscopic repair for primary inguinal hernia: a randomized controlled trial. Eur J Surg 1998;164:439–447.

49. Khoury N. A randomized prospective controlled trial of laparoscopic extraperitoneal hernia repair and mesh-plug hernioplasty: a study of 315 cases. J Laparoendosc Adv Surg Tech 1998;8(6):367–372.

50. Juul P, Christensen K. Randomized clinical trial of laparoscopic versus open inguinal hernia repair. Br Surg 1999;86(3):316–319.

51. Felix EL, Michas CA. Laparoscopic hernioplasty: totally extra-peritoneal or transabdominal preperitoneal? Surg Endosc 1995;9:984–989.

52. Ramshaw BJ, Tucker JG, Duncan TD, et al. Laparoscopic herniorrhaphy: a review of 900 cases. Surg Endosc 1996;10:255.

53. Dellemagne B, Markiewicz S, Lehaes C, et al. Extraperitoneal laparoscopic inguinal hernia repair: technique and results. Surg Endosc 1996;10:228.

54. Fielding GA. Laparoscopic hernia repair—600 cases with a median 30 month follow-up. Surg Endosc 1996;10:231.

55. Kald A, Anderberg B, Smedh K, Karlsson M. Transperitoneal or totally extraperitoneal approach in laparoscopic hernia repair: results of 491 consecutive herniorrhaphies. Surg Laparosc Endosc 1997;7(2):86.

56. Cocks JR. Laparoscopic inguinal hernioplasty: a comparison between transperitoneal and extraperitoneal techniques. Aust N Z J Surg 1998;68:506.

57. Felix EL, Harbertson N, Vartanian S. Laparoscopic hernioplasty. Surg Endosc 1999;13:328–331.

58. Friedman RL, Phillips EH. Laparoscopically-guided total extraperitoneal inguinal hernioplasty. In: Maddern GJ, Hiatt JR, Phillips EH (eds) Hernia Repair: Open vs. Laparoscopic Approaches. Philadelphia: Saunders, 1997:161–175.

59. Kashtan J, Gree JF, Parsons EQ, et al. Hemodynamic effects of increased abdominal pressure. J Surg Res 1981;30:249–255.

60. Ortegha AE, Richman MF, Hernandez M, et al. Inferior vena caval blood flow and cardiac hemodynamics during carbon dioxide pneumoperitoneum. Surg Endosc 1996;10:920–924.

61. McLaughlin JG, Scheeres DE, Dean RJ, et al. The adverse hemodynamic effects of laparoscopic cholecystectomy. Surg Endosc 1995;9:121–124.

62. Westerband A, Van DeWater JM, Amzallag M, et al. Cardiovascular changes during laparoscopic cholecystectomy. Surg Gynecol Obstet 1992;175:535–538.

63. Lowham AS, Filipi CJ, Tomanaga T. Pneumoperitoneum-related complications: diagnosis and treatment. In: Rosenthal RJ, Friedman RL, Phillips EH (eds). The Pathophysiology of Pneumoperitoneum. New York: Springer-Verlag, 1998:131–146.

64. Jones MW. Laparoscopic re-do repairs of recurrent inguinal hernias using double-mesh technique. J Soc Laparoendosc Surg 1998;2(2):175–176.

65. Fielding GA. Difficult and recurrent hernias. In: Maddern GJ, Hiatt JR, Phillips EH (eds). Hernia Repair: Open vs. Laparoscopic Approaches. Philadelphia: Saunders, 1997:183–188.

31
Laparoscopic Intraperitoneal Onlay Mesh Hernia Repair

Morris E. Franklin, Jr. and Jose Antonio Diaz-Elizondo

Rationale for Intraperitoneal Onlay Mesh (IPOM) Hernia Repair

The introduction of synthetic mesh in the 1960s offered a new tool for hernia surgery. The use of synthetic mesh for the repair of recurrent hernias, and then for the primary repair of hernias, has gradually gained acceptance among surgeons as attempts have been made to replace or reinforce a weak musculoaponeurotic layer (transversalis fascia).[1]

The surgical concept that the common pathway leading to groin hernias is a defect in the fascia transversalis is widely accepted today.[2] Replacing the deficient fascia transversalis with a nonbiodegradable layer of synthetic mesh tailored to fit and cover the hernia defect without tension is becoming the procedure of choice for repairing inguinal hernias in many patients, especially in adult males, by a growing number of surgeons.

Various techniques using synthetic mesh for hernia repairs are described in the literature.[3–6] The conventional open technique most frequently used consists of suturing, without tension, an adequate piece of mesh to the "conjoined" muscle and tendon superiorly and to the inguinal ligament inferiorly. A medially placed slit in the mesh allows for the egress of the cord, which then lies deep to the aponeurosis of the external oblique. This repair championed by Lichtenstein is attended by excellent results.[4] Duplication of the excellent results of Lichtenstein et al. has developed only sporadically, however.

The development and physiological support of the preperitoneal repair of inguinal hernias has been discussed in detail by Millelsen, Musgrove, Nyhus, and Read.[7–10] The absence of adequate structures in the preperitoneal space that could be approximated to close the hernia defect led to the abandonment of this technique without using mesh. Stoppa (in Amiens) and Rives (in Reims) rekindled interest in the preperitoneal area by using a large mesh to cover the hernia defect,[2] and this technique has gained wide acceptance in many countries for the treatment of a variety of groin hernias. In the United States its use has been generally limited to the repair of recurrent inguinal hernias.[11]

Placing a prosthetic mesh in the preperitoneal area in the case of a recurrent hernia renders unnecessary reentering previously divided planes and dissection of the spermatic cord.[12] Mesh placed preperitoneally, if adequate in diameter, will cover the area of recurrence and will also cover other potential inguinal hernia sites, including the femoral canal (Fig. 31.1). The preperitoneal placement of mesh for "first-time" and recurrent hernias has been well described in numerous publications.[2,6,13]

With the advent of laparoscopic surgery and continuous refinements in techniques occurring in this minimally invasive surgical field, the authors have tried to establish whether the principles of preperitoneal placement of prosthetic mesh could be used laparoscopically in an expeditious and safe manner by placing the mesh in an intraperitoneal position.

After an extensive developmental phase in the laboratory, we began studying the procedure in humans in early 1990. Attempts at placing a large portion of mesh (12 × 15 cm) preperitoneally required a large amount of dissection. Postoperative scrotal discomfort experienced by some patients for which we used this technique was discouraging and led us to try the much simpler intraperitoneal placement of the mesh. In this series, we arbitrarily decided not to operate on patients under 18 years of age or patients with large inguinoscrotal hernias. With experience, we have approached all hernias in this manner.

Technique

With the patient under general anesthesia, a catheter is placed in the bladder and a nasogastric tube is placed in the stomach; both are removed at the end of the procedure. The surgeon places himself on the contralateral side

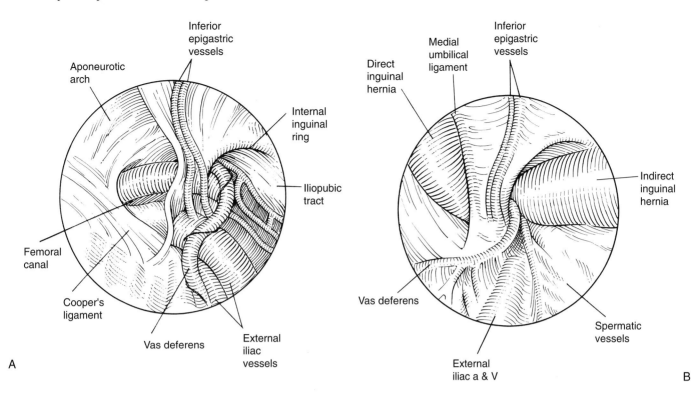

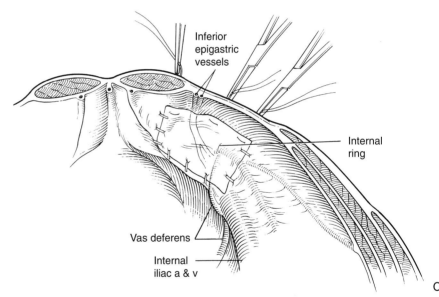

FIGURE 31.1. A. Anatomy of inguinal region. B. Inguinal hernia sites. C. Mesh placement.

of the hernia. After inflating the peritoneal cavity using a Veress needle, a laparoscope with an attached video camera is placed through a 5- to 12-mm trocar at the umbilicus. A contralateral 5-mm trocar is placed approximately 4 to 5 cm lateral to the umbilicus, just lateral to the rectus muscle. A 5-mm trocar is placed approximately at McBurney's point on the opposite side of the hernia and, on the ipsilateral side, lateral to the umbilicus. For bilateral repairs, the trocar placement is the same.

After insufflating the peritoneal cavity, the hernia site and the contralateral inguinal area are carefully inspected. For proper orientation the surgeon should recognize the median, medial, and lateral umbilical ligaments. Just below the posterior parietal peritoneum, the external iliac vein and artery, the gonadal vessels, and (in males) the vas deferens should be identified. The hidden course of the genitofemoral nerve and the approximate course of the lateral femorocutaneous nerve should be recalled and mapped, and care taken to avoid unneeded dissection in this area. The exact location of the ureter bilaterally should also be noted.

We routinely remove direct and indirect hernia sacs. Division of the sac also gives access to the preperitoneal area, where a "lipoma" of the cord, if present, can be excised. We excise the sac using laparoscopic scissors connected to an electrosurgical unit.

Progressively, by inverting the sac into the peritoneal cavity using gentle traction, the sac is incised starting 1 or 2 cm from its base at the 12 o'clock position and proceeding clockwise to about the 4 o'clock position. Excision is then completed in the appropriate direction with care taken to avoid the spermatic artery and vein, vas deferens, and the genitofemoral nerve.

Bleeding during this phase of the operation is easily controlled by electrocoagulation. Large inguinoscrotal sacs and sacs in multiple recurrent hernias often are problematic and cannot be safely removed. In these cases the sacs are ringed at the neck (incising the peritoneum circumferentially) and are left in place, as bleeding and extensive edema may ensue if these sacs are aggressively pursued.

Once the sac is removed, a piece of Prolene mesh is prepared. The size of the mesh should be such that it covers the hernia defect and extends at least 3 to 5 cm beyond its rim. We have found that a 12×15 cm portion of mesh covers most defects adequately. The folded mesh is introduced into the abdominal cavity; if the mesh is folded rather than rolled, once opened it will not have a tendency to curl and will be much easier to manipulate and hold in place. Once the mesh is unfolded, it is placed over the defect and held there with grasping forceps. The superior border of the mesh in its midportion is then tightly held against the anterior abdominal wall. A Keith needle attached to a 00 strand of Prolene is pushed through the abdominal wall and through the mesh (Fig. 31.2).

The spot where the incision is to be made and where the needle is to pierce the abdominal wall can be established by gently depressing the abdominal wall and visualizing the indentation laparoscopically. Through the same incision, a 14-gauge spinal needle is then placed through the abdominal wall and the mesh, parallel to the Keith needle. Once the Keith needle is passed through the abdomen and mesh, it is grasped, turned around, and pushed back through the lumen of the 14-gauge needle, exiting through the small skin incision. A clamp is applied to the Prolene suture at skin level, holding the mesh tightly against the abdominal wall. The same procedure is repeated at both upper corners of the mesh.

Once placed, these three sutures hold the mesh securely in place, spreading it evenly and allowing for the rest of the mesh to be precisely and easily stapled in place. Care should be taken to avoid the staples vertically

along the inferior edge of the mesh to minimize the chances of entrapping the femoral branch of the genitofemoral nerve or the lateral-femoral cutaneous nerve. Along the lower margin of the mesh, staples should be placed lightly to avoid damage to the iliac vessels and the vas deferens. A few staples are also used to fix the superior and central portion of the mesh to the anterior abdominal wall. Medially, the mesh should be secured to Cooper's ligament. Staples should not be used near the inferior and inferolateral aspect of the internal ring, for fear of injuring the structures passing through it, or over known locations of the genitofemoral and lateral femorocutaneous nerves.

The area is irrigated with saline solution and hemostasis is performed. The subcutaneous fat below the skin incisions through which the Prolene strands were placed is spread with a fine-tip hemostat, allowing them to be tied over the external oblique aponeurosis. Firm anchoring of the mesh by transabdominal sutures and staples in Cooper's ligament prevents displacement of the mesh when the abdomen is deflated and when the patient assumes the erect position. We firmly believe that it is early migration of the mesh away from its intended position that causes recurrences; therefore, we do not rely solely on staples grasping only mesh and peritoneum to hold the mesh in place. When possible, we now place omentum between the mesh and the bowel, utilizing lightly placed staples for fixation.

As the trocars are sequentially removed, the video camera examines the trocar sites to ensure that no bleed-

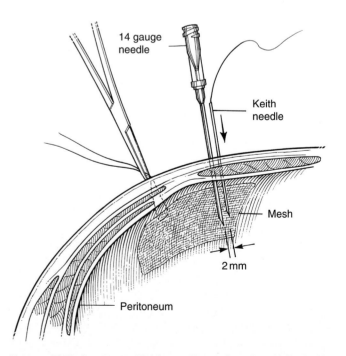

FIGURE 31.2. Suture on Keith needle used to fix mesh. A 14-gauge spinal needle is placed 2 mm away from the Keith needle.

TABLE 31.1. Demographics of patients, January 1990–June 1999.[a]

Site	Type	No. of patients	Repairs (%)
Right	Direct	23	169 (32.50%)
(n = 169)	Indirect	134	
	Pantaloon	4	
	Femoral	8	
Left	Direct	15	137 (26.35%)
(n = 137)	Indirect	118	
	Pantaloon	0	
	Femoral	4	
Bilateral			214 (41.15%)
(n = 107)			
Total		413	520 (100%)

[a] Data are for 413 patients (332 male, 81 female); weight range, 94–340 lb (average, 180.31, or 81.96 kg).

ing is present. To prevent potential herniation, all 5- to 10-mm trocar sites are closed by repairing the underlying fascia or aponeurosis with 0 Vicryl or Polysorb sutures. The patients usually are discharged the evening of surgery or the following morning.

Complications, Recurrences, and Outcomes

Our experience with laparoscopic mesh hernioplasty consists of 520 hernia repairs performed on 413 patients from January 1990 through June 1999 (Table 31.1).

Our follow-up extends for up to 84 months with a median of 68 months. There were 81 females and 332 males. The female group for the most part had unilateral hernias, as well as 12 femoral hernias; 1 of the femoral hernias was recurrent, and 4 were incarcerated. Seven females had bilateral hernias. In the male group, there were 394 hernias not previously repaired; 25 patients had recurrent hernias, and 107 patients had bilateral hernias of which 10 were bilaterally recurrent. Excluded from the study were patients under 18 years of age and, for the first 12 months, patients with large or incarcerated inguinal scrotal hernias who received standard open McVay repairs. Two patients refused laparoscopic repair and were offered McVay-type repairs.

Hospitalization at our institution for most advanced laparoscopic procedures (more than tubal ligation or diagnostic laparoscopy) is a minimum of overnight, and 388 of 413 (94.0%) of our patients were discharged in less than 23 h after surgery. Most of these patients were kept overnight at the surgeon's request and could have been discharged sooner. Twenty-five (6.0%) patients required longer hospitalization for the reasons given in Table 31.2.

We have had, to date, 5 (0.96%) recurrences after a unilateral laparoscopic mesh hernioplasty. One occurred in a nonpreviously operated hernia patient. The recurrences have been for a variety of reasons related to incorrect mesh placement, mesh too small, and poor tissue healing. All cases have had rerepairs with a combination of repairs including open, replacement and relocation of mesh, and open Stoppa repairs.

It is noteworthy that surgeons reporting their experiences with the preperitoneal placement of mesh claim that their recurrences occur early in the postoperative period, generally within the first 3 months after surgery. Few, if any, occur later.[1,12]

Follow-Up Techniques

Our follow-up extends for up to 84 months with a median of 68 months. Attempts were made to see all patients in the follow-up period, and we were very successful in this step (93%). All patients were seen by the operating surgeon at 1 week, 1 month, 3 months, 6 months, 9 months, and yearly after surgery. The patients were questioned in regard to pain, hypersensitivity, bulge, resumption of activity, and satisfaction with results.

Patients not returning for appointments were called, and most subsequently were seen (80%) or at least interviewed (13%). Seven percent of the patients (29 patients) were lost to follow-up and could not be found after 2 years (8 of these had died of cardiac and/or pulmonary disease not related to the hernia repair and 1 had died of cancer of the lung). One patient has been seen and operated by another surgeon; the complaint of recurrent hernia was found to be a residual sac but with no defect into to the abdominal cavity. The remaining 19 patients have changed address or could not be located by telephone or direct visit inquiry.

Total complications are summarized in Table 31.3.

Conclusions

Based on our present experience, it is our belief that laparoscopic approach to groin herniae in adults with the intraperitoneal onlay mesh technique stands on solid

TABLE 31.2. Hospital stay (n = 413).[a]

Reason for prolonged hospital stay (n = 25)	n	Average (days)
Cardiopulmonary	8	3
Urinary retention	7	2
Bleeding abdominal wall	3	2.5
Ileus	7	3
	25	

[a] Stay less than 23 h, 388 patients (94%); more than 23 h, 25 patients (6%).

TABLE 31.3. Complications.

Complication	n	(%)
Recurrent hernia	5	(0.96%)
Neuropraxia	12	(2.30%)
Seroma	15	(2.88%)
Testicular pain	3	(0.57%)
Infection	0	
Trocar site hernia	0	
Abdominal wall hematoma	4	(0.76%)
Neuropraxia	12	(2.30%)
Genitofemoral	3	
Lateral femorocutaneous	9	
(Pain in distribution of nerve 3)		

Note: All resolved in 3 weeks except 2: 1 resolved with cortisone injection, 1 permanent.

anatomic and physiological grounds. On the less positive side, this operation requires a general anesthetic, costs marginally more to perform than standard open repairs not using mesh, has the potential problems inherent to laparoscopy, and requires experience and skills in advanced laparoscopic surgery. The fate of the mesh placed intraperitoneally, even though proven harmless to date in the laboratory and in clinical practice, has yet to be established.

The absence of major scarring, avoiding dissection of the spermatic cord structures, the almost painless postoperative course, as well as the rapid return to unrestricted activities more than compensate for the drawbacks mentioned previously.

Literature review shows little in the way of complications (migration, carcinomatous transformation, intestinal obstruction, or erosion of the mesh into vessels) in mesh placed without other complicating factors.

We have had the opportunity to reexplore 21 patients who have undergone a laparoscopic intraperitoneal onlay mesh hernia repair. These patients were reexplored while performing a laparoscopic surgical procedure for a condition other than inguinal hernia. The findings are summarized in Table 31.4.

TABLE 31.4. Adhesions.

Reexplorations	n = 21
10 patients	Clean
6 patients	Flimsy omental aedhesions to edge of mesh
1 patient	Severe adhesions, nondissectable bowel and omentum (Gore-Tex)
4 patients	Moderately dense adhesions, all with prior surgery where adhesions were taken down to obtain exposure

TABLE 31.5. Return to activities.

Lifting activity	Less than 60 years old	Greater than 60 years old
Limited (10 lb or less)	2.5 days (1–6 days)	2.8 days (1–8 days)
Normal (10–30 lb)	3.5 days (1–15 days)	3.6 days (1–12 days)
Full (more than 30 lb)	6.8 days (1–45 days)	7.2 days (1–40 days)

Patient profile: less than 60 years of age (n = 111, 27%); more than 60 years of age (n = 402, 73%).

Patient Preparation and Postoperative Instructions

Preoperatively, the patient receives a mild colonic preparation using milk of magnesia and a soft, low-residue diet. The patient is instructed not to have anything to eat or drink at least 8h preoperatively. Skin preparation begins the night before surgery, consisting of merely a shower with an antibacterial soap. Just before surgery, the patient is shaved in the inguinoscrotal area and the trocar placement area. The surgical preparation is carried out using a solution made of iodophor and isopropyl alcohol (Duraprep). After surgery, the patient is taken to the recovery room for about 1.5h, and then is taken to a room for the rest of the day. The patient is encouraged to start sitting up and begin walking the same afternoon. Most patients are discharged less than 23h after surgery. Patients can walk, climb stairs, move freely, and eat a regular diet almost immediately. Instructions to the patient stress the importance of not straining or lifting objects heavier than 10lb for 7 days postsurgery. Gradual increase in strain and lifting capacity is achieved at the 7th to 10th day.

Evaluation of return to work is very difficult and subjective at best. Because of the great diversity in activity level among our patients, who include college students and professional athletes as well as retired gardeners, we evaluated this aspect based on each patient's concept of their readiness to return to full activity. The results are tabulated in Table 31.5.

References

1. Ijzermand JNM. Recurrent inguinal hernia treated by classical hernioplasty. Arch Surg 1991;126:1097–1000.
2. Stoppa RE, Rives JL, Warlaumont CR, et al. The use of Dacron in the repair of hernias of the groin. Surg Clin N Am 1984;64:269–285.
3. Martin R, Shureih S. The use of Marlex mesh in primary hernia repair. Surg Rounds 1983;6:52–62.
4. Rives J. Surgical treatment of the inguinal hernia with the Dacron patch. Int Surg 1967;47:360–361.
5. Lichtenstein IL, Shulman AG, Amid PK, et al. The tension free hernioplasty. Am J Surg 1989;157:188–193.

6. Rosenthal D, Walters M. Properitoneal synthetic placement for recurrent hernias of the groin. Surg Gynecol Obstet 1985;163:285–286.
7. Millelsen WP, McCready FJ. Femoral hernioplasty. Surgery (St. Louis) 1954;35:743–748.
8. Musgrove JE, McCready FJ. The Henry approach to femoral hernia. Surgery (St. Louis) 1949;26:601–611.
9. Nyhus LM, Condon RE, Harkins HN. Preperitoneal hernia repair for all types of hernia of the groin. Am J Surg 1960; 100:234–244.
10. Read RC. Preperitoneal exposure of inguinal herniations. Am J Surg 1968;116:653–658.
11. Mozingo DW, Walters MJ, Otchy DP, Rosenthal D. Properitoneal synthetic mesh repair of recurrent inguinal hernias. Surg Gynecol Obstet 1992;174:33–35.
12. Wantz GE. Testicular atrophy as a risk of inguinal hernioplasty. Surg Gynecol Obstet 1982;154:570–572.
13. Rignault DP. Properitoneal prosthetic inguinal hernioplasty through a Pfannenstiel approach. Surg Gynecol Obstet 1985;163:465–468.
14. Salerno GM, Fitzgibbons RJ, Filipi CJ. Laparoscopic inguinal hernia repair. In: Zucker KA, Bailey RW, Reddick EJ (eds) Surgical Laparoscopy. St. Louis: Quality Medical, 1991:290–291.
15. Laymen ST, Burns RP, Chandler KE, et al. Laparoscopic inguinal herniorrhaphy in a swine model. Presented at the Southeastern Surgical Congress, Atlanta, GA, June 2, 1992.
16. Arregui M, et al. Inguinal Hernia—Advances or Controversy? Oxford: Radcliffe Medical, 1994.
17. Condon RE, Carilli S. The biology and anatomy of inguinofemoral hernia. Semin Laparosc Surg 1994; 1(2):75–85.
18. Nguyen N, Camps J, Fitzgibbons R. Laparoscopic intraperitoneal onlay mesh inguinal hernia repair. Semin Laparosc Surg 1994;1(2).
19. Gadacz TR, Chase JA, Duke S. Technologic advance: technology of prosthetic material. Semin Laparosc Surg 1994;1(2):123–127.
20. MacFadyen B Jr, Mathis C. Inguinal herniorrhaphy: complications and recurrences. Semin Laparosc Surg 1994; 1(2):128–140.
21. Rosenthal D, Franklin ME Jr. Use of percutaneous stitches in laparoscopic mesh hernioplasty. Surg Gynecol Obstet 1993;176:491–492.
22. Annibali R, Camps J, Nagan R, Quinn T, Arregui M, Fitzgibbons R Jr. Anatomical considerations for laparoscopic inguinal herniorrhaphy. In: Principles of Laparoscopic Surgery: Basic and Advanced Techniques, 1st Ed. New York: Springer-Verlag, 1995.
23. Toy K, Smoot R, Carey S. Intraperitoneal Inguinal Hernioplasty: Operative Laparoscopy and Thoracoscopy, 1st Ed. Philadelphia: Lippincott-Raven, 1996.
24. Camps J, Nguyen N, Annibali R, Filipi C, Fitzgibbons R Jr. Laparoscopic inguinal herniorrhaphy: current techniques. In: Principles of Laparoscopic Surgery: Basic and Advanced Techniques, 1st Ed. New York: Springer-Verlag, 1995.

32
Laparoscopic Groin Hernia Repair: Transabdominal Preperitoneal Approach

Steven M. Yood and Demetrius Litwin

Reports of laparoscopic hernia repair by Ger[1] and Shultz[2] published in 1990 provided the momentum for the development of current techniques in laparoscopic hernia repair. Since that time, several studies have compared laparoscopic inguinal hernia repair with standard open hernia repairs. Most,[3–10] but not all,[11–13] of these studies have shown decreased pain and use of postoperative analgesics and earlier return to normal activity and work. Although most authors have shown reasonable recurrence rates with few complications,[14–20] the need for general anesthesia, increased operative time, and subsequent increased cost of the procedure has caused some delay in the full integration of laparoscopic hernia repair.[21–23] Although increased operative time is a limitation of laparoscopy initially, several authors have demonstrated that as the surgeon's experience increases, operating time and the number of complications decrease.[12,20,24]

There are three general approaches to laparoscopic hernia repair: the transabdominal preperitoneal approach (TAPP), the intraperitoneal onlay mesh repair (IPOM), and the totally extraperitoneal approach (TEP). TAPP is the focus of this chapter; IPOM and TEP are the primary focus of other chapters.

Rationale for Transabdominal Preperitoneal Approach

In the early 1990s, the transabdominal preperitoneal technique (TAPP) was described.[25,26] This approach showed promise because it was a laparoscopic procedure that adhered to the principles of the open posterior repairs, which had recurrence rates of less than 5%.[27,28] The TAPP procedure provides optimal visualization of the relevant anatomy and a comfortable working space. The important structures are easier to identify using the TAPP approach, compared to TEP and IPOM, and therefore the procedure is easier to teach. In experienced hands, the TAPP procedure can be performed with very low morbidity and a low recurrence rate.

Although the anatomy is easier to discern, some of the technical aspects of the TAPP operation are more difficult. Creating an adequate peritoneal window without tearing the peritoneum is essential. Also, closing the peritoneum completely over the mesh is crucial to avoid postoperative bowel obstruction. The potential for intraabdominal injury is present during any laparoscopic procedure, but we believe that, with the use of the open insertion technique and sound laparoscopic skills (especially with the use of electrocautery), this risk is minimal. The risk of neuralgia has been dramatically decreased over the years since laparoscopic surgeons have developed a better understanding of the pelvic anatomy and have minimized the use of staples.

Research Comparing TAPP with Other Procedures

All but one[29] of the studies that have compared TAPP with the other laparoscopic techniques are observational studies.[18,30–32] Although these studies provide important descriptive information about the performance of each procedure, they cannot be used to draw conclusions about the effectiveness of one treatment versus another because the decision about which operation to use was at the discretion of the surgeon. Because important factors such as operative times and patient outcomes are affected not only by the technique used, but also by factors associated with the patient and the physician (including surgeon experience, difficulty of repair, and comorbidities), these observational studies are subject to bias. Furthermore, a crucial point to consider when evaluating these studies is that most are retrospective comparisons in which current experience with the newer TEP procedure is compared to historical experience with the TAPP procedure. The implication of this limitation is the fact that most surgeons who attempt the TEP procedure already have had substantial experience with the TAPP repair. As a result, by the nature of the study design, studies that demonstrate superiority of TEP may actually do so because the TEP results reflect the ability of more experienced laparoscopic surgeons.

The only prospective randomized trial comparing laparoscopic hernia repair approaches is a study of the TAPP technique versus IPOM that was published in 1997 by Sarli et al.[29] The authors studied a total of 115 patients with 148 hernias (59 TAPP and 56 IPOM) over a 2-year period. The TAPP repair took an average of 71 min for a unilateral repair whereas the IPOM required an average of 53 min. There were no intraoperative complications, conversion to an open repair, or mortalities in either group. In the IPOM group there were 14 complications (25%), including 11 patients with neuralgia (20%). A total of 5 patients who had neuralgia required repeated local anesthetic infusions, 2 required removal of staples. In the TAPP group, 10 patients (17%) had complications, but only 3 patients (5%) had neuralgias and none required intervention. There were 8 recurrences (11%) over an average of 32 months in the IPOM group and none over an average of 28 months in the TAPP group. The authors recognized that their rate of neuralgia occurred primarily in the early phase of the study, before they fully understood the "triangle of pain."[33] These results prompted the authors to favor the TAPP approach.

The risk of recurrence for hernias repaired using the TAPP approach ranges from 0% to 5.0%. Recurrence risks are difficult to estimate because there are few randomized clinical trials, the risk is highly dependent upon the surgeon's experience, and long-term follow-up data are sparse. However, the TAPP procedure, when performed correctly, should be a durable minimally invasive repair with few complications.

Indications for TAPP

The laparoscopic approach is acceptable for most patients. The only absolute contraindications to the TAPP procedure are the inability to tolerate general anesthesia and a strangulated hernia with necrotic bowel. Relative contraindications such as multiple previous lower abdominal operations, an intraabdominal inflammatory process, and previous preperitoneal surgery (i.e., retropubic prostatectomy) should be carefully considered and operations on such patients performed only by experienced laparoscopic surgeons.

The procedure can be performed for indirect, direct, femoral, or combined hernias, both primary and recurrent. Incarcerated hernias can usually be reduced and repaired in a standard fashion. The operative approach is similar for all hernias.

Technique

The patient is asked to void immediately preoperatively and therefore a Foley catheter is not needed. Preoperative intravenous antibiotics (Cefazolin sodium) are given, and the mesh is soaked in a Cefazolin sodium and saline solution. Sequential compression devices are applied before the induction of general anesthesia. The patient is placed in a supine position with both arms tucked at the side, and a single video monitor is placed at the foot of the operating table. An open Hasson technique (10-mm port) is used to gain access to the abdominal cavity at the infraumbilical position. Pneumoperitoneum is then achieved and maintained at 15 mmHg. A 30°, 10-mm laparoscope is then inserted and the abdomen is explored. The patient is placed in the Trendelenburg position to allow the bowel to fall away from the pelvis. If the hernia is unilateral, a 10-mm port is placed on the side of the hernia and a 5-mm port on the contralateral side (Fig. 32.1). For bilateral hernias, two 10-mm ports are inserted laterally, slightly below the level of the umbilicus. All lateral ports should be inserted at the lateral edge of the rectus sheath. The laparoscope is then placed on the ipsilateral side of the hernia, and the surgeon operates from the contralateral side.

Once the trocars are appropriately positioned, the presence and type of hernia(s) are confirmed (Fig. 32.2). A curvilinear incision is first made in the peritoneum (Fig. 32.3) beginning laterally and extending superomedially to the level of the obliterated umbilical vessel (medial umbilical ligament). A flap of peritoneum is created medially by blunt dissection to expose Cooper's ligament (Fig. 32.4). This plane of dissection should be made so that the areolar tissue comes with the peritoneum. Laterally, the loose areolar tissue between the muscular wall and the peritoneum is stripped away in the direction of the muscular wall, leaving only the peritoneum. The dissection is carried medially until the cord structures are identified and dissected free from the peritoneal flap. An indirect sac is usually easily reduced with blunt dissection, but if the sac is large it may be transected with electrocautery.

This dissection provides an adequate preperitoneal space, and a 10 × 14 cm piece of Marlex mesh is placed into the abdomen via the umbilical port and unfurled (Fig. 32.5). The mesh is opened as flat as possible against the abdominal wall, and the indirect, direct, and femoral spaces are covered broadly (Fig. 32.6). The mesh is then stapled to Cooper's ligament and to the superomedial and superolateral corners with a stapler introduced through the umbilical port. Only four to six staples are generally required. Excessive stapling of the mesh increases the risk of nerve injury and should be avoided. Stapling the peritoneal edges together then closes the peritoneal flap. The peritoneum must be tightly opposed

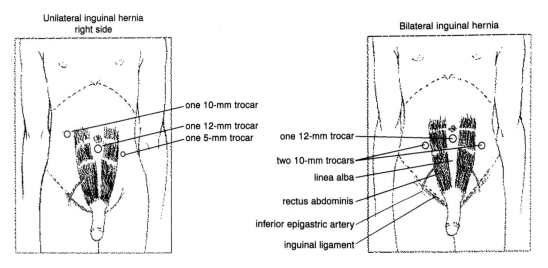

FIGURE 32.1. Trocar positions. Whenever possible, the telescope is positioned on the side of the hernia and the surgeon operates from the opposite side. (Symposium on the management of inguinal hernias: 3. Laparoscopic groin hernia surgery: the TAPP procedure. Reprinted from, by permission of the publisher, *CJS*, 1997; 40(3) pp. 192–198. © 1997 Canadian Medical Association.)

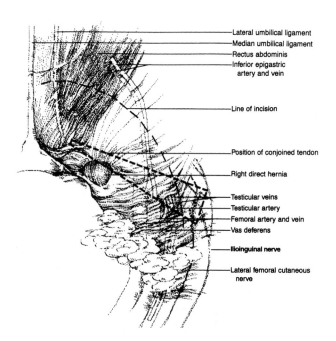

FIGURE 32.2. Posterior inguinal anatomy, showing a direct hernia. Familiarization with the anatomy from this position is of paramount importance to the laparoscopic surgeon. (Symposium on the management of inguinal hernias: 3. Laparoscopic groin hernia surgery: the TAPP procedure. Reprinted from, by permission of the publisher, *CJS*, 1997; 40(3) pp. 192–198. © 1997 Canadian Medical Association.)

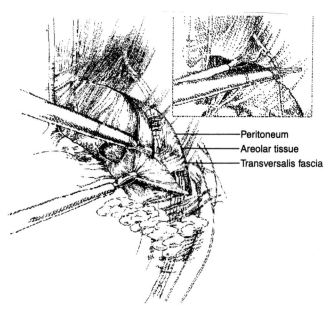

FIGURE 32.3. A curvilinear incision is made in the peritoneum, and a flap is created. Laterally, all attachments to the peritoneum are stripped off toward the abdominal wall. The superior margin (*inset*) is also stripped off the abdominal wall to create a large enough pocket for the mesh. (Symposium on the management of inguinal hernias: 3. Laparoscopic groin hernia surgery: the TAPP procedure. Reprinted from, by permission of the publisher, *CJS*, 1997; 40(3) pp. 192–198. © 1997 Canadian Medical Association.)

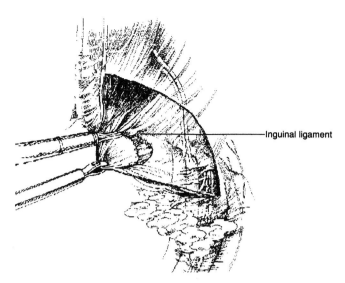

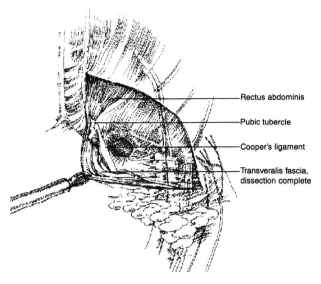

FIGURE 32.4. Medial dissection is carried out on the rectus abdominis. All fibrofatty tissue in this layer is pulled back with the peritoneum. The direct hernial sac is easily reduced with traction and blunt dissection. A reverse "pseudosac" of attenuated transversalis fascia is usually identified and pulled off the true hernial sac. (Symposium on the management of inguinal hernias: 3. Laparoscopic groin hernia surgery: the TAPP procedure. Reprinted from, by permission of the publisher, *CJS*, 1997; 40(3) pp. 192–198. © 1997 Canadian Medical Association.)

FIGURE 32.5. Adequate dissection of a preperitoneal pocket must be carried out to admit a 10 × 14 cm piece of mesh. (Symposium on the management of inguinal hernias: 3. Laparoscopic groin hernia surgery: the TAPP procedure. Reprinted from, by permission of the publisher, *CJS*, 1997; 40(3) pp. 192–198. © 1997 Canadian Medical Association.)

so that there will not be herniation between any gaps in the peritoneum.

Complications

Felix et al., reporting their extensive experience with the TAPP repair, had 9 major complications and 2 recurrences in their first 733 repairs.[30] There were 2 injuries to the small bowel and 1 bowel obstruction; all of these occurred within the first 12 months of the study. In a large multiinstitutional review of hernia recurrences, Felix et al.[34] reported on the reasons for recurrence in both TAPP and TEP repairs at major laparoscopic hernia centers. In this report, there were a total of 25 (0.46%) recurrences associated with 5163 TAPP repairs. Twelve patients recurred due to inadequate lateral fixation. In 3 of these cases, the mesh was also too small. Seven patients recurred due to inadequate medial fixation, and 6 of these also were found to have an inadequate piece of mesh. Four patients had an unrecognized hernia, and 2 had a recurrence through the keyhole in the mesh.

A summary of key studies describing major complications and recurrences using TAPP is shown in Table 32.1. Four major complications—trocar site hernia, bowel injury, bowel obstruction, and neuralgia—are discussed next.

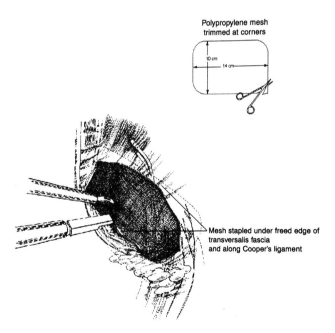

FIGURE 32.6. A standard piece of mesh is placed. It is imperative that the mesh is flat and that there is enough overlay beyond the defect. (Symposium on the management of inguinal hernias: 3. Laparoscopic groin hernia surgery: the TAPP procedure. Reprinted from, by permission of the publisher, *CJS*, 1997; 40(3) pp. 192–198. © 1997 Canadian Medical Association.)

TABLE 32.1. Summary of key studies describing complications and recurrence using the transabdominal preperitoneal approach (TAPP).

Author	Number of Hernias	Recurrence	Complications			
			Trocar hernia	Bowel injury	Bowel obstruction	Neuralgia
MacFadyen (1993)[14]	359	3 (0.8%)	Not reported	Not reported	Not reported	8 (2.2%)
Felix (1995)[30]	733	2 (0.3%)	6 (0.8%)	2 (0.3%)	1 (0.1%)	Not reported
Phillips (1995)[19]	1944	19 (1.0%)	2 (0.1%)	0	4 (0.2%)	35 (1.8%)
Fitzgibbons (1995)[18]	562	28 (5.0%)	—[a]	—[a]	—[a]	5%
Litwin (1997)[20]	632	0	3 (0.5%)	0	4 (0.6%)	11 (1.7%)

[a] Most complications reported were not stratified by type of laparoscopic approach.

Trocar Site Hernia

The risk of trocar site hernia ranges from 0.1% to 1.0%. The most common reason for this complication is failure to properly close the trocar site at the fascial level. To avoid this problem, the surgeon should first understand that all trocar sites greater than 5 mm require closure at the fascial level. This closure should either be done via laparoscopic visualization with a device such as the Endo-Closc (Tyco) or with careful closure externally, making sure to obtain good fascial closure.

Bowel Injury

Bowel injury can occur during the TAPP procedure. However, several large series have been published in which none of these complications was reported.[19,20] The most important factor to consider regarding bowel injury is that one should always remain aware of the entire operative field. Injuries can occur both within and outside the view of the laparoscope. The surgeon must visualize the insertion of each trocar and any instruments that are passed into the abdominal cavity. One must also be careful with the use of electrocautery, and if it is not working properly one must fully investigate for problems with conduction, which could lead to inadvertent bowel injury.

Bowel Obstruction

Bowel obstruction has been reported in 0.1% to 0.6% of hernias repaired. The most common reason for bowel obstruction is incomplete closure of the peritoneal window. This closure can be difficult, especially if the peritoneum is torn during the dissection. Usually, even if there is a tear, the peritoneum can be closed using the articulating stapling device. However, it may be necessary to close this window using a continuous suture.

Neuralgia

Early problems with the TAPP repair included neuralgias, usually caused by nerve entrapment by staples. This complication was a direct result of inadequate knowledge of the pelvic floor anatomy. When these complications first began appearing in the literature, more focus was directed to the anatomy from the laparoscopic point of view, and the incidence of neuralgias seems to be decreasing. The question of whether the mesh even needs fixation has been raised. In fact, Smith et al.[35] performed a prospective randomized trial comparing stapled versus nonstapled TAPP repairs and found no difference in recurrence rates. There was no significant difference with respect to operative time. There was one case of persistent neuralgia in the stapled group and none in the nonstapled group. Of note, these authors were very experienced in the TAPP repair at the time of the study, which may explain their excellent recurrence rate and low incidence of neuralgia. Their results support the use of nonstapled TAPP repairs to minimize the incidence of neuralgias. However, most surgeons remain convinced that fixation is necessary but should be kept to a minimum and should avoid the known areas of concern. The "triangle of doom," a term coined by Spaw and Spaw in 1991,[36] warns the laparoscopic surgeon of the important structures (external iliac vessels, genital branch of the genitofemoral nerve) that lie beneath the peritoneum and the transversalis fascia. Stapling should only be done medial to the vas deferens or lateral to the spermatic vessels. Also, the "triangle of pain" should be avoided, as this was the primary site of staple placement that led to neuralgia.[33] The femoral branch of the genitofemoral nerve, the femoral nerve, and the lateral famoral cutaneous nerve all lie lateral to the spermatic vessels and immediately below the fibers of the iliopubic tract. These nerves are superficial and can be damaged when staples are used below the iliopubic tract.

Mesh Rejection and Infection

Although mesh is used frequently in the repair of both open and laparoscopic hernia repairs, there are documented problems with its use. Late mesh rejection,[37] mesh infection,[38] and an intense inflammatory reaction causing colonic obstruction[39] after TAPP hernia repair have been reported but are infrequent. We recommend the use of routine preoperative Cefazolin, and we soak the mesh in a solution of normal saline and Cefazolin.

References

1. Ger R, Monroe K, Duvivier R, Mishrick A. Management of indirect inguinal hernias by laparoscopic closure of the neck of the sac. Am J Surg 1990;159(4):370–373.
2. Schultz L, Graber J, Pietrafitta J, Hickok D. Laser laparoscopic herniorrhaphy: a clinical trial preliminary results. J Laparoendosc Surg 1990;1(1):41–45.
3. Payne JH Jr, Grininger LM, Izawa MT, et al. Laparoscopic or open inguinal herniorrhaphy? A randomized prospective trial [see comments]. Arch Surg 1994;129(9):973–979; discussion 979–981.
4. Stoker DL, Spiegelhalter DJ, Singh R, Wellwood JM. Laparoscopic versus open inguinal hernia repair: randomised prospective trial [see comments]. Lancet 1994; 343(8908):1243–1245.
5. Barkun JS, Wexler MJ, Hinchey EJ, et al. Laparoscopic versus open inguinal herniorrhaphy: preliminary results of a randomized controlled trial. Surgery (St. Louis) 1995; 118(4):703–709; discussion 709–710.
6. Wilson MS, Deans GT, Brough WA. Prospective trial comparing Lichtenstein with laparoscopic tension-free mesh repair of inguinal hernia [see comments]. Br J Surg 1995; 82(2):274–277.
7. Kozol R, Lange PM, Kosir M, et al. A prospective, randomized study of open vs laparoscopic inguinal hernia repair. An assessment of postoperative pain. Arch Surg 1997;132(3):292–295.
8. Dirksen CD, Beets GL, Go PM, et al. Bassini repair compared with laparoscopic repair for primary inguinal hernia: a randomised controlled trial. Eur J Surg 1998;164(6):439–447.
9. Johansson B, Hallerback B, Glise H, et al. Laparoscopic mesh versus open preperitoneal mesh versus conventional technique for inguinal hernia repair: a randomized multicenter trial (SCUR Hernia Repair Study). Ann Surg 1999; 230(2):225–231.
10. Juul P, Christensen K. Randomized clinical trial of laparoscopic versus open inguinal hernia repair [see comments]. Br J Surg 1999;86(3):316–319.
11. Maddern GJ, Rudkin G, Bessell JR, et al. A comparison of laparoscopic and open hernia repair as a day surgical procedure. Surg Endosc 1994;8(12):1404–1408.
12. Brooks DC. A prospective comparison of laparoscopic and tension-free open herniorrhaphy. Arch Surg 1994; 129(4):361–366.
13. Aitola P, Airo I, Matikainen M. Laparoscopic versus open preperitoneal inguinal hernia repair: a prospec-

tive randomised trial. Ann Chir Gynaecol 1998;87(1): 22–25.
14. MacFadyen BV Jr, Arregui ME, Corbitt JD Jr, et al. Complications of laparoscopic herniorrhaphy [see comments]. Surg Endosc 1993;7(3):155–158.
15. Voeller GR, Mangiante EC, Britt LG. Preliminary evaluation of laparoscopic herniorrhaphy. Surg Laparosc Endosc 1993;3(2):100–105.
16. Tetik C, Arregui ME, Dulucq JL, et al. Complications and recurrences associated with laparoscopic repair of groin hernias. A multi-institutional retrospective analysis. Surg Endosc 1994;8(11):1316–1322; discussion 1322–1323.
17. Felix EL, Michas CA, McKnight RL. Laparoscopic herniorrhaphy. Transabdominal preperitoneal floor repair. Surg Endosc 1994;8(2):100–103; discussion 103–104.
18. Fitzgibbons RJ Jr, Camps J, Cornet DA, et al. Laparoscopic inguinal herniorrhaphy. Results of a multicenter trial [see comments]. Ann Surg 1995;221(1):3–13.
19. Phillips EH, Arregui M, Carroll BJ, et al. Incidence of complications following laparoscopic hernioplasty. Surg Endosc 1995;9(1):16–21.
20. Litwin DE, Pham QN, Oleniuk FH, et al. Laparoscopic groin hernia surgery: the TAPP procedure. Transabdominal preperitoneal hernia repair. Can J Surg 1997;40(3): 192–198.
21. Gilbert AI, Graham MF. Technical and scientific objections to laparoscopic herniorrhaphy. Probl Gen Surg 1995;12:209.
22. Amid PK, Shulman AG, Lichtenstein IL. Objections to laparoscopic herniorrhaphies: results aspect. Probl Gen Surg 1995;12:215.
23. Shurz JW, Cihat T, Arregui ME, Phillips EH. Complications and recurrences associated with laparoscopic inguinal hernia repair. Probl Gen Surg 1995;12:191.
24. Bittner R, Kraft K, Schmedt CG, et al. [Risks and benefits of laparoscopic hernia-plasty (TAPP). 5 years experiences with 3400 hernia repairs]. Chirurg 1998;69(8):854–858.
25. Arregui ME, Davis CJ, Yucel O, Nagan RF. Laparoscopic mesh repair of inguinal hernia using a preperitoneal approach: a preliminary report. Surg Laparosc Endosc 1992;2(1):53–58.
26. Felix EL, Michas C. Double-buttress laparoscopic herniorrhaphy. J Laparoendosc Surg 1993;3(1):1–8.
27. Nyhus LM, Pollak R, Bombeck CT, Donahue PE. The preperitoneal approach and prosthetic buttress repair for recurrent hernia. The evolution of a technique [see comments]. Ann Surg 1988;208(6):733–737.
28. Stoppa RE. The treatment of complicated groin and incisional hernias. World J Surg 1989;13(5):545–554.
29. Sarli L, Pietra N, Choua O, et al. Laparoscopic hernia repair: a prospective comparison of TAPP and IPOM techniques. Surg Laparosc Endosc 1997;7(6):472–476.
30. Felix EL, Michas CA, Gonzalez MH Jr. Laparoscopic hernioplasty. TAPP vs TEP. Surg Endosc 1995;9(9):984–989.
31. Ramshaw BJ, Tucker JG, Mason EM, et al. A comparison of transabdominal preperitoneal (TAPP) and total extraperitoneal approach (TEPA) laparoscopic herniorrhaphies. Am Surg 1995;61(3):279–283.
32. Cohen RV, Alvarez G, Roll S, et al. Transabdominal or totally extraperitoneal laparoscopic hernia repair? Surg Laparosc Endosc 1998;8(4):264–268.

33. Eubanks S, Newman LD, Goehring L, et al. Meralgia paresthetica: a complication of laparoscopic herniorrhaphy. Surg Laparosc Endosc 1993;3(5):381–385.
34. Felix E, Scott S, Crafton B, et al. Causes of recurrence after laparoscopic hernioplasty. A multicenter study. Surg Endosc 1998;12(3):226–231.
35. Smith AI, Royston CM, Sedman PC. Stapled and nonstapled laparoscopic transabdominal preperitoneal (TAPP) inguinal hernia repair. A prospective randomized trial. Surg Endosc 1999;13(8):804–806.
36. Spaw ATEB, Spaw LP. Laparoscopic hernia repair: the anatomic basis. J Laparoendosc Surg 1991;1(5):269–277.
37. Hofbauer C, Andersen PV, Juul P, Qvist N. Late mesh rejection as a complication to transabdominal preperitoneal laparoscopic hernia repair. Surg Endosc 1998;12(9):1164–1165.
38. Avtan L, Avci C, Bulut T, Fourtanier G. Mesh infections after laparoscopic inguinal hernia repair. Surg Laparosc Endosc 1997;7(3):192–195.
39. McDonald D, Chung D. Large bowel obstruction: a postoperative complication after laparoscopic bilateral inguinal hernia repair. J Laparoendosc Adv Surg Tech A 1997;7(3):187–189.

33
Laparoscopic Totally Extraperitoneal Repair for Inguinal Hernias

Jonathan D. Spitz and Maurice E. Arregui

The large number of differing operations performed for the repair of inguinal hernia attests to the fact that no perfect method currently exists. Laparoscopic herniorrhaphy began at a time when most surgeons in the United States were performing primary tissue repairs of the McVay, Bassini, or Shouldice method.[1] More recently, the tension-free anterior mesh repair championed by Lichtenstein has become the standard, with reported recurrence rates less than 1%.[2] Unfortunately, this same level of success has not been universally realized. Additionally, the various anterior repairs are associated with greater patient discomfort and longer recovery, and there is a risk of missing a contralateral or femoral defect. Laparoscopic hernia repair developed from a search for a more effective, less painful method of herniorrhaphy. The evolution of laparoscopic hernia repair has progressed from simple ring closure, to intraperitoneal onlay mesh, to transabdominal preperitoneal mesh repair (TAPP), to the totally extraperitoneal technique (TEP). The laparoscopic extraperitoneal repair represents the culmination of experience gained from earlier laparoscopic methods, and our approach functions as an uncompromising copy of the open preperitoneal large mesh repair described by Stoppa et al.[3] We have had excellent success with the suture-less laparoscopic extraperitoneal herniorrhaphy. In this chapter, we describe the pertinent fascial planes of the extraperitoneal spaces and our surgical technique. Attention is given to lessons learned in the course of our experience.

Anatomy of Preperitoneal Fascias

The technique of laparoscopic hernia repair has evolved more than any other laparoscopic procedure. This evolution is the result of a more complete understanding of the fascial anatomy of the preperitoneal spaces. The preperitoneal repair as we perform it follows a series of discrete, well-developed maneuvers based upon a thorough understanding of the region's anatomy. Our understanding of this anatomy comes from cadaveric dissections, open anterior and preperitoneal hernia repairs, and experience gained from performing transabdominal preperitoneal and totally extraperitoneal herniorrhaphy.

In repairing an inguinal hernia using a preperitoneal approach, there are several important spaces, fascial layers, and nerve and vascular structures to consider. A key principle to understand is that there is a true preperitoneal space that is distinct from the posterior rectus space (Fig. 33.1). The supposition that the posterior rectus fascia ends at the level of the arcuate line is erroneous. In fact, the posterior rectus sheath extends to Cooper's ligament, but although it is well developed above the arcuate line, it becomes attenuated caudally.[4] Blunt dissection through these fibers is required to gain entry into the true preperitoneal space. This true preperitoneal space is in direct continuity with the space of Retzius, below Cooper's ligament, within the pelvis.

Understanding that the posterior rectus sheath exists to the level of Cooper's ligament helps one visualize the relationship of the preperitoneal space, the space of Retzius, and the lateral inguinal space. To access the lateral inguinal compartment from the posterior rectus space, the anterior attachments of the posterior rectus sheath must be taken down. As with the rest of the rectus sheath, the fascia is thicker and stronger proximally, such that scissors are needed to get through. The distal portion of the posterior rectus sheath, which extends to the origin and lateral to the inferior epigastric vessels, is more attenuated and can be taken down bluntly. The lateral inguinal space is opened so that a large piece of mesh may be used.

Deep to the posterior rectus sheath is the umbilical prevesicular fascia. This thin layer is the investing fascia of the bladder and medial umbilical ligaments. It also covers the vas deferens and the other cord structures, including an indirect hernia sac if one is present. The umbilical prevesicular fascia persists as the internal spermatic fascia as the cord structures enter the inguinal canal.

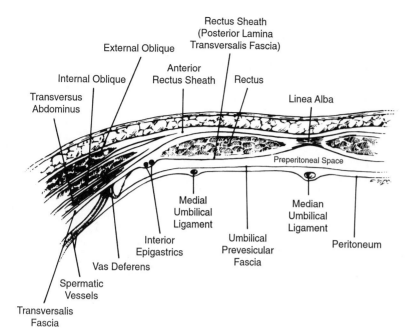

Transversus Abdominus

Internal Oblique

External Oblique

Rectus Sheath (Posterior Lamina Transversalis Fascia)

Anterior Rectus Sheath

Rectus

Linea Alba

Preperitoneal Space

Medial Umbilical Ligament

Interior Epigastrics

Vas Deferens

Spermatic Vessels

Transversalis Fascia

Umbilical Prevesicular Fascia

Median Umbilical Ligament

Peritoneum

FIGURE 33.1. Transverse view of the preperitoneal space and fascias at the level of the internal inguinal ring. Note that the posterior rectus space is separated from the preperitoneal space by the posterior rectus sheath. (Reproduced with permission from Arregui ME. Transabdominal retroperitoneal inguinal herniorrhaphy. In: MacFadyen BV, Ponsky JL (eds) Operative Laparoscopy and Thoracoscopy. Philadelphia: Lippincott-Raven, 1996.

Nerves destined for distribution to the thigh and to the abdominal wall pass in proximity to the iliopubic tract and are in jeopardy when staples or sutures are placed lateral to the internal inguinal ring (Fig. 33.2).[5,6] The so-called triangle of doom is defined medially by the vas deferens and laterally by the spermatic vessels. Within these confines lie the external iliac artery and vein, the femoral nerve, and the genital branch of the genitofemoral nerve. Outside this triangle, however, other nerves, including the femoral branch of the genitofemoral nerve and the lateral femoral cutaneous nerve, are in danger. The ilioinguinal and the iliopubic nerves do not lie below the iliopubic tract but are at risk if staples are placed anteriorly.

Indications and Patient Selection

The extraperitoneal approach has been advocated for adult patients with recurrent hernias because it avoids scar tissue from previous anterior repairs. It is also ideally suited for patients with bilateral groin defects as both sides can be repaired during a single anesthetic using the same incisions. Although there are clear advantages to the laparoscopic extraperitoneal repair for recurrent or bilateral defects, the benefits of unilateral TEP or its use for primary inguinal hernias are less clear. However, for patients with active or physical careers, there is a more rapid return to preoperative performance status with the laparoscopic repair.[7,8] Additionally, the wide dissection that we describe develops the entire myopectineal orifice so that concomitant femoral or obturator hernias are not missed and lipomas of the cord can also be identified and reduced. Because of our success with the laparoscopic

TEP, we recommend this approach to patients with recurrent or bilateral defects. All patients, however, are given the option of laparoscopic TEP if no contraindications exist.

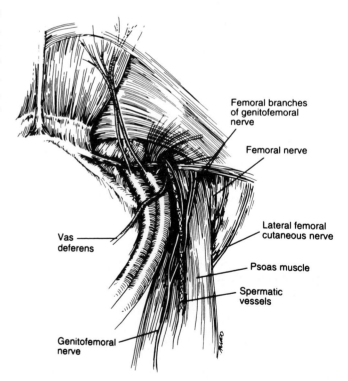

Femoral branches of genitofemoral nerve

Femoral nerve

Lateral femoral cutaneous nerve

Psoas muscle

Spermatic vessels

Vas deferens

Genitofemoral nerve

FIGURE 33.2. Nerves and vessels of the preperitoneal inguinal space. (Reproduced with permission from Arregui ME. Transabdominal retroperitoneal inguinal herniorrhaphy. In: MacFadyen BV, Ponsky JL (eds) Operative Laparoscopy and Thoracoscopy. Philadelphia: Lippincott-Raven, 1996.)

The only absolute contraindication to laparoscopic herniorraphy is the high-risk patient who is not fit for general anesthesia. For these patients, we recommend the anterior mesh repair under local anesthetic. Previous lower abdominal surgery can cause difficulty in performing the preperitoneal dissection, and early studies suggested that complications such as bladder injury or peritoneal tears were more common among these patients.[9,10] We have found, by using a blunt instrument to create the preperitoneal pocket under direct vision rather than the balloon dissector, that we have been able to avoid bowel and bladder injury. The scar tissue at the site of the previous surgery is cut with scissors to separate the peritoneum and fascia from the rectus muscle or other components of the anterior abdominal wall.

Preoperative preparation for laparoscopic hernia repair is straightforward. Patients with abnormal bowel or bladder function are routinely evaluated for colon or prostate pathology. Routine laboratory studies are not indicated for asymptomatic, clinically normal patients. The patient is instructed to refrain from eating after midnight the day before surgery, and smokers are requested to not smoke for 24h before operation. Anticoagulation or antiplatelet therapy is discontinued to allow normal hemostasis at the time of surgery.

Surgical Technique

The technique of laparoscopic extraperitoneal inguinal hernia repair may be broken down into its component parts. There are generally eight key steps in the successful completion of laparoscopic TEP: transperitoneal inspection, extraperitoneal trocar placement, dissection of the posterior rectus space, entry into the true preperitoneal space with wide dissection of the myopectineal orifice, reduction and ligation of the hernia sac or lipoma of the cord, parietalization of the spermatic cord, placement of a large mesh, and transperitoneal inspection of the mesh position.

We do not use preoperative antibiotic prophylaxis, and we ask the patient to void immediately before transport to the operating room, which obviates the need for a urinary catheter. Following the administration of general anesthesia the patient is positioned supine with the arms tucked at the sides. The abdomen and groin are prepared with standard surgical scrub, and the video monitor is positioned at the foot of the table. The operating team consists of the surgeon and one assistant or scrub nurse. The surgeon stands on the side opposite the hernia while the assistant most comfortably controls the camera from the other side of the operating table. A Veress needle at the umbilicus is used to establish a pneumoperitoneum, and, once complete, a 5-mm trocar is placed. A 30° angled 5-mm laparoscope is used to inspect the groin bilaterally

(Fig. 33.3). Anterior palpation over the external ring, massaging toward the internal ring, may reduce a clinically significant cord lipoma. If there is a previously unappreciated contralateral hernia or if the patient was thought to have bilateral hernias on a preoperative physical exam, but no peritoneal defect is identified at the time of transperitoneal inspection, then bilateral preperitoneal exploration is performed. In this latter case there may be a lipoma of the spermatic cord or a small direct inguinal hernia that is not detectable transperitoneally.

Herniorrhaphy is accomplished using a two-handed technique via three extraperitoneal trocars. The first 5-mm trocar is placed into the lateral aspect of the posterior rectus space just superior to the arcuate line on the index side. Care must be taken to avoid penetrating the peritoneum. Correct positioning is assured with the aid of the intraperitoneal laparoscopic view (Fig. 33.4). The transversely oriented arcuate line is roughly 2cm inferior to the umbilicus. Through this first trocar, a blunt-tipped grasper is used to develop the posterior rectus space by dissection of the posterior rectus sheath from the posterior aspect of the rectus muscle and the inferior epigastric vessels. Once the dissection is begun, the 5-mm laparoscope can be introduced into the posterior rectus space and the blunt dissection continued with the tip of the laparoscope. The pneumoperitoneum is released and the posterior rectus space is insufflated to 12 to 15mmHg. The posterior rectus space is developed across the midline by bluntly taking down the medial anterior attachments of the rectus sheath. Then, a second 5-mm or 10-mm extraperitoneal trocar is introduced 2cm inferior to the umbilicus. The laparoscope is repositioned to this midline port, and the blunt dissection is continued to identify the pubis and Cooper's ligament. For unilateral repair, a 5-mm extraperitoneal trocar is placed midway

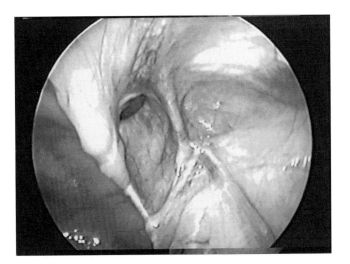

FIGURE 33.3. Transperitoneal inspection of the groin. This patient has a right direct inguinal hernia.

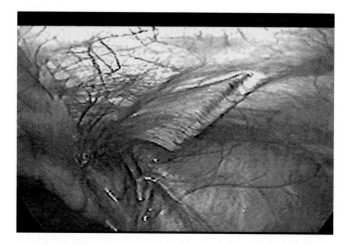

FIGURE 33.4. The intraperitoneal laparoscopic view guides placement of the first trocar into the posterior rectus space.

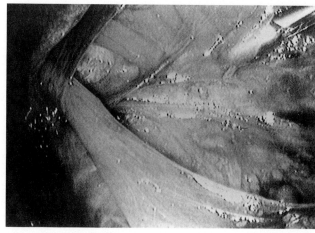

FIGURE 33.5. The umbilical prevesicular fascia is the investing fascia of the bladder. It extends laterally to cover the spermatic cord and the contained indirect hernia sac as seen here. It becomes the internal spermatic fascia as the spermatic cord enters the inguinal canal.

between the pubis and the umbilicus in the midline. If bilateral herniorrhaphy is to be performed, this trocar is placed just superior to the arcuate line on the contralateral side.

As already discussed, the posterior rectus space is distinct from the true preperitoneal space. The preperitoneal space is a direct continuation of the space of Retzius within the pelvis and is entered by bluntly breaking through the attenuated caudal fibers of the posterior rectus sheath. At the level of the umbilicus, the peritoneum and umbilical preperitoneal fascia are adherent to the posterior rectus sheath; thus, attempts to develop the potential plane at this level are met with difficulty and peritoneal tears are likely. By staying one plane more superficial and then entering the preperitoneal space within the pelvis where the posterior rectus sheath is more attenuated, it is much easier to avoid injury to the peritoneal membrane. Some surgeons rely on the disposable balloon dissector to perform the preperitoneal dissection. We have found that blunt dissection in the correct avascular plane more completely accomplishes the task without the considerable and unnecessary expense or the risk of peritoneal or visceral injury.

With the laparoscope in the infraumbilical position, the surgeon uses two blunt instruments to clear the pubis and Cooper's ligament of the attenuated adventitial attachments of the posterior rectus sheath; this allows entry into the space of Retzius. The femoral and obturator spaces can be inspected. Laterally, the anterior attachments of the posterior rectus fascia limit access into the lateral inguinal space. To place a large piece of mesh that must extend laterally beyond the internal ring, these well-developed fibers are taken down with scissors.

There is a thin fascial layer that invests the indirect hernia sac (if present), the vas deferens, and the other cord structures. This fascia is called the umbilical prevesicular fascia, and it must be opened to isolate an indirect hernia (Fig. 33.5). By gently teasing the fibers apart, the indirect sac and cord contents can be identified (Fig. 33.6). A cord lipoma is located just lateral to the cord structures. Anterior palpation over the external ring, massaging toward the internal ring, often helps to reduce the lipoma so that it may be excised. The indirect sac may be completely reduced and ligated or, if it extends well into the inguinal canal and cannot be safely reduced, it can be proximally ligated and distally divided. We routinely ligate the sac to eliminate the possibility of an internal hernia developing from the persistent peritoneal

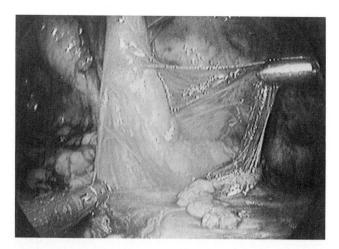

FIGURE 33.6. The umbilical prevesicular fascia (or spermatic fascia at this level) is opened by teasing the fibers apart; this is necessary to identify the indirect hernia sac.

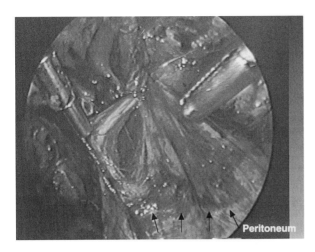

FIGURE 33.7. Parietalization of the spermatic cord. The peritoneum is mobilized posteriorly so that a large mesh can be placed. The vas deferens is being elevated by traction on the umbilical prevesicular fascia.

sac. Direct hernia sacs consist of the attenuated fibers of the transversalis fascia, which have evaginated into the inguinal canal. If the sac is large, it may accumulate fluid postoperatively and account for a persistent mass effect. To prevent this, we reduce and either ligate the sac with a looped absorbable tie or invert the sac by stitching it to Cooper's ligament.

As an alternative to the circumferential mobilization of the spermatic cord and making a slit in the mesh, Stoppa developed the technique of "parietalization" of the spermatic cord.[3] This technique involves the posterior mobilization of the peritoneum from the spermatic cord structures (Fig. 33.7). This mobilization is performed to a point proximal to the confluence of the vas deferens and the spermatic vessels at about the level where the vas deferens dives posteriorly. With such an extended exposure, the mesh can be placed between the cord structures and the peritoneum. This sandwiching of the mesh is our approach to mesh fixation, preventing it from migrating or rolling up (which is the proposed mechanism for recurrent herniation following preperitoneal mesh repair). Circumferential placement of mesh around the spermatic cord can lead to injury of the genital branch of the genitofemoral nerve or constriction of the cord vessels. The gap in the mesh can also be a site for recurrent herniation. Any tear in the peritoneum is repaired with a looped chromic tie to maintain preperitoneal insufflation and to eliminate the risk of bowel herniation through the peritoneal defect.

Once the dissection is complete, a piece of Mersilene mesh is prepared to 5 in. by 6 in. with a curved cutout for the cord structures (Fig. 33.8). It is introduced into the preperitoneal space and manipulated to widely cover the myopectineal orifice with overlap of the direct, indirect, obturator, and femoral spaces. Earlier in our experience we used Prolene mesh; however, this material is less pliable and thicker than Mersilene and consequently needed a 10-mm trocar to be introduced. Because it is stiffer the Prolene is easier to position, but there is the theoretical risk that the more rigid material will erode through the peritoneum and be exposed to the bowel, although we have never seen this happen. Mersilene is very flexible and readily adapts to the irregular configuration of the abdominal wall. The final position of the mesh extends across the midline and into the space of Retzius; it is draped across the spermatic cord and into the lateral inguinal space (Fig. 33.9). If bilateral hernias exist, then two pieces of mesh that overlap in the midline are used. No suture or staple fixation is needed with preperitoneal mesh placement because the mesh will be held in place by the intraabdominal pressure against the posterior abdominal wall until its incorporation into the tissues.

Before completion, we reinstitute the pneumoperitoneum and release the preperitoneal insufflation. We inspect the mesh in its preperitoneal position to ensure that it has not folded or moved. Once we are satisfied with the mesh position, the patient is taken out of Trendelenburg so that the bowel will fall into the pelvis. The CO_2 insufflation is evacuated, and the skin incisions are closed with subcutaneous 3-0 vicryl suture. If a 10-mm trocar is used a fascial closure is performed. Collodion (Paddock Laboratories, Minneapolis, MN, USA) applied to the trocar incisions serves as the dressing. Patients are observed in the recovery area and are typically discharged following a 1- to 3-h stay. No restrictions are placed on activity other than to avoid driving for 3 to 4 days.

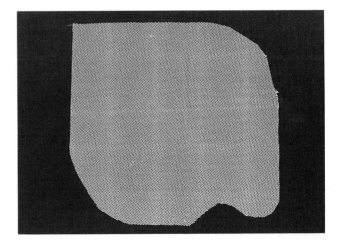

FIGURE 33.8. Mersilene mesh (5 in. × 6 in.). The superomedial corner is left square to orient the mesh.

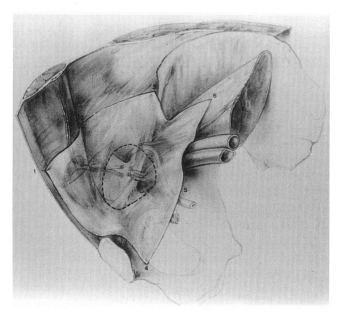

FIGURE 33.9. Correct coverage of the entire myopectineal orifice. In our repairs, we cross the midline with the medial portion of the mesh. The peritoneum will sandwich the mesh to the anterior abdominal wall. (Reproduced with permission from Wantz G. Atlas of Hernia Surgery. Philadelphia: Lippincott/Williams & Wilkins, 1989.)

Complications

Complications associated with laparoscopic herniorrhaphy have been described in a number of publications.[11–13] Most of the complications such as seroma, hematoma, local wound infection, and urinary retention are minor, transient, and common to both laparoscopic and open hernia repair. We have adopted the routine practice of either ligating or inverting the direct hernia sac to limit the space available for postoperative fluid accumulation. We also excise clinically significant cord lipomas. Transient testicular pain likely occurs from the dissection of cord structures and the associated trauma to the sympathetic innervation of the testis.[1] Careful dissection with minimal manipulation of the cord structures helps to reduce pain resulting from the trauma to those structures.

Serious complications have also been reported, and some are unique to the laparoscopic approach. Bowel obstructions can occur at the sites of trocar penetration (Richter's hernia) or through an unrecognized peritoneal defect. If, in the course of parietalization of the spermatic cord, a tear is made in the peritoneum, we close it with a looped chromic tie. The indirect hernia sac may also be a source of bowel obstruction. We ligate the indirect sac before reducing it to eliminate the possibility of an internal incarcerated hernia. Nerve injuries can occur to the genitofemoral, lateral femoral cutaneous, ilioinguinal, iliohypogastric, and the femoral nerves. These nerve injuries are usually the result of a misplaced staple. The preperitoneal hernia repair sandwiches the mesh between the peritoneum and the anterior abdominal wall. We and others have recognized that no fixation is needed.[14,15] In our series of more than 200 suture-less preperitoneal repairs, we have not realized any nerve injury. By operating in the preperitoneal space, the risk of bowel or bladder injury is theoretically reduced. However, prior lower abdominal surgery does increase the risk of hollow organ injury. The balloon dissector has also been associated with bowel, bladder, and vascular injury, especially among this group of patients.[10,16]

Recurrences

Recurrence is often considered the endpoint in the evaluation of a given hernia repair. When one considers the recurrence rate of all currently performed open repairs, it is approximately 10%.[2] In a retrospective review of 10,053 laparoscopic hernia repairs (TAPP or TEP), Felix et al. considered reasons for failure following laparoscopic hernia repair.[17] In this series, 35 patients (0.4%) developed recurrent defects during a follow-up extending from 1 month to 6 years (median, 36 months). All but 1 of the recurrences was reexplored and the cause of the failure identified as one of the following: inadequate lateral fixation of the mesh, inadequate lateral fixation compounded by too small a mesh, missed lipoma of the cord, inadequate medial fixation of the mesh to Cooper's ligament, a missed hernia, or a hernia through a keyhole in the mesh. We have found that with experience the preperitoneal dissection becomes wider and more thorough, permitting placement of a much larger mesh and eliminating the possibility of a missed defect. With a sufficiently large piece of mesh, the need for fixation with staples, tacks, or suture is avoided, and with wide parietalization of the cord there is no need to make a keyhole in the mesh.

Phillips et al. also considered the technical factors that contribute to recurrence following laparoscopic herniorrhaphy.[12] The most common reason was the use of a mesh that was too small. Less common reasons for failure were inadequate fixation and missed defects.

In a multi-institutional review of 1514 laparoscopic hernia repairs, Tetik et al. compared recurrence rates following repair by plug and patch, ring closure, intraperitoneal onlay mesh (IPOM), TAPP, and TEP.[11] The recurrence rates were 22%, 3%, 2.2%, 0.7%, and 0.4% respectively. The favorable recurrence rate associated with TEP in this series was attributed to a more complete dissection and better coverage of the entire myopectineal orifice with a large mesh.

TABLE 33.1. Disposable versus reusable instrument costs.

Disposable item	Cost	Reusable
Trocar	$93 each	$420
Balloon dissector	$175	—
Hernia stapler	$163	—
Totals	$617 (for three trocars)	NA

Source: Modified with permission from Paik PS, Anthone G: Laparoscopic appendectomy. In: Cameron JL (ed) Current Surgical Therapy. St. Louis: Mosby, 1998.

TABLE 33.3. Worker's compensation.

Number of workdays lost per 100 employees	
1972	47.9
1989	78.8
Worker's compensation	
1982	$23 billion
1990	$50 billion

Data from Bureau of Labor Statistics.
Source: From Crossland FT, Perkins JA. Disability income and loss of productivity. In: Arregui ME, Nagan RF (eds) Inguinal Hernia: Advances or Controversies? Oxford: Radcliffe, 1994.

In our series, approximately 17% of laparoscopic repairs were performed for recurrent defects following anterior repairs. Among this series of 203 herniorrhaphies, we have not realized any recurrences during follow-up extending 5 years (mean, 22 months). This success is attributed to several factors including thorough transperitoneal inspection to assess for multiple or bilateral myopectineal orifice defects, wide preperitoneal dissection with a search for a cord lipoma, placement of a large piece of mesh, and transperitoneal confirmation of correct mesh position before closure. This extraperitoneal hernia repair is the laparoscopic counterpart of Stoppa's open preperitoneal repair termed the giant prosthetic replacement of the visceral sac (GPRVS). We use a large mesh that is held in place by the intraabdominal pressure pushing against the anterior abdominal wall. No fixation is necessary. The larger mesh dimension not only repairs the current defect, but it also reinforces the entire myopectineal orifice to prevent a future hernia from an adjacent area. We routinely ligate or invert the direct hernia sac of attenuated transversalis fascia, which eliminates the dead space available for accumulation of fluid. Although not a recurrence, this fluid can cause a persistent mass effect after surgery, giving the patient the sense that the hernia was not repaired. If a hematoma or seroma occurs, ultrasound can confirm that this is not a hernia and the patient thus reassured.

Cost Considerations

Inguinal hernia repair is the second most common surgical procedure in the United States, accounting for more than 750,000 operations per year. The current climate of

TABLE 33.2. Employee replacement costs.

Category	Cost per day
Clerical	$105
Skilled blue collar	$145

Source: Reproduced with permission from Paik PS, Anthone G. Laparoscopic appendectomy. In: Cameron JL (ed) Current Surgical Therapy. St. Louis: Mosby, 1998.

health care economics demands that costs be minimized without compromising patient outcome. This fact has been a deterrent to the acceptance of laparoscopic hernia repair. However, although some specialized equipment is needed, by and large this same equipment is used in the ever-increasing applications of laparoscopic surgery. A general anesthetic is used but is safely administered on an outpatient basis. All other items such as disposable trocars, staplers, and the balloon dissector are unnecessary and add to the cost. Table 33.1 shows the costs associated with various disposable instruments at our Indianapolis facility.

An analysis of the overall cost-effectiveness of laparoscopic hernia repair must also consider, in addition to operative costs, the length of recovery time off work and the long-term recurrence rate. Tables 33.2 and 33.3 show the employee replacement and worker's compensation costs in Indiana. Several recent studies have confirmed that patients are able to return to work sooner following laparoscopic hernia repair than after open repair.[7,18,19] It is unclear at present whether the savings related to decreased pain and more rapid recovery offset the higher surgical cost of the laparoscopic approach. For employers, certainly this is an important consideration.

References

1. Arregui ME. Laparoscopic inguinal herniorrhaphy. In: Cameron JL (ed) Current Surgical Therapy. St. Louis: Mosby, 1998:1186–1191.
2. Amid PK, Shulman AG, Lichtenstein IL. Critical scrutiny of the open tension-free hernioplasty. Am J Surg 1993;165:369–371.
3. Stoppa R, Petit I, Henry X. Unsutured dacron prosthesis in inguinal hernias. Int Surg 1975;60:411–412.
4. Arregui ME. Surgical anatomy of the preperitoneal fasciae and posterior transversalis fascia in the inguinal region. Hernia 1997;1:101–110.
5. Colborn GL, Brick WG, Gadacz TR, Skandalakis JE. Inguinal anatomy for laparoscopic herniorrhaphy. Part I: The normal anatomy. Surg Rounds 1995;18:189–198.
6. Colborn GL, Brick WG, Gadacz TR, Skandalakis JE. Inguinal anatomy for laparoscopic herniorrhaphy. Part II:

Altered inguinal anatomy and variations. Surg Rounds 1995;18:223–232.

7. Payne JH, Grininger LM, Izawa MT, Podoll EF, Lindahl PJ, Balfour J. Laparoscopic or open inguinal herniorrhaphy? A randomized prospective trial. Arch Surg 1994;129:973–981.

8. Tanphiphat C, Tanprayoon T, Sangsubhan C, Chatamra K. Laparoscopic vs open inguinal hernia repair. Surg Endosc 1988;12:846–851.

9. Ramshaw BJ, Tucker JG, Mason EM, et al. A comparison of transabdominal preperitoneal (TAPP) and total extraperitoneal approach (TEPA) laparoscopic herniorrhaphies. Am Surg 1995;61:279–283.

10. Ramshaw BJ, Tucker JG, Conner T, Mason EM, Duncan TD, Lucas GW. A comparison of the approaches to laparoscopic herniorrhaphy. Surg Endosc 1996;10:29–32.

11. Tetik C, Arregui ME, Dulucq JL. Complications and recurrences associated with laparoscopic repair of groin hernias: a multi-institutional retrospective analysis. Surg Endosc 1994;8:1316–1323.

12. Phillips EH, Arregui ME, Carroll BJ, et al. Incidence of complications following laparoscopic hernioplasty. Surg Endosc 1995;9:16–21.

13. Ger R. Laparoscopic repair of groin hernias: a clinicoanatomic review. Part II. Surg Rounds 1994:395–401.

14. Van Steensel CJ, Weidema WF. Laparoscopic inguinal hernia repair without fixation of the prosthesis. In: Arregui ME, Nagan RF (eds) Inguinal Hernia: Advances or Controversies? Oxford: Radcliffe, 1994:435–436.

15. Wegner ME, Arregui ME. Laparoscopic totally extraperitoneal herniorrhaphy. Probl Gen Surg 1995;12(2):185–190.

16. Fiennes AGTW. The Kieturakis balloon dissector: an aid to the extraperitoneal approach for laparoscopic repair of groin hernias? Endosc Surg 1994;2:221–225.

17. Felix E, Scott S, Crafton B, Geis P, et al. Causes of recurrence after laparoscopic hernioplasty: a multicenter study. Surg Endosc 1998;12:226–231.

18. Liem MSL, van der Graaf Y, van Steensel CJ, et al. Comparison of conventional anterior surgery and laparoscopic surgery for inguinal hernia repair. N Engl J Med 1997;336: 22.

19. Millikan KW, Deziel DJ. The management of hernia: considerations in cost effectiveness. Surg Clin N Am 1996;76: 105–115.

34
Complications and Recurrences of Laparoscopic Hernia Repairs

Edward L. Felix

In the United States, more than 700,000 hernias are repaired each year,[1] and an increasing number of the repairs are approached laparoscopically. The initial enthusiasm for the laparoscopic approach, however, was tempered by reports of complications and recurrences.[2–4] This enthusiasm is once again justified as multiple hernia centers and practicing general surgeons around the world have reported extremely low recurrence rates and complication rates that have been equal to or lower than reported for open repairs.[5–8] The improved outcomes have been the result of an accumulation of experience and knowledge of which makes the laparoscopic approach work. Understanding which factors may lead to failure or complications has been key to improving the benchmark for laparoscopic hernioplasty. There are some situations that can be avoided altogether and others that if handled properly will result in a favorable outcome. The purpose of this chapter is to discuss these issues so that surgeons performing laparoscopic hernioplasty may benefit from the experience of others who have already faced these problems.

To better evaluate the results of laparoscopic hernia repair, one must first understand the problems that open or traditional hernia repairs have had. The worldwide morbidity of open repairs ranges from less than 1% to more than 25%, with an average recurrence rate of 10%.[9] Reports from centers or surgeons with extensive experience, however, are in the 1% to 2% range.[10] The percent of patients experiencing pain or numbness lasting more than a year after open repairs has been reported to be as great as 25%,[11] and a recent survey has demonstrated that as many as 5% of patients following hernioplasty reported postoperative discomfort to be worse than the symptoms from the original hernia.[12] Some complications that occur after laparoscopic repairs are identical to those of open traditional or prosthetic repairs; others are unique to the laparoscopic approach. In addition, each laparoscopic approach, transabdominal peritoneal (TAPP) and totally extraperitoneal (TEP), has its own inherent risks, and these are stressed in this chapter.

The Learning Curve

The early days of laparoscopic cholecystectomy taught us that even when surgeons are considered to be experts at performing a procedure using conventional open techniques, their ability to perform the same procedure with a new laparoscopic approach may fall short of the mark.[13] Our own study,[14] as well as those of others,[15,16] has shown that the complication rate after laparoscopic hernioplasty is reduced by experience. Average operative time appears to be a good measure of this experience. Stoker et al.[17] and Liem et al.[18] have shown that operative time correlates inversely with experience. In several controlled studies that have failed to show any benefit of laparoscopic hernioplasty, surgeons were early in the learning phase of the approach, as measured by operative times in excess of 60 min.[19] In contrast, our study of more than 10,000 laparoscopic hernioplasties performed by surgeons with extensive experience, more than 500 repairs per surgeon, the average recurrence rate was less than 1%.[5] The incidence of conversion from a laparoscopic approach to an open approach, or from a TEP to a TAPP approach also correlated with the complication[14] and recurrence rates.[16] The incidence, however, decreased with experience. With experience, surgeons were better able to select appropriate patients for laparoscopic repair and prevent or handle peritoneal tears during TEP procedures that otherwise would have caused conversion.

Several other studies have shown that recurrence rate as well as complication rate decrease with experience.[18,20,21] The incidence of recurrence for surgeons in these studies was decreased as experience was gained during the studies. Technical errors were a common cause of failure early in these studies but were reduced with experience.

When laparoscopic hernioplasty first began, there were an insufficient number of surgeons to mentor new surgeons who wanted to perfect the approach. Because laparoscopic hernioplasty is one of the most difficult laparoscopic procedures to master, the result was a failure of many surgeons to have a successful experience. Frustrated by poor results, these surgeons no longer utilize the laparoscopic approach. Proper training, however, can shorten the learning curve and the number of complications and recurrences.[16] In our hernia center, a stepwise teaching approach has allowed new surgeons to become experts in the laparoscopic approach to hernia repair. By borrowing from the experience of a mentor or more experienced laparoscopist and by beginning with less complicated hernias, our new surgeons have learned how to approach primary and recurrent hernias, achieving recurrence rates of less than 1% and complication rates that are comparable to open repairs.

Causes and Prevention of Recurrence

Traditionally, recurrence has been considered the most important complication of hernia repair, and understanding its etiology is the key to preventing it. The causes of recurrence have been well investigated[22] and many approaches proposed to eliminate them. Buttressing the wall with mesh to overcome intrinsic weakness or tension has been one of the most effective methods devised. Missed hernias due to failure to recognize a complex hernia at the primary operation has been shown to be the cause of recurrence in approximately 15% of failed repairs.[22,23] The laparoscopic approach, if performed properly, succeeds because it not only buttresses the wall but also virtually eliminates missed hernias.[24] Technical errors account for the other recurrences after hernia repair and appear to be the main cause of recurrence after laparoscopic repair.[5]

Review of our multicenter experience[5] with more than 7000 patients and more than 10,000 laparoscopic repairs helps explain why laparoscopic repairs recur. The TEP and TAPP approaches were equally effective in repairing inguinal hernias, if the expertise of the surgeons was equal and the appropriate approach was chosen.[25] Some patients are better repaired using a TAPP approach whereas others are better served with a TEP or even an open repair (Table 34.1). For example, approaching incarcerated hernias with a TEP technique using a balloon dissector may tear the peritoneum and lead to further complications or recurrence.[14,16] Patients with previous pelvic irradiation may have an obliterated extraperitoneal space making dissection difficult or even impossible; this may lead to recurrence from an overlooked or missed hernia. Therefore, the hernia surgeon should first decide if the patient is a candidate for a laparoscopic repair (Fig. 34.1) and then decide which repair is most appropriate for this patient according to the hernia and the surgeon's experience.

Missed hernias were found in 11% of the failures in our multicenter review, but all were seen early in the surgeon's experience. As in Phillips' review,[26] once surgeons became experienced in the laparoscopic approach, this problem was eliminated. Although no missed hernias were found after any TEP repair in our series, this approach was not immune to a similar problem, the retained or missed lipoma. One-third of the TEP repairs that failed were the result of failing to remove a lipoma from the indirect canal. It has therefore become routine to clear the iliopubic tract of fat to avoid leaving behind a lipoma that is draped over the internal ring into the canal.

In our review, inadequate lateral fixation of mesh was one of the most common causes of failure: 36% of TAPP and 22% of TEP repairs that recurred. Because of the location of major nerves, the mesh cannot be anchored with staples below the iliopubic tract; this limitation makes the mesh vulnerable to being lifted off the lateral wall, which will lead to an indirect or lateral recurrence. In the TEP repair there may be a tendency not to dissect the peritoneum far enough off the cord structures to allow the mesh to lie under the peritoneum. This problem can be prevented by completely dissecting the lateral wall. The peritoneal edge must be dissected beyond the point where the proximal edge of the mesh will lie. In addition, in the TEP approach the mesh must be held down with a grasper as the CO_2 is evacuated to prevent the mesh from being lifted by the expanding peritoneum.

In TAPP repairs, as the peritoneum is closed, the cord structures may be tented upward by the peritoneum. To prevent this, some surgeons in our study utilized a slit in the mesh that placed the mesh under the testicular vessels

TABLE 34.1. The laparoscopic approach tailored to hernia type.

	Simple	Bilateral	Large Scrotal	Incarcerated	Recurrent	Diagnostic	Pelvic incision: trans/midline
TAPP			X	X	X	X	X
TEP	X	X			X		X

TAPP, transabdominal peritoneal approach; TEP, totally extraperitoneal approach.

FIGURE 34.1. Practical scheme for choosing the surgical approach according to the surgeon's experience and complexity of the hernia.

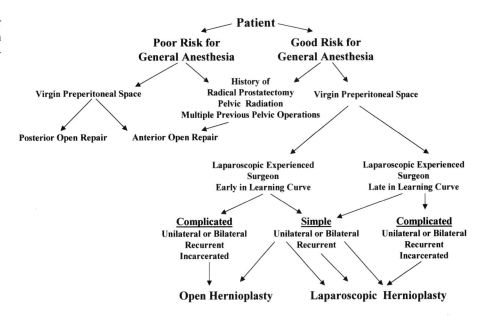

and vas deferens. This keyhole, however, was responsible for 15% of recurrences and one-third of the TEP failures. An additional mesh placed over the keyhole prevented this number from being even higher. My personal approach is now to use a keyholed mesh in only selected situations and then to cover it to prevent herniation through the opening. Other surgeons, however, continue to keyhole the mesh with good success.[15]

The size of the sheet of mesh used to cover the posterior wall was crucial in our laparoscopic repairs. If the sheet was too small, there was inadequate surface area to resist the pressure on the mesh and a recurrent hernia developed. In Phillips' report of laparoscopic failures, 60% of recurrences were due to an inadequate-sized mesh.[26] In our review, the incidence of recurrence from too small a mesh was only 29% and 90% were in TAPP repairs, most of which were performed early in the study.[5] This finding suggests that, with experience, surgeons tended to employ larger sheets of polypropylene and that it may be easier to place a larger mesh using the TEP approach, because size of the mesh was rarely a cause of failure when the TEP approach was used.

Our study included only patients who had the mesh fixed to Cooper's ligament, the transversalis fascia, and laterally above the iliopubic tract. Which fixation device was used, however, did not influence the outcome of the repair. Recently, some surgeons have advocated repairing groin hernias without fixation. The results of some investigators such as Ferzli et al.[27] and Lucas and Arregui[28] have been comparable to our results with anchored mesh. In contrast, a study from the Netherlands[29] has reported a higher incidence of recurrence, bringing into question whether fixation does reduce the chance of recurrence.[25] Eliminating fixation has been proposed to reduce cost, but if recurrence results, in less experienced hands, this cost saving will be negated. Eliminating fixation to reduce postoperative pain is probably unnecessary, as is discussed later in this chapter.

Looking at our multicenter experience over time, surgeons found that early in their experience recurrences were more likely to occur because of overlooked hernias, missed lipomas, and inadequate size of the mesh. These errors were all corrected with experience and modification of the laparoscopic technique. Ramshaw et al.,[15] in a separate study, have reported similar findings. Similar to Bendavid's experience at the Shouldice Clinic in Toronto with an open multilayered anterior approach, as experience increased and the technique evolved, the results dramatically improved.[30]

As emphasized earlier in this chapter, one must overcome the early phase of the learning curve before results comparable to those published in peer review journals can be achieved. Fortunately, understanding why the laparoscopic hernioplasty is successful in reducing recurrence and adhering to the principles outlined by the other authors of this section will decrease the length of the learning curve. The dissection of the posterior wall of the groin must be complete in every patient, exposing the direct, indirect, and femoral area in every case. All three areas must then be covered by an adequately sized mesh, and the peritoneum must lie on top of the mesh at the termination of the procedure. Patients should undergo a gradual reversal of the general anesthetic to prevent violent bucking that can lift the lower lateral end of the mesh at the end of the case. Hematomas or large retroperitoneal fluid collections should also be avoided to prevent lateral recurrences caused by lifting of the mesh.

Recognizing Recurrence

Close follow-up of patients is essential to detect recurrence after hernia repair because 40% will be asymptomatic.[31] In several reports, 25% to 50% of groin hernias that were going to fail did so within the first year of close follow-up.[32–34] In contrast, when a mesh buttressed repair was used, recurrence after the first year of observation was rare.[35] Late recurrence of a laparoscopic repair following a normal 1-year examination has rarely been reported, because the majority of recurrences after laparoscopic hernioplasty are due to technical problems that lead to early rather than late failure.[22]

Physical examination alone is usually all that is required to detect failure of a laparoscopic repair. We have not found herniograms or computerized tomography to be helpful. In contrast, an ultrasound sometimes demonstrates a fluid collection that would otherwise be mistaken for a recurrent hernia. If a recurrence is suspected, a transabdominal diagnostic laparoscopy has been used to confirm the diagnosis and initiate surgical treatment. If, on laparoscopy, the floor appears solid, but a definite impulse was palpated in the external ring on physical examination before exploration, the problem is most likely a retained lipoma; it can be removed laparoscopically by opening the peritoneum laterally or by an open approach with a small counterincision over the external ring. Again, one must be certain that the impulse is not the result of a fluid collection that can be treated with simple aspiration rather than exploration.

Treating Recurrence

Between July 1991 and September 1999, 0.4% of the 2000 hernioplasties followed prospectively have recurred during follow-up. All 8 patients have been reexplored via a laparoscopic transabdominal approach. In one case, a palpated impulse was due to an undiagnosed collection of fluid that could have been treated without surgical exploration if an ultrasound had been performed. A second patient did not have a recurrence of his hernia but has been included because he was reexplored. Five of the other 6 patients explored were successfully repaired with a transabdominal approach and have remained disease free. One patient required an open approach to repair a direct hernia with incarcerated bladder. He was undergoing his second laparoscopic exploration, at our center, of a hernia that had originally been referred to us with a failed TAPP repair. The bladder was hidden behind the mesh placed by the first surgeon. Three recurrences resulted from retained lipomas after TEP repairs. The lipoma was removed transabdominally in 2 patients and with a small anterior counterincision over the external ring in 1. Two patients had recurrence because of folding of the lateral mesh, 1 from a hematoma and the other from a lipoma.

Although not all laparoscopic recurrences can be treated laparoscopically, our experience suggests that they should initially be approached via a laparoscopic transabdominal route, as this allows the surgeon to determine the cause of recurrence as well as treat it. The peritoneum is opened, the recurrent area dissected, and mesh is added to repair the defect as needed. The peritoneum is not usually adherent to the recurrent defect because this area is virgin or, if previously dissected, is now devoid of mesh. The old mesh is not removed, unless it is causing pain (this is discussed later in this chapter). After the hernia is rerepaired, the peritoneum must be closed over the mesh, which can be accomplished by suturing the peritoneum or, in some patients, by tacking the lower edge of peritoneum to the peritonealized mesh that was left in place. If the surgeon believes that laparoscopic rerepair is too difficult or risky, an anterior mesh repair should be performed after laparoscopically evaluating the cause of the recurrence.

As previously discussed, the major causes of recurrence, that is, a missed hernia, retained lipoma, lateral or medial elevation of the mesh, and herniation through a slit in the mesh, can all be determined and repaired via a transabdominal approach no matter whether the first repair was a TAPP or TEP repair. Sometimes, however, the primary surgeon has gone so astray that exposing the recurrent defect would be dangerous. In my experience, leaving the old mesh in place and performing an anterior repair in these patients has given the best long-term results.

Overview of Complications

A recent study of patients undergoing both open and laparoscopic hernia repairs has suggested that up to 5% of patients surveyed felt that they were worse off after the hernia repair than with the hernia.[12] It is, therefore, paramount that we keep complications to a minimum no matter which approach we choose. The complication rate reported for laparoscopic repairs ranges from less than 3%[14] to as high as 20%,[36] and is similar to that reported for open repairs.[9,37] The large variation is due to the type and scope of complications considered and the expertise of the operating surgeons reviewed. As discussed earlier in this chapter, the incidence of complications is directly related to the point on the learning curve studied (Fig. 34.2). In this chapter, I confine myself to discussing only serious complications or those that, although minor, are frequent and should be recognized.

Postoperative seroma falls into the latter category. As many as 10% of patients develop a fluid collection after laparoscopic hernioplasty[38] that presents as a recurrent

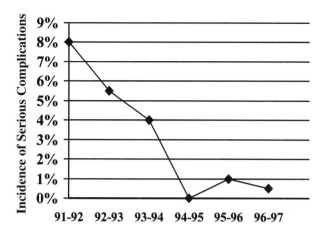

FIGURE 34.2. Learning curve for complications at Fresno Hernia Center 1991–1997: percent of serious complications per year.

mass soon after the repair and may suggest recurrence of the hernia to the patient or the unaware surgeon; it may even transmit an impulse if the patient coughs or strains. Physical examination alone usually differentiates it from a recurrent hernia. If the examiner is inexperienced, an ultrasound will confirm the diagnosis. If left alone, 90% resorb in 6 weeks. If the collection persists or is symptomatic, aspiration almost always eliminates the problem. In more than 2000 hernia repairs, only 3 patients have required surgical treatment of a persistent seroma, and no patient has developed an infection as a result of a seroma at our center.

A hydrocele presenting as an enlarged testicle or scrotal mass from 2 months to several years after a hernia repair is always alarming to the patient. The incidence of hydrocele following laparoscopic repair is the same as after open repairs and occurs in less than 1% of patients.[26] We have found that they appear no more often in patients who have had a seroma that has resolved during follow-up. It is important to warn patients preoperatively of this relatively rare complication so that they will not think the worst if it does develop. Over an 8-year period, 0.4% of our laparoscopically repaired hernias have later required surgical treatment for a hydrocele. The incidence, however, has significantly decreased since we stopped routinely using a keyhole in the mesh.[14]

There are complications following both TAPP and TEP approaches to laparoscopic hernioplasty that are related to the approach itself. The TEP repair in fact has gained popularity because it eliminates some of the potential risks of a transabdominal approach. Injuries from trocars penetrating the peritoneal cavity are now uncommon but are extremely serious complications of laparoscopic hernioplasty when they do occur. Bleeding from the inferior epigastric vessels after lateral trocar placement was once common, but this now is unusual because of the use

of 5-mm trocars and an awareness of the location of the vessels. If bleeding does occur, it can be controlled with the use of a fascia closure device (Karl Storz, CA, USA) or similar device for placing a transfascial hemostatic stitch. The inferior epigastric vessels are not immune to injury during a TEP approach. The balloon dissector can take down the vessels, which may result in bleeding from small branches. The surgeon must quickly place the other trocars and irrigate the space clear to find the source and control it with bipolar cautery.

Injury to the bowel from lyses of adhesions or the trocars themselves is the most serious complication of laparoscopic hernioplasty. The incidence of this complication is extremely low but can be reduced even further by proper selection of patients and approach (see Table 34.1, Fig. 34.1). By using a totally extraperitoneal technique, the potential for bowel injury is reduced but not eliminated.[14] If the extraperitoneal space is obliterated by previous surgery, radiation, or infection, the bowel is at greater risk if a laparoscopic approach is used. In these situations, an open approach is therefore preferred. When the bowel is incarcerated in the hernia, the transabdominal route is preferred over other approaches because this approach affords the surgeon the best view of the hernia's contents. If a totally extraperitoneal approach with a balloon dissector is used, the peritoneum and possibly the bowel may be torn as the balloon expands. In addition, dissection of the contents of the incarcerated hernia can be extremely difficult via the TEP approach because of limited space and visualization. It is important to evaluate the hernia immediately before surgery to determine whether the hernia can be reduced; this allows the surgeon to choose the proper approach and avoid inadvertent injury to the bowel or peritoneum.

Bladder injuries have been reported after both open and laparoscopic repairs. In the laparoscopic approach, it is usually due to failure to recognize that the bladder makes up part of the direct sac. Ligating the direct sac is unnecessary and can result in injury to the bladder, which presents as a delayed leak of urine from necrosis of the bladder wall. Injury from a balloon dissector during a TEP repair has also been described, but this must be extremely rare as we have not seen this complication in more than 3000 totally extraperitoneal repairs performed at our center.

Small bowel obstruction due to inadequate closure of the peritoneum has been a problem in the past when staples were used to close the peritoneum following TAPP repairs. Suture closure of the peritoneum and more widespread use of the TEP approach has made this complication rare. Schuricht, however, has stressed the importance of closing peritoneal defects following even TEP repairs by reporting one patient with a bowel obstruction following a totally extraperitoneal approach.[39]

Trocar hernias were once considered a major problem after laparoscopic hernia repair. In fact, the incidence of incisional or trocar hernias in our early experience was greater than the incidence of recurrence of the hernia repair itself.[38] When we reduced the lateral trocar size to 5mm for TAP repairs and increased the percent of TEP repairs performed, trocar hernias virtually disappeared at our center. If 10- or even 12-mm ports are used, however, a secure closure of the fascia is mandatory. There are now several commercial devices that make adequate suture closure of these wounds easier. They are all based on a technique that passes a suture through the fascia into the peritoneal cavity, allowing the surgeon to grasp the suture to pull it out the opposite fascial wall. There are even some newer trocars that make port incisions that do not need to be mechanically approximated.

Pain Following Hernia Repair

Pain following hernioplasty, open or laparoscopic, is a major problem.[12] The origin of severe or chronic pain after both TEP and TAPP approaches can be nerve injury or entrapment, the mesh itself, or even recurrence. The surgeon's approach to this complication should be dictated by the nature of the pain, its time course, and its severity. If severe pain in the distribution of a major nerve develops immediately after the hernia repair, reexploration is indicated to search for and remove an offending staple or stitch. If there is delay in seeing such a patient, exploration is still indicated.[40] In contrast, patients with minor neuralgias, parasthesias, or numbness should be observed. In general, these symptoms will improve with time. Chronic pain that does not resolve and is disabling to the patient, however, deserves surgical exploration. In my experience, patients referred with even long-standing severe pain that is localized or in the distribution of a named nerve may benefit from reoperation. Exploration should be through a transabdominal laparoscopic route. If the pain is localized, it is important to mark the area of pain before beginning the laparoscopic exploration, as this aids in correlating the operative findings with the patient's symptoms. If laparoscopic exploration identifies a tack, staple, or stitch, it can be removed laparoscopically. Relief of pain may be immediate or delayed if there is a neuritis. In some instances, a later neurectomy may be required if a neroma has formed.

Sometimes pain results not from an anchoring device placed at the primary operation but rather from the mesh itself. We have found that if polypropylene mesh curls up in the extraperitoneal space it may form an extremely

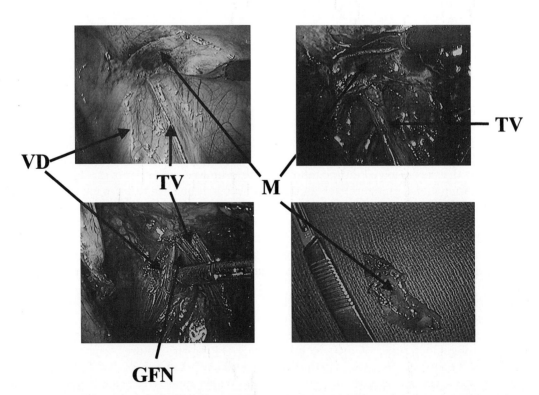

FIGURE 34.3. Curled mesh in a patient referred for 6 months of pain in the groin following a TEP repair. *Top left*: peritoneal view of curled mesh (*M*) irritating genitofemoral nerve. *Top right*: peritoneum has been opened to expose mesh and nerve. *Bottom left*: dissection freeing genitofemoral nerve (*GFN*). *Bottom right*: debrided mesh. The patient was relieved of pain 1 month after remedial surgery. *TV*, Testicular vessels; *VD*, vas deferens.

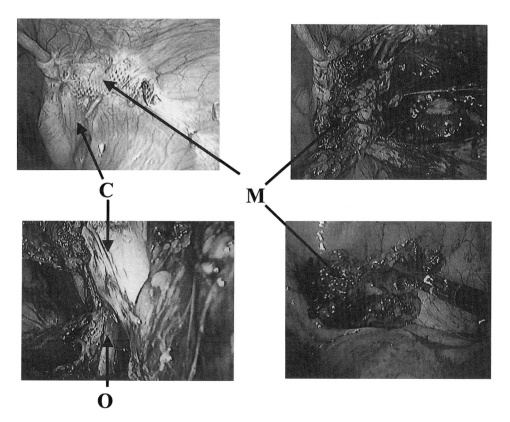

FIGURE 34.4. A female patient referred with 2 years of pain in the distribution of the obturator nerve following a TAPP repair. *Top left*: peritoneal view. *Top right*: peritoneum has been opened to expose curled mesh (*M*), which is irritating the obtu- rator. *Bottom left*: the mesh has been debrided off Cooper's ligament (*C*), exposing the obturator nerve (*O*). *Bottom right*: debrided mesh. The patient has been free of symptoms for 6 months following remedial surgery.

hard ridge that has the potential of irritating nerves or surrounding tissue (Fig. 34.3). The result is pain that is identical to that produced iatrogenically from a mis-placed staple or tack. To treat this problem the mesh must be removed and the nerve, if compressed by scar tissue, released. Usually the mesh is so hard that cautery is required to cut it free. Using this approach, we have suc-cessfully treated several patients referred to our center for postlaparoscopic pain. One patient had symptoms for more than 2 years due to compression of the obturator nerve by curled mesh. Laparoscopic debridement of the mesh (Fig. 34.4) rendered her painfree.

Most nerve injuries are preventable if certain precau-tions or steps are taken at the initial laparoscopic repair. When laparoscopic hernioplasty began, there was an out-break of serious nerve injuries because surgeons were not aware of the anatomic location of the important nerves.[37] In response, numerous articles were written instructing surgeons to avoid dissection of the "triangle of doom."[41] We now know that the real solution is knowledge of the anatomy and not placing fixation of the mesh below the iliopubic tract lateral to Cooper's ligament. Because the femoral, genitofemoral, and lateral cutaneous nerve

are all below the iliopubic tract, anchoring the mesh in this area is risky and must be avoided, which can be accomplished by visually identifying the iliopubic tract (Fig. 34.5) and by palpating the tacker or stapler against the abdominal wall with the opposite hand. In addition, cautery should be avoided in this same area if possible. To avoid curling of the lateral mesh, it should be laid smoothly against the wall and held in place with a grasper as the peritoneum expands over it if a TEP repair is performed.

The more superficial nerves, such as the ilioinguinal and iliohypogastric, previously were thought to be safe from injury during a laparoscopic repair, but these nerves can be injured by overzealous placement of staples or tacks. In thin patients, anchors placed too deeply into the wall can catch and injure the anterior nerves. The result will be a rather localized pain in the abdominal wall or pain in the sensory distribution of one of these nerves. The treatment is laparoscopic removal of the offending staple or tack if it corresponds to the area marked pre-operatively, as mentioned earlier in this section.

Several reports[18,27,42] have suggested that the way to avoid nerve injuries is to not anchor the mesh to the wall.

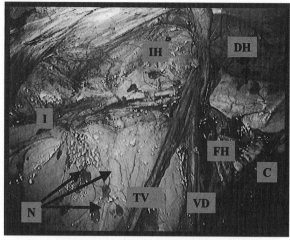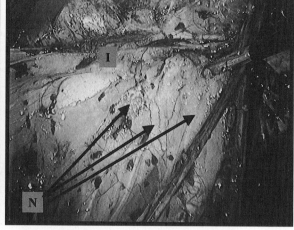

FIGURE 34.5. Extraperitoneal view of a 64-year-old male patient demonstrates the anatomy with special attention to the neural structures. *N*, Nerves; *I*, iliopubic tract; *DH*, direct hernia; *IH* indirect hernia; *C*, Cooper's ligament; *FH*, femoral hernia; *TV*, testicular vessels; *VD*, vas deferens.

I believe that this is overreaction to the problem because the incidence of pain after laparoscopic repairs with fixation is now extremely low and appears to be lower than that experienced after open repairs.[12] Not fixing the mesh may increase the recurrence rate[25,42] in exchange for only a small potential decrease in postoperative pain. The real answer is the proper use of fixation (as outlined in this section) or possibly the use of new fixatives in the future, such as cement or glue.

Conclusion

Although a randomized study from the United Kingdom has clearly demonstrated advantages associated with the laparoscopic repair, the study suggested that laparoscopic repairs be performed by specialists.[43] It pointed to rare serious complications and an increased recurrence rate in the laparoscopic group as the reason for their conclusion. In this study, however, surgeons were required to have performed only 10 cases before accruing patients in the study. Thus, this and other studies demonstrate that laparoscopic repairs should be performed by surgeons with a special interest in advanced laparoscopy and experience with more than just a few hernia repairs, but not necessarily by surgeons specializing in only laparoscopic hernia repair. Our own group as well as many others have demonstrated that excellent results can be achieved by general surgeons who are performing a variety of advanced laparoscopic procedures.[5] The key is education and supervision during the learning curve to eliminate complications that stem from inexperience. There will always be complications and recurrences after hernia repair, but by following the steps outlined by the authors in this volume and having proper guidance during one's early cases, the benchmarks established by experienced laparoscopic surgeons can be achieved.

References

1. Rutkow IM, Robbins AW. Demographic, classificatory, and socioeconomic aspects of hernia repair in the United States. Surg Clin N Am 1993;73:413–426.
2. Schultz L, Graber J, Pietrafitta J, Hickok D. Laser laparoscopic herniorrhaphy: a clinical trial preliminary results. J Laproendosc Surg 1990;1:41–45.
3. Bessel R, Baxter P, Ridell P, Watkin S, Madden G. A randomized controlled trial of laparoscopic repair as a day surgical procedure. Surg Endosc 1996;10:495–500.
4. Lukaszczyk J, Preletz R, Morrow G, Lange M, Tachovsky T, Krall J. Laparoscopic herniorrhaphy versus traditional open repair at a community hospital. J Laparoendosc Surg 1996;6:203–208.
5. Felix E, Scott S, Crafton B, et al. Causes of recurrence after laparoscopic hernioplasty. Surg Endosc 1998;12:226–231.
6. Liem M, Van der Graff, Van Steensel C, et al. Comparison of conventional anterior surgery and laparoscopic surgery for inguinal hernia repair. N Engl J Med 1997;336:1541–1547.
7. Leibl B, Schmidt J, Daubler P, Kraft K. A single institution's experience with transperitoneal laparoscopic hernia repair. Am J Surg 1998;175(6):446–452.
8. Ferzli G, Sayad P, Huie F, Hallak A, Usal A. Endoscopic extraperitoneal herniorrhaphy. A 5 year experience. Surg Endosc 1998;12(11):1311–1313.
9. MacFadyen B, Mathis C. Inguinal herniorrhaphy; complications and recurrences. Semin Lap Surg 1994;1(2):128–140.
10. Amid P, Shulman A, Lichtenstein I. Critical scrutiny of the open "tension-free" hernioplasty. Am J Surg 1993;165:369–375.

11. Cunningham J, Temple W, Mitchell P, Nixon J, Preshaw R, Hagen N. Cooperative study. Pain in the post-repair patient. Ann Surg 1995;224:598–602.

12. Gillion J, Fagniez P. Chronic pain and sensory changes after hernia repair. Hernia 1999;3:75–80.

13. Southern Surgeons Club. A prospective analysis of 1518 laparoscopic cholecystectomies. N Engl J Med 1991;324: 1073–1078.

14. Felix E, Habertson N, Varteian S. Laparoscopic hernioplasty: significant complications. Surg Endosc 1999;13:328–331.

15. Ramshaw B, Frankum C, Young D, et al. 1000 total extraperitoneal herniorrhaphies: after the learning curve. Surg Endosc 1999.

16. Wright D, O'Dwyer P. The learning curve for laparoscopic hernia repair. Semin Laparosc Surg 1998;5(4):227–232.

17. Stoker D, Spiegelhalter D, Sing R, et al. Laparoscopic versus open inguinal hernia repair: randomized prospective trial. Lancet 1994;343:1243–1245.

18. Liem M, Van Steensel C, Boelhouwer R, et al. The learning curve for totally extraperitoneal laparoscopic inguinal hernia repair. Am J Surg 1996;171:281–285.

19. Go P. Overview of randomized trials in laparoscopic inguinal hernia repair. Semin Laparosc Surg 1998;5(4):238–241.

20. Fitzgibbons R, Camps J, Cornet D, et al. Laparoscopic inguinal herniorrhaphy. Results of a multicenter trial. Ann Surg 1995;221:3–13.

21. Toy F, Moskowitz M, Smoot R, et al. Results of a prospective multicenter trial evaluating ePTFE peritoneal onlay laparoscopic inguinal hernioplasty. J Laparoendosc Surg 1996;6:375–386.

22. Felix EL, Michas CA, Gonzalez MH. Laparoscopic hernioplasty: why does it work? Surg Endosc 1997;11:36–41.

23. Ryan E. Recurrent hernias: an analysis of 369 consecutive cases of recurrent inguinal and femoral hernias. Surg Gynecol Obstet 1953;96:343–354.

24. Felix E, Michas, C, Gonzalez M. Recurrent hernioplasty. Am J Surg 1996;172:580–584.

25. Brooks D. Laparoscopic herniorrhaphy: where are we now? Surg Endosc 1999;13:321–322.

26. Phillips E, Rosenthal R, Fallas M, et al. Reasons for early recurrence following laparoscopic hernioplasty. Surg Endosc 1995;9:140–145.

27. Ferzli G, Frezza E, Pecoraro A, Ahern K. Prospective randomized study of stapled versus unstapled mesh in a laparoscopic preperitoneal inguinal hernia repair. J Am Coll Surg 1999;188(5):461–465.

28. Lucas S, Arregui M. Minimally invasive surgery for inguinal hernia. World J Surg 1999;23(4):350–355.

29. Beets G, Dirkson C, Go P, Geisler C, Baeten C, Kootstra G. Open or laparoscopic preperitoneal mesh repair for recurrent inguinal hernia? A randomized trial. Surg Endosc 1999;13:323–327.

30. Bendavid R. New techniques in hernia repair. World J Surg 1989;13:522–531.

31. Panos R, Beck D, Maresh J, Harford F. Preliminary results of a prospective randomized study of Cooper's ligament versus Shouldice herniorrhaphy technique. Surg Gynecol Obstet 1992;175:315–319.

32. Marsden A. Recurrent inguinal hernia: a personal study. Br J Surg 1988;75:263–266.

33. Read R. Recurrence after preperitoneal herniorrhaphy in the adult. Arch Surg 1975;110:666–671.

34. Schapp H, Van de Pavoordt H, Bast T. The preperitoneal approach in the repair of recurrent inguinal hernias. Surg Gynecol Obstet 1992;174:460–464.

35. Stoppa R. The treatment of complicated groin and incisional hernias. World J Surg 1989;13:545–554.

36. Tedik C, Arregui M, Dulucq J, et al. Complications and recurrences with laparoscopic repair of groin hernias. A multi-institutional retrospective analysis. Surg Endosc 1994; 8:1316–1323.

37. Payne J. Complications of laparoscopic inguinal herniorrhaphy. Semin Laparosc Surg 1997;4(3):166–181.

38. Felix E, Michas C, Gonzalez M. TAPP vs TEP laparoscopic hernioplasty. Surg Endosc 1995;9:984–989.

39. Azurin D, Schuricht A, Stoldt H, Kirkland M, Paskin D, Bar A. Small bowel obstruction following endoscopic extraperitoneal-preperitoneal herniorrhaphy. J Laparoendosc Surg 1995;5(4):263–266.

40. Seid A, Amos E. Entrapment neuropathy in laparoscopic herniorrhaphy. Surg Endosc 1994;8:1050–1053.

41. Spaw A, Ennis B, Spaw L. Laparoscopic hernia repair: the anatomic basis. J Laparoendosc Surg 1991;1:269–277.

42. Macintyre I. Does the mesh require fixation? Semin Laparosc Surg 1998;5(4):224–226.

43. The MRC Laparoscopic Groin Hernia Trial Group. Laparoscopic versus pen repair of groin hernia: a randomized comparison. Lancet 1999;354:185–189.

Part II
Laparoscopic Repair of Ventral Hernias

35
Laparoscopic Ventral/Incisional Hernioplasty

Frederick K. Toy

Ventral hernia is defined as any protrusion through the anterior abdominal wall with the exception of the inguinal area. The repair of ventral hernias, especially incisional hernias, can be one of the most challenging procedures the surgeon undertakes (Fig. 35.1A,B).

Ventral hernias include umbilical hernias, epigastric hernias, incisional hernias, and spigelian hernias. Approximately 13% of all herniorrhaphies in the United States in 1990 were ventral hernias, with a total of approximately 90,000 ventral hernia repairs per year, of which incisional hernias are by far the most common (approximately 2/3), second only to the inguinal hernia repair.[1,2]

The rate of recurrence for ventral hernias has always been very disappointing. With conventional anterior approaches, the recurrence rate is between 10% and 20%. If no prosthetic material is used, the recurrence rate is between 30% and 50%.[3,4] The potential benefits of repairing ventral hernias laparoscopically is that there are no large anterior abdominal wounds and subcutaneous flaps that require drains and lead to other complications such as seromas, hematomas, and wound infections. There is also less postoperative discomfort and reduced convalescence, and the intraabdominal pressures help to stabilize the repair, utilizing the principle of Pascal's law.

Surgical Anatomy

All abdominal surgeons understand the anatomy of the anterior abdominal wall, as viewed from the exterior. It is paramount to have a clear understanding of the anatomy of the anterior abdominal wall and inguinal region viewed from the interior before attempting to repair a ventral hernia laparoscopically.

The parietal peritoneum covers the interior of the entire abdominal wall, with the majority of its surface having no distinguishing characteristics. However, there are four specific folds radiating out from the umbilicus.

When viewed through the laparoscope, the posterior surface of the anterior abdominal wall is divided into several fossae. The most obvious of these landmarks is the falciform ligament, which drapes over the obliterated umbilical vein, also known as the ligamentum teres. This obliterated vessel passes cephalad from the umbilical annulus beneath the dense umbilical fascia for several centimeters before emerging as an obvious peritoneal fold. It courses slightly to the right of the midline toward its eventual entrance into the substance of the liver. In the midline, between the pubic bone and the umbilicus, is a fibrous band that comprises the remains of the urachus.

The fold of the peritoneum over the urachal remnant is the median umbilical ligament. Three or 4 cm lateral is another fibrous cord covered with peritoneum. This cord, which extends from the sides of the urinary bladder to the umbilicus, is the medial umbilical ligament and is the fibrous remnant of the obliterated umbilical arteries. This is an important landmark because it lies directly over the pubic tubercle. Three or 4 cm further lateral are the lateral umbilical ligaments, which are a slight protrusion of the inferior epigastric vessels and the interfoveolar ligament. Occasionally, with the bladder contracted, there are transverse folds that extend laterally from the bladder fundus to the pelvic side walls. These folds constitute a false ligament known as the transverse vesical fold.

Another important anatomic landmark in understanding the repair of ventral hernias is the linea arcuata (semicircular line of Douglas) (Fig. 35.2). Between the costal margin and the level of the anterior superior iliac spine, the aponeurosis of the internal oblique splits to enclose the rectus muscle; the external oblique aponeurosis is directed in front of the muscle and the transversus aponeurosis is directed between the muscles. Between the level of the anterior superior iliac spine and the pubis, the aponeurosis of all three muscles forms the anterior wall. The posterior wall is absent, and the rectus muscle lies in contact with the transversalis fascia. Where the

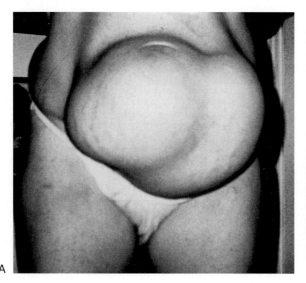
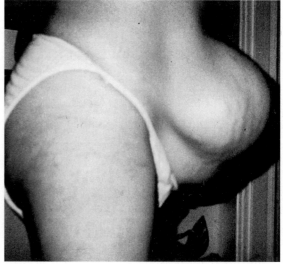

FIGURE 35.1. Giant, recurrent ×9, ventral incisional hernia repaired laparoscopically. A. Anterior view. B. Lateral view.

aponeuroses forming the posterior wall pass in front of the rectus at the level of the anterior superior iliac spine, the wall has a free, curved lower border called the arcuate line of Douglas. At this site, the inferior epigastric vessels enter the rectus sheath and pass upward to anastomose with the superior epigastric vessels. In the repair of a ventral hernia, one most have strong fixation to the anterior fascia, especially below the arcuate line of Douglas where all three aponeurotic layers make up the anterior fascia. This is why stapling alone is doomed to fail and suture fixation to the anterior fascia is necessary.

The inferior margin of the mesh must be fixed to Cooper's ligament and the iliopubic tract for secure anatomic fixation with adequate overlap of the hernia defect. For this reason, the anatomy of the pelvis, from the laparoscopic perspective, is very important for the repair of ventral hernias of the lower abdomen.

The vas deferens is covered only by peritoneum. It is usually easily identified as it exits the pelvic cavity over the pelvic brim and crosses lateral to the external iliac vein and artery obliquely. It then curves around the lateral side of the inferior epigastric vessels, where it joins the spermatic vessels. At the level of Cooper's ligament, the vas deferens lies directly over the external iliac vein and acts as a landmark for the lateral extent of exposure of Cooper's ligament. The spermatic vessels consist of the testicular artery and veins. The testicular artery is a branch of the aorta. The two testicular veins at the level of the internal inguinal ring unite to form a single vein that drains on the right side into the inferior vena cava and on the left side into the left renal vein. The spermatic vessels are covered only by the peritoneum and run along the pelvic wall over the anterior psoas muscle.

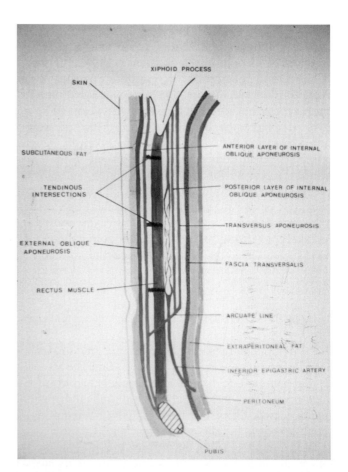

FIGURE 35.2. Lateral view of anterior abdominal wall fascia demonstrating arcuate line.

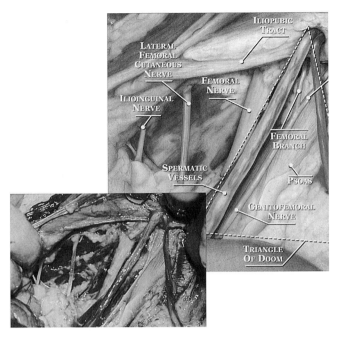

FIGURE 35.3. Laparoscopic view of inguinal area demonstrating Cooper's ligament, aberrant obturator artery, and triangle of doom.

The spermatic vessels merge with the vas deferens, forming the spermatic cord, which enters the internal inguinal ring and traverses the inguinal canal. The junction of the vas deferens and the spermatic vessels forms the apex of an imaginary triangle, termed the "triangle of doom" by Dr. Albert Spaw.[5] The external iliac artery and vein course through this triangle of doom. It is essential to identify this triangle because it is paramount not to staple or suture within this area.

Cooper's ligament (the pectineal ligament) is a strong, common, narrow tendinous ridge densely adherent to the pectineal line along the superior edge of the superior pubic ramus (Fig. 35.3). It was first described by Sir Ashley Cooper, an English anatomist and surgeon. Cooper's ligament is covered by peritoneum and subserous fascia and, when dissected, is a white, glistening, easily identified ligament. In the lower abdomen, when performing laparoscopic ventral hernioplasty, to ensure adequate fixation of the prosthetic patch it is paramount to dissect the peritoneum and fatty areolar tissue off Cooper's ligament from the pubic tubercle to the external iliac vein. Although this dissection is usually uneventful, there are two structures of which one needs to be aware. The inferior epigastric artery gives off a small branch at its origin called the pubic branch. This tiny artery runs immediately on the iliopubic tract and then courses inferiorly along the medial border of the femoral canal. It crosses Cooper's ligament and gives off a tiny branch (arteria corona mortis), which continues medially on the surface of Cooper's ligament. The pubic branch

continues inferiorly and joins the obturator artery. This tiny artery is often accompanied by several slightly larger veins. These vessels are easily cauterized during the dissection and present no problem.

In approximately 27% of the cadavers, the obturator artery origin is the first portion of the inferior epigastric artery and is quite large, 2 to 3 mm in diameter.[6] Known as an aberrant obturator artery, it courses across the femoral canal and Cooper's ligament and enters the obturator foramen with the obturator nerve. This vessel must be recognized and controlled with hemoclips to avoid considerable hemorrhage.

The inferior border of the internal inguinal ring is the iliopubic tract, an extension of the transversalis fascia that extends from its lateral attachment, the anterior superior iliac spine, to the superior pubic ramus medially. At about midway through its course, the iliopubic tract forms an interior border of the internal inguinal ring and the transition of the transversalis fascia to the anterior femoral sheath. The iliopubic tract is distinct from the inguinal ligament (Poupart's ligament), which lies anterior to it.

There are three nerves in the inguinal region with which the surgeon interested in laparoscopic hernioplasty must be familiar: the femoral, genitofemoral, and the lateral femoral cutaneous nerves (Fig. 35.4). The femoral nerve is the largest branch of the lumbar plexus and comprises the principal nerve of the anterior part of the thigh. It arises from the second, third, and fourth lumbar nerves. It emerges from the fibers of the distal, lateral border of the psoas major muscle and passes down between it and the iliacus muscle. It passes under the inguinal ligament, lateral to the femoral artery and the femoral sheath. At about 4 cm below the inguinal ligament, it terminates by dividing into anterior and posterior segments. The femoral nerve supplies all the muscles of the anterior compartment of the thigh. The anterior division gives off two branches. The cutaneous branches are (1) the medial femoral cutaneous nerve and (2) the intermediate femoral cutaneous nerves that supply the skin of the medial and anterior surfaces of the thigh, respectively. The muscular branches supply (1) the sartorius and (2) the pectineus muscle.

The posterior division gives off one cutaneous branch, the saphenous nerve, and muscular branches to the quadriceps muscles. The saphenous nerve runs downward and medially, crossing the femoral artery. It pierces the deep fascia on the medial side of the knee after emerging between the tendons of the sartorius and gracilis muscles. It then runs down the medial side of the leg, adjacent to the great saphenous vein. It passes anterior to the medial malleolus onto the foot and terminates at the base of the great toe. The muscular branch of the rectus femoris muscle supplies the hip joint; the branches of the three vasti muscles supply the knee joint.

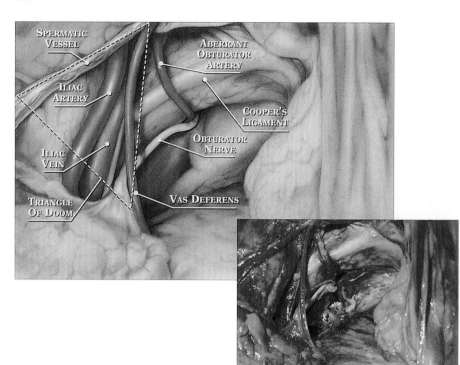

FIGURE 35.4. Femoral, genitofemoral, and lateral femoral cutaneous nerves.

The femoral nerve is in danger of injury during dissection or stapling in the area between the psoas and the groove of the iliacus muscles, dorsal to the iliopubic tract. In the average adult male, this measures approximately 9 cm lateral to the pubic tubercle. In this area, the femoral nerve is covered only by the peritoneum, subserous fascia, and the endoabdominal fascia. Injury in this area would result in a sensory deficit and pain in the dermatomes in the anteriomedial thigh. Muscular weakness, although possible, is less likely because the anterior compartment of the femoral nerve largely comprises the cutaneous branches, and the major muscular branches lie in the deep posterior division of the femoral nerve.

The genital femoral nerve arises from the first and second lumbar nerves, passes down through the psoas major muscles, and emerges on its ventral surface at the level of the third or fourth lumbar vertebrae. It is covered by the endoabdominal fascia (psoas fascia) and peritoneum. On the surface of the muscle, or occasionally within the substance of the muscle, the nerve divides into a genital and a femoral branch.

The genital branch continues caudally on the surface of the psoas muscle. It then pierces the endoabdominal fascia at the internal inguinal ring and converges with the testicular vessels, the vas deferens, to form the spermatic cord. It lies against the dorsal aspect of the cord, supplying the cremaster muscle and the skin of the scrotum. In the female, it accompanies the round ligament of the uterus. The femoral branch continues caudally on the surface of the psoas muscle, lateral to the genital branch, and passes under the inguinal ligament with the external iliac artery within the femoral sheath. It lies anterior and lateral to the artery and then pierces the sheath and fascia lata to supply the skin of the proximal part of the anterior surface of the thigh or approximately 7.5 cm below the inguinal ligament.

The genital and femoral branches may be injured when dissecting or stapling from the spermatic cord structures at the internal ring. Both these branches lie beneath the spermatic cord structures at the internal ring and travel caudally on the anterior surface of the psoas muscle. The femoral branch, however, is more lateral and may be injured if stapling is done just lateral to the spermatic vessels and dorsal to the iliopubic tract. Injury to these nerves would result in a sensory deficit or pain to the dermatomes in the scrotum and a small area on the anterior thigh, just below the inguinal ligament.

The lateral femoral cutaneous nerve arises from the second and third lumbar nerves. It emerges midway down the psoas muscle from its lateral edge and runs across the iliacus muscle obliquely toward the anterior superior iliac spine. It passes under the inguinal ligament at its lateral end and enters the thigh, where it divides into anterior and posterior branches, which supply the skin of the lateral aspect of the thigh and knee. It also supplies the skin of the lower lateral quadrant of the buttocks. This nerve can be injured when dissecting or stapling laterally near the anterior superior iliac spine and dorsal to the iliopubic tract. Such an injury would result in a sensory deficit or pain in the dermatome in the anterior lateral thigh.[7]

The Rationale for e-PTFE Dual Mesh Biomaterial

Choosing one prosthetic biomaterial over another should be made after a sound and thorough review of the experimental and clinical data available. This comparison of biomaterials is based on mechanical and biological characteristics. The mechanical characteristics are strength, fixation-retention, and durability. The biological characteristics are infectibility, adhesion formation, and erosion/fistulization.

In setting the criteria for an ideal biomaterial, strength and fixation/retention are of obvious concern, not only during the initial postoperative phase but also over the long term. A biomaterial must be able to serve its intended use over the lifespan of the patient, with no major complications. Therefore, durability is of importance as well. To evaluate strength, the various biomaterials were analyzed on a standard testing machine. Ultimate tensile strength testing demonstrates the ability of a material to withstand application of forces at high rates. The 1mm expanded polytetrafluoroethylene (e-PTFE) mesh is 2 to 14 times stronger than the polypropylene or polyester mesh materials. It should be noted that all these biomaterials have adequate tensile strength and have been superengineered for their intended application. It is a commonly stated misbelief among many surgeons that the dense fibrous incorporation of the macromesh materials is necessary to increase the strength of the repair. A large volume of study on wound repair has revealed this dense fibrous reaction forms in concentric whorls of fibrous tissue instead of the normal longitudinal fibers of fascia. This scar tissue never regains the strength of normal tissue and is converted from elastic, pliable tissue to a contracted, unelastic, brittle mass.[8–15]

The materials were also tested to determine fixation-retention values. Fixation-retention is important because of the high impact forces the material may experience in vivo (i.e., coughing, sneezing, muscle contraction, etc.). Fixation-retention testing defines the resistance of a biomaterial to the pull out of sutures or staples at very high velocity. Rectangular samples of prosthetic material were placed in the testing machine in which a pin passes through the material and the material is then pulled apart at a high velocity. The force at which the material failed was recorded. Fixation-retention for the 1-mm e-PTFE (0.9 kg/PIN) is equivalent to or several times stronger than the meshes (0.32 kg/PIN).

To evaluate durability, a test was designed to mimic the different forces that would be placed on a material in vivo over time. Muscle contraction, flexing, sneezing, and coughing can all produce significant strain on the material.

Therefore, a material must not only be strong and have adequate fixation-retention but be durable as well. The material was placed in a device similar to the fixation pullout test. A static load of 8 lb (3.6 kg) was applied, with an intermittent load of 16 lb (7.2 kg) applied every second. Each cycle was recorded until the material failed. The durability of 1-mm e-PTFE (1320.9 cycles) is considerably greater than that of the meshes (50–100 cycles).

In conclusion, considering the mechanical characteristics, the 1-mm e-PTFE is stronger, has better fixation-retention values, and is more durable than any other biomaterial available. These features, as well as good handling characteristics, make it the best biomaterial available from a mechanical standpoint.

Biological Response

Biocompatibility of an implanted material encompasses not only the nature of the response from the surrounding tissue but also the inherent characteristic of the material itself. The e-PTFE is inert, preventing significant inflammatory responses, with a microstructure that provides latticework for tissue ingrowth. Monofilament, as well as multifilament, mesh materials elicit a mild to severe inflammatory response with encapsulation of the material. It must be understood that ingrowth and encapsulation are microscopic terms. Ingrowth is characterized by infiltration of blood elements, fibrin, and proteinaceous material throughout the microstructure; this is followed by histiocytes and fibroblasts, with deposition of collagen in the interstices, providing firm anchorage. At the interface, there is fibrous tissue attachment to the material surface (i.e., e-PTFE). Encapsulation is characterized by infiltration of acellular blood elements only (fibrin, proteinaceous material). There is minimal localized attachment of tissue to material surface and no collagen deposition into the interstices. The fibrous tissue encircles the material and prevents cellular migration into the interstices. The material is isolated, and there is no incorporation by host tissue (i.e., polypropylene meshes).

During the normal healing of any wound there are three phases: inflammation, granulation tissue formation, and the rebuilding process. Natural host tissue healing events take place when an e-PTFE soft tissue patch [pore size/internodal average, 22μm (17–41μm)] is placed in a wound for the repair of a wall defect or hernia. Serous fluid and blood cells infiltrate the e-PTFE structure. White blood cells (WBCs)/leukocytes (average diameter, 14–20μm) surround and infiltrate the e-PTFE within the wound. Fibroblasts (average, 15μm wide × 50μm long) appear within the material, usually between 14 and 28 days (as early as 7 days) postoperatively and produce collagen along the e-PTFE structure and deposit collagen into the interstices of the e-PTFE. The tissue around the e-PTFE exhibits minimal contracture because of the specific orientation of the collagen fibers. The collagen fibers align in parallel with the e-PTFE surface and perpendicular to the surface within the material. Such biaxial alignment may be associated with minimal contracture of the tissues surrounding the e-PTFE. The resulting scar tissue is smooth and pliable. Other foreign implant materials (e.g., sutures and meshes, with pore sizes approximately 2–10 mm between filaments and 0–10 μm between filaments at points of contact) are also surrounded by collagen fibers and fiber bundles. These collagen fibers are parallel and concentrically aligned, encapsulating the individual mesh fibers. In contrast to the biaxial alignment of the collagen fibers with e-PTFE, the concentric alignment around the mesh filaments and the parallel alignment of the collagen fibers between the mesh filaments through the thickness of a mesh may be related to the reported distortion and scar contracture of mesh materials. In experimental studies as well as in clinical observations, e-PTFE was found to have complete fibroblastic cellular ingrowth through the interstices of the material at 8 weeks, with only minimal inflammatory reaction. With the parallel orientation of the scar tissue, the e-PTFE retained a flat orientation of graft to the fibrous tissue, forming a "neofascia." In contrast, polypropylene meshes have rapid formation of dense scar tissue with marked inflammatory tissue reaction. The fibrous tissue is concentrically aligned around the mesh fibers, causing the graft to become encased in a whorled mass of dense scar. Contracture of the scar tissue causes graft distortion and loss of anatomic position. This mechanism is believed to be a contributing factor to recurrences when polypropylene prosthetic meshes are used.

Infectibility

The incidence of wound infection with a standard ventral hernia repair has been reported to be approximately 12% to 45%.[16–19] In a large prospective multicenter study of laparoscopic ventral hernioplasty, the infection rate involving the prosthetic mesh was 1.4%.[20]

The prosthetic material in a laparoscopic hernioplasty is passed into the peritoneal cavity via a trocar site and has minimal contact with the skin, which makes the debate of infectibility somewhat irrelevant in choosing a prosthetic for laparoscopic hernioplasty. However, for wound contamination to progress to wound infection, the concentration of organisms must be 10^6 per gram of tissue for most pathogens. The host's defense system will immobilize and phagocytose and, with delay in subsequent wound healing phases, try to rid the wound of bacteria with and without the help of antibiotics.

When a prosthetic material is introduced into the wound, the concentration of microorganisms necessary to turn the wound contamination into infection significantly decreases (i.e., 10^3 per gram tissue decrease).[21] Bacteria and tissue cells are competing to reach the prosthetic material. Whichever (bacteria or tissue cell) arrives at the foreign material first will penetrate, adhere to, and populate the prosthesis to the greater degree. The host tissue defense mechanism works similarly to normal wound healing, using neutrophils and macrophages to immobilize and phagocytose foreign material and bacteria. Depending on the physical structure of the prosthesis and localized infection, the host may be able to resolve the infection.

Tissue ingrowth within the e-PTFE is important because it fills the internodal void spaces, thus limiting access for bacteria. The hydrophobic nature of the e-PTFE appears to slow initial bacterial advance into the material and inhibit "wicking" or the microorganisms. Wicking is the fluid-phase transport of bacteria. The e-PTFE structure (average pore size, 22 μm) seems to prohibit harboring of bacteria and limits the bacteria to the periphery of the e-PTFE. This reaction seems to prevent the rapid spread of infection. As a result, WBCs (neutrophil average size, 14 μm) gain ready access to the bacteria and appear to play an active role in ridding the wound of bacteria, while fibrous tissue keeps contamination localized.

In comparison, mesh materials are considered to be macroporous. Some regions between the weave filaments at points of contact are too small for WBCs and fibroblastic penetration. However, these spaces remain large enough to harbor bacteria and permit bacterial access ("wicking") along material filaments. This wicking effect can complicate and potentially inhibit the successful resolution of infection.

Elek et al. demonstrated that, when foreign bodies are present, fewer organisms are required to produce a clinical infection.[21] The foreign body acts synergistically by decreasing the concentration of bacteria necessary to produce an infection. The adherence of bacteria to a foreign body is a very complex process, involving stereospecific interaction between bacterial ligands and receptor sites on the foreign surface.[22] Sugarman showed the magnitude of the adherence is related to the type of bacteria and foreign body involved in the interaction.[23] Brown et al. demonstrated that the e-PTFE patches consistently had 100-fold fewer organisms per square centimeter than did the polypropylene meshes in the absence of antibiotics or with antibiotics administered after contamination with *Staphylococcus aureus*.[24] They concluded that e-PTFE is more resistant to the production of clinical infection if contamination occurs intraoperatively. This conclusion is supported by a great deal of clinical experience, particularly in the vascular literature, where e-PTFE has been used since 1976.[25–33] This consideration was thought to be secondary to the porous structure (22 μm) and the hydrophobic properties of e-PTFE, which result in a less hospitable nidus for bacterial adherence.

Adhesions

Adhesions may be categorized in three ways:

Fibrinous, which resolve spontaneously within a few weeks

Omental, which cause no persistent problem for the patient

Fibrous, which may form into tendinous bands capable of constricting visceral organs

The chief concern regarding peritoneal adhesions is eventual bowel obstruction. An estimated 30% of all intestinal obstructions are caused by adhesions. Experimental studies and clinical experience with full repairs of full-thickness abdominal wall defects have shown a lower incidence and grade of visceral adhesions formation or adhesion-related complications with e-PTFE when compared to mesh material.[21,33–39] Peritoneal injury and all types of foreign materials stimulate adhesion formation. In experimental studies, laparotomy incisions closed with monofilament suture had a 30% incidence of adhesions. The incidence of adhesions to e-PTFE, polypropylene mesh, and polyester mesh was 36%, 82.4%, and 100%, retrospectively. Lennox and Ellis showed that fibrinous adhesions are replaced by fibrous tissue at about 10 days, which then remain permanent.[34] This conversion is prevented by the fibrinolytic activity of the peritoneum, which is divided equally between the mesothelial and submesothelial layers.

Studies by Law and Ellis demonstrated that e-PTFE would support a continuous layer of mesothelial cells on the peritoneal surface.[35] The collagen penetration of the interstices of e-PTFE was regular and evenly distributed. The mesothelial cells would first appear at approximately 2 weeks after implantation and became a continuous layer at approximately 4 weeks. With Marlex mesh, the mesothelial cells were observed in an irregular pattern and were found only in association with fatty or omental adhesions. Law and Ellis demonstrated that adhesion formation to e-PTFE and the mesh materials is inversely related to the number of mesothelial cells on the peritoneal surface.[35] In the presence of infection, mesothelial cells are found infrequently with a reduction in fibrinolytic activity, such that the fibrinous adhesions are not removed and develop into dense fibrous adhesions that are permanent. This finding was confirmed in infected wound studies by Brown et al. and Law and Ellis, in which

there was increase in adhesions with both e-PTFE and polypropylene mesh in the presence of infection.[24,35]

If adhesions form to the e-PTFE, they usually include and originate at the line of fixation, which is a point of mechanical rigidity, tissue compression, or tissue ischemia. The adhesions to the e-PTFE have been reported to be of a filmy nature and easily dissectable. The smooth surface of the e-PTFE and associated mild foreign body response appear to provide minimal interference with peritoneal healing and neomesothelialization. The chemical nature and physical structure of mesh materials are likely factors in the formation of adhesions. Because of their rigidity and rough surface structure, meshes can irritate and injure the underlying tissue structures, causing inflammatory fibroplasia and a moderate foreign body response. The reformation of the mesothelial layer is somewhat retarded and incomplete as a result of the regular surface dense scar formation around the mesh filaments. The incidence of adhesions in experimental trials of mesh materials ranges from 80% to 90%.

Erosion–Fistulization

Erosion of abdominal viscera resulting in obstruction, abscess, and fistula formation is the cardinal determining factor for choice of prosthetic material in the peritoneal position. Experimental studies and clinical experience with polypropylene mesh are replete with complications of erosions and fistulizations.[35,39–47]

e-PTFE has been used in the peritoneal cavity for vascular bypass since 1976 and for hernia repair since 1983, with no clinical cases of bowel strangulation or fistula formation reported. In addition, e-PTFE has been used for the repair of diaphragmatic defects, slings for repair of rectal prolapse, bladder, and urethral suspension, and bands for vertically banded gastroplasties. In all these procedures, the e-PTFE is placed adjacent to hollow viscus organs, with no reports of erosion or fistulization. On the contrary, erosions and fistulization have been seen in all these procedures with the use of polypropylene meshes. The mechanism for erosion and fistula formation is similar to that for adhesion formation, with the addition of time.

Mesh materials have a moderate to severe inflammatory and foreign body response. They do not promote neomesothelialization and, therefore, cause dense fibrous adhesions. The mesh materials also have a rigid and abrasive surface. If the bowel, with its continuous wall motion (peristalsis), is densely adherent to this rigid, abrasive surface, in time the mesh will erode through the bowel wall and fistulize. On the contrary, e-PTFE is inert, has a mild inflammatory and foreign body response, and promotes rapid proliferation of mesothelial cells on the peritoneal surface. It also has a smooth, pliable, nonabra-

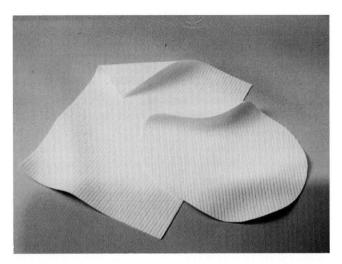

FIGURE 35.5. e-PTFE Dual-Mesh Biomaterial.

least foreign body response, has the least infectibility, has minimal adhesions, and has no reported bowel erosions or fistulizations. I believe the best biomaterial in the intraperitoneal position is e-PTFE Dual-Mesh Plus Biomaterial (Fig. 35.5).

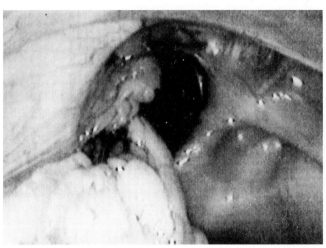

A

sive surface that does not promote erosion and fistula formation.

After reviewing the clinical and basic science data, e-PTFE mesh is superior in both the mechanical and biological categories. e-PTFE is the strongest, has the best fixation-retention strength, has the best durability, is the most inert, has the least inflammatory response, has the least foreign body response, has the least infectibility, has minimal adhesions, and has no reported bowel erosions or fistualizations.

Over the past decade, several technological advances have been made to further improve e-PTFE as a biomaterial. This material is known as Dual-Mesh Plus Biomaterial, which is e-PTFE with two distinct surfaces. The textured surface of the material has a micropore structure with an average fibril length or internodal space of greater than 17 μm, allowing for host tissue incorporation. The surface of this material should be placed adjacent to tissue where tissue incorporation is desired. The smooth surface of the material has a pore size of less than 3 μm, resulting in minimal tissue attachment. This side of the material should be positioned to the tissue or viscera where minimal tissue attachment is desired. This biomaterial is impregnated with two antimicrobial preservative agents, chlorhexidine diacetate and silver carbonate. These antimicrobial preservatives are intended to inhibit bacterial colonization of the biomaterial for up to 10 days after implantation. Zone-of-inhibition bioassays have found that this biomaterial has substantial preservative activity against the following gram-positive and gram-negative organisms (*Staphylococcus aureus, Staphylococcus epidermidis, Escherichia coli, Klebsiella pneumoniae, Pseudomonas aeruginosa*, and *Candida albicans*).

In summary, e-PTFE is the strongest, has the best fixation-retention strength, has the best durability, is the most inert, has the least inflammatory response, has the

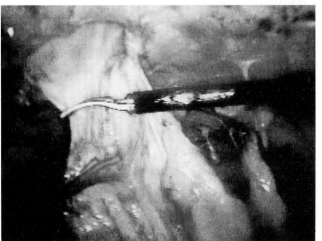

B

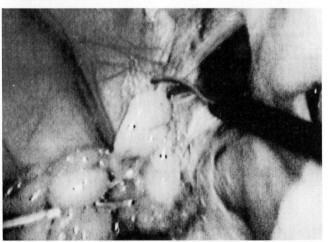

C

FIGURE 35.6A–C. Adhesionolysis.

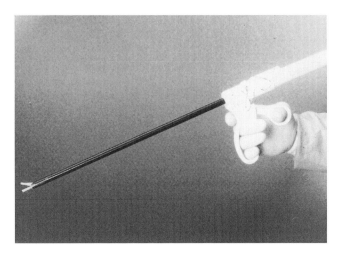

FIGURE 35.7. Ultracision Harmonic Scalpel.

Surgical Technique

The procedure is performed under general anesthesia. The patient is given antibiotic prophylaxis, and the bladder is decompressed with a Foley catheter. The stomach is decompressed with a nasogastric tube. An alternative puncture site is chosen away from the hernia defect and any abdominal incisions. A skin incision is made, and a Veress needle is inserted or an open technique is utilized. The abdomen is insufflated with CO_2. A 30° laparoscope is introduced through the same incision. Under direct visualization, additional 11-mm trocars are inserted as far lateral as possible. Adhesiolysis is performed utilizing an Endo-Babcock to provide exposure and countertraction of the hernia contents and adhesions, which are lysed with endoscopic shears (Fig. 35.6A–C). If the adhesions are dense and involve the bowel, a Ultracision Harmonic Scalpel is utilized for adhesionolysis to decrease the likelihood of a bowel injury and obtain adequate hemostasis (Fig. 35.7).

All the contents of the hernia sac are reduced into the peritoneal cavity. The hernia sac is left in situ (Fig. 35.8A,B). Additional 11-mm trocars are introduced on the opposite side laterally under direct vision. The number and position of trocar placement must be individualized. Direct vision and palpation allow identification of the edges of the hernia defect.

The edges are then drawn on the abdominal wall, and 1-mm-thick Gore-Tex dual mesh biomaterial is measured to overlap the defect by at least 3 cm in all directions and cut to the appropriate size (Fig. 35.9). Through the evolution of this procedure, it became apparent that stapling was not adequate for large ventral hernias. CV-O Gore-Tex sutures are placed and tied at all four corners, and the sutures are left approximately 6 in. long. One or two

additional sutures of 0 Ethibond (for color contrast) are placed at one edge of the patch. With the rough side of the patch up, the patch is rolled up (Fig. 35.10). The patch is grasped at one end with an Endo-Babcock clamp. One of the trocars is removed and the patch is then introduced into the abdominal cavity. Using 5-mm graspers, the free edge of the patch is grasped and the Ethibond suture is pulled unrolling the patch. This step greatly facilitates proper patch orientation. An endoscopic suture-passer is then utilized to secure the dual mesh biomaterial to the anterior abdominal wall.

The corners that are drawn on the anterior abdominal wall are then identified intraabdominally. The endoscopic suture-passer (Fig. 35.11) is then passed through a small skin incision of about 2 mm, and the sutures previously placed at the four corners of the patch are grasped with a 5-mm needle driver and loaded into the endoscopic suture-passer and pulled extracorporeally, tied, and pushed down through the subcutaneous fat to the anterior fascial layer (Fig. 35.12A,B). At this point, the patch is

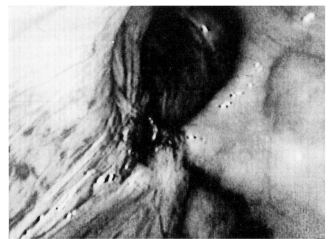

A

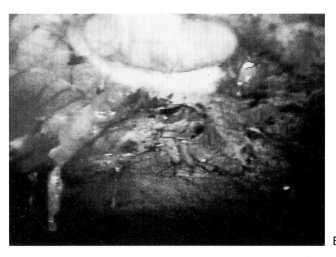

B

FIGURE 35.8A,B. Hernia defects postadhesionolysis.

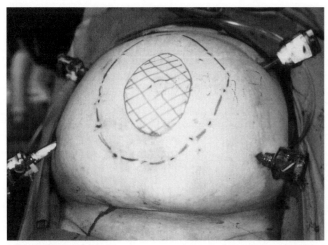

FIGURE 35.9. Defect is drawn on anterior abdominal wall and mesh size determined.

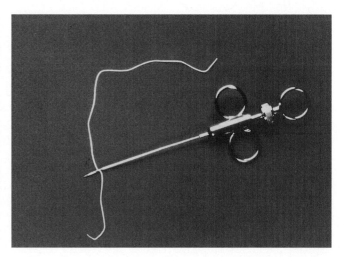

FIGURE 35.11. Endoscopic suture-passer.

then circumferentially stapled to the posterior fascial layers using the Endopath EMS Stapler; this is greatly facilitated by anterior abdominal wall countertraction.

The suturing technique was devised to obtain strong fixation to the anterior abdominal wall. Stapling is very effective on laparoscopic inguinal hernioplasties because of the ability to utilize Pascal's law, which states that pressure in a closed space, when increased, is distributed in all directions equally. If the patch is much larger than the defect, the patch is then forced up against the inner surface of the anterior abdominal wall and is stabilized in position by the very forces that tend to push the patch through the defect.

The defect-to-patch ratio for inguinal hernias where the average defects are 5cm^2 and the patch is 96cm^2 results in a patch that is 19 times larger than the defect. The defect-to-patch ratio for ventral hernias, however,

with an average defect size of 80cm^2 and an average patch size of 243cm^2, results in a patch only three times larger than the defect. When one further subdivides the ventral hernias into the very large ventral hernias, the average defect size is 336cm^2, and the average patch size

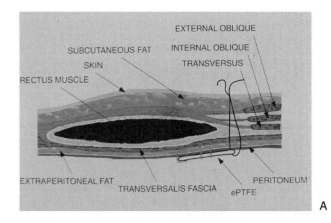

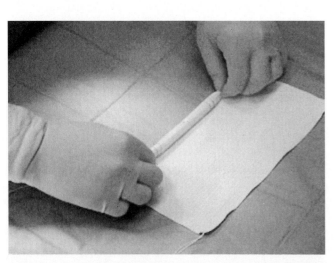

FIGURE 35.10. Mesh prepared for introduction into peritoneal cavity.

FIGURE 35.12A,B. Anatomic description of abdominal wall with patch and suture placement.

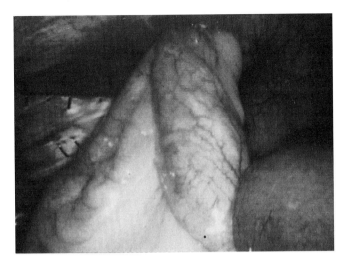

FIGURE 35.13. Trocar site (Richter's) hernia as seen through a laparoscope.

is 600 cm², making the patch only 1.8 times larger than the actual defect. With these larger defect-to-patch ratios, Pascal's principle does not stabilize the patch, and stronger anterior fascial fixation is needed, which is provided by the suturing technique. After completing the stapling circumferentially, additional nonabsorbable 0 sutures are placed circumferentially using the endoscopic suture-passer. The sutures are placed at approximately 5-cm intervals around the entire circumference of the patch.

To complete the procedure, all the trocar sites are closed. Under direct vision, the endoscopic suture-passer is passed adjacent to the trocar, angling it away from the trocar with a nonabsorbable 0 suture. The suture is then grasped with a 5-mm grasper. The endoscopic suture-passer is then passed to the opposite side of the trocar site. The suture is remounted into the endoscopic suture-passer and pulled through, creating a horizontal mattress suture around the trocar site. This technique greatly facilitates trocar site closure, especially in the obese patient. The trocar is removed and the sutures tied, completely closing the trocar site; this prevents the occurrence of trocar site (Richter's) hernias (Fig 35.13). The trocar site skin incisions are closed with 4-0 vicryl sutures, and the skin nicks are closed with steri-strips.

Conclusion

Laparoscopic ventral hernioplasty has been evaluated by a prospective, multicenter study.[20] This study reported 144 hernioplasties, 64% incisional, with a mean defect size of 98 cm². The mean operative time was 120 min with no major perioperative complications. The mean discharge from the hospital was 2.3 days, with a mean return to

normal activity of 15 days. There were 2 major infections (1.4%) that required removal of the patch; these were believed secondary to inadequate shaving of the patient and pulling hair into the suture wounds. The recurrence rate was 4.2%, with a mean follow-up duration of 355 days and a follow-up rate of 94.5%.

Clearly, the laparoscopic repair of the ventral/incisional hernia is a major addition to the surgical armamentarium for this difficult problem.

References

1. Hesselink VJ, Luijendik RW, de Wilt JHW, et al. An evaluation of risk factors in incisional hernia recurrence. Surg Gynecol Obstet 1993;176:228–234.
2. Santora TA, Roslyn JJ. Incisional hernia. Surg Clin N A 1993;73:557–570.
3. Langer S, Christiansen J. Long-term results after incisional hernia repair. Acta Chir Scand 1985;151:217–219.
4. Van der Linden FT, van Vroonhoven TJ. Long-term results after correction of incisional hernia. Neth J Surg 1988;40:127–129.
5. Spaw AT, Ennis BW, Spaw LP. Laparoscopic hernia repair: the anatomic basis. J Laparoendosc Surg 1991;1:269–277.
6. Pick JW, Anson BJ, Ashley FL. The origin of the obturatory artery. Am J Anat 1942;70:317–342.
7. Toy FK. Surgical Anatomy & Techniques for Laparoscopic Hernioplasty. Arizona: W.L. Gore & Associates, 1994:1–11.
8. Elliott MP, Juler GL. Comparison of Marlex mesh and microporous Teflon sheets when used for hernia repair in the experimental animal. Am J Surg 1979;137:342–344.
9. Madden JW, Peacock EE Jr. Studies on the biology of collagen during wound healing. III. Dynamic metabolism of scar collagen and remodeling of dermal wounds. Ann Surg 1971;174:511.
10. Peacock EE Jr, Van Winkle W Jr. Surgery and Biology of Wound Repair, 2nd Ed. Philadelphia: Saunders, 1976.
11. Douglas DM. The healing of aponeurotic incisions. Br J Surg 1962;104:273.
12. Howes EL, Soroy JW, Harvey SC. The healing of wounds as determined by their tensile strength. JAMA 1929;92:242.
13. Levenson SM, Geeve EF, Crowley W, et al. The healing of rat skin wounds. Ann Surg 1965;161:293.
14. Mason ML, Allen HS. The rate of healing of tendons. An experimental study of tensile strength. Ann Surg 1941;113:424.
15. Rovee DT, Miller CA. Experimental role of breaking strength of wounds. Arch Surg 1968;96:43.
16. Houck JP, Rypins EB, Sarfeh IJ, et al. Repair of incisional hernia. Surg Gynecol Obstet 1989;169:397–399.
17. Mueller CB. Editorial: abdominal incisional hernia—the role of wound infection. Can J Surg 1974;17:195.
18. Stoppa RE. The treatment of complicated groin and incisional hernias. World J Surg 1989;13:545–554.
19. von Smitten K, Heikel HV, Sundell B. Repair of incisional hernia by F. Langenskiold's operation. Acta Chir Scand 1982;148:257–261.
20. Toy FK, Moskowitz M, Smoot RT, et al. Results of a prospective multicenter trial evaluating the e-PTFE

peritoneal onlay laparoscopic inguinal hernioplasty. J Laparoendosc Surg 1996;6(6).

21. Elek SD, Conin PE. The virulence of *Staphylococcus pyogenes* for man: a study of the problem of wound infection. Br J Exp Pathol 1957;38:573–579.

22. Franson TR, Sheth NK, Rose HD, et al. Scanning electron microscopy of bacterial adherent to intravascular catheters. J Clin Microbiol 1984;20:500–505.

23. Sugarman B. In vitro adherence of bacterial to prosthetic vascular grafts. Infection 1982;10:2–11.

24. Brown GL, Richardson JD, Malangoni MA, et al. Comparison of prosthetic materials for abdominal wall reconstruction in the presence of contamination and infection. Ann Surg 1985;201:705–711.

25. Schmitt DD, Bandyk DF, Pequet AJ, et al. Bacterial adherence to vascular prostheses. A determinant of graft infectability. J Vasc Surg 1986;3:732–740.

26. Rosenman JE, Pearce WH, Kempezinski RF. Bacterial adherence to vascular grafts after in vitro bacteremia. J Surg Res 1985;38:648–655.

27. Voyles CR, Richardson JD, Bland KI, et al. Emergency abdominal wall reconstruction with polypropylene mesh. Ann Surg 1981;194:219–223.

28. Bhat DJ, Tellis VA, Kohlberg WI, et al. Management of sepsis involving expanded polytetrafluoroethylene grafts for hemodialysis access. Surgery (St. Louis) 1990;87:445–450.

29. Connolly JE, Brownell DA, Levine EF, et al. Complications of renal dialysis access procedures. Arch Surg 1984;119:1325–1328.

30. Gifford RRM. Management of tunnel infections of dialysis polytetrafluoroethylene grafts. J Vasc Surg 1985;2:854–858.

31. Raju S. PTFE grafts for hemodialysis access. Ann Surg 1987;206:666–673.

32. Tellis V, Weiss P, Matas A, et al. Skin flap coverage of polytetrafluoroethylene vascular access graft exposed by previous infection. Surgery (St. Louis) 1988;103:118–121.

33. Tellis VA, Kohlberg WI, Bhat DJ, et al. Expanded polytetrafluoroethylene graft fistula for chronic hemodialysis. Ann Surg 1979;189:101–105.

34. Lennox MS, Ellis H. Fibrinolysis and adhesions formation in the peritoneum. In: 2nd International Symposium on the Surgery and Biology of the Greater Omentum.

35. Law NH, Ellis H. Adhesion formation and peritoneal healing on prosthetic materials. Clin Mater 1988;3:95–101.

36. Usher FC, Gannon JP. Marlex mesh. A new plastic mesh for replacing tissue defects. Arch Surg 1959;78:131–137.

37. Boyd WC. Use of Marlex mesh in acute loss of the abdominal wall due to infection. Surg Gynecol Obstet 1977;44:251–252.

38. Saxen L, Myllarniemi H. Foreign materials and postoperative adhesions. N Engl J Med 1968;279:200–202.

39. Stone HH, Fabian TC, Turkleson ML, et al. Management of full thickness losses of the abdominal wall. Ann Surg 1981;24:543–544.

40. Schneider R, Herrington JL Jr., Granada A. Marlex mesh in repair of a diaphragmatic defect later eroding into the distal esophagus and stomach. Ann Surg 1979;45:337–339.

41. Kaufman Z, Engelberg M, Zager M. Fecal fistula: a late complication of Marlex mesh repair. Dis Colon Rectum 1981;24:543–544.

42. Voyles CR, Richardson JD, Bland KI, et al. Emergency abdominal wall reconstruction with polypropylene mesh. Short-term benefits versus long-term complications. Ann Surg 1981;194:219–223.

43. Mathes SJ, Stone HH. Acute traumatic losses of abdominal wall substances. J Trauma 1975;15:386–390.

44. Cerise EJ, Busuttil RW, Craighead CC, et al. The use of mersilene mesh in repair of abdominal wall hernias: a clinical and experimental study. Ann Surg 1975;181:728–734.

45. Dayton MT, Buchele BA, Shirazi SS, et al. Use of an absorbable mesh to repair contaminated abdominal wall defects. Arch Surg 1986;121:954–960.

46. Murphy JL, Freeman JB, Dionne PG. Comparison of Marlex and Gore-Tex to repair abdominal wall defects in rats. Can J Surg 1989;32:244–247.

47. Van da Lei B, Bleichrodt RP, Simmmermocher RKJ, Van Schilfgaarde R. Expanded polytetrafluoroethylene patch for the repair of large abdominal wall defects. Br J Surg 1989;76:803–805.

36
Laparoscopic Repair of Ventral Hernias

Guy R. Voeller

Patient Preparation

The indications for laparoscopic ventral/incisional hernia repair have been well described in the previous section. Weight loss in the obese patient before open ventral hernia repair is attempted fairly routinely in Europe. Over the years, we have tried to do the same but without much success. Most of our patients with ventral/incisional hernias are large, and weight loss before repair has been modest at best. It is probably unrealistic to assume that these patients will be able to lose significant amounts of weight. However, the wound complications observed in obese patients undergoing open ventral/incisional hernia repair are not seen in patients undergoing laparoscopic repair, so weight loss before surgery may not be as critical as it is in the open approach.

If the patient has had several previous surgeries with what is thought to be densely adherent colon involved, then I have them undergo a formal bowel preparation in case a colonic enterotomy occurs. I always tell the patient that if it is not safe to lyse adhesions or the bowel cannot be reduced safely, then an open repair will be done. I explain to them that, if an enterotomy occurs, I may or may not proceed with repair based on the type of injury, contamination, and ease of repair.

Equipment

The majority of ventral/incisional hernias can be repaired with video monitors, positioned similar to a laparoscopic cholecystectomy. However, as the hernia moves more caudad, the monitor(s) need to be moved caudad so that the surgeon works in the same direction the camera is viewing. The surgeon and assistant need to be able to approach the patient from all angles to operate from any direction. It is ideal if the arms can be tucked to the side of the patient. Often, however, this is not possible because of the large size of these patients. In these cases

one should move the operating room bed away from the anesthesiologist and drape out above the arm boards to allow the surgeon and assistant to position themselves properly.

We do not routinely use Foley catheters and nasogastric tubes. We place a Foley if it is likely that it will be a prolonged procedure or if the position of the hernia that is being repaired is very low, right at the pubic bone. In this instance, the mesh may have to be anchored to Cooper's ligament; this will require making a peritoneal flap and ensuring the bladder is out of harm's way. The Foley allows not only decompression of the bladder but in addition it can be used to instill normal saline into the bladder. Clamping the Foley allows one to distend the bladder to aid in identification during dissection. Nasogastric suction is used only if the stomach is distended or in the way during the dissection. Sequential pneumatic compression boots are placed on the legs of all patients; these are left on until the patient is ambulating.

An up-to-date video endoscopic camera, monitor, and light source are absolutely essential. A 30° or 45° angle view laparoscope is optimal to perform the operation. The angle telescope allows the surgeon to evaluate the anterior abdominal wall. The angle telescope can be turned over to manipulate the mesh and inspect the abdominal cavity. We place one 10-mm port for our initial access; however, all our working ports are either 5 mm or needlescopic. A 5-mm angle telescope thus is very useful for this procedure. The newer 5-mm telescopes offer an excellent field of vision as well as light transmission.

Atraumatic bowel graspers and very sharp scissors are required for proper dissection and to prevent injury to the viscera. The most difficult part of the dissection is lysis of adhesions and reducing viscera from the hernia. Energy sources should be used at a minimum. Monopolar cautery can be used if far away from viscera and if the proper planes are maintained, minimal blood loss should be expected. Many operators prefer the harmonic scalpel for lysis of adhesions, but this instrument gets very hot at the tip. Even with minimal thermal spread, the tip of the instrument can damage the viscera, which may not be apparent at the time of surgery. We do not use the harmonic scalpel routinely.

Suture fixation of the mesh is critical for long-term good results. We initially selected polypropylene sutures for their monofilament nature; however, their memory meant these were very difficult to work with through the laparoscope. We then selected Gore CV-0 suture because it is nonabsorbable, has no memory, and is quite easy to use through the laparoscope. To prevent internal hernia formation between the prosthetic and the peritoneal cavity, 5-mm spiral tackers are used; these allow good strong apposition of the prosthetic to the peritoneum and work much better than the staplers that were commonly used before the tacking devices became available. We use the suture-passer developed by Toy and Smoot to pass the suture through the abdominal wall. We first used a Keith needle, and other tools can be used to pass the suture; however, the Toy–Smoot suture-passer is ideal.

Polytetrafluoroethylene (PTFE) meshes are probably best suited for this laparoscopic repair. The mesh must be placed intraperitoneally, and extensive documentation shows that polyester and polypropylene meshes cause a severe inflammatory response with dense adhesion formation and the risks of bowel obstruction or fistulas. This inflammation leads to an extremely difficult reoperation if required. Over the past several years as this procedure has been developed, W.L. Gore has produced a Dual-Mesh Plus, a dual-sided mesh meant for intraperitoneal placement. One side has a very small pore size that inhibits tissue ingrowth; this side is placed against the viscera. On the other side the pore size is large enough that tissue ingrowth can occur. Obviously, this side is placed next to the peritoneal surface. In addition, the newer prosthetic has antimicrobial chlorhexidine and silver salts impregnated into the mesh.

ery requires 6 to 8 weeks. At the University of Tennessee, the Rives–Stoppa approach became the method of repair for large ventral/incisional hernias. As we began to develop the technique for laparoscopic repair, it became apparent that the technique done laparoscopically should mimic this open approach that leads to such low recurrence rates.

Hesselink et al. showed that hernias larger than 4 cm, if not repaired with mesh, have a very high recurrence rate.[3] In addition, we believe that any recurrent hernias, even if smaller than 4 cm, or any hernia in the morbidly obese, are candidates for laparoscopic repair with mesh.

It is critical that sterile technique not be compromised. We cover the skin with an Ioban protective skin drape to avoid any contact between skin flora and prosthetic. The patient should be prepped very far laterally, and draping should also be done very far laterally to allow access with trocars. Our technique of choice is the placement of a balloon-tipped blunt Hasson trocar at either costal margin as far lateral as possible, staying superior to the colon. Hasson S-shaped retractors are essential to retract each fascial and muscle layer as it is incised and separated. The peritoneum is visualized and a #11 scalpel blade incises the peritoneum; the blunt tip can then easily be placed. Trocar placement depends on hernia size and location; however, because most are midline we begin with the Hasson port, and then one or two 5-mm ports are placed to begin adhesionolysis (Fig. 36.1). These patients are quite large, and often it is easier to use one 5-mm port with your dominant hand while your nondominant hand compresses the abdominal wall to bring it down to the scissor tip or the grasper tip for dissection. The entire abdominal wall should be cleared of all adhesions to evaluate every area for possible hernia defects, which often are not appreciated preoperatively on examination. If viscera cannot be safely reduced or there is concern about bowel injury that cannot be appreciated,

Technique

The American Hernia Society has stated the Rives–Stoppa open approach for large ventral/incisional hernias should be the standard of care. It has been well documented that this repair, which places the prosthetic behind the rectus muscle and behind the fascial defect, leads to the lowest rates of recurrence.[1,2] This operation is a very large undertaking; large skin and soft tissue flaps are created, with a significant amount of dead space and a high rate of wound problems. This technique was specifically developed so that the prosthetic could be placed behind the hernia defect but kept off the viscera as the technique was described using polypropylene or polyester meshes. In addition to the high complication rate, hospital stay usually ranges from 5 to 8 days and recov-

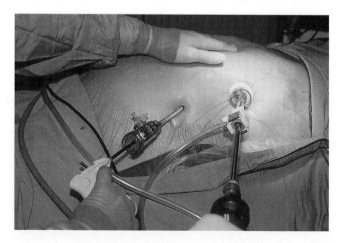

FIGURE 36.1. Initial trocar placement.

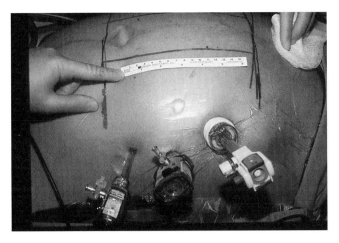

FIGURE 36.2. Border of hernia.

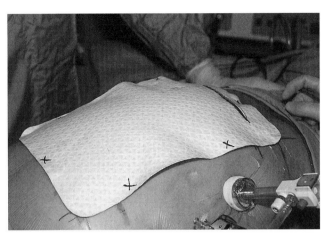

FIGURE 36.4. Suture fixation points.

the patient should be opened and a safe repair undertaken of either the viscera or the hernia. We believe if an enterotomy is created that it is safest to repair the enterotomy laparoscopically or through a very small incision and then repair the hernia another day. We have on occasion repaired a small bowel enterotomy laparoscopically and continued with repair and these patients have done well. However, we emphasize that safety is critical and if there is any question open surgery should be considered.

Once all the incarcerated viscera is reduced and all adhesions have been lysed, determine the fascial borders of the defect. Often the borders of the hernia can be evaluated simply by looking at the abdominal wall and the extent of the hernia. For example, in a long midline incision with multiple defects up and down the midline, the surgeon can look at the old scar to determine the borders of the hernia. However, if one is unsure, the hernia should be palpated preoperatively in the holding area. A technique described by Toy and Smoot also can be used, which consists of passing a spinal needle through the

abdominal wall and watching where it comes out in the peritoneal cavity in relation to the hernia defect. As the cephalad, caudad, and lateral borders are determined, these are diagrammed on the abdominal wall with a marking pen (Fig. 36.2). We then add 3 to 5cm in all directions to these dimensions, drawn on the abdominal wall (Fig. 36.3), which gives us the diagram for the needed prosthesis size. We mark the mesh to designate the top of the prosthetic; in addition, we mark X's on the mesh and on the skin at corresponding sites (Fig. 36.4) to indicate where initial stay sutures will be placed to hold the prosthetic against the abdominal wall. Gore CV-0 suture is then used to place U stitches at each of these X's on the prosthetic. The sutures are tied, leaving tails long enough to tie again once the mesh is placed intraperitoneally, and brought up through the abdominal wall. We place a hemoclip on each suture pair to facilitate grasping and passing the sutures with the suture-passer (Fig. 36.5). Five or six stay sutures are used for large patches and four for smaller patches. The mesh is then rolled from each edge

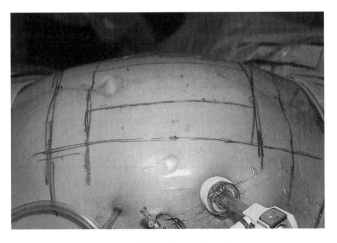

FIGURE 36.3. Size of mesh.

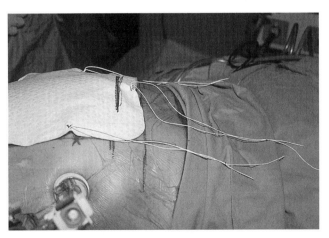

FIGURE 36.5. Hemoclip on suture pair.

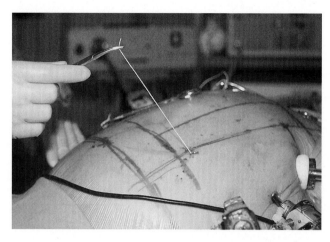

FIGURE 36.6. Sutures through the abdominal wall.

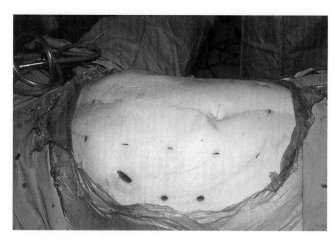

FIGURE 36.8. Final result.

toward the middle; if rolled in one continuous fashion, it is difficult to unroll once it is placed in the peritoneal cavity. Smaller pieces of mesh can be placed through the 10-mm Hasson port directly, but most large pieces require removal of the balloon-tipped Hasson by placing a grasper opposite the Hasson port through a 5-mm port placed on the opposite side. The grasper is directed out through the Hasson cannula, the Hasson cannula is removed, and the pneumoperitoneum evacuates, leaving the tip of the grasper protruding through the fascial defect of the Hasson port. The mesh is placed in the tip of the grasper and the grasper is drawn into the abdominal cavity bringing the mesh with it. Once the mesh is entirely inside the abdominal cavity, the Hasson port is reinserted and pneumoperitoneum reestablished. The laparoscope is then turned with the view looking down onto the viscera so one can view the mesh and unfurl it using two graspers placed in the middle of the mesh and pushing in opposite directions.

At each X marked on the skin, small punctures are made. The Toy–Smoot suture-passer is then used to bring each suture pair out through the entire thickness of the abdominal wall (Fig. 36.6). Both sutures of a pair come out through the same skin puncture, but through a separate fascial puncture such that there is at least a 1-cm bridge between each suture of a pair, by redirecting the suture-passer as it penetrates the fascia. Once all the sutures are brought out through the entire thickness of the abdominal wall, they are tied with the knots residing in the subcutaneous tissue. These sutures thus have anchored the mesh to the entire thickness of the abdominal wall. One must understand that the sutures are the main strength of this repair. Spiral tacks are then used to tack the prosthetic to the peritoneal surface 360° between the stay sutures to prevent internal hernia formation. One must tack in the direction of the camera; this usually requires placement of two 5-mm ports opposite the initially placed cannulas. Counterpressure on the abdominal wall is very important for good, accurate tacking. The mesh should be stretched very tightly so that when the pneumoperitoneum is evacuated there is a good solid tension-free repair without protrusion of the mesh into the hernia defect (Fig. 36.7). When tacking is complete, additional stay sutures can be placed, using the suture-passer, at 5- to 7-cm intervals. In very large hernias, sutures can be placed at even more frequent intervals. The 10-mm Hasson port can be closed laparoscopically, and we do not routinely use a drain (Fig. 36.8).

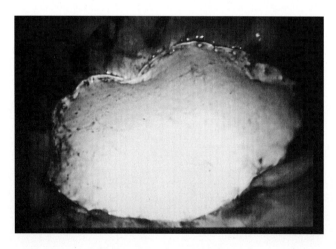

FIGURE 36.7. Mesh in place.

Postoperative Instructions to Patient

Immediately postoperatively, the patient will have much more pain than do laparoscopic cholecystectomy patients. All the peritoneal tacking and U stitches cause

TABLE 36.1. Operative data.

	Average	Range
Hernia size	100.1 cm²	1–480 cm²
Mesh size	287 cm²	24–924 cm²
Operative time	97 min	11–270 min

TABLE 36.2. Postoperative data.

Length of stay:
    Average, 1.8 days
    Range, 0–17 days
Complications, 53 (13%)
Mortality, 0
Follow-up:
    Average, 23 months
    Range, 1–60 months

significant discomfort, and narcotic analgesia is required. If the patient is to stay overnight, we use patient-controlled analgesia by the intravenous route. The pain dissipates quite quickly, however, and on the first postoperative day, oral medications are adequate to control the pain. We routinely give liquids postoperatively and advance the diet as the patient tolerates. If a significant fascial defect has been repaired, or one large hernia with a significant soft tissue excess, we place a large compression bandage over the area similar to an umbilical tape as it is used in the pediatric umbilical hernia. This compression bandage is left in place for 7 to 10 days. The patient is allowed to shower, and activity is not restricted. The discomfort that the patient experiences will limit their activities for approximately 2 weeks, and this is sufficient restriction.

We believe all patients develop a seroma between the patch and the peritoneal sac. Not all these become clinically evident but some do. Most surgeons leave the seroma as almost all disappear. I, however, aspirate large seromas on a routine basis,[4] which makes the patient more comfortable and helps them understand the bulge that remains after surgery. To date I have not caused a single infection of the prosthetic by performing aspiration of the seroma, which makes for a happier patient. In addition, I routinely take a laparoscopic picture of the hernia defect and then another picture after the patch has been placed over the defect. I show these pictures to patients to explain how the seroma forms; this gives patients an excellent idea of what is going on and helps them understand the seroma and its formation.

Outcomes and Complications

Several studies have compared laparoscopic and open incisional hernia repair.[5–7] In most of these studies the Rives–Stoppa approach was not used as the open repair of choice, which limits their relevance. However, in each study hernias were comparatively the same in both groups but hospitalization, recurrences, cost, and complications were all lower in the laparoscopic group.

Toy et al. reported preliminary data from a multicenter prospective involving 144 patients.[4] All repairs were done with PTFE as described here. The average hernia size was 98 cm². The average hospital stay was 2.3 days; this included Canadian study sites where socialized health care prolongs hospitalization. The postoperative infection rate was 3% and the recurrence rate 4%. Average return to normal activity was about 2 weeks.

Voeller et al. presented 407 laparoscopic ventral/incisional hernias at the 1999 American College of Surgeons Meeting.[8] Any patient with a hernia larger than 4 cm, any recurrent hernia, and any ventral/incisional hernia in a morbidly obese individual was entered into the study, totaling 415 patients. Eight were removed from the study because open repairs were required due to the inability to safely dissect incarcerated viscera. Body mass index in these patients was a mean of 32 kg², and 90% of the patients had previous abdominal surgery. Of the hernias in this study, 136 were recurrent, with the average number of previous repairs being 2 (range, 2–7). Table 36.1 shows the operative data, the average hernia size being 100 cm². As seen in Table 36.2, length of stay was short; there were

TABLE 36.3. Complications.

Complication	Number	Percent (%)
Prologed ileus	9	2.21
Seroma (>6 weeks)	8	1.97
Suture pain (>8 weeks)	8	1.97
Intestinal injury	6	1.47
Trocar cellulitis	5	1.23
Mesh infection	4	0.98
Hematoma/bleeding	3	0.75
Urinary retention	3	0.75
FUO	3	0.74
Respiratory distress	2	0.49
Intraabdominal abscess	1	0.25
Trocar site hernia	1	0.25

TABLE 36.4. Recurrences.

14 patients with recurrences (3.4%)
    4, infected meshes removed
    1, unsuspected bowel injury, reoperated
    6, not enough sutures used
    1, MVA with mesh disruption
6 recurrences in nonmidline hernias

few serious complications, and no deaths occurred. Our mean follow-up has been approximately 2 years with a range up to 5 years. Serious complications (Table 36.3) were a few bowel injuries and a few mesh infections. There were 14 recurrences, which compares quite favorably with the 10% to 36% range reported in the literature. As Table 36.4 shows, 28% of recurrences were due to mesh removal for infection. We have operated laparoscopically on several patients who have had a previous laparoscopic ventral/incisional hernia repair and found that any adhesions that form are very filmy and are easily lysed, compared to the dense fibrotic adhesions seen with polypropylene.

We believe that laparoscopic repair of ventral/incisional hernias has evolved to a point where it can now be done safely with a very low recurrence rate. Although techniques may differ on smaller points, it is absolutely essential that suture fixation of the prosthetic through the entire thickness of the abdominal wall be part of the surgeon's technique. Continued evaluation of recurrence rates will be important; however, the results of short-term evaluation look very promising.

References

1. Stoppa RE. The treatment of complicated groin and incisional hernias. World J Surg 1989;13:545–554.
2. Rives J, Pire JC, Flament JB, et al. Treatment of large eventrations. New therapeutic indications apropos of 322 cases. Chirurgie 1985;111(3):215–225.
3. Hesselink VJ, Luijendijk RW, de Wilt JHW, et al. An evaluation of risk factors in incisional hernia recurrence. Surg Gynecol Obstet 1993;176:228–234.
4. Toy FK, Bailey RW, Carey S, et al. Multicenter prospective study of laparoscopic ventral hernioplasty: preliminary results. Surg Endosc 1998;12(7):955–959.
5. Park A, Birch DW, Lovrics P. Laparoscopic and open incisional hernia repair: a comparison study. Surgery (St. Louis) 1998;124:816–822.
6. Ramshaw BJ, Schwab J, Mason EM, et al. Comparison of laparoscopic and open ventral herniorrhaphy. Abstract, Southeastern Surgical Congress, February 1999.
7. Holzman MD, Purut CM, Reintgen K, et al. Laparoscopic ventral and incisional hernioplasty. Surg Endosc 1997;11:32–35.
8. Voeller G, Park A, Heniford T, Ramshaw B. Laparoscopic repair of ventral and incisional hernias. Presented at American College of Surgeons, October 1999.

Section VI
Laparoscopic Procedures of the Colon and Rectum

Steven D. Wexner, MD
Section Editor

37
Laparoscopic Instrumentation

Anthony Macaluso, Jr. and Sergio W. Larach

Minimally invasive approaches to the treatment of colon disorders have been performed since 1991. Laparoscopic colon resections are technically demanding procedures, and as such were initially prohibitive for the majority of surgeons. Skills in port placement, instrumentation, and operative strategy were carefully refined and, when they were combined with surgeon experience, helped master the learning curve. Laparoscopic intrumentation is one key to help master the technically complex features of safely identifying the site of the lesion, mobilizing the appropriate segment of bowel, dissection and control of the mesenteric blood supply, and performing an anastomosis.

Laparoscopic instrumentation is important to help ensure an efficient and safe provedure. Basic laparoscopic equipment and advanced instrumentation are needed for laparoscopic colectomy procedures. This chapter reviews the basic equipment for laparoscopic colectomy with instrumentation and perspectives for future advances.

Equipment

Operating Table

An electronically operated table is preferable for the frequent changes in position needed for laparoscopic colectomy. The table is placed in Trendelenburg or reverse Trendelenburg position and titled to the left or right, allowing gravity to retract the intestines from the site of dissection.[1] The electronic table allows for quicker and smoother transition of patient position and provides a greater degree of angulation to improve intraabdominal exposure. A beanbag with Velcro attachment to the table pad helps secure the patient during steep angulation manueuvers. In addition, shoulder rolls or intravenous fluidbags taped to the table to support the shoulder also help to prevent the patient from sliding during steep Trendelenburg.

Allen stirrups (Allen Medical, Bedford Heights, OH, USA) are recommended for low lithotomy position. The lower extremities should have minimal flexion to prevent limitations of instrument motion from hitting the handles of laparoscopic instruments on the proximal thigh. The low lithotomy position is advantageous because it not only allows another area for the surgeon or assistant to stand but also aligns the surgeon with the camera and instruments for dissection of lateral fusion planes.[1]

Video Equipment

The necessary video equipment to replace the surgeon's direct visual perception and provide an image of the surgical field for safe laparoscopic surgery includes a video camera unit, the laparoscope, a light source, and monitoring and recording devices. Fundamental advances made in imaging techniques have been an important factor in allowing surgeons to perform laparoscopic colon surgery. Currently, most surgeons use two-dimensional (2-D) imaging and rely on indirect evidence of depth and position to judge spatial relationships in the peritoneal cavity. High-resolution video monitors and cameras that provide true color images, white balance, and good contrast greatly assist the surgeon to allow 2-D imaging versus three-dimensional (3-D). Three-dimensional laparoscopes are currently available; however, the 2-D imaging systems currently remain more popular.[2]

Laparoscopic cameras currently use a 0.5- to 0.67-in. silicon charge coupled device (CCD) to provide accurate dimensional detail and precise edge detection. A single-chip camera has one CCD for all colors, whereas in the three-chip camera one CCD is used for each primary color (red, yellow, and blue).[2] A three-CCD-chip camera with a resolution of about 700 to 800 lines per inch is the current state-of-the-art video camera. A signal is sent from the three-CCD chip in the camera head to a control digital signal-processing unit that processes the signal and transmits it to the video monitor or recorder.

Laparoscopes are available in various diameters and angles of visualization. The diameters range from 1.7 to 14 mm, but because laparoscopes with a diameter of 10 mm transmit approximately three times as much light as 5-mm laparoscopes, it is recommended to use a 10-mm laparoscope whenever possible.[2] An end-viewing, 0° laparoscope is easy to use but has some limitation with viewing capabilities compared to the angle-viewing scopes. The 30° laparoscope allows a wider overview with simple rotation of the scope and allows better visualization around a corner of fixed intraperitoneal structures. However, it is slightly more difficult to learn and use the 30° scope versus the 0° scope. The angle-viewing scope has more advantages, but the 0° scope is sufficient for most applications in laparoscopic colorectal surgery.

Flexible laparoscopes with optical fibers, including an irrigation channel, offer the advantages of end-viewing and angle-viewing instruments. Without loss of illumination, the visual field extends from an end view through any angle to about 120°. Thus, the scope can be positioned for maximal visualization of anatomic structures without interfering with the operating instruments. They are slightly more difficult to learn but have the distinct advantage of an irrigation channel to keep the lens clean intracorporeally and avoid frequent withdrawing of the scope to manually clean the tip.

A 10-mm, 0° rigid laparoscope (Video Hydro-Scope; Circon ACMI, Stamford, CT, USA), provides tangential irrigation of the scope lens intracorporeally and irrigation of tissue through a separate irrigation channel.[2] The advantage is cleaning of the lens intracorporeally during the surgery. The disadvantage is less light transmitted to the camera due to the additional working channels, and the scope is more difficult to clean and sterilize.

The laparosope should be warmed before insertion into the abdominal cavity so it will be at body temperature to prevent fogging. Laparoscopic warmers are commercially available, or the scope can be placed inside a heated hollow rubber dilator, or a warm water bath about 37° to 40°C may be used to keep the instrument warm. In addition, the CO_2 gas used to maintain a pneumoperitoneum is below room temperature and will cool the scope if used through the same cannula. Therefore, to prevent fogging of the lens, CO_2 should be insufflated through a port other than the one in which the laparoscope is placed. Alternatively, a heated gas high-flow system can be used (Karl Storz, Tüttlingen, Germany).

The current standard light source for most laparoscopic procedures is a 300-W xenon lamp. It is similar to sunlight, and provides an excellent transmission spectrum from ultraviolet to infrared light. The xenon light source also gives excellent field visualization. A fiberoptic cord connects the endoscope and light source. If some fibers are broken within the fiberglass cable, it will not transmit

as much light but can still be used.[2] The light source must be "white-balanced" after attachment to optimize transmission of true colors. The light source delivers intense heat and reports have been published of the drapes being ignited. Thus, the light source cable should not be left on the drapes.

A control unit processes the final signal from the camera, which is then transmitted to the video monitor or recorder. The monitors are the final component of the imaging chain and should be equal in quality to the camera system. A high-resolution camera used in conjunction with a high-resolution monitor will help deliver the best video image to replace the surgeon's direct visual perception. Color video monitors and recording devices are available with resolution of 500 lines with 256 gradations of color.[2] Copies can be stored on computer hard drives, CD-ROMs, and tapes in graphic format allowing computerized modification to create photographs or slides of the laparoscopic surgery. Videotapes of VHS or ED-Beta can also be used as recording devices for the laparoscopic colectomy.[3]

Insufflators

A high-flow insufflator capable of delivering at least 10 liters/min of gas is needed to establish and maintain a pneumoperitoneum to effectively perform laparoscopic colectomy. The gas used should be nontoxic, highly soluble in blood, colorless, incombustible, and physiologically inert.[2] Helium, argon, room air, and nitrogen oxide as well as CO_2 have been described for establishing pneumoperitoneum. Carbon dioxide is currently the most widely used to establish and maintain a pneumoperitoneum, it is highly soluble in blood and is unlikely to produce a life-threatening gas embolism if introduced into the circulatory system. The main disadvantage of carbon dioxide is absorption by the peritoneal surface, which can cause acidosis, vasodilation, and the appearance of inflamed peritoneal tissue.

There are two basic types of insufflators: pneumatic and electronic. The pneumatic insufflators only deliver gas up to 4 liters/min, which is inadequate for laparoscopic colectomy. A flow rate of 10 liters/min or greater is necessary in laparoscopic colorectal surgery because of the amount of irrigation and suctioning involved.[4] A second type of insufflator is electronically controlled in which rates of insufflation up to 30 liters/min can be obtained.

The optimal insufflator for laparoscopic colorectal surgery is electronically controlled and delivers a maximum of 30 liters/min to maintain the pneumoperitoneum and ensure it is not lost during irrigation and suctioning. The insufflator should be able to deliver at least 6 liters/min of flow at a safe pressure of no more than 12 mmHg. In addition, it should maintain an intraabdominal pressure of at least 8 mmHg with a leakage rate of approximately 1 liters/min.[2] Filtering and recirculating gas flow minimizes the potential for hypothermia.

Irrigation and Suction Devices

During advanced laparoscopic surgery a reliable combination irrigation-suction system is necessary to both irrigate rapidly and to effectively evacuate fluid or other material. A clear operating field is of paramount importance. Irrigation-suction devices provide a minimal flow rate of 1 liter/min of irrigation fluid in addition to adjustable suction with interchangeable 5- and 10-mm metallic suction tubes to remove smoke, fluid, clots, or other debris.[2] The combined system may also be insulated and equipped with electrocautery capabilities to irrigate, suction, and cauterize without having to change instruments.

A warmed isotonic solution of normal saline or lactated Ringer's is a popular choice for irrigation fluid. Some surgeons add 1000 to 3000 U heparin per liter of irrigation solution to help prevent clot formation in the tubing.[2] This concentration of heparin should not have any systemic effects; antibiotics are also occasionally added to the irrigation fluid. The irrigation is delivered via a pressure system; most commonly the presure is generated from a pneumatic device in which the irrigating solution bag is housed. However, the flow is significantly less than with a powered pressurized system. An irrigation device can be powered by CO_2 or nitrogen from the operating room wall system. The fluid is typically pressurized to 40 or 50 psi, and should have an automatic cutoff to prevent excessive CO_2 or nitrogen from entering the abdominal cavity. A combined irrigation-suction system is valuable in unforeseen bleeding or spillage of intestinal contents during laparoscopic colon surgery. Systems made of common operating room supplies are usually not sufficient and should not be used with advanced laparoscopic surgery.

Electrocautery

Monopolar electrocautery is commonly connected to dissecting instruments and scissors to assist with surgical dissection and provide hemostasis for small vessels. The electrocautery units are very familiar to surgeons and operating room personnel, simple to operate, and readily available. One disadvantage, which is discussed throughout the surgical literature but seen infrequently, is capacitance coupling. A buildup of electrical charges on the shaft of an instrument using electrocautery can promote an electrical discharge from the shaft of the instrument.[2] This problem may not be visualized in the operative field, thus causing a remote burn site injury that may go unrecognized. Capacitance coupling can be decreased by using short bursts of cautery with lower currents. Also, if the surgeon notes that expected tissue effect from cautery is not produced at the tip of the instrument, concern should be raised that an electrical discharge has occurred at a remote site. Close inspection of surfaces adjacent to the instrument shaft should be performed before proceeding with the surgery. Nevertheless, monopolar electrocautery is safe, quick, effective, familiar to operating room personnel, and is the simplest energy source currently available.

Instruments

Because there is limited access to the surgery site during laparoscopic surgery, instruments are key to assist the surgeon in the operation. There are many similar instruments currently available from different manufacturers to fulfill the purposes of laparoscopic colorectal surgery. The design of laparoscopic instruments is important: they must be of adequate length, light, easy to manipulate, easy to visualize via the laparoscopic view, and be able to rotate 360°. It is also important that the instrument can be easily manipulated with a surgeon's single hand. In the current climate of cost containment and possible disease transmission, controversial issues continue to be discussed relative to the less expensive reusable versus the more expensive disposable instruments. Continued modification and new designs of instruments are important to promote the advances of laparoscopic surgery.

The basic requirements of laparoscopic instrumentation can be divided into four main categories:

1. Instruments to establish and maintain pneumoperitoneum and to provide entry ports for surgical instruments
2. Instruments for tissue dissection and mobilization
3. Instruments for resection and anastomosis
4. Other specialized instruments for laparoscopic colorectal surgery

Instruments for Pneumoperitoneum and Access

A pneumoperitoneum can be established by using a closed, percutaneous puncture technique or an open technique with direct visualization of the peritoneal cavity. The Veress needle was invented in 1938, and is the most popular device used for the percutaneous, closed technique. Needles are available in lengths from 10 to 15 cm with an outside diameter of 1.8 mm. The Veress needle has a sharp, outer needle with a blunt-tip, spring-loaded inner stylet.[2] The blunt-tip stylet retracts during tissue resistance such as the needle passing through the abdominal wall. Once tissue resistance is absent, as when the needle enters the peritoneal cavity, the blunt stylet

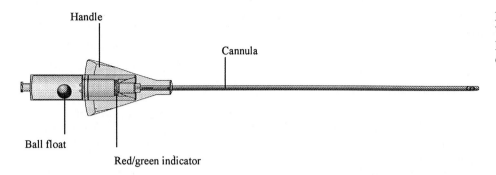

FIGURE 37.1. Endopath Ulra-Veress Needle. (Courtesy of Ethicon Endo-Surgery, Cincinnati, OH.)

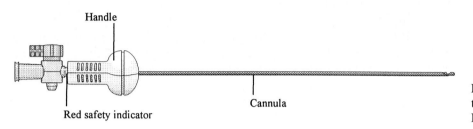

FIGURE 37.2. Endopath Pneumoperitoneum Needle. (Courtesy of Ethicon Endo-Surgery, Cincinnati, OH.)

then protects the outer sharp needle tip from damaging intraabdominal structures.

A pneumoperitoneum may then be established by insufflating gas through a lateral hole on the blunt stylet (Figs. 37.1, 37.2).

The VisiPort or Optiview is a cannula with a sharp trocar and safety shield designed for safe placement of the first trocar (Figs. 37.3, 37.4). A camera is placed into the cannula during insertion, and layers of the abdominal wall are visulized as the port is placed. The purpose is to have direct visualization during closed, percutaneous access to the abdominal cavity to prevent damage to intraabdominal structures. The port even has a handle for the palm and fingers to grasp for excellent control of the sharp trocar as it penetrates into the abdominal cavity.

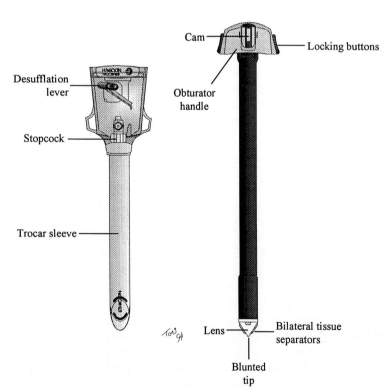

FIGURE 37.3. Endopth Optical Surgical Obturator and Sleeve. (Courtesy of Ethicon Endo-Surgery, Cincinnati, OH.)

FIGURE 37.4. Endopath Optiview with Obturator Handle. (Courtesy of Ethicon Endo-Surgery, Cincinnati, OH.)

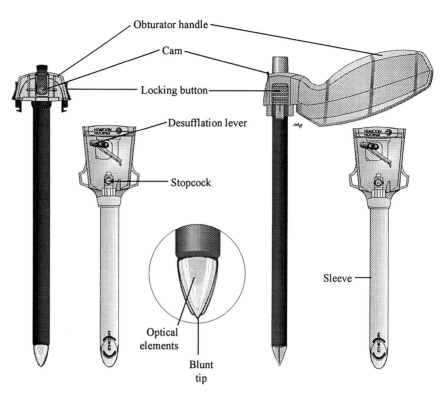

Obturator handle

Cam

Locking button

Desufflation lever

Stopcock

Sleeve

Optical elements

Blunt tip

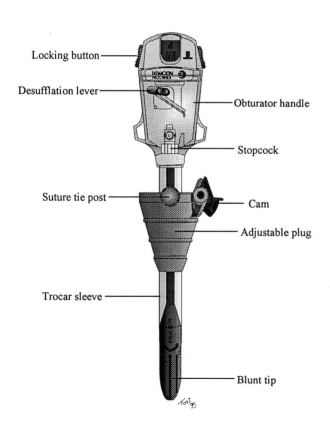

Locking button

Desufflation lever

Obturator handle

Stopcock

Suture tie post

Cam

Adjustable plug

Trocar sleeve

Blunt tip

FIGURE 37.5. Endopath Blunt Tip Surgical Trocar. (Courtesy of Ethicon Endo-Surgery, Cincinnati, OH.)

The open technique to establish pneumoperitoneum is similar to the technique used for peritoneal lavage. A small incision is made on the abdominal wall, dissection is made through the abdominal wall layers, the peritoneum is incised under direct vision, and access is gained to the abdominal cavity. Fascial sutures are typically placed to secure the cannula. A Hasson blunt-tip trocar (Fig. 37.5) is then directly and safely introduced by direct visualization into the abdominal cavity, secured to the skin and fascia, and a pneumoperitoneum is established.

There are a wide variety of cannulas and trocars currently available. The terms cannula and trocar are used interchangeably. The trocar refers to the sharp part of the instrument that is used to penetrate through the abdominal wall into the peritoneal cavity. The blade of the trocar is protected by a retractable safety shield (Figs. 37.6, 37.7). Once access to the peritoneal cavity is obtained, the trocar is then removed from the sleeve (Fig. 37.8). The remaining access device is termed a cannula or a port.[5] Cannulas may be disposable or nondisposable and range in diameter from 3 mm to 35 mm. A trumpet or flapper valve in cannulas is used to prevent gas leakage when instruments are passed through them. The trumpet valve opens and closes manually, and the flapper valve works automatically. Each cannula is built with a stopcock and Luer lock mechanism for gas insufflation. Anchoring of the cannula to the abdominal wall is important to prevent the cannula from accidental displacement during

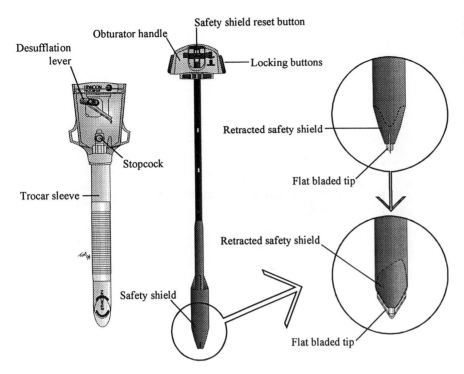

FIGURE 37.6. Endopath Dilating Tip Trocar with retractable safety shield and stability threads. (Courtesy of Ethicon Endo-Surgery, Cincinnati, OH.)

instrument withdrawal and mainpulation. Some cannulas have self-retaining sleeves that may be threaded into the fascia; others have a fascial screw to secure the position. Also, adhesive appliances fix the cannula to the abdominal wall and may seal minor leaks. Sometimes an additional heavy suture of 0-silk or 0-nylon is stitched to the skin and wrapped around the cannula to assist with stabilization.

During laparoscopic colectomy, each port must be adaptable for a variety of instruments. A 10-mm cannula is used in the infraumbilical incision and 10- or 12-mm cannulas are used in all other positions. Reducer caps allow for interchanging 5-mm instruments through larger ports (Fig. 37.9). Reducers provide needed flexibility to withdraw and interchange instruments during advanced laparoscopic surgery. The optimal cannula has good fixation to the superficial and deep abdominal wall, forms an airtight seal, and has low resistance for insertion and withdrawal of instruments. Also, a universal seal mechanism should be present to allow interchanging of different-sized instruments.

Instruments for Tissue Dissection and Mobilization

Safe tissue dissection of the colon from the surrounding intraabdominal structures, control and effective ligation of the mesenteric vessels, and atraumatic mobilization of healthy tissue is paramount in laparoscopic colon surgery. Laparoscopic instruments play a major role in tissue dissection and mobilization. The most common instruments needed are endoscopic graspers and clamps, endoscopic scissors with unipolar electrocautery, endoscopic clip appliers, harmonic scalpel, blunt dissectors, and retractors.

Endoscopic Graspers and Clamps

The grasping instruments are mainly used for handling of tissue and manipulation of the bowel. The endoscopic grasping devices are the most widely used and well-known laparoscopic tools in all types of laparoscopic surgery (Fig. 37.10). The basic endoscopic grasper has

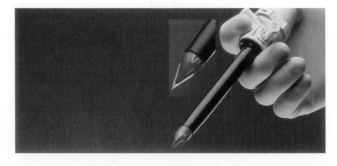

FIGURE 37.7. Trocar with retractable safety shield. (Courtesy of US Surgical Corporation, Norwalk, CT.)

FIGURE 37.8. Endopath Disposable Trocar. (1) Assembled trocar and sleeve, 1. retractor, side view; (2) Single patient use trocar obturator, 1. shield reset button, 2. locking buttons, 3. blade shield, 4. obturator handle; (3) Single patient use trocar sleeve housing, 1. stopcock, 2. external threads; (4) Reusable trocar sleeve, 1. internal threads, 2. stability threads. (Courtesy of Ethicon Endo-Surgery, Cincinnati, OH.)

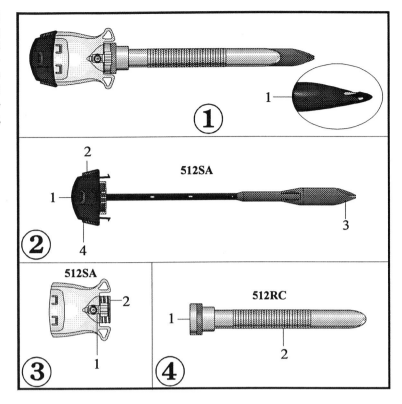

handles connected to the instrument shaft and center rod that are attached to the grasper jaws. The handles are squeezed together or opened apart, thereby allowing the jaws to close or open accordingly.[2] Some earlier, resuable graspers have one grasper jaw that is fixed to the instrument shaft and a single-action jaw to open or close. Today, most endoscopic grasper jaws are hinged for dual-action jaw control. Dual-action jaws are necessary for

laparoscopic colorectal surgery, and are important for fine grasping and tissue dissection. In addition, a curved or articulated tip may give better control to grasp tissue.

Endoscopic graspers are either traumatic or atraumatic to tissue depending on the blade tip. Traumatic graspers generally have blades with teeth at the tip that provide a firm and sure grip of the tissue. However, the teeth are more prone to tear and damage tissue versus the

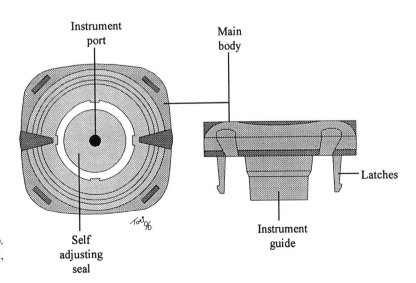

FIGURE 37.9. Endopath One-seal Reducer Cap. (Courtesy of Ethicon Endo-Surgery, Cincinnati, OH.)

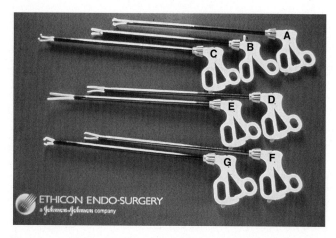

FIGURE 37.10. Endopath Endoscopic Bowel Instruments: *A*, Babcock; *B*, scissors.; *C*, right angle; *D*, curved Kelly; *E*, atraumatic bowel clamp; *F*, Allis; *G*, anvil grasper. (Courtesy of Ethicon Endo-Surgery, Cincinnati, OH.)

Endoscopic Babcock clamps are important instruments in laparoscopic colorectal surgery and perform multiple functions (Fig. 37.12). The atraumatic, long blades and wide jaw span are safe and effective for intestinal manipulation. They are currently available in 5-mm and 10-mm sizes; however, the larger clamp offers a better grip than does the 5 mm. The Babcock clamp can be used as a grasper to move small and large intestine for better exposure and to firmly clamp the bowel for retraction during dissection. It is imperative to apply the maximum force necessary to hold the tissue firmly, then activate the locking mechanism to prevent excessive pressure to the bowel. Also, simultaneous pulling, torquing, and twisting of the clamped intestine may cause the clamp to slide and create mesenteric rents and serosal tears. Thus, careful handling of inestinal tissue, whether using endoscopic Babcock clamps or atraumatic graspers, is important. The endoscopic Babcock clamp is also useful to firmly hold the intestine during extraction through the abdominal wall for extracorporeal resection of the bowel or to create an ileostomy or colostomy.

atraumatic graspers, which generally have smooth blade tips.[2] Graspers have a holding mechanism to lock the jaws closed that is easily activated and released with a trigger (Fig. 37.11). If the grasper is locked and the tissue is simultaneously pulled and torqued, the result may be avulsed or torn tissue. Some atraumatic graspers are designed with long, blunt blades with a serrated inner side of the blade, as well as a wide jaw span to maintain a relatively safe grip of a sufficient amount of tissue. It is important to realize certain tissues are better handled with traumatic grasping devices for a sure grip such as the omentum, abdominal side wall, adhesions, or mesentery; however, it is mandatory to use atraumatic graspers to manipulate the intestine and mesenteric vessels. In fact, the intestine should only be handled by noncrushing endoscopic Babcock clamps if at all possible, because any type of graspers, traumatic or atraumatic, have been shown to cause serosal tears.

Endoscopic Scissors

Scissors are important instruments for tissue dissection in laparoscopic colorectal surgery. They are available as microscissors with small blades, hook scissors, and curved scissors (Figs. 37.13, 37.14). The most common scissors have a 5-mm-diameter shaft, are 31 cm long, and have 16-mm-long blades with an 8-mm jaw span. They are well insulated so that electrical current can safely be used and are commonly disposable. Reusable scissors require the tips to be changed, cleaned, and sharpened periodically, which may dull the blades. New, larger scissors with a 10-mm-diameter shaft have longer blades for faster blunt dissection and transection. However, the length of the instrument shaft is the same, and fine dissection is more difficult compared to smaller scissor blades. The optimal

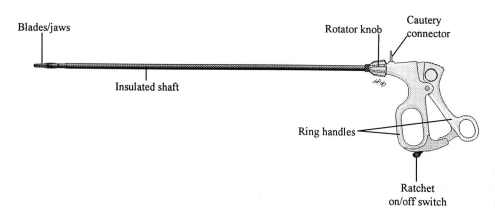

FIGURE 37.11. Endopath 5-mm Blunt Grasper. (Courtesy of Ethicon Endo-Surgery, Cincinnati, OH.)

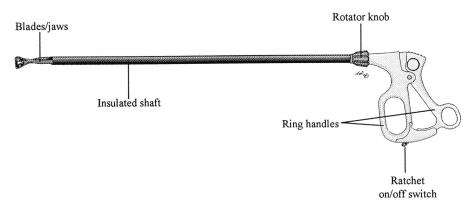

FIGURE 37.12. Endopath 10-mm Babcock Grasper. (Courtesy of Ethicon Endo-Surgery, Cincinnati, OH.)

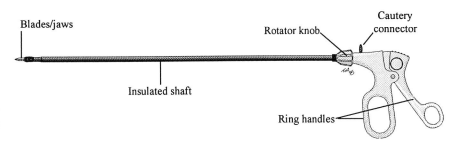

FIGURE 37.13. Endopath Microscissors. (Courtesy of Ethicon Endo-Surgery, Cincinnati, OH.)

scissors for advanced laparoscopic surgery have sharp blades and a blunt tip for sharp and blunt dissection, easily rotate 360° along the longitudinal axis of the shaft, and connect to unipolar electrocautery for tissue dissection.

Endoscopic Clip Appliers

Endoscopic clip appliers are mainly used for vascular control of mesenteric vessels. They are available as a reusable, single-clip applicator (Fig. 37.15) or as a

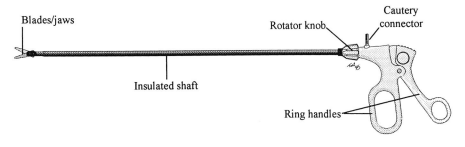

FIGURE 37.14. Endopath Curved Scissors. (Courtesy of Ethicon Endo-Surgery, Cincinnati, OH.)

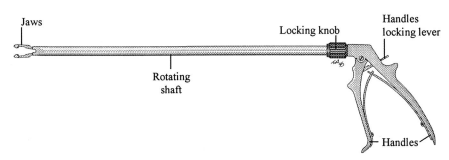

FIGURE 37.15. Endoscopic Single Clip Applier. (Courtesy of Ethicon Endo-Surgery, Cincinnati, OH.)

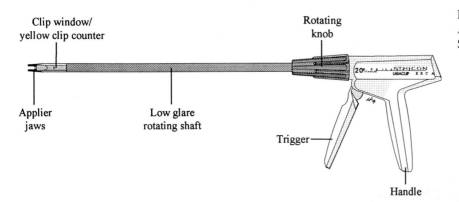

Clip window/
yellow clip counter

Rotating
knob

Applier
jaws

Low glare
rotating shaft

Trigger

Handle

FIGURE 37.16. Endoscopic Multiple Clip Applier. (Courtesy of Ethicon Endo-Surgery, Cincinnati, OH.)

disposable, automatic multifire rotating clip applicator (Fig. 37.16) that can fire up to 20 clips.[2] A large 10-mm automatic clip applier is most commonly used for laparasopic colorectal surgery, although a new 5-mm clip applier is currently manufactured. Clips are made of absorbable polyglycolic acid and polydioxane, stainless steel, or titanium.[2] The distance between the clip legs before application is 4.5 mm. During application, the tips of the legs close first to trap the tissue, followed by the body of the clip. Thus, it is important to completely visualize the tips of the instrument before engaging to prevent inadvertent clipping of surrounding tissue. The clips are 11 mm in length and crimp securely to ligate vessels up to 4 mm in diameter.

After careful dissection and isolation of mesenteric vessels, two proximal clips and one distal clip are typically applied. The distance between clips should allow adequate room to comfortably transect the vessel, and to place additional clips on the proximal or distal vessels, if needed, to complete hemostasis. Clips should not be crossed during application because this decreases their strength and may lead to bleeding. Also, twisting or placing tension and rubbing the vessel should be avoided as this may cause misfire or, worse, transect the vessel before the clip is securely applied.

Endoscopic clips should be applied easily and effectively to control hemostasis after isolation of the vessels. The 360° rotating shaft allows safe placement of clips in a variety of situations. Absorbable clips are now available but only in a single clip applicator, which is time consuming. Current controversy involves the uncertainty of tissue inflammation and adhesions caused by clips. There are no current clear clinical data to support whether titanium, absorbable, or stainless steel clips cause more adhesions. Although stainless steel clips are stronger than titanium, titanium clips do not interfere with either CT or MRI.[2]

Ultrasonic Scalpel or Shears

Ultrasonic instruments use longitudinal mechanical waves with a frequency greater than 20,000 cycles per second as an energy source for tissue dissection. Ultrasonic waves can selectively fragment tissue based on water content. Fat or the parenchyma of the liver has a high water content and is fragmented with low power, whereas nerves or blood vessels have low water content and will not be damaged. The mechanical energy from the directly applied ultrasonic vibration is converted to thermal energy and thus uses coagulation to dissect tissue. The ultrasonic scalper or shears use piezoelectric elements to convert electrical energy into mechanical waves of various frequencies and lengths. The ultrasonic energy is then converted to heat in the tissue, and the coagulation causes collagen molecules in adjacent tissue to denature. Because the tissue is heated but not the scalpel, there is minimal smoke production or accumulation of debris on the instrument.

The ultrasonic scalpel unit consists of a generator and a handpiece (Fig. 37.17). The generator supplies an electrical signal to the handpiece that is then converted to mechanical energy by an acoustic transducer within the handpiece.[2] An acoustic mount in the handpiece amplifies the frequency produced by the transducer, and a maximum vibration of approximately 55.5 kHz is delivered directly to the blade. The blade itself also has an additional amplifier to increase the mechanical vibration,

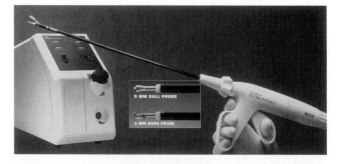

FIGURE 37.17. Endoscopic Ultra Shears. (Courtesy of US Surgical Corporation, Norwalk, CT.)

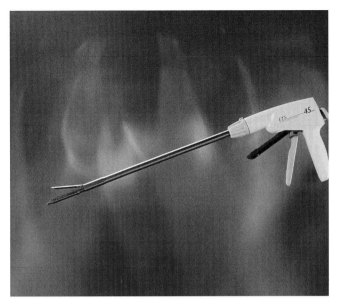

FIGURE 37.18. Ultracision. (Courtesy of Ethicon Endo-Surgery, Cincinnati, OH.)

tissue. The main advantage of the ultrasonic shears is dissection of fatty tissue such as mesentery or omentum with excellent hemostasis.

The ultrasonic shears is a valuable tool for the surgeon performing advanced laparoscopic surgery. The grasping jaws allow an extra instrument to manipulate and dissect tissue before coagulation. The endoscopic scissors can coagulate and cut tissue, but are not graspers which is sometimes limiting to the operator. One jaw blade of the ultrasonic shears can bluntly dissect tissue planes; coagulation of the desired tissue can then easily be performed without changing instruments. The ultrasonic shears provides the two-handed advanced laparoscopic surgeon the freedom to have a tissue grasper, blunt dissector, coagulation device, and cutting device all within one instrument. The current disadvantages of the ultrasonic scalpel and shears is cost of the equipment and the longer time needed to coagulate tissue. However, both the authors and the editor believe the multipurpose use of this single instrument decreases overall operative room time, and that when properly used it is the most important instrument in laparoscopic colorectal surgery.

Blunt Dissectors and Retractors

Endoscopic retractors are seldom used in laparoscopic colorectal surgery but should be readily available. Researchers are currently investigating new products because retraction of the mobile intestine is a major challenge. Change in patient position with tilting of the operating table and use of grasping instruments are the most common current techniques for retraction of the intestine. A single-finger retractor or an articulating fan retractor are available but generally do not provide adequate exposure (Fig. 37.19). In addition, loops of small intestine may become trapped between the fingers of the fan retractor and cause potential bowel injury. A fan retractor is more appropriate for fixed organs such as the liver. An endoscopic snare device to retract divided large intestine was initially used in laparoscopic colorectal surgery but has recently come into disfavor because grasping instruments and gravity provide adequate exposure in most cases.[2] Exposure is a key to any operation,

and the direct effect on tissue depends on the type of blade selected. A sharp hook, dissecting hook, ball coagulator, and a coagulating spatula are the choice of blades. The blunt side of the blade allows good coagulation of tissue, whereas the sharp edge of the blade is better for cutting.

Ultrasonic shears act as a clamp and coagulator using ultrasonic energy in tissue dissection and mobilization (Fig. 37.18). The tip of the ultrasonic shears has two portions: a stationary side, which supports the grasped tissue, and the vibratory side that transmits ultrasonic energy to the tissue. After the tissue is grasped and clamped, ultrasonic energy then coagulates the tissue between the blades. A sharp blade allows better cutting of the tissue; however, a rounded blade provides more complete coagulation. The coagulation of tissue is also dependent on the power setting; decreased power reduces cutting quality but improves hemostasis.[2] The surgeon also directly controls the cutting and coagulation effect by using the handgrip to vary the pressure applied to the

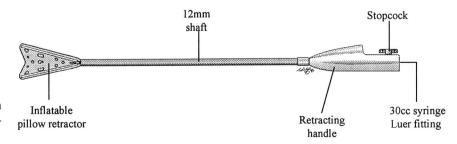

FIGURE 37.19. Inflatable Large Organ Retractor. (Courtesy of Ethicon Endo-Surgery, Cincinnati, OH.)

Inflatable
pillow retractor

12mm
shaft

Retracting
handle

Stopcock

30cc syringe
Luer fitting

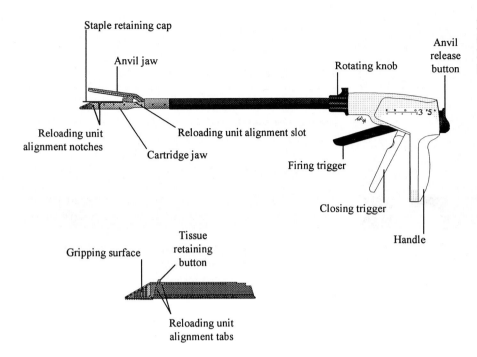

FIGURE 37.20. Endopath EZ 35 Endoscopic Linear Cutter. (Courtesy of Ethicon Endo-Surgery, Cincinnati, OH.)

especially laparoscopic surgery, and if the patient is obese, has a limited peritoneal cavity, or has distended intestine, conversion to an open procedure is sound surgical judgment.

Blunt dissection is not commonly recommended in laparosopic colon surgery. Mobilization and dissection of the colon and mesentery typically is performed sharply with scissors or with coagulation. Blunt dissecting instruments such as a Kittner dissector or a blunt grasping instrument are rarely used. In the technique of hand-assisted laparoscopic surgery, the hand can be used as a safe blunt dissecting instrument similar to open surgery.

Instruments for Resection and Anastomosis

After adequate tissue dissection and mobilization of the colon, the intracorporeal resection includes mesenteric vessel division and laparoscopic division of the bowel wall. The anastomosis may be performed either intra- or extracorporeally. Laparoscopic instruments for resection and anastomosis include endoscopic staplers, endoscopic clip appliers, needle holder, knot pusher, anvil grasper, and grasping instruments. Extracorporeal resection and anastomosis uses standard open techniques.

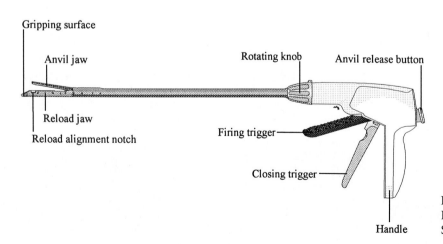

FIGURE 37.21. Endopath ETS Endoscopic Linear Cutter. (Courtesy of Ethicon Endo-Surgery, Cincinnati, OH.)

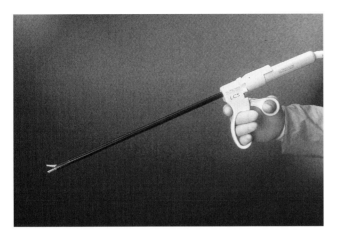

FIGURE 37.22. Endopath ETS 45 Endoscopic Linear Cutter. (Courtesy of Ethicon Endo-Surgery, Cincinnati, OH.)

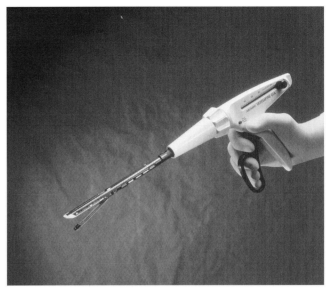

FIGURE 37.23. Autosuture Versafire GIA. (Courtesy of US Surgical Corporation, Norwalk, CT.)

Endoscopic staplers have been marketed since 1991. The Multifire Endo GIA (US Surgical Corporation, Norwalk, CT, USA) was one of the first endoscopic staplers introduced. It is a 30-mm stapler applied through a 12-mm cannula with a triple row of staggered staples on either side of the blade track. The knife blade stops one and a half staples short of the end of the staple line, allowing both ends of the intestine to close in an everted mucosa-to-mucosa fashion. Endoscopic staplers have cartridges for normal-thickness tissue, thick tissue, and vascular applications that can be used for dividing the mesentery as well as major vascular trunks (Figs. 37.20, 37.21). Three reloads are permitted, after which a new stapler device must be employed. Endoscopic stapler manufacturers subsequently developed a 60-mm Endo GIA through a 15-mm cannula (US Surgical Corporation), and a 60-mm Endopath ELC endoscopic linear cutter through an 18-mm cannula (Ethicon Endosurgery).

Manufacturers of laparoscopic instruments have greatly improved the versatility of endoscopic staplers. Currently, multiple types of stapling units such as straight versus roticulating in 2.0- to 4.8-m sizes are available. The length of the stapler jaw can vary from 30 to 45 mm (Fig. 37.22) and up to 60 mm, all via a 12-mm cannula (Fig. 37.23). A 90-mm linear cutter is currently being tested through an 18-mm cannula. The most advantageous recent advance is the development of the roticulating endoscopic stapling unit (Fig. 37.24). This design allows more versatility and flexibility in performing a 90° transection of the bowel rather than an angled staple line traversing the colon. When laparoscopically transecting the bowel, especially the proximal rectum, it is sometimes difficult to align the straight endoscopic GIA in a perpendicular cutting line across the intestine. The roticulating endoscopic GIA allows for better alignment of the

stapler across the intestine to avoid an angled staple line. The Endo GIA Universal Roticulator by US Surgical Corporation and the ETS Flex Endopath GIA by Ethicon Endosurgery (Fig. 37.25) are currently the two most popular and new stapling units on the market. This development represents the importance of continued advancement and research in laparoscopic instrumentation to improve the technical aspects of the surgical procedure.

Intracorporeal laparoscopic resection of the bowel wall is performed with an endoscopic GIA stapler. The mesenteric vessels and major vascular trunks are controlled via multiple options, including electrocautery, coagulation with ultrasonic vibration, endoscopic clip appliers, endoloop pretied ligatures, or endoscopic staplers with a vascular cartridge.[1] The peritoneum of the mesentery is typically incised with electrocautery, small vessels are usually coagulated, and the major vascular

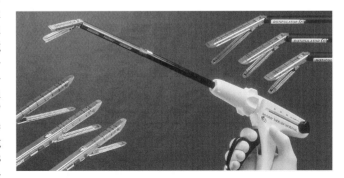

FIGURE 37.24. Autosuture Endo GIA Universal Roticulator. (Courtesy of US Surgical Corporation, Norwalk, CT.)

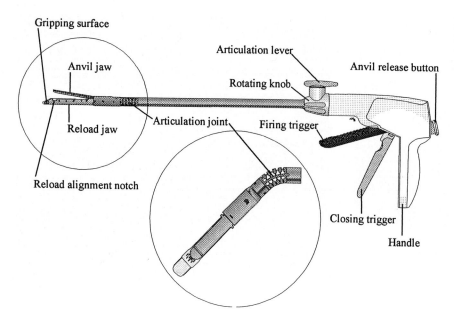

FIGURE 37.25. Endopath ETS Flex Endoscopic Articulating Linear Cutter. (Courtesy of Ethicon Endo-Surgery, Cincinnati, OH.)

trunks are controlled with surgical clips or a vascular stapler. A flexible or roticulating endoscopic stapler with a vascular cartridge allows for a perpendicular ligation and division of the vasculature. An intracorporeal functional end-to-end anastomosis of intestine can be fashioned from the proximal and distal ends using a linear endoscopic stapler. Another option is to perform a hand-sewn intracorporeal laparoscopic anastomosis using a spring-loaded needle holder (Fig. 37.26) or the Szabo–Berci matched pair of needle holders. The knots can be tied intracorporeally or extracorporeally using a knot pusher to replace the surgeon's fingertip to ade-

quately secure the knot to the tissue. Endoknot pretied suture and improved intracorporeal knot-tying techniques such as the Ethicon Suture Assistant are also available (Fig. 37.27). The time required and the degree of difficulty in performing an intracorporeal anastomosis has led most surgeons to combine an intracorporeal mobilization and resection, with or without mesenteric division, with an extracorporeal anastomosis.

Standard open techniques are typically employed for laparoscopic right colon resection. The right colon and hepatic flexure are laparoscopically mobilized, the mesenteric vessels are usually ligated and divided, and

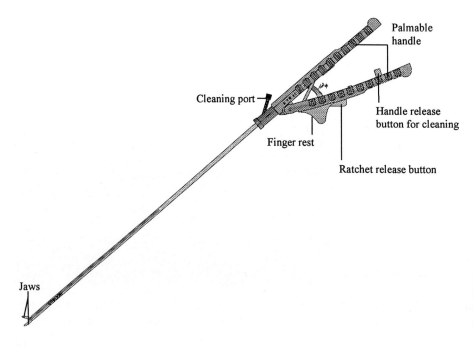

FIGURE 37.26. Endopath Endoscopic Reusable Needle Holder. (Courtesy of Ethicon Endo-Surgery, Cincinnati, OH.)

FIGURE 37.27. Endopath Suture Assistant. (Courtesy of Ethicon Endo-Surgery, Cincinnati, OH.)

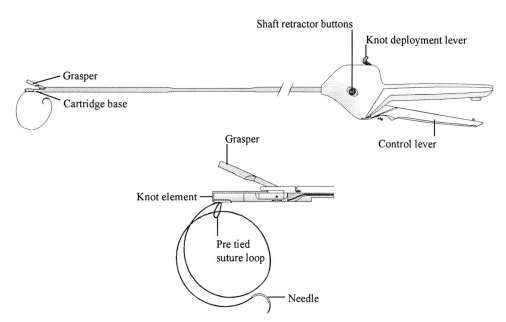

out onto the abdominal wall. A wound protector is placed to aid in prevention of wound infection and tumor implantation. The bowel is resected near skin level, and a pursestring device is used to secure the anvil of a circular stapler to the proximal limb. The prepared proximal limb is then returned to the abdominal cavity where the anastomosis can be performed under direct vision through the existing abdominal incision. Alternatively, the incision is closed, the pneumoperitoneum reestablished, and the anastomosis performed laparoscopically. A circular stapling device (Fig. 37.29) is inserted transanally and the trocar extended through or adjacent to the midportion of the staple line of the distal limb.

the resection and anastomosis is performed extracorporeally using standard GIA and TA staplers (Fig. 37.28). A via drape or wound protector drape is used to protect the abdominal wall from contamination, as well as for prevention of tumor implantation.[1]

For left colonic resections where the anastomosis will be at the distal sigmoid or rectum, a double-stapling technique is preferred. The left colon is divided intracorporeally with an endoscopic GIA stapler, and the mesenteric vessels are usually divided and ligated with a vascular cartridge on the endoscopic GIA stapler. One port site is then enlarged, the pneumoperitoneum temporarily decompressed, and the proximal colon is brought

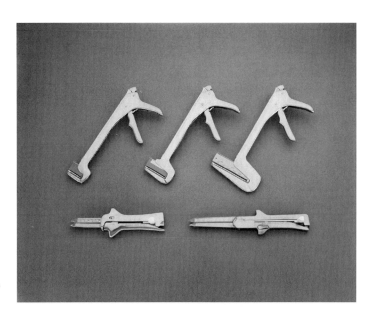

FIGURE 37.28. Standard GIA and TA stapling instruments. (Courtesy of US Surgical Corporation, Norwalk, CT.)

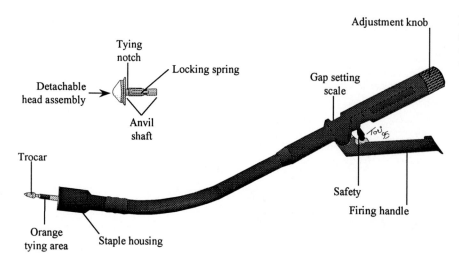

FIGURE 37.29. Endopath Stealth Endoscopic Curved Intraluminal Stapler. (Courtesy of Ethicon Endo-Surgery, Cincinnati, OH.)

A laparoscopic anvil grasper (Ethicon Endosurgery) is specifically designed to grasp the secured anvil to assist connection to the shaft of the circular stapling device and connect the proximal and distal limbs. A Babcock grasping instrument or a right-angle instrument (Fig. 37.30) may be used if an anvil grasper is not available. The circular stapler is then fired and activated, and two anastomotic doughnuts should be removed and inspected to ensure complete rings of tissue (Fig. 37.31). The pelvis is then filled with saline and the proximal lumen carefully occluded with a laparoscopic Babcock clamp. Air is insufflated into the rectum via a bulb syringe or a proctoscope to ensure the anastomosis has no air leak. An additional advantage of the proctoscope is visual inspection of the anastomosis.

Other Specialized Instruments

Hand-assisted laparoscopic colorectal surgery is becoming more popular. The technique allows surgeons to use their favorite instrument, the hand. The Pneumosleeve (Dexterity, Blue Bell, PA, USA) is a new device that allows the surgeon to place one hand into the abdominal cavity while preserving the pneumoperitoneum. Difficult dissection in laparoscopic colorectal procedures such as diverticulitis is made easier, faster, and more confident using the surgeon's experienced hand. The multiple advantages include tactile sensation, dissection along natural tissue planes, atraumatic retraction of organs such as small and large intestine or uterus, three-dimensional (3-D) perception with the hand as a guide for quick orientation, and better agility to orient tissues for suturing or placing tissue in the jaws of linear staplers. Because a small incision, usually 5 to 7 cm, is needed for specimen removal in laparoscopic surgery, the Pneumosleeve takes advantage of the incision from the onset of surgery.

The Pneumo Sleeve Set contains two pneumosleeves, one base with incision template, a wound protractor, sterile lubricant, and one pneumo dome. After application of the template on the abdominal wall, an incision cut to fit the surgeon's glove size is made. The Wound Protractor (Dexterity) is placed and provides a combination wound protector and incision retractor. The

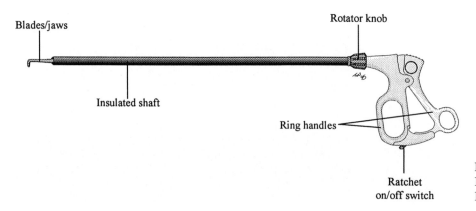

FIGURE 37.30. Endopath Right Angle Dissector. (Courtesy of Ethicon Endo-Surgery, Cincinnati, OH.)

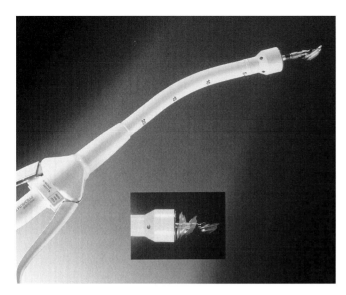

FIGURE 37.31. Autosuture CEEA circular stapler. (Courtesy of US Surgical Corporation, Norwalk, CT.)

surgeon's hand is placed in the pneumosleeve, lubricated, and then inserted into the abdominal cavity through the incision template and wound protractor while maintaining pneumperitoneum. If a surgeon has large hands and the patient has a small peritoneal cavity, it is difficult to have good visualization with laparoscopic surgery.

In conventional open colorectal cancer surgery, the liver, porta hepatis, and paraaortic tissues are assessed with bimanual palpation or intraoperative ultrasound to clinically stage the cancer before resection. Intraoperative ultrasound has been clinically shown to have high sensitivity and specificity in detecting hepatic lesions.[2] Because ultrasound is inexpensive and quickly performed, it is becoming the method of choice to evaluate the liver and surrounding tissues in colorectal cancer surgery.[2] Laparoscopic ultrasound probes with rigid or flexible tips are inserted through a 10-mm cannula under direct laparoscopic vision. A 5- to 7.5-mHz probe allows good resolution and visualization of the liver with linear or sector scanning modalities.

Port site hernias are being reported with increasing frequency in laparoscopic surgery. As a general rule, port sites greater than 5 mm should have fascial closure. With advanced laparoscopic surgery, closure of a 10- or 12-mm port site would require extending the skin incision. Port site closure devices have been used since the beginning of laparoscopic surgery, but the technical results are discouraging. Currently, the Storz needle port site fascial closure device (Karl Storz Endoscopy-America, Culver City, CA, USA) is effective and popular. Under laparoscopic guidance, a needle-shaped grasper is introduced around the fascia of the port site and a suture is passed full thickness into the abdominal wall on both sides of the port site for suture closure.

Conclusion

Laparoscopic colon and rectal surgery is a challenging and technically demanding procedure. The research and development of advanced laparoscopic instrumentation allows the possibility of current surgical techniques. Laparoscopic instrumentation is the key to performing safe and effective surgery. Yet, further advancements are still needed to optimize complete intracorporeal surgery. Some future improvements include a high-resolution camera with lens washer that does not limit vision, better atraumatic grasping instruments for the intestine, decreased cost, and eventual decreased diameter of instruments to fit 5-mm port sites. As technology improves, advanced laparoscopic surgery may incorporate three-dimensional viewing, virtual reality, robotics, or human interface technology. Nevertheless, laparoscopic instrumentation plays a vital role in advanced laparoscopic colon and rectal surgery, and further research and development is imperative.

References

1. Simmang C, Rosenthal, D. Tools for laparoscopic colectomy. Semin Colon Rectal Surg 1994;5:228–238.
2. Milsom JW, Bohm B. Laparoscopic Colorectal Surgery. New York: Springer-Verlag, 1996;
3. Smith LE, Gordon PH. Laparoscopic colon and rectal surgery. In: Gordon PH, Nivatvongs S (eds) Principles and Practice of Surgery for the Colon, Rectum, and Anus. St. Louis: Quality Medical, 1999:1337–1379.
4. Ballantyne GH, Begos DG. Operating room setup. In: Jager RM, Wexner SD (eds) Laparoscopic Colorectal Surgery. New York: Churchill Livingstone, 1996:105–126.
5. Corman ML. Colon and Rectal Surgery, 4th Ed. Philadelphia: Lippincott-Raven, 1998:1001–1032.

38
Laparoscopic Appendectomy

W. Keat Cheah and Peter M.Y. Goh

Kurt Semm from Switzerland performed the first laparoscopic appendectomy in 1980 and introduced it as an alternative form of treatment to open appendectomy.[1] However, the procedure was not widely received until the increased popularity of laparoscopy in general surgery in the late 1980s, following the overall success of laparoscopic cholecystectomy. Laparoscopic appendectomy is now more popular because of improvements in video equipment and laparoscopic instruments and because some prospective reviews favor laparoscopic over conventional open appendectomy.

Patient Selection

Virtually any patient with a diagnosis of suspected appendicitis can potentially undergo laparoscopic appendectomy. This broad indication applies to most patients who are young and healthy. However, there is a small group of patients in whom laparoscopy should be avoided, including patients who are severely septic for whom a laparotomy is indicated; those individuals who have had previous lower abdominal surgery and developed adhesions in which laparoscopy may be impeded; patients with severe lung disease in whom carbon dioxide pneumoperitoneum may exacerbate their condition; and women with advanced pregnancy where laparoscopy is suboptimal. Laparoscopy is particularly beneficial in female patients with equivocal right iliac fossa pain in whom pelvic diseases mimic appendicitis in presentation. In such instances, laparoscopy avoids an unnecessary gridiron incision and allows therapeutic gynecological laparoscopy to take place. It is also beneficial in obese patients because a large incision and potential wound infection are avoided.

Preoperative Preparation

The preoperative preparation for laparoscopic appendectomy is similar to that for open appendectomy. During consent taking, the procedure is explained to the patient, who is also informed of the potential for conversion to open appendectomy. In the female patient, a menstrual history is taken and the beta-hCG level is determined to detect any unsuspected pregnancy. Intravenous fluids and antibiotics (Cephalosporin and Metronidazole) are started, and intramuscular analgesia (Pethidine) is given.

Surgical Procedure

General anesthesia with muscle relaxation and endotracheal intubation are administered. The patient is placed supine with the left arm by the side because the surgeon and the camera assistant both operate standing on the patient's left side. For the female patient, a bladder catheter is inserted to decompress the bladder so that the pelvis can be clearly viewed; the catheter can be removed at the end of the operation. An operating table with capacity to tilt to the Trendelenburg and right-side-up positions is used so that the abdominal contents gravitate away from the cecum and appendix. The patient is draped from the umbilicus to the pubis to expose the lower and lateral abdomen.

General Laparoscopy

Entry into the peritoneal cavity is made by the open method through a 1-cm infraumbilical incision. A 10- or 12-mm cannula is inserted and carbon dioxide is insuf-

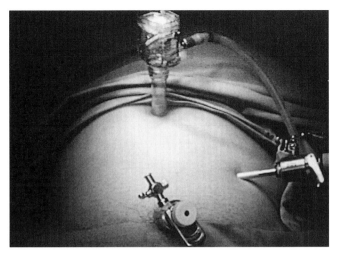

FIGURE 38.1. Port placement.

flated to a maximum pressure of 12 mmHg to achieve pneumoperitoneum. A 30°, 10-mm diameter laparoscope is inserted; if fogging of the lens occurs, an antifog solution can be applied to the lens. A general laparoscopy of the entire abdomen is performed, including an assessment of the degree of peritonitis from the spread of purulent peritoneal fluid. Next, two 5-mm ports are inserted through small incisions. The lower midline port is inserted just above the pubic hairline under laparoscopic vision with care not to injure a distended bladder. The left lateral port is inserted at the lateral edge of the rectus muscle equidistant from the other two ports, following transillumination of the abdominal wall by the laparoscope to avoid puncturing the inferior epigastric vessels. This port placement allows the surgeon to operate in a comfortable position with both arms close to the body (Fig. 38.1). A pair of atraumatic bowel grasping forceps with long jaws is inserted through the lower port, which the surgeon holds with the left hand to grasp the appendix. A pair of curved dissecting forceps is placed through the left port (Fig. 38.2). If it becomes obvious the appendix is not inflamed, a careful search is made for other pathology such as cecal diverticulitis, terminal ileitis, Meckel's diverticulitis, small bowel mesenteric adenitis, and, in the female, for salpingitis, ovarian cyst rupture or torsion, or endometriosis.

Mobilization of the Appendix

The omentum that is frequently adherent to the inflamed appendix can be gently teased away with the graspers to expose the tip of the appendix. The relatively healthy and not the necrotic part of the appendix should be gently grasped with the atraumatic grasper to avoid avulsing the specimen. The appendix is raised to the anterior abdominal wall to apply some tension so that gentle blunt dissection can clear adherent tissue. The dissection continues to the base of the appendix (Fig. 38.3). Often the tip of the appendix is not visualized because of its variable location. In these instances, the initial step is to locate the ileocecal junction as a guide to the more constantly located appendiceal base, which is 2 cm lateral and inferior. When the cecum is raised, the base can be readily identified even if the tip is not. The base of the appendix is grasped, and gentle dissection is undertaken toward the tip. If the appendix is adherent to the lateral wall, then the attachment is divided close to the appendix with care to prevent perforation.

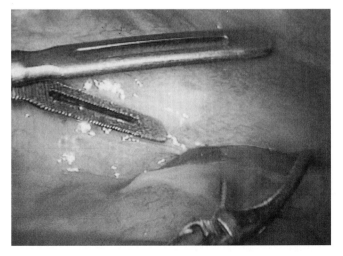

FIGURE 38.2. Curved dissecting forceps are placed through the left port.

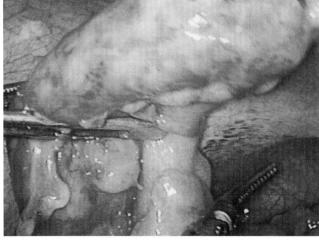

FIGURE 38.3. Dissection continues to the base of the appendix.

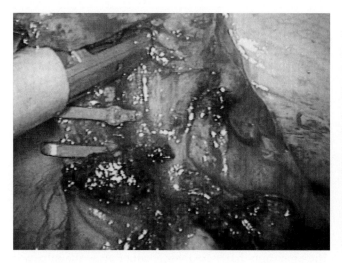

FIGURE 38.4. A 55-mm Ligaclip applicator is applied through the lateral port with an atraumatic grasper in the lower port holding the appendix.

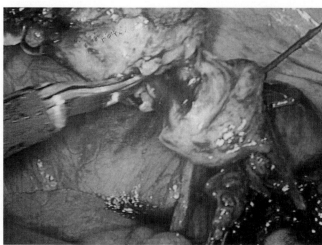

FIGURE 38.6. The appendix is cut with scissors, leaving a 6-mm stump above the lower loop.

Division of the Mesoappendix and Appendix

There are a few safe methods of dividing the mesoappendix.

Ligaclipping the Appendicular Artery

The mesoappendicular fat is incised with diathermy, starting at the middle of the free edge and working toward the base of the appendix. The reason for starting at the midlevel of the mesoappendix is that if the artery is

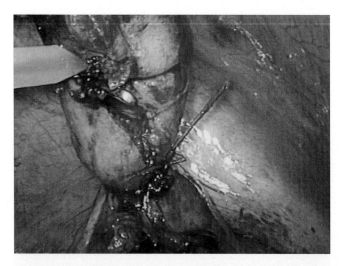

FIGURE 38.5. The mesoappendicular fat is cleared from the base of the appendix by inserting a pretied vessel loop through the lateral port, encircling the base, and placing another loop approximately 1 cm cephalad.

accidentally injured and bleeds, there is enough arterial length for control without fear of retraction. The fat is gently teased toward the base with the grasping forceps or divided with scissors as necessary; care is taken to avoid injury to the appendicular artery. Once the artery is isolated by clearance of the surrounding fat, the 5-mm ligaclip applicator is applied through the lateral port, with the atraumatic grasper in the lower port holding the appendix (Fig. 38.4). One or two secure clips are necessary at the base of the artery and one distal, leaving sufficient space for division of the artery.

The next step is to clear the mesoappendicular fat from the base of the appendix so that it can be safely ligated. This step is done by inserting a pretied vessel loop through the lateral port, encircling the base, and placing another loop approximately 1 cm cephalad (Fig. 38.5). The appendix is then cut with scissors, leaving a 6-mm stump above the lower loop (Fig. 38.6). It is not necessary to diathermy the tip of the stump because the heat energy that is concentrated at the most constricted point of ligature may cause injury and sloughing of the stump. We do not routinely invert the stump because it does not offer any added advantage.

Tying the Mesoappendix and Appendix

It is also possible to ligate the mesoappendix with intracoporeal or extracorporeal tying with 2/0 polyglactin sutures. This maneuver is accomplished by using a curved grasping forcep to create a window in the mesoappendix adjacent to the base of the appendix. The suture can then be delivered through the window and sutured (Fig. 38.7). This technique is repeated for the appendix, and both structures are divided between the site of ligatures.

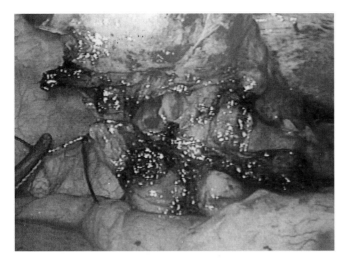

FIGURE 38.7. To ligate the mesoappendix, a suture is delivered through a window in the mesoappendix, adjacent to the base of the appendix, and sutured.

Using Bipolar Diathermy

Bipolar diathermy can be safely used to coagulate the mesoappendix (Fig. 38.8). There is minimal lateral spread of heat energy, thus avoiding damage to surrounding tissues. In contrast, unipolar diathermy disperses energy and can cause damage if used for prolonged periods. However, unipolar cautery can be effectively used for short periods of time. Following bipolar coagulation to the appendicular artery, which causes it to thrombose, it is then cut leaving some length of artery stump as a precaution. In the event of hemorrhage, further bipolar diathermy can be applied or a ligaclip can be securely placed at the base of the artery. An alternative method of using bipolar diathermy is to remove the mesoappendix from the appendix along its length. The process commences at the tip and proceeds to the base, taking care not to perforate the appendix, thus avoiding the artery altogether. The appendix is ligated with the loops and divided as previously described.

Stapler Division

To use endo-stapling, the view must be changed to a 5-mm laparoscope through the lateral port. The 12-mm stapler is inserted through the umbilical port and, if the appendix together with the mesoappendix is not excessively thick, then an endoscopic linear cutter stapler can be closed over the entire structure at the base of the appendix and engaged to divide it (Fig. 38.9). To ensure optimal hemostasis at the edge of the staple line, a vascular stapler is used. However, it is not advisable to apply diathermy to the edge because of potential sloughing. If the mesoappendix is too thick for firing of the stapler in one engagement, then multiple cartridges may be used. This method is done by creating a window in the mesoappendix adjacent to the base of the appendix, dividing the mesoappendix with a vascular cartridge, and then dividing the appendix with an intestinal cartridge. It is important to divide the appendix at its base, the junction between the appendix and the cecum; otherwise, the excessive length of stump left behind could cause recurrent appendicitis. The stapling technique is our preferred method of dividing the appendix because it is safe (leaving three rows of titanium clips), rapidly, and easily

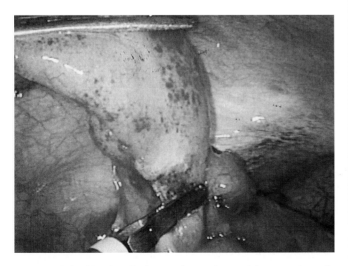

FIGURE 38.8. Bipolar diathermy is used to safely coagulate the mesoappendix.

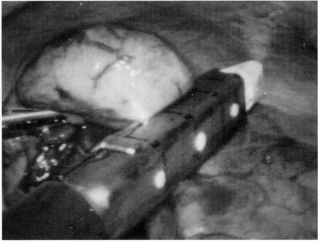

FIGURE 38.9. If the appendix and mesoappendix are not excessively thick, an endoscopic linear cutter stapler can be used over the entire structure at the base of the appendix and engaged to divide it.

effected, and it is useful in difficult situations as discussed later in this chapter.

Removing the Appendix

The view is changed to the 5-mm laparoscope through the lateral port, while the lower port grasper continues to gently hold the appendix to prevent it from dropping into the peritoneal cavity. If the appendix is not thickened, a 10-mm grasper inserted through the umbilical port holds the mesoappendix at the base of the appendix. Again, the tip should not be manipulated as breakage at this inflamed, friable point is possible. Ultimately, the specimen is removed through the port with the valve held open. There is no contact with the abdominal wall, thus reducing the incidence of wound infection. If the appendix cannot be removed because of its thickness, then an endo-bag is inserted, the appendix is placed into it, and the bag is closed and then removed together with the port (Fig. 38.10). The port is reinserted and pneumoperitoneum is re-established. A microbiological swab of the appendix is sent for culture.

Irrigation and Closure

The 10-mm laparoscope is reinserted, and the 5-mm irrigator inserted through the lateral port is used to wash the cecal area with a copious volume of saline until the effluent becomes clear. If there is contamination in other quadrants, then the laparoscopic approach has an advantage over the other techniques of being able to adequately view and lavage other areas, especially the pelvis. Occasionally more than 3 liters of saline are needed depending on the degree of contamination; pressurized

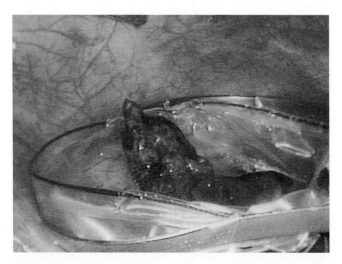

FIGURE 38.10. An endobag is used to remove a thick appendix.

irrigation to dislodge fibrin can be used for more efficient cleansing. At the end of the procedure, the patient is placed head up and the fluid that gravitates to the pelvis can be suctioned. A suction drain is placed in the pelvis through the lower port if a perforation is present. A final verification for hemostasis and secure placement of the ligature or clip is made. The two 5-mm ports are removed under vision to detect any bleeding from the abdominal wall or epigastric vessels. The umbilical wound is closed with a figure-of-eight 0-polyglactin suture, the wounds are cleaned with antiseptic solution, and the skin is closed with subcuticular 4/0 suture. The wounds are then infiltrated with bupivicaine.

Postoperative Management

Oral fluids can usually be taken on the next day when bowel sounds return, although perforation may cause ileus, thus retarding this schedule. When tolerated, a soft diet is introduced. Intramuscular analgesia such as pethidine or morphine is given initially, followed by oral analgesia. Antibiotics are continued for a few days only in perforated cases. The drain, if present, can be removed when the aspirate is minimal or nonpurulent, usually in 1 to 2 days. Most patients are fully ambulatory and are discharged from the hospital by the second postoperative day.

Needlescopic Appendectomy

Needlescopic appendectomy uses instruments with diameters of approximately 3 mm, much smaller than the 5- and 10-mm instruments used in other procedures, and thus becomes even less invasive than conventional laparoscopic surgery. The port and needlescope in the umbilicus are 3 mm in diameter, as are the other two ports, and placed in the same positions as described earlier. Because of the fragile nature of the instruments, they need to be handled with care to prevent bending or breakage. The view with the 3-mm scope is narrower than the 5-mm view but with new optical systems it is clear enough for adequate dissection (Fig. 38.11). The mesoappendix is divided using 3-mm bipolar diathermy and scissors, and the appendix is ligated with mini-pretied vessel loops. Following division of the appendix, it is brought close to the umbilical wound and retrieved with artery forceps through the wound. The advantages of this procedure are that the wounds are even smaller than conventional laparoscopy, with the potential of less pain, and only the umbilical wound is closed with suture; the rest of the wounds are closed with tape. It is most applicable when surgery is achieved early for an appendix that is minimally inflamed. This method is not encouraged in

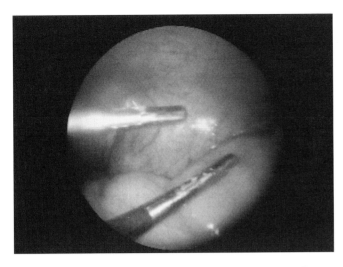

FIGURE 38.11. View from a 3-mm scope during dissection.

situations where the appendix is very inflamed or perforated, where maximum dissection and irrigation is required.

The Difficult Appendix

Certain situations require maneuvers in addition to the conventional laparoscopic appendectomy steps described earlier.

Retrocecal Appendix

If the appendix cannot be identified after exposing the ileocecal junction, then it is likely to be retrocecal or retroileal. In this situation, the cecum and ascending colon must be mobilized from the lateral abdominal wall by dividing the lateral attachments with blunt dissection and scissors, similar to the mobilization for a hemicolectomy. The atraumatic bowel grasper in the lower port is essential for this process by gently retracting the colon; the irrigator can also be used as a blunt dissector. The concealed appendix can be revealed adherent to the cecum and should be gently separated from it by blunt dissection. It is imperative to avoid injury to the retroperitoneal structures such as the right ureter or iliac vessels by judicious use of the diathermy.

Unexposed Appendix Tip

Occasionally, the base of the appendix is identified but it is not possible to retrieve the tip because of adherence to deeper tissues. In this situation, it may be unwise to continue to try to forceably deliver the appendix for fear of avulsing the tip and leaving it behind to form a source of infection and abscess. It is much safer to first divide the base with either a stapler or loops, and then dissect toward the tip by carefully dividing the mesoappendix close to the appendix. Eventually, the entire appendix can be removed. In the event of an avulsed appendix, the tissues and bowel in the vicinity need to be separated and all necrotic tissues removed. The area is copiously irrigated, and one or more drains are placed.

Necrotic Appendiceal Base

When the inflammation extends to the base of the appendix and involves part of the cecum, it is safer to use the endo-stapling device to divide the appendix by placing the jaws of the stapler below the necrotic area and removing the appendix with part of the cap of the cecum. More than one staple cartridge may be needed. Due to the multiple rows of titanium clips, this procedure is safer than are the other techniques described. Alternatively, if stapling is not available, then the necrotic segment can be excised and the healthy cecal edges approximated with intracorporeal suturing.

In difficult situations where all methods fail to successfully remove the appendix, then conversion to an open procedure is necessary as a safety measure, usually in cases in which the appendix is either not identified or encased in severe adhesions. This use of the laparoscope, known as assisted laparoscopy, is still helpful in irrigating the areas inaccessible to the open incision and in guiding the surgeon to place the incision just over the appendix, thus minimizing the wound size.

Laparoscopic Compared to Open Appendectomy

Laparoscopic appendectomy is valuable for the following reasons.

1. It is a useful tool for more accurate diagnosis of abdominal pain.[2,3] In situations where the appendix appears grossly normal, the laparoscope can detect other pathologies, especially in the female pelvis, more accurately than an examination through a small gridiron incision. A decision can then be made as to whether the appendix should be removed. This advantage is in contrast to open appendectomy, where pelvic examination is limited and a normal-looking appendix is invariably removed when no other pathology is detected.

2. If other pathologies exist, then treatment can often be achieved by therapeutic laparoscopy. Other laparoscopic or laparoscopic-assisted procedures include oophorectomy, ileocolic resection, Meckel's diverticulectomy, and sigmoid colectomy.

3. The main advantages over open appendectomy lie in the smaller wounds, and in removing the appendix without directly contaminating the wound, thus providing better pain management, lesser wound infection, and faster recovery to normal. These three benefits are the predominant advantages, as determined from a recent meta-analysis of randomized trials comparing laparoscopic and open appendectomy.[4]

4. The laparoscopic method allows more superior capacity to irrigate the peritoneum in all areas of the abdomen.

5. In contrast to the open technique, the much smaller wounds may lower the risk of adhesions, infection, dehiscence, and herniation.[5]

6. It is as safe as open appendectomy.

7. It has a cosmetic advantage over open appendectomy.

8. It is a good base for laparoscopic training.

These benefits may be offset by the following reasons.

1. The initial operative experience includes a learning curve and leads to longer operating times, but with experience this difference disappears. Similarly, the setup of the laparoscopic equipment may add additional time; however, the overall time may not be affected.

2. The laparoscopic instruments are costly, particularly if disposable ones are used; this disadvantage can be minimized by using reusable instruments. Also, the young patient who returns to work faster than after open appendectomy may accumulate societal cost savings to offset the cost of the instruments.

3. The pneumoperitoneum may be deleterious in generalized peritonitis, but this problem has not been proven with localized appendicitis.

4. A higher rate of abscess following laparoscopic appendectomy when compared to open methods has been intimated but not proven.

Conclusion

Because acute appendicitis is a common condition, laparoscopic appendectomy has become a commonly performed procedure. It offers the surgeon a minimally invasive method of removing the appendix and offers the patient certain advantages over open appendectomy. It is our preferred method of appendectomy, especially in young females and in obese patients, regardless of age or sex.

References

1. Semm K. Endoscopic appendicectomy. Endoscopy 1983;15: 59–64.
2. Kum CK, Sim E, Goh P. Diagnostic laparoscopy: reducing the number of normal appendectomies. Dis Colon Rectum 1993;36:763.
3. Barrat C, Catheline JM, Rizk N, Champault GC. Does laparoscopy reduce the incidence of unnecessary appendicectomies? Surg Laparosc Endosc 1999;9:27–31.
4. Garbutt JM, Soper NJ, Shannon WD, Botero A, Littenberg B. Meta-analysis of randomized controlled trials comparing laparoscopic and open appendectomy. Surg Laparosc Endosc 1999;9:17–26.
5. Kum CK, Ngoi SS, Goh PMY, Tekant Y, Isaac JR. Randomized controlled trial comparing laparoscopic and open appendectomy. Br J Surg 1993;80:1599–1600.

39
Laparoscopic Right Hemicolectomy

Juliane A. Miranda-Rassi and Jay J. Singh

Removal of both benign and malignant lesions of the distal ileum, cecum, ascending colon, and hepatic flexures can be managed by right hemicolectomy (Table 39.1). Depending upon the nature of one's practice and referral patterns, the most common indications are neoplasia and inflammatory bowel disease. This chapter focuses upon the laparoscopic performance of right colonic resection. Laparoscopic right hemicolectomy is distinctly different from ileocolic resection as the latter involves removal of the distal ileum and cecum and avoids extensive mobilization of the transverse colon; this more limited procedure is best for Crohn's ileitis or palliative resection of metastatic cecal lesions. Standard right hemicolectomy, whether performed by laparotomy or by laparoscopy, is the procedure of choice for malignant lesions of the right colon, cecum, ileocecal valve, or appendix, as well as any infiltrative or inflammatory processes that preclude a lesser resection; it entails complete mobilization of the terminal ileum and right colon to the level of the midportion of the transverse colon. In addition to the technical issues, this chapter focuses on the results of laparoscopic right hemicolectomy for various indications and the controversies surrounding this approach.

Preoperative Evaluation

As with conventional surgical procedures, patients undergoing laparoscopy should have a thorough medical evaluation with special emphasis on their pulmonary and cardiac status. In general, the patient must be able to withstand a potentially lengthy operative procedure with multiple position changes. It is important to realize that a patient who cannot tolerate a laparotomy cannot undergo a laparoscopic colon resection as the likelihood of conversion is inherent. Preoperative workup should include a complete blood count and chemistries; a coagulation profile is included if the patient has a history of bleeding. The exact localization and full evaluation of any pathology to be removed may require contrast enemas, CT scans, or complete endoscopic evaluation. General endotracheal anesthesia with adequate muscle relaxation is fundamental, as is avoidance of nitrous oxide as an inhalation anesthetic agent, because this substance may lead to small bowel dilatation.

Preoperative Preparation

Preparation for laparoscopic colon surgery is identical to that used for laparotomy.[1] The evening before operation, patients are given 90 ml sodium phosphate-based oral solution (Fleet phosphosoda; CB Fleet, Lynchburg, VA, USA). It has been demonstrated, in two prospective randomized studies, that this preparation is better tolerated by patients than the traditional 4-liter polyethylene glycol-based solution with equal efficacy of bowel cleansing.[2,3] Oral and broad-spectrum parenteral antibiotics are administered before the surgery, and all patients provide consent for formal laparotomy and intraoperative colonoscopy, should either be necessary. Heparin is administered, with the use of sequential compression stockings, as antithrombotic measures. After the induction of general anesthesia, a nasogastric tube and an indwelling bladder catheter are inserted to minimize the risk of trocar injury to the stomach and the bladder, respectively.

Patient Positioning

The patient is positioned in the supine modified lithotomy position in Allen stirrups (Allen Medical, Bedford Heights, OH, USA). The patient must be on a table that can quickly and easily be manipulated into many positions and should be secured so that shifting does not occur even at extremes of vertical and lateral tilt. Ideally,

TABLE 39.1. Indications for right colon resection.

Benign colorectal disease
  Colonoscopically nonresectable villous and villotubular adenomas
  Lipomas, leiomyomas
  Inflammatory bowel disease
  Diverticular disease
  Typhilitis
  Volvulus
  Posttraumatic stricture

Malignant colorectal disease
  Palliation of metastatic cancer
  Adenocarcinomas
  Carcinoid tumors

the arms should be safely secured to the patient's sides. Flexion at the knees and hips should be no greater than 15° to facilitate instruments and movements. Any greater flexion can interfere with port and instrument use in the lower quadrants of the abdomen. The lithotomy position offers greater flexibility in placement of the surgeon, assistants, and instruments and allows transanal endoscopy and stapler insertion.

Surgical Technique

The abdomen is prepped and draped in the standard fashion to provide wide exposure in case a laparotomy is required. A small incision that will snugly fit a 10- or 12-mm trocar is made above or below the umbilicus for the insertion of the Veress needle. Suspicion of adhesions in patients who have had prior abdominal surgeries should encourage the use of the "open" Hasson technique.[4] When using the Veress needle, correct placement must be verified by tactile sensation, by hearing the needle penetrate the abdominal cavity, and by placement of a drop of sterile water at the top of the needle that should easily enter the abdominal cavity. After creation of a 15mmHg pneumoperitoneum with CO_2 insufflation, the needle is removed from the abdomen and a 10- or 12-mm trocar is placed through the umbilical incision. This port site will be primarily employed by the camera, as all subsequent maneuvers are undertaken under direct visualization. A 30° laparoscope can be employed with a standard 0° instrument to enhance visibility in the pelvis and around the flexures where the angles are more acute. Efficient use of these angled scopes requires a great deal of expertise.[4] The placement of ureteric catheters should be undertaken in patients with a history of inflammatory conditions, prior pelvic surgery, sepsis, or radiation; either ordinary or illuminated stents may accelerate the identification of the ureters.

For right colon resections, two or three 10- or 12-mm ports are commonly required; these are placed in the

umbilicus, the left paraumbilical area, and the left lower quadrant (Fig. 39.1). Under direct visualization, the lateral ports should be placed outside the left rectus muscle to avoid injuring the epigastric vessels and to allow more control over both dissection and vascular ligation. If necessary, a fourth port can be added in the right lower quadrant, in the suprapubic region, or high in the left upper quadrant. Nevertheless, the exact port site placement depends more on the patient's body habitus, type of resection, and operative findings. Adhesions from prior appendectomy, hysterectomy, or cholecystectomy can impose a significant hindrance and flexibility in the placement, and thus the use of these ports should not be underestimated. It is noteworthy that all ports should be at least 10-mm in diameter. Laparoscopic colorectal surgery is a multiquadrant process that often demands frequent repositioning of the instruments. More important, the surgeon should be able to place the 10-mm camera in any port, as needed.

The routine use of monitors, one on each side of the patient, remains the current standard of viewing the procedure. The operating room is configured so that the monitors can be easily moved should the surgeon require a change of position during the procedure. For right hemicolectomy, the surgeon typically stands either on the left side of the patient, next to the assistant, or between the patient's legs.

After the pneumoperitoneum is established and the first port is placed in the transumbilical incision, the camera is passed through the 10- to 12-mm trocar and the abdomen is thoroughly examined. The liver and the pelvis should be scanned for any evidence of associated or unrelated pathology. A steep Trendelenburg position

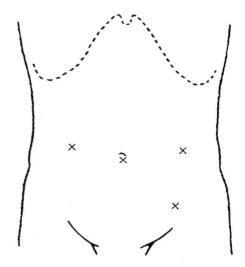

FIGURE 39.1. Port site placement for laparoscopic right colon resection.

should facilitate complete visualization of the liver to exclude metastases in the case of colon cancer or any unassociated problems such as gallstones. Placing the patient in reverse Trendelenburg will move small bowel loops out of the pelvis so that any coexistent pelvic pathology may be assessed. The small bowel should also be carefully examined using the hand-over-hand technique, with gentle maneuvers to avoid any injury. At this time, all abdominal wall adhesions are sharply divided under direct vision to permit the safe placement of the remaining ports.

The resection should begin with mobilization of the cecum. The patient is placed in reverse Trendelenburg position with the left side of the table tilted down. The small bowel is usually retracted to the left, and the left ureter is identified. Delicate grasping of the terminal ileum and cecum provide traction so that the surgeon can divide the retroperitoneal attachments of the right colon. Either the harmonic scalpel or electrocautery may be utilized for this purpose; however, improved hemostasis and visibility have been advantages of the former (Wexner Salum, 1998; personal communication). Retraction is facilitated by using the companion port so that the surgeon is "two handed." After the cecum is mobilized, the right colon is grasped proximally and distally, and medial retraction allows exposure of the line of Toldt; this avascular plane is then divided. At this time, the iliac vessels, duodenum, and right ureter should be identified. While the table is still tilted to the left, the head of the table should be raised for hepatic flexure mobilization. Frequent use of vascular clips may be necessary at this stage of the procedure because vessels of a larger caliber at the flexure may be safely controlled with the harmonic scalpel or cautery.

After the entire right colon is mobilized, vascular ligation and anastomosis may be undertaken, either completely intracorporeally or extracorporeally for the laparoscopic-assisted technique. In the latter setting, the intended specimen is delivered through an extension of the umbilical incision; this portion of the procedure should take place with the patient and table in the horizontal position. The camera should be placed into the left-sided port, and an atraumatic grasper is placed through the umbilical port onto the cecum. Extension of the umbilical incision and entrance into the peritoneal cavity is facilitated by incising or cauterizing along the shaft of the trocar. A small wound drape may be placed at this time to protect the wound edges before withdrawal of the port, grasper, and cecum as one unit. The rest of the specimen is then removed, and division of the vascular supply and bowel anastomosis are rapidly and safely completed outside of the peritoneal cavity. Currently, this laparoscopic-assisted method is favored over the total intracorporeal approach because of the latter's greater technical difficulty, increased time and cost, decreased safety, and increased potential for contamination. Ultimately, an incision must be created to retrieve the specimen. After extending the umbilical incision, the mesentery is ligated between clamps, ensuring placement of suture ligatures in the proximal end of each vessel. This method is very useful, especially for the thickened friable mesentery found in patients with Crohn's disease. The anastomosis may be completed in the usual fashion; the mesenteric defect is repaired, and the bowel is returned into the abdomen. The pneumoperitoneum must be reestablished after the incision is closed to verify hemostasis and anastomotic integrity.

Results and Controversies

The primary advocates of laparoscopic right hemicolectomy for the treatment of colorectal disease are those surgeons who use this technique with frequency and thus are in a position to realize its many potential benefits. Subjective advantages such as improved cosmesis and decreased pain are difficult to measure and depend heavily on the patient's expectations. Objective parameters such as decreased length of ileus, shorter hospital stay, and earlier resumption of normal activity are more easily quantified. The majority of studies have been either retrospective or prospective and nonrandomized; thus, the significance of their findings must be tempered when advocating guidelines for laparoscopy for these indications. The achievement of better cosmetic results has been reported by many authors.[5,6] Alabaz et al.[5] reported that only 13 (42%) patients had "good" or "excellent" cosmesis after open surgery for Crohn's disease whereas 14 (88%) patients in the laparoscopy group had the same feeling ($p < 0.004$). The same paper reported a significantly shorter hospital stay (6.9 ± 0.9 days) and an earlier return to work ($3.7 + 1.3$ weeks) than after laparotomy (8.2 ± 1.1 weeks).

Talamini et al.[7] reported their 2-year experience with 20 patients who underwent laparoscopic-assisted surgery for ileocolic Crohn's disease compared to 36 patients who underwent the same types of resection by laparotomy. The authors did not study cosmesis, yet the laparoscopic-assisted incision had a mean of 3.9 (range, 3–5) cm through which resection and anastomosis was completed. When comparing laparoscopy to laparotomy, the minimally invasive group had significantly less blood loss (147 versus 243 ml; $p < 0.05$), earlier return of bowel function (3.7 versus 5.1 days; $p < 0.05$), a shorter hospital stay (5.9 versus 8.1 days; $p < 0.005$), fewer morphine equivalents used for postoperative pain (159 versus 307; $P < 0.005$), and better surgical recovery index (13.1 versus 20.3; $p < 0.05$). The authors were able to achieve these significant advantages for laparoscopy (214 versus 207 min).

Crohn's disease appears to be an ideal indication for laparoscopic right hemicolectomy because of the benefit to this relatively young group of patients with regard to early return to normal activity, which may translate into improved productivity and self-esteem. In addition, many patients with Crohn's disease may require more than one resection in their lifetime. There is some indication that adhesion formation is decreased after laparoscopy when compared to laparotomy.[8,9] If so, patients who require multiple procedures may benefit from easier second or even third operations and possibly decreased incidences of future adhesive obstruction.

Crohn's disease is not the only indication for laparoscopic right hemicolectomy. Patients with large, sessile, endoscopically irretrievable polyps may also be good candidates for a laparoscopic procedure. Regarding these indications, better cosmesis, faster recovery, decreased postoperative pain, and earlier return to preoperative activity have been reported as compared to laparotomy.[10,11] However, its potential disadvantages include longer operative time and a shorter specimen. Chen et al.[12] compared a group of 71 patients who underwent laparoscopy for the treatment of benign disease with the same number of patients submitted to laparotomy to assess disability in terms of the number of postoperative days until return to partial activity, full activity, and work. The patients, assessed by a questionnaire, seemed to have an earlier return to baseline activity and work in the laparoscopy group. Laparoscopic-assisted right hemicolectomy seems to be a reliable procedure, although deep vein thrombosis,[13] bleeding,[14] and anastomotic leak have all been reported.[15]

Although the treatment of benign colonic disease by laparoscopic right hemicolectomy has become acceptable, the same cannot be said about the use of this technique for the treatment of potentially curable colon cancer. The primary concern is if laparoscopy offers the same oncologic standards as laparotomy. The efficacy of the technique is based upon four aspects of the surgery: margins of resection, number of retrieved lymph nodes, alteration of the immune system, and port site recurrence. An adequate distal margin is seldom problematic in right hemicolectomy. The number of lymph nodes retrieved in the specimen furnishes quantitative criteria to compare laparotomy to the laparoscopic procedure. Jacobs et al.[16] compared the number of lymph nodes recovered by laparoscopic right hemicolectomy with that of laparotomy and failed to identify a significant difference. Although the number of lymph nodes harvested from the mesentery of resected specimens depends on some aspects other than surgical ability such as individual anatomic variations, thickness of mesentery, and pathologist dissection, the benefit of resecting as many lymph nodes as possible has been shown, mainly regarding recurrence.[17,18]

The rationale sustaining the use of laparoscopy to treat colon cancer is that this procedure would not cause as great a derangement in the immune system. Both animal and human studies have shown that laparoscopic surgery affects the cellular and the humoral immune system to a lesser extent than does laparotomy.[19,20] Perhaps the most important and unsolved problem in laparoscopic surgery for colon cancer is port site recurrence (PSR). Its etiology is uncertain, and some associated factors may be aerosolized cancer cells,[21,22] contamination of instruments, ischemia at port sites,[23] and technical factors.[24] So long as these and other doubts regarding the use of laparoscopy for the treatment of potentially curable malignancies are unresolved, these techniques should be offered only to patients enrolled in peer-reviewed, externally monitored, prospective randomized trials.

References

1. Wexner SD, Beck DE. Sepsis prevention in colorectal surgery. In: Fielding LP, Goldberg SM (eds) Operative Surgery: Colon, Rectum and Anus, 5th Ed. London: Butterworth Heineman, 1993.
2. Oliveira L, Wexner SD, Daniel N, et al. Mechanical bowel preparation for elective colorectal surgery. A prospective, randomized, surgeon-blinded trial comparing sodium phosphate and polyethylene glycol-based oral lavage solutions. Dis Colon Rectum 1997;40(5):585–591.
3. Cohen SM, Wexner SD, Binderow SR, et al. Prospective, randomized, endoscopic-blinded trial comparing precolonoscopy bowel cleansing methods. Dis Colon Rectum 1994;37(7):689–696.
4. Hasson HM. A modified instrument and method for laparoscopy. Am J Obstet Gynecol 1971;110:886–887.
5. Alabaz O. Iroatulam AJN, Nessim A, Weiss EG, Nogueras JJ, Wexner SD. Comparison of laparoscopic-assisted and conventional ileocolic resection for Crohn's disease [abstract]. Surg Endosc 1997;11:190.
6. Dunker MS, Stiggelbout AM, van Hogezand RA, et al. Cosmesis and body image after laparoscopic-assisted and open ileocolic resection for Crohn's disease. Surg Endosc 1998;12(11):1334–1340.
7. Talamini MA, Moesinger RC, Kaufman H, Kutka M, Harris M, Bayless T. Laparoscopic assisted bowel resection for Crohn's disease: the best of both worlds [abstract]. Gastroenterology 1997;4:A1478.
8. Reissman P, Teoh TA, Skinner K, Burns JW, Wexner SD. Adhesion formation after laparoscopic anterior resection in a porcine model: a pilot study. Surg Laparosc Endosc 1996;6(2):136–139.
9. Joo JS, Agachan F, Wexner SD. Laparoscopic surgery for lower gastrointestinal fistulas. Surg Endosc 1997;11(2):116–118.
10. Sands LR, Wexner SD. The role of laparoscopic colectomy and laparotomy with resection in the management of complex polyps of the colon. Surg Oncol Clin N Am 1996;5(3):713–721.

11. Joo JS, Amarnath L, Wexner SD. Is laparoscopic resection of colorectal polyps beneficial? Surg Endosc 1998;12(11);1341–1344.

12. Chen HH, Wexner SD, Weiss EG, et al. Laparoscopic colectomy for benign colorectal disease is associated with a significant reduction in disability as compared with laparotomy. Surg Endosc 1998;12(12):1397–1400.

13. Millikan KW, Szczerba SM, Dominguez JM, McKenna R, Rorig JC. Superior mesenteric and portal vein thrombosis following laparoscopic-assisted right hemicolectomy. Report of a case. Dis Colon Rectum 1996;39(10):1171–1175.

14. Verzaro R, Twoh T-A, Wexner SD. Laparoscopic colorectal surgery: risk factors for local recurrences. Reg Cancer Treat 1994;7:183–187.

15. Monson JR, Darzi A, Carey PD, Guillou PJ. Prospective evaluation of laparoscopic-assisted colectomy in an unselected group of patients. Lancet 1992;340(8823):831–833.

16. Jacobs M. Laparoscopic colon resection: the Miami experience. In: Laparoscopic Colon and Rectal Seminar Syllabus. Cincinnati: Ethicon Endo-Surgery, 1992.

17. Toyota S, Ohta H, Anazawa S. Rationale for extent of lymph node dissection for right colon cancer. Dis Colon Rectum 1995;38(7):705–711.

18. Bernstein M, Wexner SD. Laparoscopic resection for colorectal cancer: a USA perspective. Semin Laparosc Surg 1995;2(4);216–223.

19. Allendorf JD, Bessler M, Kayton ML, et al. Increased tumor established and growth after laparotomy vs laparoscopy in a murine model. Arch Surg 1995;130(6):649–653.

20. Bouvy ND, Marquet RL, Jeekel H, Bonjer HJ. Impact of gas(less) laparoscopy and laparotomy on peritoneal tumor growth and abdominal wall metastases. Ann Surg 1996;224(6):694–700.

21. Fritsch S, Gossot D, Lesourd A, Laborde F, Poupon MF. Experimental abdominal wound metastases following laparoscopic versus open resection for colonic malignancy. Surg Endosc 1997;11:552.

22. Hewett PJ, Thomas WM, King G, Eaton M. Intraperitoneal cell movement during abdominal carbon dioxide insufflation and laparoscopy. An in vivo model. Dis Colon Rectum 1996;39(suppl 10):S62–S66.

23. Tseng LNL, Bouvy ND, Kazemier G, Marguet RL, Bonjer HJ. "Port site" metastases: the role of local ischemia and chimney effect [abstract]. Surg Endosc 1997;11:556.

24. O'Rourke N, Price PM, Kelly S, et al. Tumor inoculation during laparoscopy [letter]. Lancet 1993;342:368.

40
Laparoscopic Transverse Colectomy

Laurence R. Sands and Michael D. Hellinger

Accepted indications for laparoscopic transverse colectomy include benign polyps and endoscopically irretrievable masses. At our institution, malignant neoplasms of the transverse colon are considered for laparoscopic resection only in those patients who have metastatic disease and are to be palliated. In these cases, a laparoscopic colonic sleeve resection with an extracorporeal anastomosis may be performed. However, an isolated transverse colectomy is rarely indicated. Most often, lesions of the hepatic flexure and the proximal transverse colon are incorporated in a right hemicolectomy with an ileocolic anastomosis, whereas lesions of the midportion or distal transverse colon often are treated with an extended right hemicolectomy. An extended right hemicolectomy or left hemicolectomy may best treat a lesion at the splenic flexure. Both operations, however, require mobilization of the splenic flexure.

Laparoscopic colectomy has certainly been shown to be a feasible operation. However, operative times have been reported to be longer with this approach, with an average time of 227 min in one particular study.[1] In addition, reported conversion rates to laparotomy vary from 3% to 24%.[2–4] It has also been shown that the conversion rate as well as morbidity may be greater in obese than in asthenic patients.[5–7] Nonetheless, the transverse colon is certainly amenable to laparoscopic resection. Various techniques for laparoscopic transverse colectomy have been described, including the use of abdominal wall lifting bars and eliminating the use of pneumoperitoneum.[8] In any case, regardless of the technique employed, the operation requires the mobilization of both the hepatic and splenic flexures, both of which are demanding and technically challenging advanced laparoscopic procedures.

In addition, transverse colectomy requires high or proximal ligation of the middle colic vessels, which may be confused with the superior mesenteric artery (SMA). Accidental division of the superior mesenteric artery is a devastating and disastrous complication that requires prompt recognition, attention, and immediate repair. In addition to the SMA, there are other anatomic considerations in resection of the transverse colon, including proximity of the duodenum, the pancreas, the spleen, and the omentum. Injury to any of these organs can occur during this operation. Mobilization of the renocolic, liencolic, and gastrocolic ligaments must all be performed in this resection as well. Therefore, the surgeon should be familiar with laparoscopic colon surgery as well as the laparoscopic equipment before performing this procedure. This chapter discusses the procedure and provides several technical points related to the mobilization of both flexures and resection of the transverse colon.

Patient Positioning

The patient is positioned in the lithotomy position with the legs placed in stirrups. The legs are positioned with the thighs horizontally in line with the abdomen to diminish interference with the manipulation of the laparoscopic instruments. Both arms are adducted to the sides of the patient to facilitate movement of the instruments. The modified lithotomy position allows the surgeon to perform portions of the procedure from between the legs. In addition, this position allows transanal access for intraoperative colonoscopy to assist in localization of lesions.

Initial Setup and Port Placement

After the induction of general anesthesia and endotracheal intubation, the patient is properly positioned and a bladder catheter and orogastric tube are placed for bladder and gastric decompression, respectively. The television monitors are placed at the head of the patient on both sides to allow both the surgeon and the assistant a good view of the procedure (Fig. 40.1).

SURGICAL TEAM POSITION

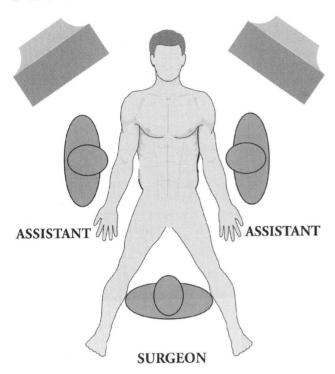

ASSISTANT   ASSISTANT

SURGEON

FIGURE 40.1. Operating room setup.

trocar is placed in the right upper quadrant and is primarily used for retraction.

The traditional approach to laparoscopic transverse colectomy has been to start the dissection by mobilizing the superior portion of the left colon and then the splenic flexure. This method has been preferred because the splenic flexure mobilization is the most difficult and time-consuming portion of the procedure.[10] This order allows the surgeon the opportunity to convert the procedure to a laparotomy early in the course of the operation should the need arise from difficulties with this part of the operation. Once again, this sequence has not been our standard approach to this procedure for several reasons. First, we prefer to have the colon tethered at the sidewalls to provide additional countertraction on the transverse colon during mobilization to assist the surgeon. Second, our preference is to undertake the easier portions of the operation first, so that if conversion to a laparotomy is necessary, we may then only need to perform a limited incision because most of the mobilization will have already been performed.

We, therefore, begin the dissection with the patient in slight reverse Trendelenburg position with the surgeon positioned between the patient's legs. The camera is placed via the umbilical port, and superior retraction of

The initial 12-mm trocar is placed via the open technique just cepahalad to the level of the umbilicus through a small midline incision. Alternatively, a Veress needle may be used in those patients who have not had prior surgery. The position of this needle is always confirmed with the saline drop test to ensure that it is intraperitoneal. The abdomen is insufflated to 15 mmHg pressure. Recent data suggest fewer postoperative pulmonary complications with insufflation to slightly lower intraabdominal pressures.[9] Exploration of the abdominal cavity is initiated with the aid of the laparoscope, and a determination of feasibility and resectability is then made.

Classically, the remaining three 12-mm trocars are placed under direct vision (Fig. 40.2). The second and third trocars are placed symmetrically on opposite sides of the abdomen, in the midclavicular line, lateral to the rectus sheath, and at the level of or slightly superior to the level of the umbilicus. The fourth port is placed in the left anterior axillary line just superior to the level of the umbilicus.

Alternatively, our preference has been to place the trocars according to Figure 40.3. Once again, all the trocars used are 12 mm in size to facilitate repositioning of the equipment. This approach places the two midabdominal ports lateral to the rectus sheath and just inferior to the level of the umbilicus. In addition, a fourth

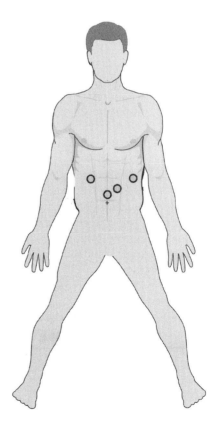

FIGURE 40.2. Port placement.

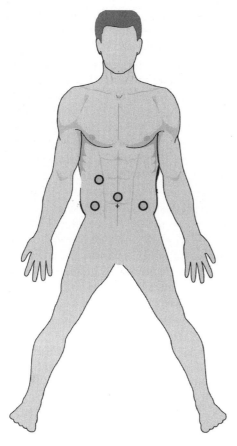

FIGURE 40.3. Alternative port placement.

Colonic Devascularization

At our institution, the next part of the operation consists of devascularization of the transverse colon. Most sources actually describe this manuever as the final step before exteriorizing the specimen and creating the anastomosis.[9] We believe that this is best accomplished early in the operation while the surgeon works on the midportion of the transverse colon.

This maneuver, which entails ligation of the middle colic artery, represents the most crucial part of the procedure. The surgeon must be certain of the anatomy at this point to properly ligate the correct structure. As previously mentioned, this vessel may be confused with the superior mesenteric artery with disastrous consequences. Identification of the middle colic artery may be made especially difficult in those patients with a thick, fat-filled mesentery. Unfortunately, the technique of mesenteric transillumination is rarely of any great help in laparoscopic surgery, although some authors have reported success with this technique.[11] Retracting the transverse colon superiorly provides mild tension on the middle colic vessels, which facilitates identification of this vessel. Additional techniques using laparoscopic ultrasound have been described in properly identifying this important vessel.[12]

After the omentum is completely dissected from the transverse colon, it is lifted superiorly above the stomach. The surgeon remains between the legs of the patient and the patient is placed in greater reverse Trendelenburg position. The lesser sac is completely freed from the transverse colon mesentery to allow careful and direct visualization of the middle colic vessels. The transverse colon is then lifted superiorly along with the omentum to provide tenting of the middle colic vessels. Having the colon tethered at the flexures aids the surgeon by providing the necessary tension in helping to properly identify these vessels. Mesenteric windows are made on either side of the vessels with either the cautery scissors or the harmonic scalpel. A right-angled laparoscopic instrument placed via the right-sided port may also assist in ligating the correct vessels. A proximal ligation of the middle colic artery is performed with the use of the vascular endoscopic linear cutter or alternatively with intracorporeal suturing techniques. The mesentery is then opened laterally in both directions with the cautery scissors, and the hepatic flexure is approached next.

the omentum is provided from the right upper quadrant port and the left-sided port. We start the procedure by preserving and lifting the omentum superiorly off the transverse colon and dissecting in this avascular plane to open the lesser sac. This dissection is carried out laterally in both directions with either cautery scissors or the ultrasonic scalpel (Ethicon Endo-Surgery, Cincinnati, OH, USA). One advantage of the ultrasonic scalpel is the absence of smoke, thereby allowing the surgeon clear visibility without having to constantly release smoke and air pressure from the abdominal cavity. Another advantage of this instrument is that there is no thermal injury to adjacent structures as can occur with cautery; it can also provide excellent hemostasis. If one decides, however, to resect the omentum, then this structure must be divided with the use of clips and possibly endoscopic linear cutters. Once again, the ultrasonic scalpel may be helpful in resecting and dividing the omentum. Care must be taken to ensure preservation of the gastroepiploic vessels at the greater curve of the stomach.

Hepatic Flexure Mobilization

The camera may be kept at the umbilical port site. The patient is now rotated to the left side and kept in reverse Trendelenburg position. The assistant is repositioned to the right side of the patient. Instruments placed by the assistant via the right upper quadrant port and the right-sided port may be used for medial retraction of the hepatic flexure. The surgeon will use the left-sided port for dissection and may continue the operation from between the patient's legs or move to the left side of the patient. After the colon is appropriately retracted medially and inferiorly by the assistant, the white line of Toldt on the right side is mobilized with cautery scissors and the hepatocolic ligament is divided. The dissection is completed to the level of the greater omentum that was dissected off the transverse colon in the steps just described, and the dissection of the gastrocolic ligament is completed. On mobilizing the right colon off the retroperitoneum, the duodenal sweep is clearly identified and protected from injury. The splenic flexure is approached next.

Splenic Flexure Mobilization

The patient is kept in the reverse Trendelenburg position and tilted to the right side. The surgeon may stay between the patient's legs or may move to the right side of the patient. The right-sided port is used for dissection and the right upper quadrant port is used for retraction. The assistant retracts the splenic flexure medially and inferiorly from the left-sided port, and the dissection begins on the left side of the colon mobilizing the white line of Toldt on this side with cautery scissors. The white line of Toldt is completely mobilized at the superior aspect, and the splenic flexure is thereby mobilized. The renocolic and lienocolic ligaments are completely divided. Once the flexure is mobilized, medial retraction and a gentle sweeping motion are used to ensure that the lateral structures are adequately mobilized and are protected out of harm's way. Of course, extreme care should be taken to prevent a splenic injury, as in the case with an open colectomy. Bleeding in this area may be difficult to control via the laparoscope and could result in conversion to a laparotomy. The dissection is completed by joining the splenic flexure mobilization with the mobilization of the gastrocolic ligament over the left side of the transverse colon. The entire transverse colon is now freely mobile and may be resected by exteriorizing this segment of bowel.

Resection and Anastomosis

An incision is made in the midepigastrum; this incision may be performed either transversely or as a midline incision. The bowel is then exteriorized with the use of a wound protector or with the assistance of retractors.

Either a stapled side-to-side anastomosis or a handsewn anastomosis may be fashioned as would be done during a laparotomy. There should be adequate mobility of the colon, and this anastomosis should be done without any obvious tension. The mesenteric defect may be closed or left widely open. The completed anastomosis is returned to the abdominal cavity, and the incision is closed. The abdomen is reinsufflated, and the bowel is once again inspected to ensure that there has been no twist of the bowel and that the anastomosis appears patent. The remaining ports are removed under direct vision, and the fascial defects are closed.

Conclusion

Laparoscopic resection of the transverse colon is a procedure that clearly requires advanced skills. Recently, there have been data to support some of the advantages of the laparoscopic approach, including shorter length of hospitalization, earlier return to baseline activity, earlier return to work, and lessened overall disability.[13] Therefore, we believe that laparoscopic transverse colectomy should be familiar to the surgeon, even though the indications for this procedure are somewhat limited. However, transverse colon mobilization, resection, and anastomosis may be a component of other more frequently indicated colorectal procedures.

References

1. Musser DJ, Boorse RC, Madera F, et al. Laparoscopic colectomy: at what cost? Surg Laparosc Endosc 1994;4:1–5.
2. Phillips EH, Franklin M, Carroll BJ, et al. Laparoscopic colectomy. Ann Surg 1992;216:703–707.
3. Zucker KA, Pitcher DE, Martin DT, et al. Laparoscopic-assisted colon resection. Surg Endosc 1994;8:12–18.
4. Ortega EA, Peters JH. Physiologic alterations of endosurgery. In: Peters JH, DeMeester TR (eds) Minimally invasive surgery of the foregut. St. Louis: Quality Medical, 1994.
5. Dean PA, Beart RW Jr, Nelson H, et al. Laparoscopic assisted segmental colectomy: early Mayo Clinic experience. Mayo Clin Proc 1994;69:834–840.
6. Falk PM, Beart RW Jr, Wexner SD, et al. Laparoscopic colectomy: a critical appraisal. Dis Colon Rectum 1993; 36:28–34.
7. Saida Y, Yamaguchi T, Chen W, Weiss EG, Nogueras JJ, Wexner SD. Is obesity a high risk factor for laparoscopic colorectal surgery? Presented at the 100th Anniversary Meeting and Tripartite Meeting, May 1–6, 1999, Washington, DC.
8. Nisii H, Hirai T, Ohara H, Masuda Y. Laparoscopic-assisted colon surgery by abdominal wall lifting with newly developed lifting bars. Surg Endosc 1997;11(7):754–757.
9. Schwenk W, Bohm B, Witt C, Junghans T, Grundel K, Muller J. Pulmonary function following laparoscopic or conven-

tional colorectal resection: a randomized controlled evaluation. Arch Surg 1999;134:6–13.

10. Larach SW, Plasencia G, Jacobs M, Caushaj PF. Transverse colectomy. In: Jacobs M, Plasencia G, Caushaj P (eds). Atlas of Laparoscopic Colon Surgery. Baltimore: Williams & Wilkins, 1996:77–94.

11. Schirmer BD. Laparoscopic colon surgery. Surg Clin N Am 1996;76(3):571–583.

12. Franklin ME. Laparoscopic surgery of the colon and rectum. In: Arregui ME, Fitzgibbons RJ Jr, Katkouda N, McKerman JB, Reich H (eds) Principles of laparoscopic surgery: basic and advanced techniques. New York: Springer-Verlag, 1995:300–308.

13. Chen HH, Wexner SD, Weiss EG, et al. Laparoscopic colectomy for benign colorectal disease is associated with a significant reduction in disability as compared with laparotomy. Surg Endosc 1998;12:1397–1400.

41
Laparoscopic Left Hemicolectomy and Sigmoidectomy

Karl A. Zucker

Following the success and excitement surrounding laparoscopic biliary tract surgery in the late 1980s and early 1990s, surgeons were easily encouraged to apply this technology to the treatment of other organ systems, including the large intestine. Initial reports of laparoscopic and laparoscopic-assisted colon surgery for both benign and malignant disease first appeared in 1991.[1-3] Since then, laparoscopic colon resection has been successfully performed for the treatment of a wide spectrum of disease processes of the large bowel. These indications include large benign polyps not amenable to colonoscopic resection, invasive malignancies, inflammatory lesions, and even patients presenting with acute or recurrent volvulus.[1-5] Early clinical studies have repeatedly echoed the benefits of the laparoscopic technique, citing a safe and effective procedure, improved postoperative pain management, diminished effects on pulmonary function, faster postoperative recovery, and shorter hospitalizations.[1,6,7] The only aspect of laparoscopic surgery that has not shown to be an advantage when compared to conventional surgery is cost, particularly operating room expenses. This difference is undoubtedly due to the high charges passed on to the patient for the use of disposables as well as the longer operating times reported by most surgeons. Although most surgeons believe that the shortened hospital stay and more rapid recovery more than make up for these additional charges, this belief has been difficult to prove.

Another area of continuing controversy has been the use of laparoscopic surgery for patients with localized, and presumably curable, cancers of the colon. Several case reports have been published describing trocar site and wound recurrences of malignancies following laparoscopic surgery.[8-10] This controversy has resulted in most surgeons adopting a very cautious approach when describing laparoscopy to their patients as an option for the surgical treatment of proven or even suspected colon cancer. A number of prospective trials that have been conducted or are ongoing have been designed to examine this issue.[11-16]

Although definitive answers are not yet available, these studies appear to support the contention that the incidence of port site metastasis is not as high as some of the early reports suggested; such metastases may be more related to the stage of disease or the individual surgeon's operative technique rather than to laparotomy itself.

In this chapter, a description of left hemicolectomy and sigmoidectomy is presented. These procedures can be the most technically challenging laparoscopic operations that most surgeons perform. Several techniques have been described for mobilizing and resecting the splenic flexure, descending colon, sigmoid, and rectum. A steep learning curve for mastering these maneuvers exists because of the complexity of skills needed for these operations. These hurdles, however, can be overcome provided the basic skills of endoscopic surgery are mastered.

Preoperative Evaluation, Patient Preparation, Positioning, and Equipment

Patient selection is of paramount importance for all surgeons contemplating a laparoscopic approach for any pathological condition of the colon. Relative contraindications to attempting laparoscopy include morbid obesity, cirrhosis (especially with associated portal hypertension), uncorrectable coagulopathies, severe acute inflammatory diseases, a history of multiple prior abdominal surgeries, or previous radiation treatment to the pelvis. An informed consent with the patient should include a discussion of the benefits and controversies of laparoscopic colon surgery as well as the possible need for conversion to laparotomy and the use of intraoperative colonoscopy.

The preoperative workup of any patient undergoing colon surgery should be the same regardless of the surgical approach. The only special consideration for the individual scheduled for laparoscopic surgery is ensuring that the surgeon can identify the site of pathology at the time of operative intervention. The loss of tactile sensation with laparoscopic surgery stresses the importance of other localizing techniques, especially if the lesion is small and located in a very mobile portion of the bowel. Lesions can be evaluated by barium enema or colonoscopy before surgery. Barium enemas are not always a part of the routine preoperative evaluation for colon cancer, especially in this era of widespread colonoscopy. Unfortunately, the very nature of colonoscopy results in some distortion of the large bowel anatomy, which can cause some problems when predicting the exact location of a small neoplasm. In contrast, x-rays can provide the surgeon with a specific anatomic location of the lesion. Alternatively, the lesion can be marked with colored dye or India ink during colonoscopy to make the area transmurally visible during surgery. If there remains any question as to the ability of the surgeon to identify the lesion, he or she should be prepared to perform intraoperative colonoscopy to confirm the location of the pathology. Intraoperative colonoscopy is best performed after the establishment of pneumoperitoneum and placement of all the anticipated trocars. One member of the surgical team can then straighten out loops of bowel while at the same time carefully occluding the lumen of the more proximal colon. These maneuvers then allow the endoscopist to rapidly advance the colonoscope to the site of the pathology without distending the proximal bowel. After the lesion is identified, the surgical team can mark the location by placing an endo-loop or a vascular clip on the adjacent epiploic fat.

Individuals scheduled for elective laparoscopic colon surgery should undergo a preoperative mechanical bowel preparation 24 h before the scheduled surgery, typically with 90 ml sodium phosphate[17] or 4 liters polyethylene glycol.[18] In addition, both oral and parenteral broad-spectrum antibiotics are administered. All patients should

TABLE 41.1. Equipment needs.

One and, preferably two, high-resolution video monitors
Two high-flow insufflators
A high-resolution video camera, preferably one of the newer three-chip devices
An angled laparoscope
Atraumatic bowel grasping forceps
Atraumatic endoscopic retractors
Angled dissector
Clip appliers
Laparoscopic cannulas that will accommodate all instruments used
Suction/irrigation probes
An energy device for dissection and/or coagulation, such as a Tri-Polar forceps or an ultrasonic scalpel
Appropriate stapling devices for dividing the bowel and/or completing the anastomosis
Devices for protecting the wound
Laparoscopic needle holders/drivers
Pretied laparoscopic sutures

be advised to refrain from aspirin or other platelet-inhibiting products for at least 14 days before surgery.

Patient positioning depends largely on the location of the bowel being removed and whether there is any anticipated need for intraoperative endoscopy. I prefer to avoid the lithotomy position as often the flexed thighs interfere with the mobility of the laparoscopic instruments through the lower ports. Instead I prefer the split-leg position, which is also commonly used for laparoscopic surgery of the foregut (Fig. 41.1). This position enables an assistant to stand between the patient's legs and also allows for access to the lower GI tract if intraoperative colonoscopy is needed. The patient should be well secured to the operating room table because most surgeons utilize a number of different positioning schemes such as a steep, reverse Trendelenburg or left tilt-up.

It is my policy to routinely employ pneumatic compression devices on every patient undergoing laparoscopic colon surgery. If the individual is at an increased risk for thrombosis, low-dose subcutaneous heparin or low molecular weight heparin may be administered. Furthermore, a stent may be inserted in one or both ureters in selected patients. This procedure should be done if there is a strong preoperative suspicion of anatomic distortion. However, if such conditions are present, the surgeon should carefully consider the appropriateness of laparoscopic surgery, especially if they have limited experience with this technique. The best guideline is to maintain the same indications for stent placement for laparoscopy and for laparotomy.

Equipment Needs

As with most advanced laparoscopic procedures, it is important that the surgeon have the appropriate endoscopic and videoscopic instrumentation to safely complete the procedure (Table 41.1).

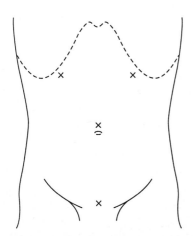

FIGURE 41.1. Suggested sites for trocar placement.

Obviously, specific instrument needs largely depend on the surgeon's preference as well as the techniques used to complete the laparoscopic procedure. The surgeon should try to anticipate every possible operative scenario and the equipment needed to avoid potential problems such as retraction/exposure, bleeding, and enterotomy. One step that should be emphasized is the simultaneous use of two high-flow insufflators. An insufflation rate of 20 liters per minute is really measured as CO_2 leaving the exit port on the machine. By the time the gas passes through the tubing, filters, and insufflation port of the cannula, the actual rate of gas flow is lowered to only 6 or 7 liters per minute under the best of circumstances. If the surgeon should encounter even moderate bleeding, the aspiration probe used to clean the operative field can also rapidly deflate the pneumoperitoneum, thereby hindering visibility and control of the hemorrhage. In my experience, the use of two insufflators helps maintain adequate pneumoperitoneum under such circumstances. Also, if one gas cylinder should empty during the operation, the surgeon can continue working instead of waiting for a new cylinder to be located, connected, and opened.

Surgical Technique

For right-handed surgeons, I recommend standing on the patient's right side with the assistant located on the opposite side of the operating room table. The patient's right arm should be tucked next to the side to provide the surgeon ample maneuverability to mobilize the splenic flexure, descending colon, sigmoid, and rectum. Video monitors are usually placed at the head of the bed on the patient's left side to facilitate viewing during mobilization of the splenic flexure and at the foot of the bed.

The first operative maneuver in any laparoscopic procedure is to gain access to the peritoneal cavity and establish a pneumoperitoneum. Most surgeons use one of two techniques to accomplish these goals: (1) the percutaneous approach utilizing a specialized insufflation or Veress needle or (2) an open technique technique whereby the surgeon uses a 2- to 3-cm incision to enter the peritoneal cavity under direct vision. The latter approach generally requires some sort of modified cannula to seal this larger fascial opening around the sheath. The method used depends on surgeon preference and patient factors. If the abdomen is markedly distended or there is a history of prior surgery near the site chosen for initial access, many surgeons prefer the open technique. Another consideration is that an enlarged fascial opening is required, in nearly all patients undergoing laparoscopic colectomy, for specimen extraction and completing the anastomosis. Ideally, the same opening can be used for both establishing the pneumoperitoneum and completing the colectomy.

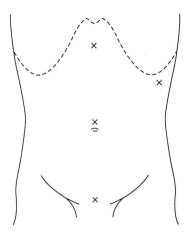

FIGURE 41.2. Alternate sites for trocar placement.

After distending the abdominal cavity with carbon dioxide, a laparoscope is introduced to confirm the presence of an adequate pneumoperitoneum and to exclude any possible visceral injuries. I prefer a 30° to 45° angled laparoscope because of the greater visibility afforded by such devices. Accessory cannulas are then inserted depending on the region of colon targeted for surgery. These ports should be placed under direct vision to minimize the risk of injury. Several schemes for trocar site placement have been described, and each surgeon should probably adopt one with which he or she feels most comfortable. The most important concept to remember is to avoid placing the trocars too close to the operative region and to place them far enough apart so that the motion of one instrument does not hinder the movement of any other devices. Trocar placement for these procedures includes positions at or near the umbilicus, above the pubic symphysis, in the left anterior axillary line in the midabdomen, and in the right midclavicular line just below the costal margin. Alternate trocar placements can include the left midclavicular line just below the costal margin and below the xiphoid process to the left of the falciform ligament (Figs. 41.1, 41.2). Care must be taken that the trocars are the proper size for the introduction of all necessary instrumentation into the operative field, including staplers, clip appliers, specimen bags, and retractors.

Intraoperative success for laparoscopic surgery is founded upon many of the same principles used in conventional laparotomy. These tenets include traction and countertraction, proper identification of the anatomy, including the avascular planes, and minimal manipulation of the region of pathology. However, several new techniques and operative maneuvers are also unique to the field of laparoscopy. For example, the use of gravity to assist by tilting the operative table allows ports and instruments to be available for other uses. The use of both hands for synchronous laparoscopic manipulations and adapting to viewing a three-dimensional field from a two-dimensional screen with the inherent loss of depth perception and alterations in color and lighting are important adjuncts to master. Additional skills are familiarity with intracorporeal knot tying and the use of an angled laparoscope. All laparoscopic-assisted colon procedures have several common principles: (1) localization of the lesion, (2) mobilization of the colon, (3) devascularization of the specimen, (4) isolation of the specimen without spillage (dividing the bowel), (5) protection of the wound during specimen retrieval, and (6) completion of the anastomosis (either intra- or extracorporeal).

After localizing the lesion as previously described, mobilization of the colon begins by dividing natural attachments to the lateral abdominal wall, retroperitoneum, and other adjacent organs. These attachments can be divided using either monopolar or bipolar electrocautery or the ultrasonic scalpel. Dissection usually begins at the sigmoid colon. The bowel is gently grasped with an atraumatic forceps and retracted toward the midline (Fig. 41.3). Special attention should be paid to minimize the risk of injury while holding the bowel. This admonition is especially pertinent for laparoscopic procedures because the semirigid abdominal wall can act as a fulcrum and magnify the traction force applied to the internal structures. I prefer to use an atraumatic, Babcock-like clamp and place it all the way around the intestine so that the jaws of the instrument are actually applying more pressure against the adjacent mesentery. Dissection begins along the peritoneal reflection and proceeds cephalad and caudad. I prefer a curved scissors for this maneuver. If the dissection proceeds in the right plane, there should be minimal or no bleeding. The operating room table should be placed in a steep Trendelenburg with a rotation to the right to help "drop" the small bowel away from the operative field. After dividing the lateral peritoneal attachments, an Endo-Sponge (DeRoyal, TN) can be used to gently mobilize the colonic mesentery away from its retroperitoneal attachments. This sponge is supplied in a pretied, tubular shape that is easily introduced through a 10- or 11-mm cannula. Ideally, the descending colon, sigmoid, and attached mesentery should be dissected enough to allow retraction well over to the right side of the abdominal cavity. As the distal descending colon and sigmoid are medially mobilized, it is important to identify both ureters, which should be done early, before any bleeding and staining of the tissues. The same landmarks used for identification in laparotomy are used during laparoscopy. If necessary, the ureter may have to be laterally mobilized to avoid inclusion within the transected specimen. If there is some concern about the location or integrity of a ureter, conversion to a laparotomy should be considered.

Adequate mobilization of the specimen may require mobilizing the splenic flexure and portions of the transverse colon if they encompass the lesion or if additional length is necessary for a tension-free reconstruction. This mobilization must proceed with caution so as to prevent trauma to the spleen. Usually this maneuver requires at least four laparoscopic cannulas. If extensive mobilization of the splenic flexure is required, it is advisable to move the patient into a steep reverse Trendelenburg position with the right side tilted down so that the small bowel drops away from the operative field. The surgeon may even decide to stand between the patient's legs to directly face the upper abdomen and video monitor. The omentum should be retracted away from the operative field so that the surgeon has a good view of the splenic flexure. Gentle, caudad traction on the colon helps expose its attachments to the lower pole of the spleen as well as to any of the perisplenic tissues. Most of these attachments can be safely divided with either a bipolar instrument or an ultrasonic scalpel. Vessels larger than 4

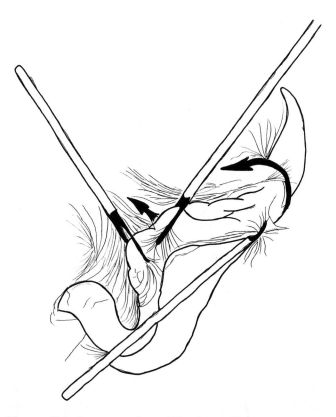

FIGURE 41.3. Laparoscopic mobilization of the sigmoid colon. Placement of the laparoscopic clamp to minimize the risk of injury to the bowel wall.

point distal to the lesion is accomplished by retracting the rectum laterally, anteriorly, and cephalad. The ureters should once again be visualized and their course followed to the trigone of the bladder. The plane between the mesorectum and Waldeyer's fascia can be opened with bipolar cautery or the ultrasonic scalpel. The mesocolon is usually quite short and relatively avascular compared to the mesentenic attachments of the descending and sigmoid colon. If performing a proctectomy for benign disease, the surgeon should try to preserve the sympathetic nerves. The plane of dissection should be kept medial to the fascia and anterior to the sacral promontory. With these maneuvers the seminal vessels should be easily visible and can be used as an additional guide to avoid injury to these nerves.

After completely mobilizing the appropriate segments of colon, the next step is to devascularize the specimen. The mesentery of the colon is then placed under tension to create a "bow-stringing" effect that is helpful in identifying the named vasculature to the specimen. These larger vessels are then dissected so that a window is created around the pedicle and divided close to their origin with either clips, staples, or sutures (Fig. 41.5).

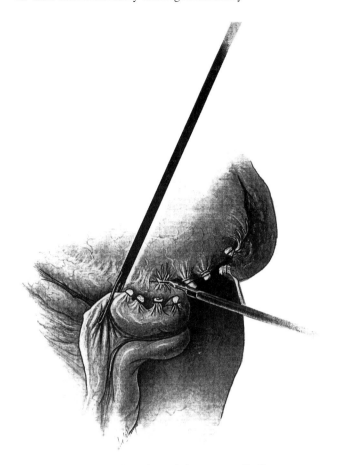

FIGURE 41.4. Dissection of the gastrocolic ligament.

to 5mm should probably be clipped before division. Care must be taken to avoid injury to the spleen as well as the inferior border or tail of the pancreas. Once again, this fulcrum effect of the abdominal wall may result in far more traction on the tissues attached to the lower pole of the spleen than is appreciated by the surgeon. Some surgeons have described using the colonoscope to retract the splenic flexure.[19] This technique has some appeal as the endoscope may already be in the operating room for localization purposes, but once again the endoscopist must try to minimize the air used to distend the bowel.

Complete mobilization of the splenic flexure may also require some separation of the gastrocolic ligament (Fig. 41.4). The distal transverse colon is retracted medially and caudad and, if necessary, the greater curvature of the stomach is grasped and elevated. Retraction of the stomach will help avoid inadvertent dissection of the transverse mesocolon. These maneuvers should expose the gastrocolic ligament and allow the surgeon to divide the vessels with bipolar cautery, clips, or ultrasonic scalpel.

For distal sigmoid or rectal lesions it may be necessary to mobilize both the bowel and the mesentery caudal to the peritoneal reflection. Dissection of the rectum to a

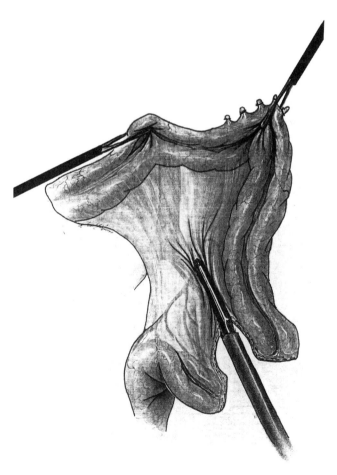

FIGURE 41.5. Isolation and transection of the mesenteric vessels.

Before dividing these vessels, it is important that the surgical team again confirm the location of the ureter(s). The remaining mesentery is then divided with cautery or the ultrasonic scalpel. Depending on the indication for surgery, this mesenteric dissection may take place near the bowel wall or lower, near the root of the mesentery, so that a more en bloc resection is achieved.

The next step is to divide the bowel so that the specimen can be removed; this can be accomplished intracorporeally or after completely eviscerating the mobilized segment of bowel. The technique used depends on location and the actual disease process requiring surgical intervention. For benign lesions located in the sigmoid or distal descending colon, the surgeon can, in most cases, mobilize the bowel so that it can be brought through a 3- to 6-cm fascial opening. I now prefer to enlarge the umbilical fascial/trocar site as this method minimizes trauma to the rectus muscles. Alternatively, an opening can be made just above the pubic symphysis, or a left

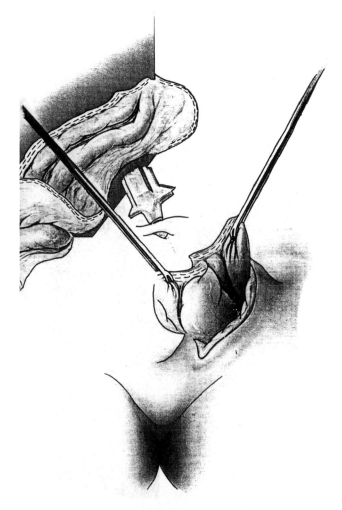

FIGURE 41.6. In some cases, an enlarged fascial opening allows the specimen to be removed and the anastomosis completed outside the abdomen.

midabdominal or lower quadrant muscle splitting incision may be used (Fig. 41.6). Once outside the abdomen, the surgeon can confirm the localization of the pathology and then divide the bowel with either conventional instruments or staplers. The anastomosis is also completed outside the abdomen and may be handsewn or stapled depending on the surgeon's preference. If necessary, any significant mesenteric defect should be closed. The bowel is then placed back into the peritoneal cavity and the fascial defect closed. The abdomen is once again distended so the surgical team can examine the anastomosis and check for any bleeding or remaining mesenteric defects.

The extracorporeal method of resection and anastomosis may not be possible if the distal margin of resection involves the rectum that cannot be mobilized above the skin. Therefore, for most left-sided lesions, the mesenteric dissection, division of bowel, and anastomosis must be completed within the peritoneal cavity. The mesentery is divided as described earlier. Bowel segments are usually divided using a 30- to 60-mm laparoscopic linear stapler; the stapler cartridges are selected depending on the thickness of the tissue being divided and stapled. After isolating the specimen, an enlarged fascial opening is still necessary to remove the specimen. If operating on a patient with possible localized malignancy, an impenetrable barrier is placed within the extraction site incision during manipulation and removal of the specimen to protect the wound against tumor implantation.

For sigmoid colectomy or anterior resection of the rectum, the most popular method of completing the anastomosis is a laparoscopic-assisted technique employing a circular stapler guided through the anus and rectum (Fig. 41.7). The bowel and mesentery are intracorporeally divided and extracted via an umbilical or right illiac fossa fascial opening. Through the same opening, the proximal bowel segment is eviscerated and prepared for a stapled anastomosis. This step usually entails dissecting the attached distal mesentery so that, when fired, the staples penetrate the bowel wall and not surrounding fat. The anvil of the circular stapler is positioned within the proximal bowel segment and a pursestring suture placed to secure it within the lumen. The colon is returned to the peritoneal cavity, the fascial opening closed, and the pneumoperitoneum reestablished. The shaft of the circular stapler is transanally introduced up to the end of the distal bowel segment. With light pressure against the intestinal wall, the trocar within the shaft is slowly extruded until it pierces the bowel wall. Under laparoscopic guidance, the anvil of the stapler is connected to the trocar of the circular stapler. A special anvil-grasping instrument is available to help perform this maneuver (Endo-Alis Clamp; Ethicon Endosurgery, Cincinnati, OH, USA). The circular stapler is then fired and the integrity of the anastomosis is verified by inspection of

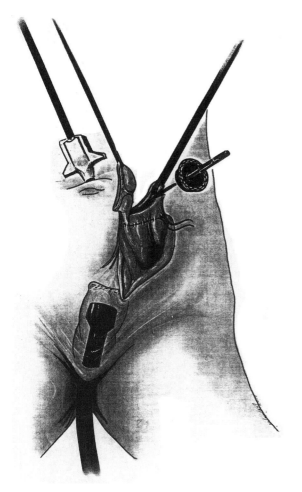

Figure 41.7. For a low anterior anastomosis, a circular stapler can be introduced via the anus.

both tissue doughnuts. I prefer to distend the segment of bowel incorporating the anastomosis with air while flooding the peritoneal cavity/pelvis with saline. A flexible sigmoidoscope or colonoscope can be used to both distend the colon and visually inspect the anastomosis. If air bubbles are seen, the anastomotic leak must be identified and repaired. If necessary, a small laparotomy can be made directly over the anastomosis for reinforcement or revision. Laparoscopic inspection of the anastomosis and operative field is then conducted to further assess the anastomosis and to verify hemostasis. All fascial openings larger than 5mm in diameter are closed.

Abdominoperineal Resection and Diverting Colostomy

The abdominal portion of an abdominoperineal resection may be laparoscopically undertaken using the techniques and principles previously described.[20] The small bowel is mobilized out of the pelvis using a steep Trendelenburg position and occasionally a fan-type retractor. The bladder is bluntly dissected free from the bowel after dividing the peritoneum over the anterior rectum. The posterior and lateral attachments of the proximal and middle third of the rectum are divided using a combination of sharp and blunt dissection. The proximal and middle hemorrhoidal vessels are ligated and divided or simply cauterized with the tripolar forceps. A transanally placed probe or sigmoidoscope can assist in dissection of the rectum. The proximal margin of resection is divided using a laparoscopic stapling device, and the specimen is removed through a standard perineal incision. The perineal dissection should avoid entering the peritoneal cavity until the abdominal dissection has been completed as this will result in rapid loss of the pneumoperitoneum. A lower abdominal trocar site may be utilized for the stoma if properly preoperatively selected.

A diverting colostomy for an obstructing lesion with resection or an unresectable lesion may be performed with laparoscopic assistance.[21] Again, one or two trocar sites should be placed so that they may be used for location of a stoma. A vertical opening is made in the mesentery to allow both ends of the colon to reach the anterior abdominal wall without tension. This distance will be considerably less once the pneumoperitoneum is released, and then both ends may be brought through separate fascial openings or the distal limb left in situ.

Laparoscopic-Assisted Polypectomy

Laparoscopic surgery can also be used for segmental or sleeve resections of large or broad-based polyps that are not amenable to colonoscopic removal.[22,23] The latter concerns include very large or sessile polyps as well as the possible location of the lesion. With a combined laparoscopic/colonoscopic approach to such polyps, most patients can be spared an open laparotomy for sleeve resection of the involved segment of colon.

The patient should undergo a full mechanical and antibiotic bowel preparation. The operating room should be set up for both colonoscopy and laparoscopy. The patient's legs need to be separated to allow for unhindered lower GI access. Ideally, a videoscopic colonoscope is used so that both the endoscopic and the laparoscopic surgeon can visualize the intraluminal lesion as well as the peritoneal cavity. Before introducing the colonoscope, the surgical team can fully mobilize the segment of large bowel containing the polyp. The atraumatic clamp is placed on the colon proximal to the site of the lesion. The colonoscope is then introduced and slowly advanced. Minimal insufflation of the bowel lumen will help maintain an adequate laparoscopic view of the operative field. The surgical team can use atraumatic

Babcock-like clamps to straighten out kinks or loops of the large bowel so that the colonoscope will be easier to maneuver toward the polyp. After visualizing the lesion, the next step is to place an endoscopic cautery loop around the entire polyp or in a piecemeal fashion. Often, the surgical team can help maneuver the segment of colon so that a previously inaccessible polyp is now easily excised via the colonoscope. As the polyp is being removed the surgical team can monitor the serosal surface to see if there are any signs of a full-thickness injury.

If the polyp is still inaccessible despite laparoscopic mobilization, or is simply too large, or penetrates deep into the wall of the colon, the surgical team may then elect to open the colon and perform laparoscopic-guided polypectomy. The colotomy is then closed with sutures or by application of the endoscopic linear stapler. Alternatively, a laparoscopic-assisted sleeve resection can be performed as described earlier. Before completing the operative procedure, the lumen can be distended with gas while flooding the serosal surface with saline. Bubling would indicate a remaining defect that should be addressed.

Franklin and Balli recently reported 48 laparoscopic-guided polypectomies in 34 patients.[22] Only 4 patients required a full-thickness colotomy and polypectomy; the remaining polyps were removed via the colonoscope. All patients were kept overnight in the hospital, and no postoperative complications were noted.

Special Considerations When Operating on Patients with Localized Cancer

The development of appropriate techniques for laparoscopic and laparoscopic-assisted colon resection for localized adenocarcinoma of the colon requires that accepted principles of conventional bowel resection be followed. These steps include avoidance of tumor spill, minimizing direct manipulation of the tumor, obtaining adequate resection margins, and harvesting adequate lymph nodes for appropriate staging. This last maneuver is particularly important now that effective immunochemotherapy is available for selected individuals with regional disease. Intraoperative staging with evaluation of the liver, omentum, peritoneum, and remaining colon for synchronous lesions can be accomplished using both laparoscopic evaluation and intraoperative ultrasound. In addition, preoperative staging with standard contrast and noncontrast x-rays as well as CT scanning has proven to be fairly accurate in detecting both local spread and metastatic disease. Lesions selected for laparoscopic-assisted resection have included T1 to T3 lesions but typically not T4 lesions. Although there have been reports of individuals undergoing laparoscopic resection for cancers fixed or fis-

tulizing into adjacent tissues, most of these cases are probably better approached via a conventional laparotomy. However, patients with evidence of metastatic disease are considered to be excellent candidates to undergo palliative laparoscopic resection or diverting colostomy.

An area of tremendous controversy concerns tumor recurrence at trocar sites used during the initial tumor resection. These port site recurrences have not been limited to regions where the tumor was extracted from the abdominal cavity. Recurrences have also included remote trocar sites where no instrumentation had come in direct contact with the tumor or was used as the site of tumor extraction. Port site implants have been observed in both early- and advanced-stage tumors and following both potentially curable and intentionally palliative resections. Several factors may be related to these recurrences, including increased local tissue trauma, augmentation of tumor nutritional supply by local hyperemia, and alterations in the host's immune status.[8–10]

In addition, the pneumoperitoneum created by insufflating carbon dioxide (CO_2) may create a more optimal pH environment that assists tumor cell implantation. Possible mechanisms for trocar site recurrences include spread of tumor cells by direct contact, exfoliation of cells by laparoscopic manipulation, spread of airborne tumor cells by the circulating pneumoperitoneum, or spread of malignant cells intraluminally or by transvenous circulation. Direct spread of cancer cells by contact with wound edges does not explain recurrences at lateral trocar sites; pneumoperitoneum has been shown to increase port site recurrences in an animal model. Shedding of tumor cells and local tissue trauma during laparoscopic procedures may be another possible explanation; however, this does not completely explain the patterns of recurrences seen to date. Similarly, intraluminal or hematogenous spread does not correlate with trocar site recurrences.

Animal studies offer conflicting data on wound recurrence as related to pneumoperitoneum.[24,25] It is also difficult to draw conclusions from isolated case reports of trocar site implants. Since their initial descriptions, several retrospective series have reported varying prevalences from single and multiple institutions, ranging from none to as high as 21%.[11–13,26] If the recurrence rates of conventional surgery are more carefully examined, interesting patterns emerge. The incisional wound is claimed to be the site of tumor implants in up to 0.6% of recurrences after laparotomy.[27] More recently, several studies have compared laparoscopic colon surgery for cancer with laparotomy. These studies show equivalent pathological data for specimens retrieved with definite clinical benefits seen with the laparoscopic procedure, including improved pain relief, shorter lengths of stay, less blood loss, fewer complications, and quicker return of bowel function and return to normal activities. Because laparoscopic colon surgery is a relatively recent advancement, follow-up from these studies has been limited, ranging from 2 to as long as 5 years. Nevertheless, there appears to be similar overall survival, local recurrence, and mortality. Specifically, there did not seem to be an increased trocar site recurrence seen for patients undergoing laparoscopic colon resections (0.5%–1.7%).[13–16] Nevertheless, it is appropriate to include these patients in an appropriate trial comparing laparoscopic and conventional surgery. If no such study is readily available or if the patient refuses to participate, the surgeon should discuss this controversy and document this discussion in the medical records.

Results and Postoperative Care

Following laparoscopic colon surgery, patients experience an earlier return of gastriointestinal function than those individuals undergoing open surgery.[27] Whether a laparotomy or a laparoscopic resection has been performed, most surgeons remove the naso- or orogastric tube at the end of the operation. Most patients are able to tolerate an oral diet by the first or second day after surgery and are offered liquids almost routinely the day following surgery. If liquids are tolerated, the diet is rapidly advanced to solids. The rather subjective length of stay has also been shown to decrease by as much as 3 to 5 days following laparoscopic colectomy as compared to laparotomy.[11,13,15,27] Patients undergoing laparoscopic resections have less perceived pain and lower narcotic requirements as compared to patients undergoing laparotomy. Patients undergoing laparoscopic surgery also have equivalent results as compared to laparotomy with regards to perioperative mortality, length of specimen resected, adequacy of margins, and number of lymph nodes collected. Improved postoperative T-cell-mediated immunity, lymphocyte function, and neutrophil chemotaxis have also been seen after laparoscopic surgery.[7]

Return to normal activity is based on each individual patient, depending upon their age, normal occupation, and motivation. Patients should not drive while taking postoperative narcotic medications, and heavy lifting should also be avoided for at least 6 weeks after surgery.

Complications

Several series of laparoscopic colectomy have been reported in the literature that have described the numerous complications which can occur with these procedures. For the most part, the same complications associated with laparotomy have also occurred during laparoscopic colectomy; these include ureteral injuries, inadvertent enterotomies, anastomotic leaks, postoperative strictures or even actual obstruction at the anastomosis, herniation through the mesenteric defect, and intraabdominal abscess.[27–32] Some of the earlier clinical series reported very high laparoscopic-associated complications (greater than 30%) and rates of conversions (greater than 40%).[33–35] These preliminary studies simply confirmed that there is a steep learning curve associated with minimally invasive colon surgery. Later publications have shown that, with experienced surgeons, laparoscopic surgery is associated with a significant decrease in both major and minor postoperative complications as well as shorter hospital stay.[36,37] Most clinical investigators have also shown that laparoscopic surgery has a much smaller intraoperative blood loss than comparable open procedures and that there is far less compromise in postoperative pulmonary function.[38,39] Operative times for laparoscopic colon procedures are undoubtedly longer than comparable open operations.[36] Initially, this was thought to be because of the steep learning curve, with some early authors reporting times in excess of 8h.[33] However, as the surgeon's experience with laparoscopy grows, operative times have decreased significantly. Operative times ranging from 45 to 90min are now not uncommon in uncomplicated cases.

An overall in-hospital cost savings with laparoscopic surgery may not initially occur because the decreased length of stay is offset by high intraoperative costs, due to the high charges for laparoscopic disposable devices and the longer operative times discussed earlier. However, greater cost savings may be realized as operative times decrease and costs of laparoscopic instrumentation decrease as a result of production and economic market forces driven by competition. Additionally, return to usual activities and work is much quicker with a laparoscopic approach.[36,40] This advantage has been underreported as a cost benefit to both society and the business community and thus has been poorly recognized. As there is increased concern by employers regarding the loss of productivity related to sick leave taken by their employees, factors such as the method of surgery used will play a greater role in the managed care market.

Conclusion

Laparoscopic colon surgery has been performed in the United States since 1990. Nearly all the principles of colonic resection for surgery can be followed through a laparoscopic approach. In experienced hands, laparoscopic surgery has been shown to offer patients real advantages in decreased postoperative pain, shorter hospitalization, better cosmesis, and a quicker return to normal activity. As a result, this procedure has been enthusiastically embraced by many clinicians as a reasonable treatment option for benign colonic disorders or as a palliative procedure in those unfortunate individuals with distant metastatic cancer. In contrast, a very cautious approach has been taken when considering patients with localized cancer as possible candidates for laparoscopic surgery. Although adequate proximal and distal margin requirements are easily achieved and lymph node retrieval is similar to open surgery, sporadic reports of tumor implants at the trocar sites have clearly raised a red flag. As a result, there has been a greater emphasis on enrolling patients in prospective randomized trials to determine the appropriateness of laparoscopic intervention in such patients, including a large, multicenter trial funded by the National Cancer Institute. Smaller prospective clinical series focused on this issue have already appeared.[40–43] These investigations regarding laparoscopic colon resection for cancer have been very encouraging. Long-term follow-up data from these and other prospective randomized trials are required to definitively resolve the current controversies. Until these results are available, laparoscopic colectomy for the treatment of cancer should be limited to those institutions with established protocols to provide adequate follow-up for these patients.

Adequate proximal and distal margin requirements can be achieved, although large and bulky lesions may be indications for laparotomy. Some investigators believe that lymph node retrieval is similar to laparotomy, whereas others have found that the laparoscopic approach yields fewer nodes within the resected specimen; the clinical significance remains to be determined. There is no statistically significant difference in the rate of survival between regional lymph node dissection and extended regional node dissection off the periaortic nodes. Several factors that are controlled by the pathologist which affect the yield of lymph nodes recovered from the specimen have as great an effect on survival and prognosis as the surgical level of mesenteric resection. The laparoscopic approach for resection of colon carcinomas is a viable, effective procedure, with definite advantages for the patient as well as potential future cost benefits.

References

1. Jacobs M, Verdeja JC, Goldstein HS. Minimally invasive colon resection (laparoscopic colectomy). Surg Laparosc Endosc 1991;1(3):144–150.
2. Cooperman AM, Katz V, Zimmon D, Botero G. Laparoscopic colon resection: a case report. J Laparoendosc Surg 1991;1(4):221–224.
3. Saclarides TJ, Ko ST, Airan M, Dillon C, Franklin J. Laparoscopic removal of large colonic lipoma. Dis Colon Rectum 1991;34:1027–1029.
4. Miller R, Roe AM, Eltringham WK, Espiner HJ. Laparoscopic fixation of sigmoid volvulus. Br J Surg 1992;79:435.
5. Reissman P, Salky BA, Pfeifer J, Edye M, Jagelman DG, Wexner SD. Laparoscopic surgery in the management of inflammatory bowel disease. Am J Surg 1996;171:47–51.
6. Schwenk W, Bohm B, Witt C, Junghans T, Grundel K, Muller JM. Pulmonary function following laparoscopic or conventional colorectal resection. Arch Surg 1999;134:6–12.
7. Kuntz C, Wunsch A, Bay F, Windeler J, Glaser F, Herfarth C. Prospective randomized study of stress and immune response after laparoscopic versus conventional colonic resection. Surg Endosc 1998;12:963–967.
8. Fusco MA, Paluzzi MW. Abdominal wall recurrence after laparoscopic-assisted colectomy for adenocarcinoma of the colon. Dis Colon Rectum 1993;36:858–861.
9. Walsh DC, Wattchow DA, Wilson TG. Subcutaneous metastasis after laparoscopoic resection of malignancy. Aust N Z J Surg 1993;63:563–565.
10. Ota DM, Nelson H, Weeks JC. Controversies regarding laparoscopic colectomy for malignant disease. Curr Opin Gen Surg 1994:208–213.
11. Milsom J, Bohm B, Hammerhofer KA, Fazio V, Steiger E, Elson P. A prospective, randomized trial comparing laparoscopic versus conventional techniques in colorectal cancer surgery: a preliminary report. J Am Coll Surg 1998;187: 46–57.
12. Bokey EL, Moore WE, Keating JP, Zelas P, Chapuis PH, Newland RC. Laparoscopic resection of the colon and rectum for cancer. Br J Surg 1997;84:822–825.
13. Lacy AM, Garcia-Valdecasas JC, Pique JM, et al. Short-term outcome analysis of a randomized study comparing laparoscopic vs open colectomy for colon cancer. Surg Endosc 1995;9:1101–1105.
14. Ortega AE, Beart RW, Steele GD, Winchester DP, Greene FI. Laparoscopic Bowel Surgery Registry: preliminary results. Dis Colon Rectum 1995;38(7):681–686.
15. Stage JG, Schulze P, Overgaard H, Andersen M, Rebsdorf-Pedersen VB, Nielsen HJ. Prospective randomized study of laparoscopic versus open colonic resection for adenocarcinoma. Br J Surg 1997;84:391–396.
16. Vukasin P, Ortega AE, Greene FL, et al. Wound recurrence following laparoscopic colon cancer resection: results of the American Society of Colon and Rectal Surgeons Laparoscopic Registry. Dis Colon Rectum 1996;39(10): S20–S23.
17. Cohen SM, Wexner SD, Binderow SR, et al. Prospective, randomized, endoscopic-blinded trial comparing precolonoscopy bowel cleansing methods. Dis Colon Rectum 1994;37(7):689–696.
18. Oliveira L, Wexner SD, Daniel N, et al. Mechanical bowel preparation for elective colorectal surgery. A prospective, randomized, surgeon-blinded trial comparing sodium phosphate and polyethylene glycol-based oral lavage solutions. Dis Colon Rectum 1997;40(5):585–591.
19. Reissman P, Teoh TA, Piccirillo MF, Nogueras JJ, Wexner SD. Colonoscopic-assisted laparoscopic colectomy. Surg Endosc 1994;8:1352–1353.
20. Sackier JM, Berci G, Hiatt JR, Hartunian S. Laparoscopic abdominal perineal resection of the rectum. Br J Surg 1992;79:1207–1208.
21. Lyerly HK, Mault JR. Laparoscopic ileostomy and colostomy. Ann Surg 1994;219(3):317–322.

22. Franklin ME, Balli JE. Laparoscopic management of difficult colonic polyps. In: Zucker KA (ed) Surgical Laparoscopy, 3rd Ed. Philadelphia: Lippincott/Williams & Wilkins, 2000.

23. Smedh K, Skullman S, Kaid A, Anderberg B, Nystrom P. Laparoscopic bowel mobilization combined with intraoperative colonoscopic polypectomy in patients with an inaccessible polyp of the colon. Surg Endosc 1997;11: 643–644.

24. Jacobi CA, Ordemann J, Bohm B, et al. The influence of laparotomy and laparoscopy on tumor growth in a rat model. Surg Endosc 1997;11:618–621.

25. Wu JS, Brasfield BS, Guo LW, et al. Implantation of colon cancer at trocar sites is increased by low pressure pneumoperitoneum. Surgery (St. Louis) 1997;122:1–7.

26. Hughes ESR, McDermott FT, Polglase AI, Johnson WR. Tumor recurrence in the abdominal wall scar tissue after large-bowel cancer surgery. Dis Colon Rectum 1983;26: 571–572.

27. Zucker KA, Pitche DE, Martin DM, Ford S. Laparoscopic assisted colon resection. Surg Endosc 1994;8:12–18.

28. Wexner SD, Cohen SM, Johansen OB, Nogueras JJ, Jagelman DG. Laparoscopic colorectal surgery: a prospective assessment and current prospective. Br J Surg 1993;80:1602–1605.

29. Franklin M, Ramos R, Rosenthal D. Laparoscopic colonic procedures. World J Surg 1993;17:51–56.

30. Guillou PJ, Darzi A, Monson JRT. Experience with laparoscopic colorectal surgery for malignant disease. J Surg Oncol 1993;2:43–49.

31. Quattlebaum JK, Flanders HD, Usher CH. Laparoscopic assisted colectomy. Laparoscopic assisted colectomy. Surg Laparosc Endosc 1993;3:81–87.

32. Kawamura YJ, Sunami E, Masaki T, Muto T. Transmesenteric hernia after laparoscopic-assisted sigmoid colectomy. J Surg Laparosc Surg 1999;3(1):79–81.

33. Larach SW, Salomon MC, Williamson PR, Goldstein E. Laparoscopic assisted colectomy. Experience during the learning curve. Coloproctology 1993;1:38–41.

34. Reissman P, Cohen S, Weiss EG, Wexner SD. Laparoscopic colorectal surgery: ascending the learning curve. World J Surg 1996;20(3):277–281.

35. Falk PM, Beart RW Jr, Wexner SD, et al. Laparoscopic colectomy: a critical appraisal. Dis Colon Rectum 1993; 36(1):28–34.

36. Chen HH, Wexner SD, Weiss EG, et al. Laparoscopic colectomy for benign colorectal disease is associated with a significant reduction in disability as compared with laparotomy. Surg Endosc 1998;12(12):1397–1400.

37. Talamini ME, Moesinger PC, Kaufman H, Kutka M, Harris M, Bayless T. Laparoscopic assisted bowel resection for Crohn's disease. The best of both worlds. Gastroenterology 1997;4:A1478.

38. Muckleroy SK, Ratzer ER, Fenoglio ME. Laparoscopic colon surgery for benign disease: a comparison to open surgery. J Surg Laparosc Surg 1999;3(1):33–37.

39. Schwenk W, Bohm B, Witt C, Junghans T, Grundel K, Muller JM. Pulmonary function following laparoscopic or conventional colorectal resection: a randomized controlled evaluation. Arch Surg 1999;134(1):6–12.

40. Ing R, Jacobs M, Placencia G. Laparoscopic colectomy for cancer. In: Zucker KA (ed) Surgical Laparoscopy, 3rd Ed. Philadelphia: Lippincott/Williams & Wilkins, 2000.

41. Franklin ME Jr, Rosenthal D, Norem RF. Prospective evaluation of laparoscopic colon resection versus open colon resection for adenocarcinoma. A multicenter study. Surg Endosc 1995;9(7):811–816.

42. Bouvet M, Mansfield PF, Skibber JM. Clinical, pathologic, and economic parameters of laparoscopic colon resection for cancer. Am J Surg 1998;176(6):554–558.

43. Smedh K, Skullman S, Kald A, Anderberg B, Nystrom P. Laparoscopic bowel mobilization combined with intraoperative colonoscopic polypectomy in patients with an inaccessible polyp of the colon. Surg Endosc 1997; 11(6):643–644.

42
Laparoscopic-Assisted Anterior Resection

Brian J. Mehigan, John E. Hartley, and J.R.T. Monson

Excellence in surgical technique is of particular importance in the treatment of rectal cancer. The only hope of cure for such patients lies in adequate surgery, and wide variations in success, both within institutions and between individual surgeons, are apparent.[1] Routine excision of the intact mesorectum during resection of cancers of the mid- and lower rectum has resulted in the lowest rates of local recurrence ever reported.[2] These standards, established by Heald and coworkers, are those against which any new technique should be measured. Many surgeons have therefore argued that, given the concern over the safety and efficacy of laparoscopic technology, carcinoma of the rectum should be excised only by specialist colorectal surgeons using conventional techniques.[3] However, others suggested that the excellent magnified views obtained deep within the pelvis with laparoscopy may facilitate sharp excision of the mesorectum and preservation of the pelvic nerves while offering the potential advantages of minimally invasive surgery. We describe in this chapter our current technique of laparoscopic-assisted anterior resection with total mesorectal excision. A totally laparoscopic anterior resection utilizing a triple stapled or handsewn anastomosis has been described.[4] However, we are yet to be convinced that the extra time and effort required for such an anastomosis is worthwhile; in addition such an approach creates problems with regard to mode of specimen delivery. Although resected specimens can be transanally delivered, this method requires unphysiological dilatation of the sphincters and, for malignant lesions, has a theoretical risk of tumor seeding.

Indications

Although not universally accepted, contraindications to the laparoscopic approach include these:

1. Specific contraindication to laparoscopy
2. Doubtful resectability (or reconstructability; vide infra)
3. Multiple previous abdominal incisions

If possible, the decision regarding sphincter sacrifice in low rectal cancer should be made before surgery as the laparoscopic approach lacks tactile sensation and therefore does not permit trial dissection and palpation to ascertain reconstructability. If the decision cannot be made, then a laparotomy should be scheduled rather than potentially needlessly sacrificing the anal sphincters. It is undoubtedly better to subject 99 patients to laparotomy then to wrongly excise a single anus.

Withholding the foregoing contraindications, the indications for laparoscopic anterior resection are essentially the same as for open surgery. In our experience, totally laparoscopic total mesorectal excision has proved feasible for carcinoma of the middle and lower rectum in slightly more than 50% of patients; predicting those patients with preoperative assessment has not proven possible with current techniques.[5]

Patient Preparation

Our preoperative assessment includes physical examination, liver function tests, carcinoembryonic antigen assay, liver ultrasound, pelvic and liver MRI scan, sigmoidoscopy, and biopsy. Examination under anesthesia is often required to determine tumor height and resectability and should be undertaken when there is any concern over reconstructability. Complete preoperative evaluation of the colon with either full colonoscopy to the cecum or barium enema is necessary to avoid missing synchronous tumors. Anesthetic assessment must take into account the patient's suitability for prolonged laparoscopy because significantly longer operative times are a feature of the laparoscopic approach.[5,6] Standard practices of bowel preparation, thromboembolic prophylaxis, and perioperative antibiotics apply.

Surgical Technique

Patient Positioning

Under general anesthesia, the patient is positioned in a modified Lloyd–Davis position in which the legs are held almost straight (because the legs when flexed at the hips tend to intrude upon the laparoscopic instruments) and the arms are adducted. Placing the patient on a beanbag and using an operating table capable of steep and reverse Trendelenburg positions, as well as right and left rotation, are advisable to allow for the many adjustments required to gravitate the small bowel out of the operating field at various stages of the procedure. A urinary catheter and nasogastric tube are inserted to help guard against trocar injury to the viscera. The abdomen and perineum are prepared and draped in the usual manner.

Instrumentation

Videolaparoscopy facilities with at least two monitors are required. A 30° telescope in addition to a conventional 0° telescope can be helpful in rectal dissection and in splenic flexure mobilization. Standard 10-mm ports are required, with one port site extended to 12 mm to admit a 30-mm endoscopic linear cutter. Laparoscopic instrumentation is constantly improving, but we consider certain instruments essential (Table 42.1).

The laparoscopic-assisted technique permits division of the rectum at the pelvic floor using a conventional stapling device via the specimen delivery incision and proximal division of the descending colon with a linear cutter. The endoscopic equivalents of these instruments require ports of 15 mm or greater and, in our opinion, are not yet of sufficient maneuverability to allow confident division of the rectum at the pelvic floor.

TABLE 42.1. Essential instruments for laparoscopic anterior resection.

1. Two Babcock-type bowel grasping instruments
2. Curved disposable scissors
3. Linear stapling device with vascular cartridges
4. Multifire endoscopic clip applicator
5. Long laparoscopic scissors for low pelvic dissection
6. Suction irrigation device
7. Laparoscopic fan retractor

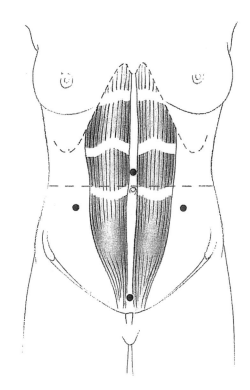

FIGURE 42.1. Suggested configuration of trocars for laparoscopic-assisted anterior resection.

Surgeon and Trocar Positioning

The surgeon commences work on the patient's right-hand side. Pneumoperitoneum is created using an open technique via a vertical supraumbilical incision, and initial laparoscopy is performed. Subsequent trocars must be positioned under direct vision to avoid injury. Positioning of subsequent trocars varies slightly depending on the patient's body habitus, but the configuration shown is usually sufficient (Fig. 42.1). To allow flexibility in camera and instrument positioning, 10-mm ports are used at all locations; one of these incisions is subsequently extended to 12 mm to permit entry of the linear cutter. An attempt is made to locate the right iliac fossa port at the site marked for a defunctioning ileostomy, should that become necessary, and to site the suprapubic port, if used, where it may be incorporated into the subsequent Pfannenstiel incision.

Surgical Technique

Preliminary laparoscopy is first performed paying particular attention to the pelvic organs. There is a critical angle of Trendelenburg, varying from patient to patient, beyond which the small bowel will fall out of the pelvis. Any

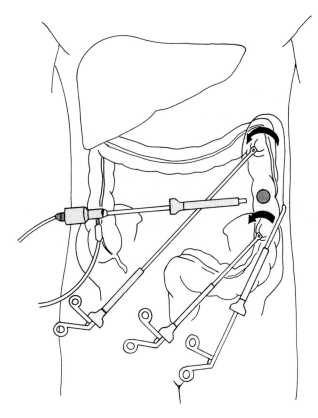

FIGURE 42.2. Incising along the lateral peritoneal reflection of the sigmoid colon.

adhesions between the small bowel and the pelvic structures must therefore be divided at an early stage. The table is then returned to neutral position and the remainder of the peritoneal cavity examined. We routinely perform laparoscopic ultrasound of the liver at this stage.[7]

Mobilization of the sigmoid colon is now commenced. This maneuver is most readily performed with the patient in steep Trendelenburg position and rolled right-side down.[8] The surgeon stands on the right-hand side opposite the assistant. The apex of the sigmoid loop and the rectosigmoid are held with Babcock clamps by the assistant, and the surgeon, while applying countertraction with an atraumatic grasper, incises the lateral peritoneal reflection of the sigmoid along the white line of Toldt using electrocautery scissors (Fig. 42.2).

The mobilized sigmoid is then elevated by the assistant and the medial aspect of the sigmoid mesocolon is dissected. The inferior mesenteric artery and vein are thus identified and skeletonized by medial to lateral dissection. The left ureter is identified through the window in the mesocolon in a similar medial to lateral dissection to avoid the risk of inadvertent damage to a "tented-up" left ureter approached from the lateral side. We have not found ureteric stents to be advantageous, and their placement adds time to an already lengthy procedure. Atten-

tion is then turned to the vascular pedicle, where the skeletonized inferior mesenteric artery and vein are individually divided near their origin using a vascular cartilage of a 30-mm endoscopic linear cutter, which places three rows of staples on each side of the incision (Fig. 42.3).

The sigmoid mobilization is now carried proximally to the splenic flexure. The splenic flexure is fully mobilized to the midtransverse colon in all patients having total mesorectal excision. The lateral sigmoid dissection is continued distally down over the pelvic brim and along the left pelvic sidewall to the midline in either the rectovesical or rectovaginal pouch, all the while pushing the mesorectum medially.

Mobilization of the rectum is continued by carrying the dissection of the vascular pedicle downward over the aortic bifurcation keeping anterior to the parietal peritoneum and the sympathetic nerves. With the patient still in steep Trendelenburg position, the patient's right shoulder is now rolled upward and the surgeon stands on the left-hand side of the table. The critical angle of Trendelenburg is of vital importance in keeping the small bowel out of the operating field. The assistant standing opposite the surgeon grasps and elevates the sigmoid and proximal rectum with Babcocks. In the female, the uterus or fallopian tubes can be stapled or sutured temporarily to the abdominal wall (Fig. 42.4). The surgeon applies countertraction to the retroperitoneum and incises the parietal peritoneum over the sacral promontory to carefully enter the plane between the mesorectum anteriorly and the presacral nerves posteriorly. This avascular presacral areolar tissue constitutes the "holy plane" of rectal cancer surgery (Fig. 42.5). The plane is developed in this way down into the pelvis incising the peritoneum along the right pelvic sidewall until the midline is reached in the

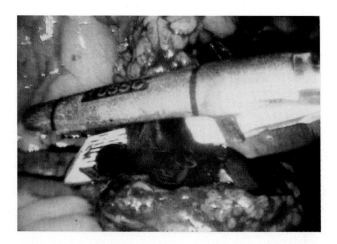

FIGURE 42.3. High ligation of the inferior mesenteric artery using an endoscopic linear cutter.

rectovesical or rectovaginal pouch. Like the left ureter, the right ureter must also be identified and preserved. During this phase of the procedure, the laparoscope is often best used via a right-sided port because the mobilized rectum when lifted out of the pelvis tends to obscure the view from the subumbilical port. The right-sided plane of dissection is finally connected to that on the left through the presacral space, avoiding the left ureter. The lateral ligaments can be safely divided with cautery.

Having connected the peritoneal incisions from the left and the right sides of the pelvis, the surgeon retracts the rectum toward the sacrum by grasping the cut edge of the peritoneum with a Babcock clamp and continues the anterior dissection following the plane of Denonvilliers' fascia, utilizing a fan retractor to provide anterior countertraction on the bladder or the vagina. If this final part of the dissection cannot be completed safely laparoscopically, it is prudent to undertake it through the Pfannenstiel incision rather than to oncologically compromise the entire operation.

Full laparoscopic mobilization of the splenic flexure and high ligation of the inferior mesenteric vein provide a sufficiently mobile descending colon to permit tension-free anastomosis at the pelvic floor. A low Pfannenstiel-type incision of 7 to 10 cm is performed for specimen delivery, bowel transection, and stapled reanastomosis under direct vision. The laparotomy phase of the surgery should be carried out in exactly the same fashion as any anterior resection by laparotomy. We prefer the 30-mm linear stapler for rectal transection at the level of the pelvic floor and a 28-mm or 31-mm circular stapler for end-to-end anastomosis following the construction of a 7-cm colonic J pouch.[9] The pelvis is irrigated, and the anastomotic integrity is tested. The fascia of all ports should be closed under direct vision to prevent injury and herniation.

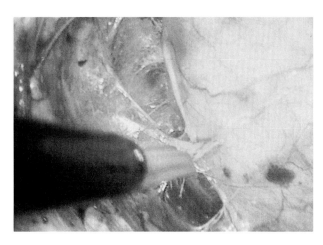

FIGURE 42.5. Magnified view of the intact mesorectum during sharp laparoscopic dissection.

Conclusion

We have described one method of approaching this procedure. The laparoscopic-assisted method combines the benefits of laparoscopic mobilization with the advantages of bowel division and reanastomosis under direct vision; the incision also allows a degree of flexibility in the most crucial area, allowing the available option of rectal dissection by laparotomy. The available data suggest that, in terms of histological parameters and early survival and recurrence, the laparoscopic procedure is comparable to laparotomy.[5,6,8] The laparoscopic-assisted approach requires an incision of 7 to 10 cm and therefore may not yield the benefits of minimally invasive surgery. However, the magnified views provide excellent visualization of the pelvic nerves and the potential for better postoperative functional outcome requires further prospective assessment.

References

1. Phillips R, Hittinger R, Blesovsky L, et al. Local recurrence following "curative" surgery for large bowel cancer: I. The overall picture. Br J Surg 1984;71:12–16.
2. MacFarlane J, Ryall R, Heald R. Mesorectal excision for rectal cancer. Lancet 1993;341:457–460.
3. O'Rourke N, Heald R. Laparoscopic surgery for colorectal cancer. Br J Surg 1993;80:1229–1230.
4. Azagra JS, Goerben M, Gilbart E, et al. Anterior resection: the total laparoscopic approach. In: Monson JR, Darzi A (eds) Laparoscopic Colorectal Surgery. Oxford: Isis Medical Media, 1995:38–55.
5. Hartley JE, Qureshi A, Farouk R, et al. Total mesorectal excision: assessment of the laparoscopic approach. Dis Colon Rectum, 2001;44:315–321.

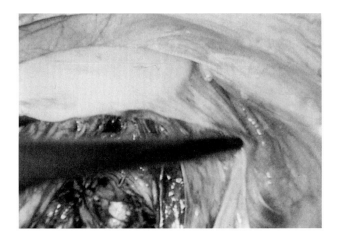

FIGURE 42.4. Uterus sutured to the anterior abdominal wall to provide traction during laparoscopic rectal dissection.

6. Tate JJ, Kwok S, Dawson JW, et al. Prospective comparison of laparoscopic and conventional anterior resection. Br J Surg 1993;80:1396–1398.

7. Hartley JE, Kumar H, Drew PJ, et al. Laparoscopic ultrasound for the detection of hepatic metastases during laparoscopic colorectal cancer surgery. Dis Colon Rectum 2000;43:320–324.

8. Lord SA, Larach SW, Ferrara A, et al. Laparoscopic resections for colorectal carcinoma. A three year experience. Dis Colon Rectum 1996;39:148–154.

9. Hallbook O, Pahlman L, Krog M, Wexner SD, Sjodahl R. Randomized comparison of straight and colonic J pouch anastomosis after low anterior resection. Ann Surg 1996; 224(1):58–65.

43
Laparoscopic Abdominoperineal Resection

Ara Darzi and Jared Torkington

Case Selection and Preoperative Preparation

The introduction of operative techniques that aim to conserve the anal sphincter mechanism has led to a reappraisal of the indications for excision of the rectum. The indications for laparoscopic abdominoperineal resection should be identical to those for conventional open procedures. The resection of rectal tumors that are less than 4 to 5 cm from the dentate line therefore provide the principal indication for this technique.

The most important preoperative consideration is whether to submit the patient to an abdominoperineal resection or an anterior resection. During conventional surgery, the final decision may be made intraoperatively, with the benefit of a trial pelvic dissection; as such, it is commonplace to appropriately counsel the patients before surgery. There is no such opportunity during the laparoscopic approach, as the abdominal surgeon is unlikely to visualize the tumor if the aforementioned strict selection criteria are applied. The surgeon must therefore be certain as to the intended resection before surgery. Preoperative counseling by the stoma therapist is mandatory in all patients consenting to abdominoperineal resection, and the patient's notes should be accordingly marked. The patient must also be aware of the possibility of conversion to a laparotomy and must give consent for this eventuality.

There are no conclusive data as yet on the morbidity or mortality rates associated with the laparoscopic approach, but knowledge of the principles of laparoscopy can assist the surgeon with recommendations regarding case selection. A laparoscopic approach in patients with significant cardiorespiratory compromise cannot be advocated. In such patients, the decrease in venous return consequent on the pneumoperitoneum may lead to a significant reduction in cardiac output. Second, the technical problems associated with laparoscopy in the grossly obese or those with previous lower abdominal surgery justifiably influence both preoperative and intraoperative decision making. Neither of these factors constitutes an absolute contraindication to the laparoscopic approach, but those inexperienced in this field would do well to avoid abdominoperineal resection in such patients because the pelvic dissection in particular is likely to prove technically demanding.

Equipment and Instrumentation

During the past few years, the engineering and design of equipment used for laparoscopy has been changing rapidly. Purchase of equipment is based on acceptable quality versus budget constraints. The best way to select equipment is to use it in the operating room and give all potential users the opportunity to evaluate it.

Laparoscopes

The laparoscope must deliver a high-quality image to be safe and effective for dissection and identification of bleeding points. Little has changed from the rod-lens system introduced in the early 1950s. Laparoscopes are available in all diameters, but the 10-mm size is used routinely in laparoscopic colorectal surgery, with either a 30° viewing angle (authors' preference) or a 0° angle (editor's preference).

Insufflators

Insufflation machines should be able to generate a flow of at least 10 liters per minute. Carbon dioxide (CO_2) is usually used because it is not combustible and is readily absorbed. The machine should have automatic pressure and flow regulators to maintain a constant intraperitoneal pressure.

Power Instruments

Cutting and dissecting may be achieved using water jet, electricity, laser, or an ultrasonic scalpel. Ultrasonic scalpels and shears use high-energy ultrasonic vibrations to mechanically denature proteins and tissue, thus sealing vessels and closing cavitation. Cutting coagulation requires vibration frequencies of 55,000. As cells are selectively fragmented leaving nerves, ducts, and larger blood vessels, the cell debris and liquid are suctioned away. The inability to coagulate large vessels necessitates the need for clips, ligatures, and electrocoagulation. In an attempt to minimize this failure with larger vessels, ultrasonic shears with blunt stationary jaws and sharp vibrating blades have been developed.

Operating Instruments

Retractor

Colonic surgery requires movement from one side of the abdomen to the other. To achieve this mobility while maintaining good vision, it is necessary to retract the adjacent organs, especially the small bowel. The positioning of the table allows gravity to direct organs dependently, while the pneumoperitoneum helps push and hold organs away. Some local retraction will also be required. Retraction should be blunt and should be with atraumatic tips and blunt edges. Unfortunately, for an instrument to fit through a cannula, it must be bladelike.

Graspers

For the purpose of colonic surgery, grasping forceps are necessary to push, pull, and dissect. Although forceps are available with traumatic, or atraumatic tip designs, the atraumatic jaws required to avoid colon injury are most often needed. Generally, the shafts can be rotated 360° to direct the tip appropriately.

Clip Applicators

Clips are used to secure larger vessels. The clip applicators may be single loaded or multifire. Generally, the single-loading devices are reusable and the multifire devices are disposable. In colon resection, multiple clips are needed, and therefore a multifire clip applicator is appropriate.

Staplers

Laparoscopic linear staplers apply a row of staples and cut between them. The staples may be 3 or 6 cm long. The 6-cm staples only fit through a 50-mm cannula and the 3-cm stapler fits through a 12-mm cannula. These staplers are used to transect the bowel and to divide the inferior mesenteric vessels in abdominoperineal resections.

Operative Procedure

Preoperative Preparation

The mechanical and antibiotic preparation of the colon is the same as that for an open abdominoperineal resection. Generally, this entails the use of laxatives, most commonly including sodium phosphate enemas; oral polyethylene glycol solutions are used much less frequently. In some patients, the laparoscopic procedure is converted to an open procedure, and the informed consent should reflect that provision.

Patient Positioning

The table is equipped with a device to hold the patient in place, even when marked tilting of the table is necessary. A beanbag torso holder and shoulder braces work well. The patient is placed in the modified lithotomy position with the legs in stirrups. The perineum is placed just off the inferior end of the table to allow access to the perineal part of the operation. The patient's legs are positioned so that the surgeon or the assistant can stand between the legs. The hips and knees are flexed less than usual to avoid impediment to the surgeon's arm movements and to keep the patient's thighs from obstructing the movement of instruments. The legs are wrapped in compression stockings to enhance blood flow.

Laparoscopic Abdominoperineal Resection

The Abdominal Stage

Under general anasthesia, the abdomen and perineum is prepared and draped and the anus is closed with a purse-string suture. Carbon dioxide pneumoperitoneum at a pressure of 15 mmHg is then achieved using a closed or open technique. A 10-mm trocar is inserted, and a 10-mm laparoscope is introduced through the port. Visceral injury can only be consistently avoided if all subsequent trocars are inserted under direct vision (Fig. 43.1).

Preliminary laparoscopy is now performed paying attention first to the pelvic organs. There is a critical angle of Trendelenburg varying from patient to patient, beyond which the small bowel will fall out of the pelvis. Any adhesions between the small bowel and pelvic structures prevent this occurring and they must therefore be divided at any early stage in the procedure. The table is then returned to the neutral position and the remainder of peritoneal cavity is examined. In particular, the liver must be carefully examined for the presence of metastases.

Elevation and retraction of the sigmoid and mobilization of the rectum are facilitated by early ligation and

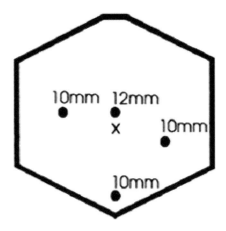

FIGURE 43.1. Schematic representation of sites and sizes of ports.

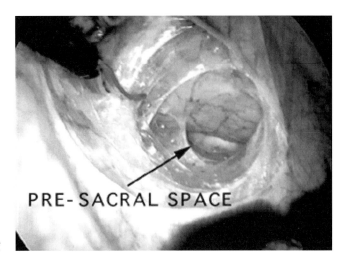

FIGURE 43.2. Dissection in the "holy plane" with the mesorectum anteriorly.

division of the inferior mesenteric pedicle, a maneuver that also helps reduce blood loss during the subsequent pelvic dissection. Because we perform this operation almost without exception for malignancy, it is our practice to identify and skeletonize these vessels near their origin. Once the vessels have been skeletonized, they are divided using an endoscopic 3-mm stapling device.

Sigmoid mobilization is most readily performed with the patient in the steep Trendelenburg position and rolled to the left. The surgeon stands on the right of the table opposite the assistant. The apex of the sigmoid loop and the rectosigmoid are held with Babcock tissue forceps by the assistant. The surgeon, while applying countertraction with some form of grasping instrument, incises the lateral peritoneal reflection of the sigmoid colon along the white line of Toldt. As this maneuver progresses, the mesosigmoid is pushed gently toward the midline. This lateral incision is continued over the pelvic brim and along the left pelvic sidewall to the midline, in either the rectovesical or rectovaginal pouch. Identification of the left ureter at an early stage in this procedure is of paramount importance if iatrogenic injury is to be avoided. In thin patients, it may be readily visible through the transparent posterior parietal peritoneum.

Mobilization of the rectum is continued by carrying the foregoing dissection into the avascular areolar tissue of the presacral plane, the so-called holy plane (Fig. 43.2). The plane is developed in this way down to the pelvis, incising the peritoneum along the right pelvic sidewall, until the midline is reached in the rectovesical or rectovaginal pouch. The right ureter must be identified and preserved.

Having connected the peritoneal incision from the left and right side of the pelvis, the surgeon retracts the rectum toward the sacrum by grasping the cut edge of the peritoneum with a Babcock clamp. The fascia of Denonvillier is then incised, and after this plane is opened the dissection is completed by the perineal operator (Fig. 43.3). In females, a finger in the vagina can be used to provide anterior retraction. The assistant retracts the rectum out of the pelvis laterally, with two Babcock clamps from the opposite side of the table to the surgeon. The lateral ligaments are then divided by electrocautery or clips, under direct vision. The dissection now proceeds easily down to the level of the middle rectum. If meticulous attention is paid to hemostasis, this rectal dissection can be carried out all the way down to the level of the levators under direct vision. The perineal operator is then well positioned to complete the dissection from below.

Having completed this mobilization, the proximal colon must be transected before the perineal dissection is commenced. It would be impossible to complete this

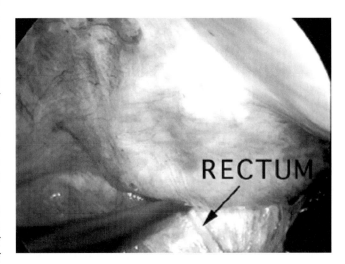

FIGURE 43.3. Continuing the anterior dissection.

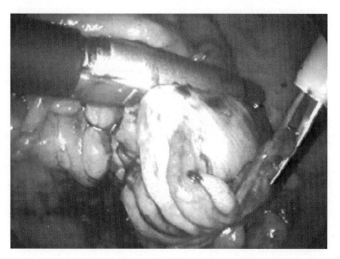

FIGURE 43.4. Division of the colon using a stapling device.

safely without an adequate pneumoperitoneum. The colon is elevated and held with a Babcock clamp, and an Endo GIA is used to transect the rectum. Two firings might be required in some cases to complete the division of the bowel (Fig. 43.4).

Perineal Stage

The perineal stage is then started in the same way as described in an open abdominoperineal resection.

Constructing the Colostomy

Before the bowel is transected and with full pneumoperitoneum, the mobilized colon is grasped with a Babcock clamp and brought up to the abdominal wall. Provided this is easily achieved, the colon can be divided safely in the knowledge that a tension-free end colostomy can be constructed once the abdomen has been deflated. After transection of the bowel, it is our practice to leave a Babcock clamp attached to the blind stapled proximal end; this can then be brought out to the left iliac fossa port site at the end of the procedure. The port site is first enlarged by excising a disk of skin followed by the subcutaneous fat down to the rectus sheath, which is also enlarged. After the perineal and abdominal wounds are closed and dressed, the staple line is opened and the colostomy is sutured in the standard manner.

Postoperative Care

The postoperative care of patients who have undergone laparoscopic abdominoperineal resection is, in essence, identical to that of patients who have been subjected to open resection. Thus, antibiotic prophylaxis is administered, the nasogastric tube is removed on the night of surgery, and oral fluids are commenced on the first postoperative day.

Chest physiotherapy should be routine and the patient should be mobilized as soon as possible. Thromboembolic prophylaxis must be continued until the patient is fully mobile. The patient is discharged when he is tolerating a normal diet and managing a colostomy.

44
Laparoscopic Stoma Creation and Reversal

Lucia Oliveira

The creation of a stoma is a common procedure in a colorectal or general surgery practice. The ideal method for the performance of this procedure is basically surgeon dependent. However, certain principles are important regardless of the technique, such as choosing and preparing the appropriate site for the stoma, using adequate supplies and material for stoma fixation and care, and providing enterostomal therapy education.[1] Furthermore, reversal for a stoma, which may be created under special circumstances such as sigmoid resection for severe diverticulitis, is also routinely performed. For reversal of a stoma and restoration of bowel continuity, the anastomosis can be performed manually or mechanically. Like most other operations involving the gastrointestinal (GI) tract, these procedures may be performed either by laparotomy or laparoscopy.[2,3] "Simpler" laparoscopic colorectal procedures, such as sigmoid colectomy, the creation and reversal of stomas, and right hemicolectomy, have been shown to offer distinct advantages as compared to laparotomy.[4,5]

Stoma Creation

The indications for stoma creation are shown in Table 44.1. The main advantages of performing a stoma by laparoscopic surgery include the absence of an incision, the ability to view the entire cavity, the staging of disease, and the ability to lyse adhesions and obtain biopsies. Furthermore, visualization of the intestinal loop as it is brought through the stoma site helps ensure appropriate orientation of the mesentery and bowel. Because no incision is required, postoperative pain is minimized and an early return of patient activities is expected. Finally, another advantage of laparoscopic stoma creation, as compared to laparoscopic colectomy, is the need for relatively few instruments (Table 44.2).

Procedure

Patients are operated on under general anesthesia, in the supine modified lithotomy position in Allen stirrups (Allen Medical, Bedford Heights, OH, USA) after a full mechanical bowel preparation and prophylactic oral and parenteral antibiotic administration.[6] Ideally, the operation should be performed with at least two monitors, with the surgeon standing opposite the intended side of the stoma creation. The ideal stoma site is preoperatively chosen, as is the segment of bowel to be used for the stoma. The author's preference is to create a loop ileostomy whenever possible.[7] However, in some situations, an end descending colostomy is preferred. Transverse loop colectomies and any right-sided colonic stomas are assiduously avoided due to their high complication rates and management difficulties.

The establishment of pneumoperitoneum can be performed using either a Veress needle or by the open technique. The open technique should be selected for patients who have had previous surgery, in whom adhesions are expected. The second trocar is placed at the intended stoma site. Regardless of the type of stoma created, laparoscopy offers numerous advantages as compared to both laparotomy and trephine stoma. First, adhesions can be safely divided. Second, in patients with a history of carcinoma, exploration and biopsy of any suspicious areas can be undertaken. If malignancy is found, it may be resected, or if this is deemed inappropriate, then at least fecal diversion proximal to the lesion can be ensured. Third, in patients with Crohn's disease, the bowel can be caudally inspected and any radiographically undetected strictures treated by either resection or strictureplasty. Again, fecal diversion can be ensured as proximal to any disease. Last, anatomic orientation of the bowel and mesentery can be ensured. Although transanal endoscopy can help ensure appropriate rotation of a trephine ileostomy, the techniques are more difficult in

TABLE 44.1. Indications for fecal diversion.

Fecal incontinence
Trauma
Radiation proctitis
Perineal sepsis
Crohn's disease
Colonic inertia
Anal stenosis
Unresectable rectal cancer
Kaposi's sarcoma
Cervix carcinoma with rectovaginal fistula
Spinal trauma; paraplegia

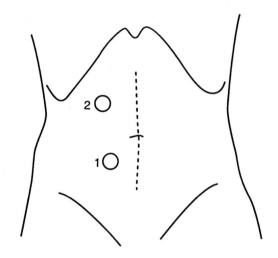

FIGURE 44.1. Babcock clamp delivers the most distal portion of the loop ileostomy (ileum) through the trocar.

cases of a trephine ileostomy. The possibility of conversion to laparotomy should always be discussed as part of the informed consent procedure. Consent for and the availability of intraoperative colonoscopy should always be expected.

Loop Ileostomy

The loop ileostomy is usually placed in the right lower quadrant through the rectus sheath (Fig. 44.1), where the trocar will allow a Babcock clamp to gently grasp and deliver the most distal segment of the ileum that can be delivered without tension. The port is withdrawn over the Babcock clamp shaft, which is maintained within the port sleeve well within the abdomen. An adequate fascial opening can be secured by incising the fascia along the insulated shaft of the Babcock clamp and then performing a digital dilatation (Fig. 44.2). Exteriorization of the loop is then facilitated with partial deflation of the pneumoperitoneum. The camera is used to both visualize the procedure and ensure adequate orientation of the bowel

and its mesentery (Fig. 44.3). An optional third port can be used if extensive adhesions require division or if mobilization is required. After exteriorization, the loop can be gently grasped with a Babcock clamp and subsequently anchored with a supporting rod (Fig. 44.4). Finally, closure of the camera port site incision with interrupted

TABLE 44.2. Instruments required for laparoscopic stomas.

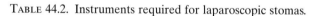

Creation:
  2 10-mm trocars
  1 12-mm trocar
  1 5-mm trocar
  1 endoscopic Babcock clamp
  1 plastic rod for loop ileostomy/colostomy
  1 endoscopic biopsy forceps
  1 endoscopic 30-mm stapler

Reversal of Hartmann's procedure:
  3 10-mm trocars
  1 5-mm trocar
  1 33-mm trocar
  1 endoscopic scissors
  1 endoscopic Babcock clamp
  1 endoscopic anvil grasper
  1 circular stapler (29 or 33mm)

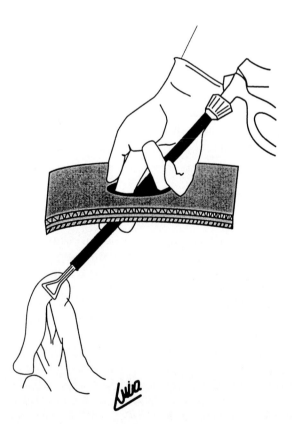

FIGURE 44.2. Digital dilatation of the stoma site.

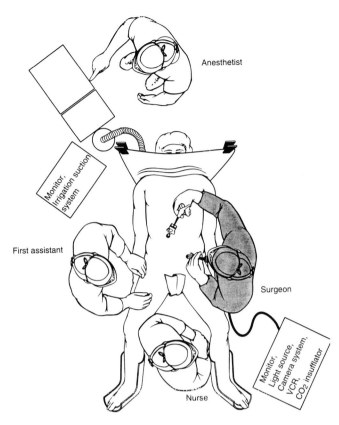

FIGURE 44.3. Position of the equipment and the personnel for ileostomy.

absorbable sutures and maturation of the ileostomy are undertaken. A subcutaneous infiltration of a solution of Marcaine (0.5%) at the camera port site incision can be used for analgesia.

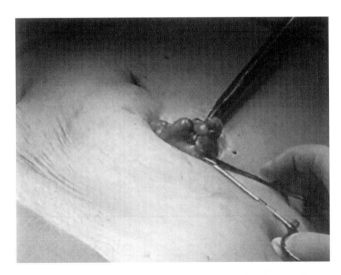

FIGURE 44.4. Loop ileostomy after exteriorization anchored with supporting rod.

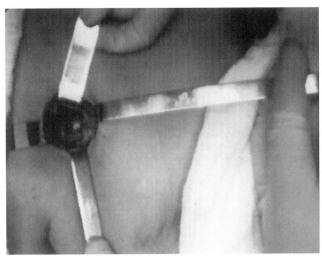

FIGURE 44.5. Excision of skin necessary to create sigmoid colostomy.

Loop Colostomy

A loop colostomy is difficult to manage as it is usually large and, if right sided, has a very liquid effluent. There is a high risk of parastomal hernia and stomal prolapse. Nonetheless, on rare occasions it may be the only type of stoma to form. Even in this setting we prefer a divided loop to allow maturation as an end transverse colostomy. The distal limb can be either completely closed or left open and matured in the antimesenteric corner as described by Pearl et al.[8] For the creation of a colostomy, the camera should be placed on the opposite side of the stoma, allowing enough space for both the Babcock clamp and the camera. The patient may also be placed in the steep Trendelenburg position to allow isolation of the segment of transverse colon that will be most easily delivered as a stoma. A complete inspection of the cavity is crucial to avoid involvement of the small bowel in the pelvis, especially if the diversion is created for pelvic malignancy. In cases of obstruction, gentle manipulation of the bowel is mandatory to avoid tearing the distended loops. If adhesions are present, a third port may be necessary, usually at the suprapubic quadrant; this procedure is similar to that previously described.

For a loop sigmoid colostomy, the procedure can start with the excision of the disk of skin necessary for stoma formation at the stoma site (Fig. 44.5). The first port is then inserted using an open technique. A pursestring suture is placed around the opening in the posterior sheath (Fig. 44.6), and an 18- or 33-mm trocar is inserted into the peritoneal cavity (Fig. 44.7); the pneumoperitoneum is established. The abdominal cavity is inspected and the second trocar (10 or 12 mm) is inserted lateral to the rectus sheath, opposite to the stoma site. The camera

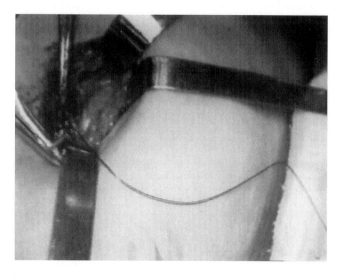

FIGURE 44.6. Pursestring suture around opening in the posterior sheath.

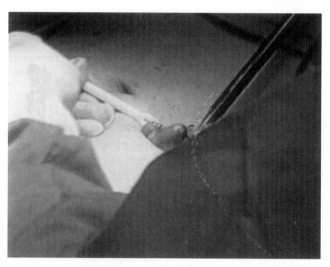

FIGURE 44.8. A Babcock or Allis clamp is used to correctly position the stoma and a plastic rod is inserted.

is then placed at this second port, and a Babcock clamp is inserted at the stoma site port to grasp the sigmoid colon. The whole procedure is performed under direct vision, and the loop is brought through the abdominal wall; care must be taken to avoid torsion of the mesentery (Fig. 44.8). Once the sigmoid colon is exteriorized by the laparoscopic Babcock clamp, the instrument should be held in a fixed position and grasped by its shaft rather than its handles (Fig. 44.4). A conventional Babcock or Allis clamp can then help to correctly position the stoma, and a plastic rod is inserted (Fig. 44.8). The stoma is then matured (Fig. 44.9).

End Colostomy

Creation of an end colostomy often requires mobilization of the left colon and division of the loop with a linear stapler. The procedure should always start with a meticulous inspection of the entire pelvic cavity, especially if malignant disease is the cause for diversion; the small bowel may be attached to the pelvic mass or the distal ileum may be obstructed. The Babcock clamp is used to gently grasp and orient the sigmoid loop which is then held in a fixed position. Dividing the loop with a conventional linear stapler at the skin level allows easy formation of the end sigmoid colostomy. Alternatively, an intraperitoneal division with a laparoscopic linear stapler

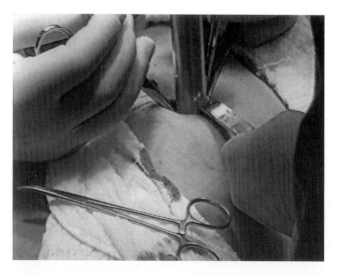

FIGURE 44.7. An 18-mm or 33-mm trocar is inserted into the peritoneal cavity.

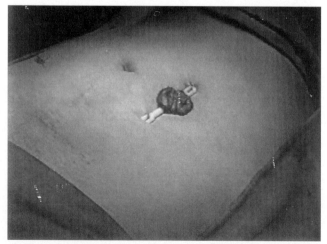

FIGURE 44.9. The stoma is matured.

can be undertaken; a third port will be necessary to introduce an endoscopic linear cutter. After division of the colon, the proximal end is delivered through the stoma site and conventionally matured; the distal end may be matured as a mucous fistula or left in the abdomen.

Stoma Reversal

Regardless of the indication for a temporary end stoma, the principles of the stoma closure are the same as for any laparoscopic procedure. It is crucial to avoid inadvertent lesions during establishment of pneumoperitoneum, placement of trocars, and manipulation of the bowel. During reoperation, adhesions should be expected and may complicate isolation of the bowel. It is always prudent to convert to a laparotomy to avoid impending complications rather than to subsequently convert because of complications.

Laparoscopic surgery is not necessary to reverse loop stomas, as they can be more easily and quickly closed using conventional methods. However, whenever inspection of the abdominal cavity or obtaining biopsies is required, laparoscopic techniques may be more easily used. Moreover, laparoscopic reversal of end stomas, such as an end sigmoid colostomy due to a Hartmann's procedure, or an end ileostomy due to right hemicolectomy for Crohn's disease, may be advantageous[9]; laparoscopy should always be considered in these situations.

Reversal of Hartmann's Procedure

Laparoscopic reversal of Hartmann's procedure has become an option for restoration of bowel continuity, by avoiding a second laparotomy, which may be associated with higher morbidity and disability rates. Before restoration of bowel continuity, it is important to exclude previously undiagnosed pathology such as concomitant malignancy or new pathology such as a stricture. The patients are prepared as for any abdominal procedure with a standard mechanical bowel prep, including phosphate enemas of the rectal stump and prophylactic antibiotics. Preoperative endoscopy and radiographic assessment of both proximal and distal segments are advisable to exclude pathology such as residual sigmoid diverticulitis; rigid or flexible proctoscopy should be performed to verify that the entire distal sigmoid has been resected, leaving behind a rectal stump approximately 15 cm long. Absence of diverticuli at the cephalad aspect of the Hartmann's pouch should be confirmed by endoscopic as well as radiographic evaluation. A water-soluble contrast enema is an excellent method to delineate the residual stump. The patient is placed in a modified lithot-

omy position with Allen stirrups. Intraoperative ureteric stent insertion can be helpful, especially when the first operation was performed because of acute diverticulitis or when extensive pelvic or retroperitoneal inflammation is expected. The possibility of conversion to a laparotomy is always discussed with the patient as part of the informed consent procedure.

The operation begins with dissection and complete mobilization of the stoma by conventional surgical technique. Under direct vision, adhesions are lysed and the edges of the stoma are trimmed; the anvil of a 33-mm stapler is introduced and secured with a pursestring suture of 0 polypropylene. Subsequently, the proximal end of the colon is introduced into the abdominal cavity. The fascial edges at the stoma site are then grasped with Kocher clamps and as much adhesiolysis as possible is accomplished under direct vision. A 10-mm midline port is then introduced under direct vision; great care must be taken to resect any residual diseased proximal sigmoid colon before anvil introduction. Although it is not necessary to resect all diverticular-bearing colon, it is imperative to remove all muscular hypertrophied segments. In general, confirmation of the ease of the 33-mm-diameter circular stapler anvil is sufficient to ensure that supple, compliant disease-free bowel has been utilized. Next, the stoma site is either closed or occluded with a 33-mm port. After insufflation, the abdominal cavity is completely inspected, and additional adhesions are lysed. The patient is placed in a Trendelenburg position to prevent the small bowel from entering the pelvic cavity. Two or three additional ports are placed as shown in Figure 44.10. Mobilization of the left colon and splenic flexure may be necessary and can be performed using electrocautery scissors or the ultrasonic scissors. The rectal stump must be well visualized and freed from any adhesions.

At this point an assistant may perform a rigid proctoscopy to facilitate identification and dissection of the rectal stump. The stump should be tested for integrity with rigid or flexible proctoscopic confirmation of the intended anastomotic height. Laparoscopic verification should confirm the position to correspond to the level of the sacral promontory or caudad to this point. Transanal visualization should again ensure absence of any distal sigmoid on the cephalad aspect of the rectum. If any distal sigmoid remains, it must be resected as for a standard sigmoid colectomy. Choices for mesenteric transection include the harmonic scalpel, diathermy with clips, or an endoscopic linear cutter with a vascular cartridge. The remaining distal sigmoid can and must be resected with an endoscopic linear cutter. The additional bowel can be withdrawn through the prior stoma site. If a 33-mm port was placed, the residual specimen may fit through that port or alternatively the port may need to be removed and then replaced. If bowel is delivered through this site, wound protection should be utilized.

Alternatively, if this site was closed, it could be reopened for delivery of this specimen and then reclosed, protecting the edges during actual specimen extirpation. It is critical to resect this residual sigmoid as the recurrence rate approximately triples, comparing coloproctostomy with colodistal sigmoidostomy anastomoses.[10]

Regardless of whether the newly closed stump is utilized for anastomosis, this stump should be tested for integrity by either proctoscopic air insufflation while the pelvis is filled with water during laparoscopic visualization or by povidine iodine irrigation through the proctoscope with laparoscopic visualization for leakage. The method is less important than the performance of the task. If a leak is detected, it can often be used as the point through which the trocar is made to protrude to fashion the anastomosis. However, alternatives include resection and reclosure of the stump as already described, or suture or staple fixation of the defect. Regardless of which of these three alternatives is employed, the anastomosis should be retested for integrity if the identified defect is not to be used for a trocar introduction. Once all the adhesions have been freed, the small bowel safely delivered from the pelvis, and the rectal stump verified for absence of attached sigmoid and for closure integrity, preparation is made for the anastomosis. The patient

remains in the Trendelenburg position, the previously introduced anvil and the proximal bowel are reidentified, and a modified Allis anvil grasping clamp is introduced through a left paraumbilical port. At this point in the operation, it is easiest to facilitate circumferential visualization of the anastomosis by placing the camera through the right iliac fossa port. The stapler is carefully introduced by the perineal operator so that the cartridge rests flush with the apex of the Hartmann's pouch. The trocar is then made to carefully protrude, after which the anvil is reattached. Great care is taken to ensure appropriate orientation of the mesentery and the bowel in construction of this tension-free anastomosis. The stapler is thus closed.

If the Hartmann's closure was more distal than the level of the sacral promontory, transperineal digitation of the vagina with laparoscopic visualization may be helpful to ensure exclusion of the vagina during stapler closure. The anastomosis is fashioned under direct manual and visual guidance of both the abdominal and perineal fields, after which the stapler is gently removed. The proximal and distal doughnuts are carefully inspected. The pelvis is then irrigated with fluid sufficient to cover the anastomosis while the proximal bowel is gently occluded with a noncrushing clamp. Endoscopic evaluation is then performed to again check the level of the anastomosis, to help the appearance of the mucosa proximal and distal to the anastomosis, and to verify the hemostasis and patency of the anastomosis and the absence of air leakage. All port sites are closed, and the colostomy site may be either completely or partially closed or left open for healing by secondary intention.

Discussion

Although the laparoscopic techniques used for creation of stomas are some of the simplest laparoscopic colorectal procedures, those involving stoma reversal can be some of the most difficult. Specifically, because of extensive adhesions, the anticipated rate of conversion for laparoscopic Hartmann's reversal may greatly exceed that for laparoscopic segmental colectomy. Certainly this has been the author's experience within the first 400 laparoscopic colorectal procedures. Most of the publications on laparoscopic fecal diversion to date have been brief case reports of patients in whom a laparoscopic loop ileostomy or colostomy was undertaken[11–20] (Table 44.3). However, more recently, Hollyoak et al.[20] reported a series of 40 patients who underwent laparoscopic stoma creation as compared to 15 patients who had stoma construction by laparotomy. Although the study was not prospectively randomized, morbidity and mortality were reduced in patients who underwent laparoscopic stoma creation. Oliveira et al. evaluated 32 patients who under-

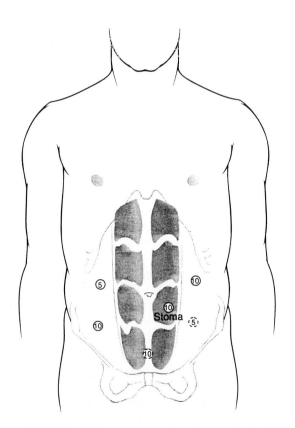

FIGURE 44.10. Port placement for reversal of Hartmann's procedure.

TABLE 44.3. Laparoscopic stoma series.

Author	Year	n	Loop ileostomy	Loop colostomy	Loop colostomy
Lange[11]	1991	1	—	1	—
Romero[12]	1992	1	—	—	1
Khoo[13]	1993	1	1	—	—
Roe[14]	1994	4	1	3	—
Lyerly[15]	1994	4	1	2	1
Fuhrman[16]	1994	17	2	8	7[a]
Jess[17]	1994	1	1	—	—
Ludwig[18]	1996	24	16	2	6
Oliveira[19]	1997	32	25	4	3
Hollyoak[20]	1998	—	40	—	—

[a] Part of abdominoperineal resection.

went laparoscopic stoma creation.[19] Conversion was required in 5 patients with a history of previous abdominal surgery. In fact, the presence of extensive adhesions from previous surgery has been the most difficult aspect of laparoscopic stoma creation, although not a contraindication. One of the most important aspects observed in our series was the creation of a sufficient fascial opening at the stoma site and adequate orientation of the stoma loop to avoid stoma outlet obstruction. Accordingly, we recommend a fascial incision at the stoma site to avoid narrowing of the loop.

Certainly, a prospective randomized trial would be necessary to adequately answer all the questions regarding the ideal method of performing a stoma, including the use of the trephine stoma.[21] However, the literature demonstrates that laparoscopic creation of stomas is a safe, simple, and relatively inexpensive procedure, compared to other more complex laparoscopic colorectal operations. It allows complete visualization of the abdominal cavity during the procedure as well as while the bowel loop is brought through the stoma site; biopsy specimens can be obtained and staging of malignant disease can be performed; and in selected cases such as Crohn's disease or partial bowel obstruction, it is possible to inspect the loops and choose the best segment for a stoma.

The small incision of a trephine stoma may prevent adequate visualization of the cavity and safe mobilization of the ideal loop of bowel. In addition, all the advantages related to the laparoscopic method, such as abdominal cavity inspection, biopsy, orientation of the bowel loops under direct visualization, and staging of the malignant disease, are not possible with the trephine method.

Conclusion

Laparoscopic stoma creation and reversal has multiple advantages over the conventional techniques: an excellent view of the entire cavity, staging of diseases, thorough evaluation of the entire small bowel and colon, enterolysis, and biopsy. The rapid recovery that can be expected after laparoscopic stoma creation can also be seen after laparoscopic stoma reversal. The avoidance of reopening a laparotomy incision coupled with the potential for less handling of the bowel despite equally extensive enterolysis may contribute to these advantages. Both laparoscopic stoma creation and reversal should be considered in every patient scheduled to undergo these procedures. With very rare exceptions, patients are offered these operations by laparotomy instead.

References

1. Celestin LR. Appliances and accessories. The Surgery and Management of Intestinal Stomas. Buttermarket, England: Wolfe Medical, 1987:115–129.
2. Molenaar BH, Bijnen AB, Ruiter P. Indications for laparoscopic colorectal surgery. Surg Endosc 1998;12:42–45.
3. Milsom JW, Bartholomaus B (eds) Laparoscopic Colorectal Surgery. New York: Springer-Verlag, 1996.
4. Monson JRT, Darzi A, Carey PD, Guillou PJ. Prospective evaluation of laparoscopic-assisted colectomy in an unselective group of patients. Lancet 1992;340:831–833.
5. Wexner SD, Johansen OB. Laparoscopic total abdominal colectomy. Dis Colon Rectum 1992;35:651–665.
6. Oliveira L, Wexner SD, Daniel N, et al. Mechanical bowel preparation for elective colorectal surgery: a prospective, randomized, surgeon-blinded trial comparing sodium phosphate and polyethylene glycol-based oral lavage solutions. Dis Colon Rectum 1997;40:585–591.
7. Wexner SD, Taranow DA, Johansen OB, et al. Loop ileostomy is a safe option for fecal diversion. Dis Colon Rectum 1993;36:349–354.
8. Pearl RK, Prasad ML, Orsay CP, Abcarian H, Tan AB. A survey of technical considerations in the construction of intestinal stomas. Am J Surg 1985;51(8):462–465.
9. Reissman P, Wexner SD. Laparoscopic Hartmann's procedure and Hartmann's reversal procedure. In: Phillips EH, Rosenthal RJ (eds) Operative Strategies in Laparoscopic Surgery. New York: Springer, 1995:251–257.
10. Benn PL, Wolff BG, Ilstrup DM. Level of anastomosis and recurrent colonic diverticulitis. Am J Surg 1986; 151(2):269–271.
11. Lange V, Meyer G, Schardey HM, Schildberg F. Laparoscopic creation of a loop ileostomy. J Laparosc Surg 1991; 1(3):307–312.
12. Romero CA, James KM, Cooperstoner LM, et al. Laparoscopic sigmoid colostomy for perianal Crohn's disease. Surg Laparosc Endosc 1992;2(2):148–151.
13. Khoo REH, Montrey J, Cohen MM. Laparoscopic loop ileostomy for temporary fecal diversion. Dis Colon Rectum 1993;36:966–968.
14. Roe AM, Barlow AP, Durdey P, et al. Indications for laparoscopic formation of intestinal stomas. Surg Laparosc Endosc 1994;4(5):345–347.
15. Lyerly HK, Mautt JR. Laparoscopic ileostomy and colostomy. Ann Surg 1994;219:317–322.

16. Fuhrman GM, Ota DM. Laparoscopic intestinal stomas. Dis Colon Rectum 1994;37:444–449.

17. Jess P, Christianese J. Laparoscopic loop ileostomy for fecal diversion. Dis Colon Rectum 1994;36(37):721–722.

18. Ludwig KA, Milson JW, Garcia-Ruiz A, et al. Laparoscopic stoma procedures. Dis Colon Rectum 1996;39:285–288.

19. Oliveira L, Reissman P, Wexner SD. Laparoscopic creation of stomas. Surg Endosc 1997;11:19–23.

20. Hollyoak MA, Lumley J, Stitz RW. Laparoscopic stoma formation for fecal diversion. Br J Surg 1998;85:226–228.

21. Anderson ID, Hill J, Vohra R, et al. An improved means of fecal diversion: the trephine stoma. Br J Surg 1992;79: 1080–1081.

45
Polyps

Yoshihisa Saida

Polyps are one of the most common indications for laparoscopic surgery (Table 45.1). As polyps increase in size to greater than 2 cm in diameter, the difficulty of colonoscopic polypectomy increases and its safety decreases.[1] Although it is possible to excise some of these large polyps by piecemeal technique, this approach presents several disadvantages, including compromise of pathological staging of the lesion, an increased risk of perforation, and difficulties in hemostasis. A flat-elevated polyp, however, has a higher malignant potential than do pedunculated or sessile polyps.[2]

Colonic or rectal polyps that cannot be safely removed by colonoscopic or transanal techniques can be laparoscopically resected. Moreover, cases in which the probability of residual carcinoma (after colonoscopic polypectomy) is high are good indications for laparoscopic colorectal segmental resection. When the margin of polypectomy is positive for adenoma, a colonoscopic procedure may be required for rebiopsy of the lesion. However, if subsequent pathological findings are of concern, then laparoscopic colorectal segmental resection may be advisable.

Some authors have advocated laparoscopic treatment of a polyp by a colotomy and polypectomy,[3] by laparoscopic-assisted colonoscopic polypectomy,[4,5] or by colonoscopic-assisted intracorporeal laparoscopic wedge resection.[6] However, laparoscopic colorectal segmental resections are the most common and best accepted procedures for the appropriate treatment of colorectal polyps.[7,8] Although the lesser procedures such as colotomy or wedge resection may improve postoperative recovery time and substantially reduce disability,[9–11] they may not be adequate for cure of invasive neoplasia; they are mentioned here only to be condemned. Laparoscopic colectomy for large adenomatous neoplasms is both a feasible and a reasonable objective that offers more oncologically appropriate treatment. The rate of malignancy for villous adenomas is 8.3% to 41%, compared with 2.1% to 4.8% for all colorectal adenomas.[12] There-

fore, large villous adenomas must be removed by an oncologically acceptable segmental resection rather than a suboptimal procedure.

Several authors have reported good results with acceptably low morbidity and a low conversion rate in laparoscopic-assisted resection for colonic adenomatous polyps.[8,13–17] The overall mean length of hospitalization in these studies ranges from 4.1 to 9.1 days (Table 45.2). We performed laparoscopic surgery for polyps in 51 of the first 308 patients (16.6%) who underwent laparoscopic colorectal surgery between August 1991 and December 1997; during that time, polyps were the second most common indication for laparoscopic surgery, following Crohn's disease, in 60 patients (19.5%).[10] All patients underwent segmental resection for polyps; the mean length of hospitalization was 6.5 days.

Critical Components

Marking

Before any polyps can be treated with laparoscopic surgery, their location must be identified using one of the following methods.

Intraoperative Colonoscopy

After establishment of the pneumoperitoneum and initial exploration, the terminal ileum is gently occluded with an atraumatic bowel clamp. The colonoscope is then advanced into the colon under laparoscopic guidance. The light intensity of the laparoscope is decreased so that the colonoscope can be observed as it traverses the colon. The laparoscopic surgeon may then mark the location of the polyp with clips, sutures, or cautery. Intraoperative colonoscopy is frequently used during laparoscopic colectomy for precise localization of smaller, nonpalpable colonic lesions. However, the colonoscope may also be

397

TABLE 45.1. Possible indications for laparoscopic surgery for colorectal polyps.

Polyp cannot be safely removed by colonoscopic techniques (>2 cm)
Ployps with submucosal invasion
Polyp with positive margin of severe dysplasia
Polyp with other adenoma components

used to provide traction during the laparoscopic mobilization of the splenic and hepatic flexures.[18]

Preoperative Colonoscopic Injection of Dye

Preoperatively marking the intestinal wall adjacent to the polyp (ideally within 72 h before surgery) is performed by colonoscopic injection of sterile India ink through a sclerotherapy needle. Before injection of ink, a small amount of saline should be injected to lift the mucosal and submucosal layers and avoid perforating the serosa with the dye, which may cause distorted visualization. Also, complications of inadvertent intraperitoneal injections have been reported.[19,20] Other compounds, such as indocyanine green, have been utilized for the same purpose.[21] Previous dye injection avoids the potential of intestinal distension that can occur with intraoperative colonoscopy. Because it is impossible to know whether a lesion is on the mesenteric margin (in which case the dye cannot be laparoscopically visualized), injections at 90° intervals around the circumference of the band of the polyp should be undertaken. However, if there is any doubt about the polyp location, intraoperative colonoscopy is mandatory before resection.

Preoperative Contrast Enema

A preoperative contrast enema can provide a good indication of polyp location. Although the technique provides a good road map, it may not be accurate enough to allow intraoperative resection guidance.

Preoperative Preparation

Preoperative preparation for laparoscopic surgery of a polyp is the same as for any other laparoscopic procedure.[22] All patients receive a standard mechanical cathartic bowel preparation with a low dose of sodium phosphate. Both oral and parenteral antibiotic prophylactic preparations are also employed.[23,24] After the induction of general endotracheal anesthesia, a nasogastric tube and an indwelling bladder catheter are placed to minimize the risk of trocar injury to the stomach and bladder, respectively. There is an increased risk of deep venous thrombosis,[25] probably due to an increased level of CO_2 in the blood, from stasis resulting from positioning in reverse Trendelenburg, and from increased intra-abdominal pressure. Heparin or enoxaparin sodium injection therapy, as in laparotomy, may help prevent the occurrence of deep venous thrombosis. Additionally, the legs of patients are fitted with pneumatic compression antithrombotic stockings (PAS) to help prevent venous stasis and deep vein thrombosis.[26,27]

As a prerequisite for laparoscopic surgery, a thorough investigation should include a careful assessment of the risk of cardiac compromise when the abdomen is inflated under pressure of pneumoperitoneum as the preload is decreased and the afterload is increased. The respiratory compromise is usually less of a problem, but bleeding disorders must also be considered. It must be remembered that conversion to laparotomy is always a possibility so that the candidate for laparoscopic surgery should be a potential candidate for laparotomy as well. As such, both the patient and operating room should always be prepared so that, if necessary, conversion to laparotomy can be made without delay.

Port Placement

Port placement in laparoscopic colorectal surgery is as important as incision location length during laparotomy. The selection of port sites should depend on the proposed operation. Basically, these ports should be close enough together that instruments can easily reach the operative field in a straight visual line (Fig. 45.1). However, it is important that the instruments not clash within the peritoneal cavity, like "sword-fighting." An umbilical port is usually required. It should be noted, however, that there is no ideal port placement schema, because factors such as body habitus and the individual preferences of the surgeon affect site selection. For this reason, we prefer not to place all ports before starting the dissection but rather to add ports as needed after an anatomic assessment has been made.

Mobilization and Vascular Control

Before beginning the mobilization, a thorough visual inspection of the intraperitoneal contents is performed and adhesions are carefully lysed. These maneuvers are accomplished by a combination of gentle traction and

TABLE 45.2. Laparoscopy for adenomatous polyps.

Source	Total patients (n)	Polyps (n)	Length of stay, mean days (range)
Wexner et al.[8]	140	16	6.5 (4–12)
Zucker et al.[13]	65	14	4.1 (3–8)
Lumley et al.[14]	240	25	5 (3–35)
Tucker et al.[15]	114	14	4.8 (NS)
Gellman et al.[16]	104	20	5.7 (NS)
Jansen[17]	51	8	9.1 (4–29)

NS, not stated.

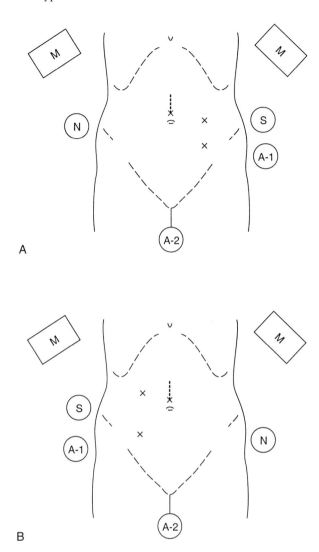

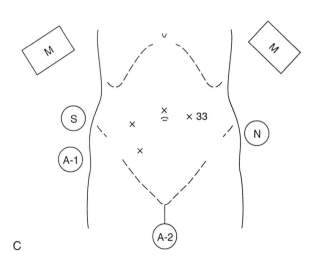

FIGURE 45.1. Suggested port, personnel, and equipment for (A) cecal polyp, (B) transverse colon polyp, and (C) left colonic polyp. *S*, surgeon; *M*, video monitor; *N*, nurse; *A-1*, first assistant; *A-2*, second assistant.

ultrasonic scalpel dissection (Ethicon Endosurgery, Cincinnati, OH, USA). We prefer the ultrasonic scalpel to either electrocautery or the laser for several reasons, including high power of coagulation, less smoke, which is important for clear visualization, lower potential of injury to adjacent organs, and lower cost.[28] Table positioning and retraction can help facilitate exposure. For example, when mobilizing the hepatic flexure, reverse Trendelenburg position and a table tilt to the left can help maintain loops of small bowel away from the operative field.

To expose its retroperitoneal attachments, the colon is gently grasped with noncrushing intestinal clamps and is medially reflected. Mobilization from the retroperitoneum is then accomplished by dividing along the avascular line of Toldt, using a combination of blunt and sharp dissection; the ultrasonic scalpel is particularly helpful at this stage of the operation. When the flexures are reached, larger vessels may be controlled either by the ultrasonic scalpel or with laparoscopic hemoclips. Detachment of the omentum from the transverse colon can usually be accomplished with the ultrasonic scalpel along the avascular plane between the two structures. Alternatively, it can be divided caudal to the gastroepiploic vessels.

Once full mobilization has been accomplished, the mesenteric vascular supply is divided. When the proximal ligation of mesenteric vessels is not required, this step may be performed in an extracorporeal fashion, along with the extracorporeal anastomosis. Intracorporeal vascular division is performed by skeletonization of the vessels and double ligation with surgical clips, sutures, or a 30-mm vascular cartridge on an endoscopic linear cutter stapler.

Anastomosis

After full intracorporeal mobilization and mesenteric vessel division, a small incision (usually 3–5cm) is made in the abdominal wall by enlarging the port. The mobilized colon is delivered; vessel ligation is accomplished unless previously intracorporeally performed; the bowel is divided; the specimen is retrieved intact; and an anastomosis is created. For the proximal colon (cecum, ascending, transverse, descending), the extracorporeal stapled side-to-side anastomosis is recommended as described in detail elsewhere.[29] For the sigmoid colon and rectum, intracorporeal anastomosis by an anastomotic device is in the usual manner.

References

1. Ballantune GH. Polypectomy. In: Ballantune GH, Leahy PF, Modlin IM (eds) Laparoscopic Surgery. Philadelphia: Saunders, 1994.

2. Watanabe T, Sawada T, Kubota Y, et al. Malignant potential in flat elevations. Dis Colon Rectum 1993;36:548–553.

3. Sacclarides TJ, Ko ST, Airan M. Laparoscopic removal of a large colonic lipoma. Report of a case. Dis Colon Rectum 1991;34:1027–1029.

4. Hensman C, Luck AJ, Hewett PJ. Laparoscopic assisted colonoscopic polypectomy: technique and preliminary experience. Surg Endosc 1999;13(3):231–232.

5. Beck DE, Karulf RE. Laparoscopic-assisted full-thickness endoscopic polypectomy. Dis Colon Rectum 1993; 36(7):693–695.

6. Shallman RW, Shaw TJ, Roach JM. Colonoscopically-assisted intracorporeal laparoscopic wedge resection of a benign right colon lesion. Surg Laparosc Endosc 1993;3:482–484.

7. Cohen SM, Wexner SD. Laparoscopic right hemicolectomy. In: Lezoche E, Paganini AM, Cuschieri A (eds) Minimally Invasive Colorectal Surgery. Milan: Documento Editoriale, 1994:23–26.

8. Wexner SD, Reissman P, Pfeifer J, Berstein M, Geron N. Laparoscopic colorectal surgery. Analysis of 140 cases. Surg Endosc 1996;10:133–136.

9. Alabaz O, Iroatulam AJN, Chen HH, Weiss EG, Wexner SD. Laparoscopic ileocolic resection with anastomosis for benign disease. Chir Laparosc 1997;3:219–222.

10. Saida Y, Sumiyama Y, Nagao J, Takase A. Low postoperative stress, early oral nutrition, and mobilization of laparoscopic operation for colon in comparison with traditional open approach. J Jpn Soc Coloproctol 1996;49:1087–1092.

11. Wexner SD, Cohen SM, Johansen OB, Nogueras JJ, Jagelman DG. Laparoscopic colorectal surgery: a prospective assessment and current perspective. Br J Surg 1993; 80:1602–1605.

12. Galadluk S, Fazio VW, Jagelman DG, et al. Villous and tubulovillous adenomas of the colon and rectum. Am J Surg 1987;153:41–47.

13. Zucker KA, Pitcher DE, Martin DT, Ford RS. Laparoscopic-assisted colon resection. Surg Endosc 1994;8:12–18.

14. Lumley JW, Fielding GA, Rhodes M, Nathanson LK, Siu S, Stitz RW. Laparoscopic-assisted colorectal surgery: lessons learned from 240 consecutive patients. Dis Colon Rectum 1996;39:155–159.

15. Tucker JG, Ambroze WL, Orangio GR, Duncan TD, Mason EM, Lucas GW. Laparoscopically assisted bowel surgery. Analysis of 114 cases. Surg Endosc 1995;9:297–300.

16. Gellman L, Salky B, Edye M. Laparoscopic assisted colectomy. Surg Endosc 1996;10:1041–1044.

17. Jansen A. Laparoscopic-assisted colon resection. Ann Chir Gynaecol 1994;83:86–91.

18. Reissman P, Teoh TA, Piccirillo M, Nogueras JJ, Wexner SD. Colonoscopic-assisted laparoscopic colectomy. Surg Endosc 1994;8:1352–1353.

19. Coman E, Brandt LJ, Brenner S, et al. Fat necrosis and inflammatory pseudotumor due to endoscopic tattooing of the colon with India ink. Gastrointest Endosc 1991;37: 65–68.

20. Park SI, Genta RS, Romeo DP, et al. Colonic abscess and focal peritonitis secondary to India ink tattooing of the colon. Gastrointest Endosc 1991;37:68–71.

21. Hammond DC, Lane FR, Mackeigan JM, Passinault WJ. Endoscopic tattooing of the colon: clinical experience. Am J Surg 1993;59:205–210.

22. Wexner SD, Beck DE. Sepsis prevention in colorectal surgery. In: Fielding LP, Goldberg SM (eds) Operative Surgery: Colon, Rectum and Anus, 5th Ed. Oxford: Butterworth Heinemann.

23. Cohen SM, Wexner SD, Binderow SR, et al. Prospective randomized endoscopic-blinded trial comparing pre-colonoscopy bowel cleaning methods. Dos Colon Rectum 1994;37:659–696.

24. Oliveira L, Wexner SD, Daniel N, et al. Mechanical bowel preparation for elective colorectal surgery. Dis Colon Rectum 1997;40:585–591.

25. Guillou OJ, Darzi A, et al. Experience with laparoscopic colorectal surgery for malignant disease. J Surg Oncol 1993; 2(suppl 1);43–49.

26. McCammon R. Anesthetic and positional complications. In: Jager RM, Wexner SD (eds) Laparoscopic Colorectal Surgery. New York: Churchill Livingstone, 1996:45–53.

27. Schwenk W, Bohn B, Fugener A, Muller JM. Intermittent pneumatic sequential compression of the lower extremities prevents venous stasis during laparoscopic cholecystectomy. A prospective randomized study. Surg Endosc 1998; 12:7–11.

28. Moreira H Jr, Yamaguchi T, Choi J, Sardinha C, Billotti V, Wexner S. Safety of sodium hyaluronate-based membrane (Seprafilm™) after bowel injury: a prospective randomized trial. Dis Colon Rectum 1998;41:A6–A7.

29. Jager M, Wexner SD. Laparoscopic Colorectal Surgery. New York: Churchill Livingstone, 1996.

46
Colonic Carcinoma

Emina Huang and R. Larry Whelan

Laparoscopic-assisted techniques for colon resection, although currently considered the gold standard for cholecystectomy and gastroesophageal reflux procedures, have not yet replaced laparotomy. In no other area is the controversy regarding this approach as heated as in the area of the minimal access approach to colonic carcinoma. Currently, long-term randomized data regarding survival and recurrence rates are lacking. Additionally, with some investigators reporting port site tumor incidences as high as 21%,[1] most surgeons have been less than enthusiastic about minimally invasive colectomy for cancer. Proponents note that numerous recent clinical series include wound tumor incidences of 0% to 1% and that most reports have documented short-term benefits. Largely in an effort to determine the long-term survival and recurrence rates, including the incidence of abdominal wound tumors, several randomized and prospective trials have been initiated. The largest trial to date is the National Cancer Institute's Clinical Outcomes of Surgical Therapies (COST) Trial, which thus far has enrolled more than 600 patients. In addition to long-term outcome data, the randomized trials will also answer questions regarding short-term results, adequacy of resection, and the length of surgery. Since its introduction in 1991, laparoscopic colectomy techniques have evolved considerably and have been modified, especially in regard to cancer resection. A sizable number of animal and human studies have been undertaken that consider the impact of laparotomy and CO_2 pneumoperitoneum on tumor growth and abdominal wound tumors, as well as methods of avoiding these recurrences.

Definitions

Because there is no universally accepted nomenclature regarding minimally invasive colectomy and because the extent of the operation laparoscopically performed, as well as the names used to describe these operations, may vary considerably from surgeon to surgeon, it is crucial that the terms used in this chapter be well defined. A laparoscopic-assisted colon resection (LACR) entails full mobilization of the colon and at least partial intracorporeal resection of the bowel before making the "assisted" incision. The intracorporeal portion of the procedure usually includes proximal division of the main vascular bundle of the segment in question. The incision for specimen removal and facilitation of anastomosis is usually no larger than 5 to 8 cm. On the left side, an intracorporeal double-stapled anastomosis is usually undertaken after the proximal anvil has been extracorporeally placed, whereas on the right side an extracorporeal anastomosis is performed. A fully laparoscopic procedure involves transanal removal of the specimen and is not recommended by most surgeons. A laparoscopic-facilitated procedure involves a larger incision, greater than 8 cm long, through which mobilization and resection may be completed, and the anastomosis fashioned.

Hand-assisted laparoscopic operations, which are not discussed in this chapter, are undertaken with one hand in the abdomen while the abdomen is insufflated. Proponents believe that the operation can be significantly shortened and simplified with the help of the intraabdominal hand. According to these definitions, hand-assisted laparoscopic procedures would most likely fall into the laparoscopic-facilitated category because an incision of at least 8 cm is needed to insert the hand of most surgeons.

Contraindications

Patients with very large tumors may not be good candidates because such lesions are more difficult to safely manipulate laparoscopically and require a sizable incision for specimen removal regardless. A true laparoscopic-assisted resection in this instance may not be a wise choice; however, a hybrid procedure, which is described next, may be an option for some of these lesions. Tumors that are thought to have invaded adjacent organs (T4 lesions) are not candidates for LACR because it may not be possible to laparoscopically perform the required en bloc removal of the lesion and attached adjacent organ(s) with clean margins. As per the COST study criteria, patients with transverse colon lesions are not candidates for laparoscopic colectomy. It was initially thought that transverse colectomy was too difficult because both flexures need to be mobilized and the middle colic vessels divided. It is now clear that this operation, although difficult, is feasible provided the surgeon has the prerequisite skills. Presently, only elective resection for potentially curable colon cancer in select patients is being undertaken in the study. Emergency procedures for obstructing, perforated, or acutely bleeding lesions are not advised thus far. A history of previous abdominal surgery is a relative contraindication at the surgeon's discretion. In these cases, the initial trocar should be placed by a carefully performed incision distant to all scar(s). If the surgeon cannot obtain enough working space to perform the operation, then conversion will be necessary. It is wise to carefully assess the situation after the first 30 to 45 min of the operation. If adhesiolysis is imminent at that point, then it is probably best to convert to laparotomy, to avoid lengthy enterolysis. Patients with severe pulmonary disease or cardiac disease (class 4 status, American Society of Anesthesiology) are not considered as candidates for the laparoscopic colectomy trial because of concerns that they cannot tolerate a prolonged CO_2 pneumoperitoneum. The use of an abdominal wall lifting device, an alternative gas for insufflation (e.g., helium), or a hybrid approach that includes lifting devices and a low-pressure pneumoperitoneum are minimally invasive exposure alternatives for this difficult patient group.

Rectal Cancer Resections

The use of the laparoscope for curative rectal resection is outside the purview of the present North American randomized prospective trial. Laparoscopic abdominoperineal resection (APR), although challenging, is feasible in many patients, as is anterior resection. Although some surgeons are performing minimally invasive resections for distal and proximal rectal cancers, most are not attempting laparoscopic-assisted resection of midrectal cancers. Such lesions require full rectal and mesorectal mobilization to the levators from above as well as distal division of the rectum deep in the pelvis. The latter task is very hard to accomplish given the technical limitations of current stapling instruments. Similarly, in the opinion of the authors, laparoscopic coloanal sphincter-saving procedures are ill advised. A phase 1

study to analyze laparoscopic rectal resection is underway with the goal of creating a randomized rectal cancer trial.

Although a true laparoscopic-assisted rectal resection remains controversial, a hybrid procedure that includes laparoscopic splenic flexure mobilization and, possibly, proximal division of the main sigmoidal vessels followed by a lower abdominal laparotomy and rectal resection may be a reasonable option. In most cases, this approach obviates the need for the supraumbilical extension of the midline incision that is usually necessary for the sole purpose of mobilizing the flexure to allow a tension-free anastomosis. In the authors' opinion, the patient still benefits substantially if the supraumbilical incision is avoided even though a 10- to 15-cm infraumbilical incision has been made. This type of hybrid procedure is also a reasonable option in patients with large colonic tumors or tumors that may be fixed. For example, if a large cecal tumor is thought to be invading the abdominal sidewall, laparoscopic flexure mobilization and, possibly, division of the ileocecal vascular bundle is followed by an 8- to 12-cm incision through which the tumor and portion of sidewall are resected and the operation is completed.

Port Placement

Judicious port placement facilitates performance of the procedure with the fewest possible ports and minimal clashing of instruments causing interference. Ideal port placement allows the surgeon to work in the same direction as the camera is pointed for most of the case. Right colectomy can usually be performed with four ports; however, most left-sided resections require five ports, in the authors' experience. The size of the ports to be placed depends almost entirely on the chosen method of vascular control (monopolar or bipolar cautery, ultrasonic shears, staplers, clips, ties, or other) and the type of laparoscopic equipment available. The goal is to use as many 5-mm ports as possible because the 10- to 12-mm ports require fascial closure and are more traumatic. Most surgeons utilize a 10-mm telescope, although some of the newer 5-mm telescopes may prove adequate for colectomy. A 12-mm port will be needed if a laparoscopic linear stapling device is to be used. Ultrasonic shears and devices of 5 mm now on the market, if available, obviate the need for the 10-mm ports required for the original 10-mm ultrasonic instruments. Similarly, adequate 5-mm atraumatic bowel graspers are now available that can be used in place of 10-mm Babcock clamps or other 10-mm graspers.

Port placement must be individualized based on the patient's body habitus and the segment of the bowel to be removed. A midline supra- or infraumbilical port is almost always utilized as the telescope port. Usually, this port is to be placed first except when the patient has had prior incisions in this area. The lateral abdominal ports are ideally placed lateral to the rectus abdominus muscle to avoid injuring the epigastric vessels. This pattern usually provides access to both the flexures and at least the proximal part of the pelvis. However, in patients with a very broad abdomen or a long xyphoid-to-pubis distance, it may not be possible to reach the flexure with the ports in this configuration. In these patients it may be useful to place the lateral ports in a more medial location so as to increase the reach through that port; rarely, a sixth port may be required.

Exfoliated viable tumor cells are, most likely, present in the abdomen during these procedures and may reside in the free intraperitoneal fluid, on the ports and instruments, on serosal surfaces, or in the CO_2 gas as an aerosol. Port dislodgement during a case allows a tumor cell-contaminated port tip or instrument to contact the port wound, thus providing an opportunity for tumor cell seeding. Desufflation, either intentional or accidental, may also provide transportation for liberated tumor cells to the port wounds. Thus, instead of "bleeding" ports via the insufflation stopcock to decrease the level of pneumoperitoneum, suctioning via a centrally placed suction/irrigation device is advised. To prevent inadvertent dislodgement of the ports, as well as sudden desufflation, and to maintain the intraabdominal location of the ports, different methods of port anchoring have been utilized. Screw grips that can be attached to the ports facilitate this immobilization; however, grips do not provide adequate protection against dislodgement. In addition to the grips, the authors advise using a skin suture placed near the port entry site that is loosely tied, then looped several times around the insufflation armature, and then secured with a small clamp.

Tumor Localization

Once pneumoperitoneum has been established and the ports placed, the location of the tumor must be confirmed before mobilization and resection. Large lesions can usually be located without much difficulty by carefully balloting and palpating the bowel with a Babcock clamp or other instrument. The bowel must be very carefully handled at this stage to avoid inadvertently traumatizing the tumor. Once it is located, clips can be placed proximal and distal to the lesion to mark the segment. Preoperative colonoscopic tattooing, with India ink or other dyes, is an alternate means of marking the site of lesions. A preoperative barium enema can also identify the general location of the tumor. However, despite these measures, it may not be possible to locate the tumor at surgery. In these instances, intraoperative colonoscopy is necessary and, for this reason, a colonoscope should be

available for all laparoscopic colonic cases. When the lesion is localized, the segment can be marked with either a laparoscopically placed clip or suture. When performing colonoscopy in this setting, it is important to prevent small bowel distension, which can occur if the ileocecal valve is incompetent. An atraumatic laparoscopic clamp can be used to occlude the bowel proximal to the colon exam. It is easier to occlude the terminal ileum than the colon because of the considerably larger diameter of the latter and the tendency of the distended distal colon to dislocate the occluding clamps. One disadvantage to occluding the distal ileum is that, at the conclusion of the exam, the colonoscope must be inserted, at least to the distal ascending colon, to fully decompress the colon before withdrawal.

Mobilization and Devascularization

Once the tumor has been localized, one of two different approaches may be used to mobilize and devascularize the segment in question. The first method entails early devascularization followed by medial to lateral mobilization of the bowel. The second technique utilizes a more standard lateral to medial dissection and mobilization followed by devascularization. The former method embraces a number of the components of Turnbull's "no touch" technique, most notably early devascularization and avoidance of early tumor manipulation. Although Turnbull's method has never been shown to be associated with significantly better results than that of the more standard lateral to medial approach, it has been embraced by many laparoscopic surgeons for two basic reasons. First, they claim this method is easier, as the exposure obtained during laparoscopy lends itself to initial division of the principal vascular bundle and a medial to lateral approach. The lateral attachments serve to retract the specimen laterally and thus facilitate the medial dissection. Leaving the colon in place also allows the surgeon orientation when necessary. The last step is the division of the "white line of Toldt." Second, in the authors' opinion, many laparoscopic cancer surgeons are obsessed with avoiding the spillage or liberation of tumor cells from the primary tumor that might increase the chances of a port tumor or other intraabdominal recurrence.

It is not necessary to fully adhere to Turnbull's method to derive significant benefit from the medial to lateral approach. If only the main vascular pedicles are divided early in the operation, the procedure will still be facilitated. On the left side, in the process of dividing the main sigmoidal vessels, the left ureter and the gonadal vessels must be identified near the iliac fossa as the rectosigmoid mesentery is posteriorly mobilized. On the right side, preparation for division of the main ileocolic vessels will have fully exposed the duodenum and right upper quadrant retroperitoneum. Once the main vascular bundle has been divided, even if subsequent conversion to laparotomy is necessary, the laparotomy will have been greatly facilitated. The segment to be removed is considerably more mobile once the main vessels have been divided. The details regarding the technique of colon resection are found elsewhere in this volume and are not repeated here, with the exception of brief descriptions of how to divide the main vascular bundles on the left and right at the beginning of the case.

The avascular "clear space" between the ileocolic and the middle colic vessels is readily exposed by gently anteriorly retracting the distal ascending colon and the proximal transverse colon with the patient in reverse Trendelenburg and the left side of the table down. The duodenum can usually be seen through the thin layer of peritoneum in this area. A window in this clear space is made immediately anterior to the duodenum. The ileocolic bundle is immediately caudal to this window and is readily seen by retracting either the cecum or the distal mesentery near the cecum, upward and toward the right lower quadrant. The bundle is isolated and thinned by dividing the peritoneum proximal to and overlying the vessels close to their origins and by carefully dissecting, in a blunt fashion, lateral to these vessels. This dissection allows entry to the window already created anterior to the duodenum. A linear stapler with a vascular cartridge is then used to divide and secure the bundle. At this point, the remaining ileal mesentery or the right branch of the middle colic artery can be dissected and divided, thus completing the mesenteric division; alternatively, the bowel can be mobilized.

To expose and isolate the main sigmoidal vessels, the rectosigmoid colon is anteriorly retracted through the left-sided ports and the patient is placed in Trendelenburg position with the right side of the table down. The dissection is begun at the base of the right side of the rectosigmoid mesentery at the sacral promontory level. The main vessels may be readily visible in thin patients with the bowel retracted as already described. The peritoneum is scored along the base of the mesentery caudad into the pelvis for 3 to 5 cm; it is usually easy to locate the avascular plane between the mesentery and the presacral tissues. Once it is identified, the dissection is continued toward the left side. It is important to stay immediately adjacent to the vessels to avoid the hypogastric nerves. The left ureter and gonadal vessels are then exposed through this right-sided approach, and the colon mesentery is carefully dissected away from these structures. Next, the main vascular bundle is defined by retracting the bowel anteriorly and inferiorly. The peritoneum on the right side of the mesentery overlying the vascular bundle is proximally scored and a mesenteric window created on the proximal side of the bundle through a combination of careful sharp and blunt dissection. The bundle is thinned and then divided with a linear stapler at the desired level. It is possible to dissect further proximally to expose the origin of the inferior mesenteric artery (IMA) if ligation close to the origin of the IMA is desired.

Not every patient or tumor lends itself to the medial to lateral approach. The more accepted lateral to medial mobilization followed by mesenteric devascularization may be more appropriate in some cases and can be accomplished while adhering to standard surgical oncologic principles. Regardless of the approach, it is crucial that the tumor be localized and direct contact with the tumor avoided. It is also important that sufficient bowel be mobilized before specimen removal that a tension-free anastomosis can be constructed. It is the authors' practice to routinely fully mobilize the splenic flexure and at least the left half of the transverse colon for left-sided lesions and to similarly mobilize the hepatic flexure and right half of the transverse colon for all right colonic neoplasms.

Specimen Retrieval

A plastic specimen bag or wound protector should be used for all laparoscopic cancer resections to decrease the chances of shedding tumor cells into the wound. If the specimen has been fully detached, then it can be placed in a bag. Once the enlarged port incision has been made, the bag can be maneuvered into and through the wound. To facilitate extraction of the specimen, the externalized portion of the bag can be opened, and either end of the specimen can be located and grasped within the bag and then pulled through the bag-lined wound.

If the bowel specimen remains attached at either one or both ends, then a bag will not work well because the open end of the bag cannot be fully closed and may slide off before the specimen is extirpated. The authors advise using either a commercially available or a self-made plastic wound protector in this situation. If homemade, a plastic sleeve about 3 to 4 in. in height, cut from a sterile camera bag or other plastic bag, is placed in the enlarged wound. Several small slits approximately 1 in. in length can be made on the end that is put into the abdomen so that the specimen does not get caught on the sleeve when being withdrawn. Care must be taken to ensure that the entire depth of the wound is covered by the plastic sleeve, and two medium-sized retractors are used to hold the bag in place. With the retractors in place, the specimen is then withdrawn through the center of the sleeve. To facilitate locating the specimen and for removal before desufflation, a laparoscopic loop tie is placed on the specimen, well away from the tumor, and the long end of the suture can be delivered through the port to be enlarged. A

Babcock clamp can also be gently placed on the specimen via the same port for the same purpose.

It can be frustrating and exasperating to extract a fully mobilized segment of bowel through the wound. Large epiploicae, a fatty mesentery, a twisted piece of bowel, or a piece of omentum may thwart facile extraction. The plastic sleeve wound protector and retractors can also trap a piece of the specimen in the abdomen or between the retractor and the edge of the wound. When difficulty is encountered during removal, the surgeon should place a finger into the abdomen via the wound and sweep it around the specimen searching for the cause of the problem. Reorientation of the specimen or delivery of a previously excluded piece of the specimen will usually permit the safe removal of the bowel segment. If these efforts fail, then the wound must be enlarged. Despite the fact that much of the point of minimally invasive colectomy is to avoid a large incision, it is critical that a sufficiently large incision be made that the specimen can be safely removed. A 6-cm tumor is likely to be traumatized or fractured if extracted via a 4-cm wound. The primary concern of the surgeon should be to atraumatically remove the tumor-containing bowel segment, not to make the smallest possible incision.

Facilitation and Performance of Anastomosis

If a laparoscopic transanal double-stapled circular EEA-type anastomosis is anticipated after extracorporeal placement of the proximal anvil, then the proper orientation of the proximal bowel will be intracorporeally determined. If an extracorporeal anastomosis is planned, however, proper orientation of the proximal and distal bowel ends that are to be joined is critical. When working through a small wound, it can be very difficult to know when one of the bowel ends is twisted. The surgeon might face several different scenarios once the specimen has been removed. The extent to which the bowel resection was intracorporeally undertaken may determine the specific dilemma. The three possible situations (with respect to the bowel) at the time of specimen removal are (1) a fully resected and detached specimen, (2) a bowel segment that remains attached at one end (either proximally or distally), and (3) a mobilized (and possibly devascularized) segment of bowel that remains in continuity both proximally and distally.

The first situation permits easy removal of the specimen but makes proper orientation of the ends of the bowel to be subsequently anastomosed more difficult. Faced with two ends of bowel extruding from a small wound, it is hard to tell if one or both ends are twisted. The best way to avoid this problem is to intracorporeally suture the proximal and distal bowel ends together in the

proper orientation before enlargement of the wound. This step ensures that the bowel will not be twisted when the ends are delivered through the wound for anastomosis. If this maneuver was not accomplished before wound enlargement, then the surgeon must first locate the two ends within the abdomen to be externalized. The two ends can be "tagged" with loop ties or sutures before desufflation and the long ends of the suture delivered through the port to be enlarged. After the bowel is externalized, the divided edge of the mesentery is traced back into the abdomen with a finger, as far as possible along the proximal and distal ends of the bowel. If any doubt remains about bowel orientation, then the wound should be enlarged until proper alignment can be confirmed.

If the bowel has not been intracorporeally divided, either proximally or distally, orientation of the bowel ends once resection has been completed should not be a problem. However, the extraction process in this situation is more difficult because there is no cut end to bring into the wound; instead, a folded length of bowel and mesentery must be brought through the wound. Although this approach is best for assurance of appropriate limb orientation, it may require a larger wound for safe extraction.

In the last scenario, the bowel has been intracorporeally divided in a single place and the specimen is still attached to the intact gut at one end. In this situation it is usually not difficult to properly orient the attached end. The other end, which is free, can be twisted, however. Once outside, the cut edge should be traced as described and the orientation determined.

Tumoricidal Irrigation

A number of practices have been devised over the years in an effort to decrease the chances of intraabdominal and bowel suture line tumor recurrences. As an example, Turnbull's "no touch" method included intraluminal colonic irrigation with a tumoricidal solution. The laparoscopic era rejuvenated this awareness regarding liberated viable tumor cells in the abdominal cavity because of the many early reported port wound tumors. It has been well established that tumor cells can often be recovered from blood or fluid from both the specimen and the abdominal cavity at the time of colectomy for cancer. Therefore, it is reasonable to destroy these liberated tumor cells before they have the opportunity to implant and develop into tumor recurrences. A variety of tumoricidal solutions have been devised for this purpose. The surgeon can utilize tumoricidal solutions in three places during colectomy: (1) the colon lumen, (2) the abdomen, and (3) the abdominal wounds.

Intraluminal irrigation with tumoricidal agents before resection of the bowel or anastomosis, as mentioned, has been practiced by some surgeons for decades. The goal is to destroy any viable free tumor cells that may be present in the bowel lumen. The most popular agents include chlorhexidine, mercuric perchloride, and povidone-iodine and water.[2,3] Although these irrigation agents have been tested in vivo, randomized human trials have not been undertaken. It makes sense to perform the irrigation before resection so that the bowel proximal to the lesion is exposed to the solution. This irrigation can be accomplished either transanally with a bulb syringe or catheter for left-sided lesions, or through a colonoscope.

Shed tumor cells may also be present in the abdominal cavity or the wounds. Intermittent, thorough irrigation and suction with saline during the procedure is advised and should (at least in theory) reduce the number of tumor cells left in the abdomen at the end of the operation. The following have been studied during animal experiments: (1) povidone-iodine, (2) taurolidine, (3) chlorhexidine, (4) methotrexate, and (5) 5-fluorouracil.[4-7] The most effective, based on current animal study results, appear to be taurolidine and a diluted povidone-iodine solution. The former agent is not commercially available in the United States but is used in Europe and elsewhere. The latter method is being used by an unknown number of laparoscopic surgeons in the United States.

The tumoricidal effects of povidone-iodine have been well established both in vitro and in vivo.[1,3,8] In one study, povidone-iodine was shown to have an effective cytotoxic property even at a dilution of 1:1000.[1] Toxicity from peritoneal povidone-iodine irrigation depends on three factors: concentration, amount, and length of exposure. Acute toxicity from a single intraperitoneal lavage with povidone-iodine is rare; there are only three reported cases. One patient developed tachydysrhythmia,[9] and two patients developed sclerosing encapsulating peritonitis following irrigation with full-strength povidone-iodine (10%), most of which was left inside the abdomen.[10] In 1979, Sindelar and Mason reported the only randomized controlled clinical trial in which intraperitoneal povidone-iodine lavage was evaluated. In this study, 168 patients with bacterially contaminated abdomens were randomized to control, saline irrigation, or povidine-iodine irrigation. The povidine-iodine irrigation group underwent 60-s intraperitoneal irrigation with 1 liter 1% povidine-iodine, after which more than 90% of the irrigant, on average, was recovered. A significantly decreased intraabdominal abscess rate was noted in the povidine-iodine group; none of the patients developed complications related to the povidone-iodine irrigation.[11]

It is the authors' practice to irrigate both the abdomen and the wounds during both laparotomy and laparoscopic cases with a dilute solution of povidone-iodine (1%; 9:1 dilution of the commercially available solutions). The solution is allowed to dwell for 1 min and then is suctioned from the abdomen. The abdomen is then irrigated with several liters of saline. Although admittedly anecdotal, no complications relating to the use of dilute povidone-iodine irrigation, as just described, have been noted in more than 100 consecutive laparoscopic-assisted colectomies.

Adequacy of Resection

Reasonably, surgeons have questioned whether a comparable resection of bowel and mesentery could be accomplished using laparoscopic methods when compared to laparotomy. Most nonrandomized studies have compared a current laparoscopic colectomy series to an historical group of patients after laparotomy. Most of these analyses have failed to demonstrate any significant differences in either the size of the specimens or the average number of lymph nodes harvested. However, such studies are less than ideal because patient selection bias, which is likely to be present in many of the early series, favors the laparoscopic groups. However, preliminary results from two small internally controlled nonpeer-reviewed randomized prospective trials from the Cleveland Clinic Foundation and Barcelona, Spain, have failed to demonstrate any significant benefits relative to specimen size, proximal or distal margins, length of resected mesentery, or number of harvested lymph nodes between the laparotomy and laparoscopic groups.[12,13] Together, these two trials involved more than 300 patients. In conclusion, the data, thus far, suggest that a skilled laparoscopic surgeon can perform an adequate oncologic resection.

Long-Term Results

Unfortunately, the 5-year results from the small externally monitored prospective randomized trials mentioned earlier are not yet available. The preliminary local recurrence and survival results from the Barcelona randomized trial with a mean follow-up of more than 2 years are similar for the open and the minimally invasive colectomy groups.[13] A preliminary report involved a consecutive series of patients who underwent either laparoscopy (191) or laparotomy (224) from two different institutions[14]; the length of follow-up varied from 30 to 37 months. The groups were well matched for age, sex, and tumor stage. There were no significant differences in survival, local and distant recurrence rates, or disease-free survival when the two groups were compared by stage. Other recently presented nonrandomized uncontrolled studies of laparoscopic colectomy patients have anecdotally demonstrated 5-year survival and local recurrence rates within the range of results from previously published series of laparotomies. In summary, to date, survival and recurrence rates after laparoscopic colectomy appear to be in the same range as those after laparotomy. Significant improvements have been noted; the 5-year results from the peer-reviewed externally monitored prospective randomized trials are awaited. The surgeons who have thus far reported equivalent results are all technically acclaimed laparoscopists. Therefore, their results may not be representative of those of the average community surgeon. Even these experts were only able to find equivalence, and not superiority, of laparoscopy as compared to laparotomy.

Port Site Tumors

The majority of general and colorectal surgeons have refrained from performing laparoscopic colectomy for cancer because of concerns regarding port site tumors. In large part, these tumors were also the driving force that led to the randomized trials presently under way. The literature contains reports regarding at least 50 patients who have developed tumors at a port site or at the wound used for specimen extraction. Although most tumors have occurred in patients with Dukes' C or D lesions, some lesions have occurred in patients with Dukes' A and B lesions. The reported incidence of abdominal wound tumors following laparoscopic colectomy varies from 0% to 21%.[1] It is important to note that abdominal wound tumors may develop after laparotomy: the incidence of incisional tumors in two large retrospective reviews ranged from 0.6% to 0.68%.[15,16] The majority of the early publications regarding port site tumors were case reports and small series that represented the initial experiences of surgeons with laparoscopic-assisted colectomy. In larger series published in the past several years, the incidence has ranged from 0% to 1.3%.[17] However, the true incidence is presently unknown. The randomized trials already mentioned should provide the best data. The preliminary reports from the single center randomized trials carried out at the Cleveland Clinic Foundation and in the Barcelona trials report a 0% to 1% incidence of report wound tumors.[12,13] Again, these results represent single surgeon series and may not be reflective of general practice.

In summary, recent human studies have reported port wound tumor incidences of 0% to 1.2%. The etiology remains unclear, although many laparoscopic surgeons believe that surgical technique is the most important variable in the recurrence of these tumors. Traumatization of the tumor via direct handling of the tumor-bearing segment during mobilization or at the time of specimen extraction appears to be one of the means by which tumor cells become separated from the primary lesion. Animal studies suggest that the CO_2 pneumoperitoneum may also play a role in the formation of these tumors.

Immunological and Oncologic Consequences of Minimally Invasive Colectomy

Laparotomy results in suppression of cell-mediated immune function. Animal and human studies have demonstrated, through study of a variety of parameters, that there is significantly less cell-mediated immunosuppression following pneumoperitoneum and laparoscopic procedures than after the equivalent laparotomy.[18–22] A human study that measured delayed-type hypersensitivity (DTH) responses before and after colectomy by both laparoscopy and laparotomy demonstrated a significant decrease in the mean area of postoperative DTH responses after laparotomy when compared to their preoperative responses. Conversely, the pre- and postoperative responses in the laparoscopic group were not significantly different.[23] Other animal studies have demonstrated that a full-length sham laparotomy when postoperatively compared to CO_2 pneumoperitoneum is associated with increased tumor growth and an increased incidence of tumor establishment.[24] More specifically, tumor cell turnover has been shown to be increased and apoptosis decreased after laparotomy.[25,26] In light of these results, it seems reasonable to wonder if preservation of immune function and avoidance of a large laparotomy wound might convey some oncologic benefit to minimally invasive colectomy patients. In theory, local intraabdominal recurrence rates may be lower and long-term survival rates higher after laparoscopic colectomy than after laparotomy. Despite these attractive theories, there is no human evidence to support the concept that a significant benefit in survival or recurrence rates exist after laparoscopic colectomy.

Training

The early port site tumor experience has made it abundantly clear that curative colectomy for colon cancer should be attempted only after laparoscopic colectomy techniques have been mastered on patients with benign colonic disorders. Laparoscopic-assisted colon resection for colon cancer is challenging for the following reasons: (1) it requires working in two or three quadrants of the abdomen; (2) the bowel must be mobilized and devascularized; (3) a sizable specimen must be removed; and (4) an anastomosis often must be fashioned. Laparoscopic appendectomy and colostomy formation are reasonable early cases that allow the surgeon to gain experience handling bowel and mastering the two-handed technique. Elective segmental sigmoid colectomy for uncomplicated diverticular disease and inflammatory bowel disease as well as rectopexy and sigmoid resection for rectal prolapse are reasonable second-tier cases that provide an opportunity to learn bowel mobilization and devascularization techniques as well as laparoscopic double-stapled transrectal circular end-to-end anastomotic methods. Palliative colon resection for those patients with known metastatic disease may also be resonable at this point. The last cases to be attempted are the curative cancer resections and the large benign neoplasms that are not amenable to endoscopic removal. Unless endoscopic ultrasound has been done to confirm absence of invasive cancer (via demonstration of penetration through the submucosal layer of the bower wall), these cases should be cautiously treated because they may harbor areas of invasive cancer.

The randomized trials in progress will, it is hoped, answer the important outstanding questions regarding the safety and efficacy of laparoscopic methods for the curative treatment of colon cancers. In the opinion of the authors, until these results are available, surgeons performing these minimally invasive operations should do so in the setting of an externally monitored, peer-reviewed prospective randomized trial.

References

1. Berends FJ, Kazemier G, Bonjer HJ, Lange JF. Subcutaneous metastases after laparoscopic colectomy [letter]. Lancet 1994;344:58.
2. Umpleby HC, Williamson RC. The efficacy of agents employed to prevent anastomotic recurrence in colorectal carcinoma. Ann R Coll Surg Engl 1994;662:192–194.
3. Docherty JG, McGregor JR, Purdie CA, et al. Efficacy of tumoricidal agents *in vitro* and *in vivo*. Br J Surg 1995; 82:1050–1052.
4. Jacobi CA, Ordemann J, Bohm B, Zieren HU, Sabat R, Muller JM. Inhibition of peritoneal tumor cell growth and implantation in laparoscopic surgery in a rat model. Presented at International Meeting of Animal Laparoscopic Researchers in Frankfurt, Germany, 1997.
5. Neuhaus SJ, Watson DI, Ellis T, et al. Efficacy of cytotoxic agents for the prevention of laparoscopic port site metastases [abstract]. Surg Endosc 1998;12(8):515.
6. Lee SW, Gleason NR, Woodring J, et al. Peritoneal irrigation with betadine solution following laparoscopic splenectomy significantly decreases port tumor recurrence in a murine model [abstract]. Dis Colon Rectum 1998; 41(4):A24.
7. Schneider C, Reymond MA, Tannapfel A, et al. Port site metastases can be largely prevented [abstract]. Surg Endosc 1998;12(5):517.
8. Lucarotti ME, White H, Deas J, et al. Antiseptic toxicity to breast carcinoma in tissue culture: an adjuvant to conservation therapy? Ann R Coll Surg Engl 1990; 72:388–392.
9. Glick PL, Guglielmo J, Tranbaugh RF, et al. Idoine toxicity in a patient treated by continuous povidone-iodine mediastinal irrigation. Ann Thorac Surg 1985;39:478–480.
10. Keating JP, Neill M, Hill GL. Sclerosing encapsulating peritonitis after intraperitoneal use of povidone iodine. Aust N Z J Surg 1997;67:742–744.
11. Sindelar WF, Mason GR. Intraperitoneal irrigation with povidone-iodine solution for the prevention of intra-abdominal abscesses in the bacterially contaminated abdomen. Surg Gynecol Obstet 1979;148:409–411.
12. Milsom JW, Bohm B, Hammerhofer KA, et al. A prospective, randomized trial comparing conventional techniques in colorectal cancer surgery: a preliminary report. J Am Coll Surg 1998;187:46–54.
13. Lacy AM, Delgado S, Garcia-Valdecasas JC, et al. Port site metastases and recurrence after laparoscopic colectomy. A randomized trial. Surg Endosc 1998; 12(8):1039–1042.
14. Franklin ME, Rosenthal D, Abrego-Medina D, et al. Prospective comparison of open versus laparoscopic colon surgery for carcinoma: five year results. Dis Colon Rectum 1996;39(suppl 10):s35–s46.
15. Hughes ESR, McDermott FT, Polglase AL, et al. Tumor recurrence in the abdominal wall scar after large-bowel cancer surgery. Dis Colon Rectum 1983; 26(9):571–572.
16. Reilly WT, Nelson H, Schroeder G, Wieand HS, et al. Wound recurrence following conventional treatment of colorectal cancer. Dis Colon Rectum 1996;39:200–207.
17. Fleshman JW, Nelson H, Peters WR, et al. Early results laparoscopic surgery for colorectal cancer: retrospective analysis of 372 patients treated by Clinical Outcomes of Surgical Therapy (COST) Study Group. Dis Colon Rectum 1996;39:s53–s58.
18. Trokel MJ, Bessler M, Treat MR, Whelan RL, Nowygrod R. Preservation of immune response after laparoscopy. Surg Endosc 1994;8(12):1385–1388.
19. Allendorf JD, Bessler M, Whelan RL, et al. Better preservation of immune function after laparoscopic-assisted vs. open bowel resection in a murine model. Dis Colon Rectum 1996;39(suppl 10):s67–s72.
20. Griffith JP, Everitt NJ, Lancaster F, Boylston A, et al. Influence of laparoscopic and conventional cholecystectomy upon cell-mediated immunity. Br J Surg 1995; 82:677–680.
21. Horgan PG, Fitzpatrick M, Couse NF, Gorey TF, Fitzpatrick JM. Laparoscopy is less immunotraumatic than laparotomy. Minim Invasive Ther 1992;1:241–244.
22. Decker D, Schondorf M, Bidlingmaier F, Hirner A, von Ruecker AA. Surgical stress induces a shift in the type-1/type-2 T-helper cell balance, suggesting downregulation of cell-mediated and upregulation of antibody-mediated immunity commensurate to the trauma. Surgery (St. Louis) 1996;119:316–325.
23. Whelan RL, Franklin M, Donahue J, et al. Postoperative cell-mediated immune response is better preserved after laparoscopic versus open colectomy in humans: a preliminary study [abstract]. Surg Endosc 1998; 12(4).
24. Allendorf JD, Bessler M, Kayton M, et al. Tumor growth after laparoscopy and laparotomy in a murine model. Arch Surg 1995;130:649–653.

25. Allendorf JD, Bessler M, Whelan RL, et al. Differences in tumor growth after open versus laparoscopic surgery are lost in an athymic model and are associated with differences in tumor proliferative index. Surg Forum 1996; XLVII:150–152.

26. Lee SW, Gleason NR, Ssenymanturno K, Woodring JV, Bessler M, Whelan RL. Colon cancer tumor proliferative index is higher and tumor cell death rate is lower in mice undergoing laparotomy vs. insufflation. Surg Endosc 1998;12(5):514.

47
Laparoscopic Total and Subtotal Colectomy

Mara R. Salum and Eric G. Weiss

Laparoscopic total and subtotal colectomy are procedures that have been proven to be feasible for a variety of diseases (Table 47.1). Nevertheless, the potential benefits of laparoscopic surgery, such as improved cosmesis, reduced postoperative pain, shorter length of hospitalization, and faster return to normal activity,[1,2] may be overcome by higher complication rates and longer lengths of surgery.

Patient Preparation

The preoperative preparation of the patient for laparoscopic surgery is essentially the same as for open procedures.[3] The patient is given a full bowel preparation, which includes a mechanical preparation and both preoperative oral and perioperative intravenous antibiotics. The patient's consent is always obtained for both a laparoscopic and open procedure because conversion may be necessary. Consent for a stoma is also obtained when indicated. The stoma therapist marks the ileostomy site using standard enterostomal therapy guidelines.[4] Moreover, if preoperative studies reveal retroperitoneal sepsis, extensive inflammation, or a phlegmon overlying one or both ureters, ureteric stents are typically placed, as discussed with more detail in Chapter 56.

The patient, under general endotracheal anesthesia, is positioned on the operating table in a modified lithotomy position with the legs in Allen stirrups (Allen Medical, Bedford Heights, OH), abducted and flattened; the hips and knees are flexed to a maximum of 15° to allow free rotation of the laparoscopic instruments. It is imperative that the thighs are lower than the abdominal wall so as not to interfere with use of the instruments. In addition, this position allows intraoperative colonoscopy and access to the anus for introduction of a circular stapler for construction of an ileorectal anastomosis or ileal pouch anal anastomosis. All patients require indwelling bladder catheters and gastric decompression before the establishment of the pneumoperitoneum. The arms are positioned at the sides, and a beanbag or other fixation device is useful to prevent patient movement with steep positioning required for laparoscopy. Deep venous thrombosis prophylaxis should also be undertaken with pneumatic compression stockings and Enoxaperim (Lovenox, Rhone Polenc). The abdomen is prepped and draped in the usual sterile fashion, carefully providing wide exposure for trocar placement.

A periumbilical or transumbilical incision is made with the patient in a steep Trendelenburg position. The pneumoperitoneum is established through a Veress needle inserted into the peritoneal cavity; alternatively, the Hasson "open" technique can be used in patients who have had previous abdominal surgery. If the closed technique is chosen, the surgeon should be familiar with both the manual tactile sense that the needle has entered the peritoneal cavity and the typical noise of the retracting needle tip as it enters the peritoneal cavity. A water drop test should be performed, and low-pressure, high-flow insufflation should be easily achieved. After the pneumoperitoneum is established with CO_2 to a pressure of 15mmHg, the Veress needle is removed and a 10- or 12-mm trocar is placed through this site. The 10-mm, 0° diameter camera is inserted, and the peritoneal cavity is inspected. All the other working ports are placed under direct visualization. For laparoscopic colorectal surgery, almost all ports are 10 or 12mm in size to allow removal and introduction of all instruments, cameras, and staples through any port. A variety of positions are required to allow gravity to displace the loops of the bowel from the operative field. The patient, therefore, should be secured to the operating table with atraumatic straps or with the use of a vacuum beanbag.

Subtotal Colectomy

After the pneumoperitoneum is established, 10- to 12-mm ports are placed in each of the four abdominal quadrants, lateral to the rectus abdominis muscles. Placing all

TABLE 47.1. Indications for laparoscopic total and subtotal colectomy.

Subtotal colectomy
1. Crohn's disease (IRA, end ileostomy)
2. Colonic inertia (IRA)
3. Ulcerative colitis (IRA)
4. Familial adenomatous polyposis (IRA)

Total colectomy
1. Ulcerative colitis (IPAA)
2. Familial adenomatous polyposis (IPAA)
3. Crohn's disease (end ileostomy)

IRA, ileorectal anastomosis; IPAA, ileal pouch anal anastomosis.

ports initially allows for rapid and continuous instrument exchange throughout the procedure. With the patient placed in steep left-side-down and Trendelenburg position, the right colon is mobilized along the white line of Toldt. Traction on the right colon is provided by a combination of gravity and Babcock-type noncrushing clamps applied to the serosal surface of the colon. The avascular plane is developed with both blunt and sharp use of the Harmonic Scalpel (Ethicon Endosurgery, Cincinnati, OH, USA). The right ureter is identified and reflected posteriorly and laterally. The dissection is carried cephalad toward the hepatic flexure, exposing the third portion of the duodenum with dissection of the same bowel mesentery to that level and then to the transverse colon. The gastrocolic omentum, when feasible, is separated from the superior surface of the transverse colon. The colon is grasped with one clamp and the omentum with the other, and the avascular plane is dissected, separating the two structures. The transverse colon dissection is a phase of the procedure that should be carried with great attention because of the extreme mobility of this segment and the tendency of the omentum to hang over the operative field. The gastroepiploic vessels are carefully identified and preserved. The patient is then placed in a steep right-side-down Trendelenburg position, and the identical mobilization is undertaken on the left side. Specifically, the white line of Toldt is incised on the left side, up to and around the splenic flexure. The left ureter is identified and reflected away posteriorly and laterally. The inferior mesenteric vein and inferior mesenteric artery are identified and divided using an endoscopic linear cutter with a vascular (white) cartridge. The middle colic vessels are then divided similarly. The right iliac fossa port is exchanged, using the Seldinger technique exchange, for an 18-mm port through which the longer 60-mm stapler is introduced. The rectosigmoid is divided at the rectosigmoid junction, and the supraumbilical port site is extended to a 3- to 5-cm incision through which the colon is delivered and the terminal ileum transected, as well as the right

colic artery. Alternatively, a small Pfannenstiel incision can be made or, if a Brooke ileostomy is to be fashioned, the specimen may be delivered through a preoperatively marked incision in the right iliac fossa, which will subsequently function as the ileostomy site. If an ileorectal anastomosis is to be constructed, the anvil of a circular stapler is introduced and fixed into the ileum with a pursestring suture. The ileum is returned to the peritoneal cavity, the port site of extraction is closed, and pneumoperitoneum is reestablished. A circular stapler is transanally passed, and the camera is moved to the right iliac fossa; the stapler is fired. As with conventional surgery, the integrity of the anastomosis is verified for leakage by air testing by immersing it in saline and proximally occluding the bowel with an atraumatic clamp and instilling air transanally.

Total Colectomy

To perform a laparoscopic-assisted total colectomy, five 10- or 12-mm ports are utilized in the same fashion as described for subtotal colectomy. The white line of Toldt of the ascending and descending colon is incised, the hepatic and splenic flexures are mobilized, and the gastrocolic omentum is dissected in the same manner as previously detailed in this chapter. The presacral space is entered posterior to the rectosigmoid junction at the sacral promontory and dissection is undertaken in the avascular plane, proceeding distally to the levator muscles. The Waldeyer's fascia is then incised using an ultrasonic scalpel. The dissection then proceeds laterally, eventually separating the rectum from the vagina.

The proctectomy is performed with the patient in steep Trendelenburg position to allow for gravity retraction of the small bowel from the pelvis. Anterior retraction of the bladder can be achieved by suspending it with a suture through the abdominal wall. The vagina and the uterus can be retracted anteriorly with a transvaginal uterine levator or by insertion of the assistant's finger. The exposure and visualization are excellent in this procedure because the magnification and placement of the laparoscope deep in the pelvis allows close-up identification and preservation of the nerves.

After division of the superior hemorrhoidal artery, the rectum is mobilized dissecting the presacral loose areolar tissue plane. The lateral attachments can be preferably divided by the Harmonic scalpel (Ethicon). After achieving complete mobilization of the rectum to the level of the levators, the perineal phase commences. This portion is performed in the intersphincteric plane. The procedure is performed for benign disease, and one can take advantage of decreased perineal wound complications associated with the preservation of the external sphincter.[5] The entire colon can be removed through the perineal incision, after which a moist sponge is used to temporarily seal the wound and reinstate the pneumoperitoneum. The pelvis is explored with the use of the laparoscope to ensure hemostasis, and a suction-irrigation drain is placed with the technique described by Reissman et al.[6] The stoma is then matured, and the perineum is closed in layers.

Alternatively, if a restorative procedure is indicated, an ileal pouch anastomosis is performed. After full mobilization of the entire colon as previously described, a small Pfannenstiel incision incorporating the two lowest port sites is made; this allows completion of the colectomy in a standard fashion including the mesenteric division, if desired. Therefore, the proctectomy, pouch creation, and ileal pouch–anal anastomosis are performed under direct vision in the standard fashion, as described elsewhere.[7] We perform the anastomosis using the double-stapled technique and usually complete the procedure with a diverting loop ileostomy. One of the port sites is generally used as a stoma site, which is preoperatively marked. However, before exteriorization of the loop of bowel, the fascia at the stoma site should be incised under direct vision to achieve an adequate opening. The opening created even by a large trocar is insufficient and can cause a postoperative stoma outlet obstruction.[8]

Although some criteria exist to determine which patients should undergo diversion, these have not yet been clearly defined or studied in a randomized trial. First, patient selection is critical, which includes various parameters such as the general health of the patient and associated comorbidity such as nutritional status, presence of anemia, advanced age, current steroid use, or use of other immunosuppressant drugs. Intraoperative considerations are also important, including absence of tension, adequate vascularization of the anastomosis, lack of intraoperative complications, and satisfactory intraoperative testing of the integrity of the anastomosis.

There are reports of completely intracorporeal ileal pouch anal anastomosis where the colectomy is done laparoscopically including the vessel ligature, and the specimen is removed through the anus before the laparoscopic creation of the pouch. However, removal of the colon through the anus, although very appealing to a surgeon not experienced in anal physiology, can severely damage the sphincter mechanism.[9]

Patients have the nasogastric tube removed immediately after surgery, begin a clear liquid diet on the first postoperative day, and then advance to a regular diet within the next 24 to 48h, as tolerated.[10] Patients are discharged home after having tolerating a regular diet and having had at least one bowel movement.[11]

A limited number of reports and series of these advanced procedures are found in the literature. Table 47.2 lists a variety of published series of laparoscopic total and subtotal colectomy. As one can see, very few procedures have been reported, and it is difficult to draw conclusions given the small numbers. However, the procedures are feasible and can be performed. We abandoned these procedures in 1993 due to a threefold increase in complications compared to segmental laparoscopic procedures.[13] Our experience, however, may not

TABLE 47.2. Results of laparoscopic total and subtotal colectomy.

Author/year	Number of patients	Procedure	Length of surgery, min (mean)	Morbidity (%)	Conversion (%)	Postoperative hospitalization, days (mean)
Wexner et al. 1992[12]	5	Subtotal colectomy	230	0	0	9.2
Schmitt et al. 1994[13]	22	TAC + IPAA	240	55	—	8.7
Thibault and Poulin 1995[14]	4	TAC	438	—	—	10
Reissman et al. 1996[8]	72	Subtotal colectomy (30) Ileocolic resection (30) Loop ileostomy (6) Ileorectal anastomsis (3) Duodenal bypass (3)	174	18	10	6.5
Milsom et al. 1997[15]	16	Subtotal colectomy	232	12.5	0	5
Hildebrandt et al. 1998[16]	89	Ileocecal resection (45) Anastomotic resection (14) Small bowel resection (4) Hemicolectomy (12) Subtotal colectomy (9) Loop ileostomy (4) Adhesiolysis (1)	173.7	12.3	11.2	13.3
Hildebrandt et al. 1998[17]	5	TAC + IPAA	362.5	0	0	14.5
Araki et al. 1998[18]	10	Subtotal colectomy	282	—	—	—

TAC, total abdominal colectomy; IPAA, ileal pouch anal anastomosis.

mimic all surgeons' experience. We performed these procedures early in our laparoscopic experience before we had ascend the learning curve. Now, perhaps, with more than 400 procedures performed in our department, revisiting these procedures seems appropriate.

Conclusions

Total abdominal colectomy with either ileostomy or ileal pouch anal anastomosis is a natural extension of segmental colectomies performed laparoscopically. Although technically demanding and requiring significant expertise, these procedures may be performed in selected individuals. Exact selection criteria are not available, and the technique should be applied on a case-by-case basis.

References

1. Bauer JJ, Harris MT, Grumbach NM, Gorfine SR. Laparoscopic-assisted intestinal resection for Crohn's disease. Dis Colon Rectum 1995;38:712–715.
2. Fleshman JW, Fry RD, Birnbaum EH, Kodner JJ. Laparoscopic-assisted and minilaparotomy approaches to colorectal diseases are similar in early outcome. Dis Colon Rectum 1996;39:15–22.
3. Wexner SD, Beck DE. Sepsis prevention in colorectal surgery. In: Fielding LP, Goldberg SM (eds) Surgery of the Colon, Rectum and Anus. Oxford: Butterworth-Heinemann, 1993.
4. Teoh TA, Reissman P, Weiss EG, Verzaro R, Wexner SD. Enhancing cosmesis in laparoscopic colon and rectal surgery. Dis Colon Rectum 1995;38:213–214.
5. Lubbers EJ. Healing of the perineal wound after proctectomy for nonmalignant conditions. Dis Colon Rectum 1982;25:351–357.
6. Reissman P, Cohen SM, Weiss EG, Wexner SD. Simple technique for pelvic drain placement in laparoscopic abdominoperineal resection. Dis Colon Rectum 1994;37:381–382.
7. Wexner SD, James K, Jagelman DG. The double-stapled ileal reservoir and ileoanal anastomosis: a prospective review of sphincter function and clinical outcome. Dis Colon Rectum 1991;34:487–494.
8. Reissman P, Salky BA, Pfeifer J, Edye M, Jagelman DG, Wexner SD. Laparoscopic surgery in the management of inflammatory bowel disease. Am J Surg 1996;171:47–51.
9. Morgan R, Patel B, Beynon J, Carr ND. Surgical management of anorectal incontinence due to internal sphincter deficiency. Br J Surg 1997;84:226–230.
10. Reissman P, Teoh TA, Cohen SM, Weiss EG, Nogueras JJ, Wexner SD. Is early oral feeding safe after elective colorectal surgery. Ann Surg 1995;222(1):73–77.
11. Binderow SR, Cohen SM, Wexner SD, Schmitt SL, Nogueras JJ, Jagelman DG. Must early oral intake be limited to laparoscopy? Dis Colon Rectum 1994;37(6):584–589.
12. Wexner SD, Johansen OB, Nogueras JJ, Jagelman DG. Laparosocpic total abdominal colectomy. A prospective trial. Dis Colon Rectum 1992;35:651–655.
13. Schmitt SL, Cohen SM, Wexner SD, Nogueras JJ, Jagelman DG. Does laparoscopic assited ileal pouch anal anastomosis reduce the length of hospitalization? Int J Colorect Dis 1994;9:134–137.
14. Thibault C, Poulin EC. Total laparoscopic proctocolectomy and laparoscopic-assisted proctocolectomy for inflammatory bowel disease: operative technique and preliminary report. Surg Laparosc Endosc 1995;5:472–476.
15. Milsom JW, Ludwig KA, Church JM, Garcia-Ruiz A. Laparoscopic total abdominal colectomy with ileorectal anastomosis for familial adenomatous polyposis. Dis Colon Rectum 1997;40:675–678.
16. Hildebrandt U, Schiedeck T, Kreissler-Haag D, et al. Laparoscopically assisted surgery in Crohn disease. Zentralbl Chir 1998;123:357–361.
17. Hildebrandt U, Lindeman W, Kreissler-Haag D, Feifel G, Ecker KW. Laparoscopically-assisted proctocolectomy with ileoanal pouch in ulcerative colitis. Zentralbl Chir 1998;123:403–405.
18. Araki Y, Isomoto H, Tsuki Y, Matsumoto A, Yasunaga M. Clinical aspects of total colectomy: laparoscopic versus open technique for familial adenomatous polyposis and ulcerative colitis. Kurume Med J 1998;45:203–207.

48
Ileocolic Resection

Bruce Belin and Steven D. Wexner

Indications

Crohn's disease if amenable to treatment with laparoscopic ileocolectomy because of the frequent involvement of the terminal ileum. Frequently, stricture, phlegmon, or even abscess and fistula are components of the disease process. Even with these associated conditions, laparoscopic resection is generally an elective procedure.

Crohn's disease poses special challenges to the laparoscopist. Patients are frequently malnourished and immunosuppressed, with inflamed friable thickened tissue and adhesions from prior operations. They are often young, anxious to quickly return to full activity, interested in a good cosmetic outcome, and able to cease taking medication for their disease. Surgical indications are no different whether the procedure is undertaken by laparotomy or laparoscopy.

Although patients can derive significant benefit from laparoscopic ileocolic resection, the procedure can be technically demanding. Although resections for minimal disease (without fistula or abscess) are most easily accomplished by laparoscopy, the benefit may be less significant than that found after more difficult dissections in more advanced cases.[1] In this latter setting, patients may have a large fixed mass, a fistula, adhesions, or thickened mesentery.[2] Although these challenges can lengthen the operation and increase the chance of conversion to laparotomy, ultimately these patients derive great benefit as measured by a decrease in length of stay, less postoperative discomfort, and fewer postoperative adhesions.[3–6]

Preoperative Preparation

Preoperative measures are identical whether the procedure is performed by laparotomy or laparoscopy. Preoperative evaluation starts with a complete history and physical exam. In particular, the patient should be queried with respect to the use of steroids, immunosuppression, and past hospitalizations. Pertinent past radiographs, operative reports, discharge summaries, and pathology slides should be obtained and reviewed. Special attention should be paid to nutritional evaluation such as recent changes in the patient's diet, weight, and bowel function. Basic laboratory workup should include a complete blood count as well as prothrombin time, partial thromboplastin time, and a basic electrolyte panel. Further evaluations, including electrocardiogram, chest x-ray, and further metabolic workup (albumin and prealbumin), are performed as needed. Both colonoscopy with biopsies, including examination of the terminal ileum, and small bowel followthrough, or enteroclysis, are routinely performed to evaluate distribution and severity of intraluminal disease.[7] Furthermore, a CT scan is frequently performed to delineate any extraluminal phlegmonous disease or retroperitoneal ureteric displacement or compression. Arrangements are made if resuscitation or preoperative nutrition is required; enteral nutritional support is preferred when there is adequate small bowel function.

Before surgery, patients are counseled about autologous blood donation and advised to avoid aspirin and nonsteroidal anti-inflammatory drugs for 14 days before surgery. Even if the probability of a stoma is low, this contingency is always discussed; the patient meets an enterostomal therapist for education and site selection. The possibilities of intraoperative colonoscopy and conversion to laparotomy are discussed. Patients are consented for these eventualities (stoma, colonoscopy, and laparotomy) as well as for intraoperative ureteric catheter localization, which is especially useful in cases of iliac fossa phlegmon, abscess, or if a fistula is identified.[8] In case unsuspected proximal strictures are discovered, the patient should understand the principles for strictureplasty. An informed consent is given to the patients to ensure that they and their family are knowledgeable about the various risks, benefits, alternatives, and complications of surgery.

On the day before surgery, the patient undergoes bowel preparation with 45 ml sodium phosphate (Fleets Phosphosoda; CB Fleet, Lynchburg, VA, USA) at both 6 P.M. and midnight, each followed by ten 10-ounce glasses of water. One gram each of Flagyl and Neomycin is given at 1, 2, and 10 P.M. to decrease the bacterial load of the colon. The patient is kept NPO after midnight before surgery and is admitted the morning of surgery unless otherwise indicated. At that time, perioperative systemic antibiotics are given, usually 2 g Cefotan on call to the operating room and for two postoperative doses, assuming normal renal function and no known medical allergies. Stress dose steroids, such as hydrocortisone 100 mg, is given on call to the operating room and tapered postoperatively if the patient has been on daily steroid medications during the past 6 months. Before induction of general endotracheal anesthesia, pneumatic compression stockings and subcutaneous heparin (Lovenox, 40 mg; Rhone-Poulenc Rorer, Collegeville, PA, USA) are utilized for deep venous thrombosis prophylaxis.

Positioning

Under general endotracheal anesthesia, the patient is placed in a modified lithotomy position with the lower extremities in Allen stirrups (Allen Medical, Bedford Heights, OH, USA), abducted and flattened; the hips and knees are flexed to a maximum of 15° to allow free rotation of the laparoscopic instruments. This position enables intraoperative colonoscopy (if needed) and increases flexibility of positioning ports and equipment. A bladder catheter and orogastric tubes are inserted before the start of pneumoperitoneum.

Operative Preparation

We routinely perform cystoscopy and bilateral ureteric catheter placement for ileocolic resection in both the laparoscopy and laparotomy setting (Table 48.1). This

TABLE 48.1. Equipment.

Trocar/ports, 10 and 12 mm
30° scope
Suction irrigation
Three-chip camera
Endo Babcock or atraumatic grasper
Beanbag: Velcro to bed
Allen stirrups
Thromboguards
Secure for airplaning/Trendelenburg
10-mm cautery scissors or Harmonic (ultrasonic) scissors (Ethicon Endosurgery, Cincinnati, OH, USA)

step facilitates the identification of the right ureter, as the degree of inflammation cannot always be anticipated, even if a CT scan was obtained. The catheter can be easily identified when an instrument is swept over the tissue.

The abdominal wall is prepared and draped in the standard fashion exposing from zyphoid to pubis and the width of the abdominal wall between the iliac spines. The camera, electrocautery, insufflation line, and irrigation equipment are all prepared and secured on the field. Should conversion be required, the table is prepared with instruments for laparotomy. Pneumoperitoneum is created with the Hasson "open" technique if the patient is thought to have adhesions to the abdominal wall, bowel obstruction, or prior laparotomy. Alternatively, the Veress needle is inserted; placement is verified by an audible "click" and by the flow of sterile saline into the peritoneal cavity through the needle. If resistance to flow is encountered, the Veress needle should be replaced or the trocar should be placed by open technique.

The CO_2 pneumoperitoneum should be achieved in a slow, gradual manner until the intra-abdominal pressure reaches 15 mmHg. The surgeon should observe the insufflation rate and pressure to recognize any abnormal compliance indicative of improper positioning of the Veress needle. If a gas warmer is part of the insufflator unit, it may increase the resistance in the insufflation tubing and should not be mistaken for needle malposition. Reassurance of proper insufflation can be accomplished by examining for dull tympani of the peritoneal cavity during insufflation. The Veress needle is removed after pneumoperitoneum is created and replaced by a 10- to 12-mm trocar. The 10-mm-diameter camera is then inserted and the peritoneal cavity inspected; table positioning facilitates exposure.

A 10- or 12-mm port is placed in the left abdomen at the level of the umbilicus with care to avoid the epigastric vessels. Transillumination of the abdominal wall with the laparoscope usually permits visualization and avoidance of these potentially troublesome vessels; a third port is placed in the left lower quadrant. Trocars should be placed at least 10 cm apart to avoid "sword fighting." This additional port is particularly useful in obese patients.

Careful inspection of the entire small bowel is an essential part of the procedure. Despite preoperative evaluation, findings at this point may necessitate conversion to a laparotomy if the anatomy is unclear or if the pathology cannot be satisfactorily treated by laparoscopy. The bowel is evaluated with two Babcock clamps in a bimanual fashion, running the bowel in a hand-over-hand manner; alternatively, the small bowel may be progressively exteriorized for evaluation. Although this method carries a lower risk of clamp injury, it can result in mesenteric laceration, venous stasis, and hematoma formation from drawing a thick mesentery through a narrow fascial aperture. We prefer the former inspection technique—

grasping only the bowel that will be in the resection specimen. "Skip" areas of disease may be identified with stricture or thickening of the bowel wall. These regions do not mandate conversion to laparotomy because they can be delivered for evaluation and either resection or strictureplasty through the extended umbilical trocar incision after mobilization is complete.[9] They should, however, be marked with clips to facilitate subsequent identification. Regardless of the method of evaluation, the bowel must be handled with care to avoid inadvertent enterotomies.

The patient is placed in Trendelenburg and left-side tilted-down position. A 10-mm-diameter disposable Babcock clamp is used to retract the right colon. Dissection of the mesentery is initiated at the inferior lateral border of the cecum along the white line of Toldt at the lateral retroperitoneal reflection. The appendix is retracted superiorly and medially, and dissection using the harmonic scalpel through the left inferior port is initiated. The smokeless division of tissue using the harmonic scalpel avoids the need for venting the peritoneal cavity and avoids inadvertent cautery injury to other tissues in contact with the device. The ureter is routinely identified during the mobilization as it may be medially displaced into the inflammatory mass. A common error is to enter a plane too lateral such that the retroperitoneum is entered beneath the ureter and the duodenum is inadvertently cauterized. Although obese patients may pose certain difficulties, alternatively cachectic patients may have very thin mesentery that is easily traversed. If difficulty if encountered in identification of the proper plane, the harmonic scalpel may be utilized from the left upper abdominal trocar. After mobilization of the hepatic flexure, the proximal transverse colon is addressed. This step is best performed after the right colon has been mobilized in the appropriate plane to avoid the portal and pancreaticoduodenal vessels. Nonetheless, large vessels may be encountered between the omentum and the hepatic flexure. These vessels are best divided between clips or with the harmonic scalpel. The endpoint for dissection is the duodenum, encountered after full mobilization of the cecum superiorly and of the hepatic flexure medially.

Adequate mobilization can be verified by retracting the terminal ileum and proximal transverse colon to the umbilical trocar. Intracorporeal mesenteric vascular division and ligation can be achieved by creating windows in the avascular areas of the mesentery followed by vascular pedicle ligation with clips, pretied vascular loops, or vascular staples. However, these measures are potentially hazardous because of the thickened friable mesentery; the intracorporeal technique is both cumbersome and time consuming. Therefore, it is our preference to perform the mesenteric division, bowel resection, and anastomosis in an extracorporeal fashion. Given the lack

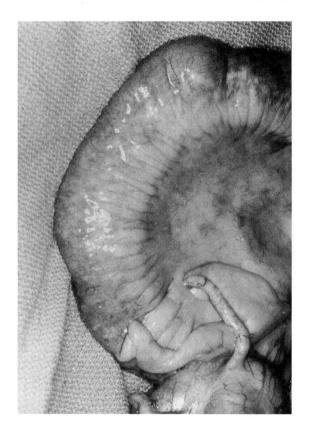

FIGURE 48.1. Delivery of diseased terminal ileum onto field after laparoscopic mobilization.

of demonstrable benefit from intracorporeal mesenteric division and colonic resection, we perform this in an extracorporeal fashion.[10] Specifically, a Babcock clamp is gently placed on the cecum through the umbilical port, and the umbilical incision is lengthened to about 5 cm. A plastic wound drape is inserted along the shaft of the Babcock clamp, after which the terminal ileum is extracorporealized (Fig. 48.1). Care should be taken never to apply any undue tension to the mesentery to avoid avulsion of major vascular structures. Instead, the umbilical incision should be lengthened as needed. All suspicious areas of the small bowel are inspected and palpated. Strictureplasty or additional resections may be performed if needed. The mesentery is then divided in the standard manner.

Reapproximation of the mesenteric defect is initiated before division of the bowel to decrease the risk of inadvertently twisting the mesentery. The resection is completed using a linear cutter stapler at the proximal and distal extents of resection. The specimen is retrieved from the operating table and opened to confirm diagnosis and grossly disease-free margin. A side-to-side, functional end-to-end anastomosis is then completed using a 75-mm linear cutter stapler (Fig. 48.2). The anastomosis

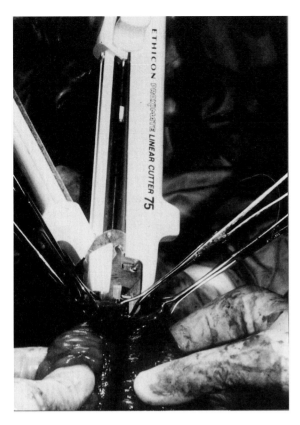

FIGURE 48.2. Extracorporeal stapling of ileocolic anastomosis.

is then irrigated and aspirated with saline, and carefully inspected to ensure meticulous hemostasis and absence of any Crohn's disease. The staple line is reinforced if needed to secure optimal hemostasis. The apical enterotomy is then reapproximated with a linear stapler. Again, the staple line is inspected for hemostasis and suture-reinforced as needed. The closure of the mesenteric defect is then completed with care to avoid any mesenteric vessels. After completion, the anastomosis is returned to the peritoneal cavity and any additional areas of disease are treated as necessary. Ultimately, pneumoperitoneum is reestablished after closure of the infraumbilical incision. The peritoneal cavity is inspected for hemostasis, mesenteric closure, and bowel orientation.

After resection is complete and the specimen has been removed, the fascia at each port site should be reapproximated either using a laparoscopically guided endosuture device or by simply retracting the skin edges while reapproximating the fascia. The ureteric catheter and orogastric tube are removed in the operating room while the bladder catheter remains in place. Figure 48.3 shows the appearance of the abdominal wall at the completion of surgery.

Postoperative Care

The postoperative management is identical to that for standard laparotomy. Patients spend 12 to 24h in a monitored bed; a complete blood count and a basic electrolyte panel are drawn on the first postoperative morning. Patients are usually mobilized on the first postoperative day, after which the bladder catheter is removed. A clear liquid diet is commenced on the first postoperative day independent of the laparoscopic approach and advanced as tolerated with documentation of return of bowel function as evidenced by the passage of flatus and stool. Nasogastric tubes are placed only if patients develop gastric dilatation or have more than two episodes of emesis. Discharge criteria are no different from patients having undergone laparotomy. Discharge to home is considered when patients have tolerated a solid food diet for at least 24h and have passed at least one bowel movement.[11]

Results

Although initial results of laparoscopic procedures focused on the possibility to successfully complete a procedure with a new modality of treatment, the focus

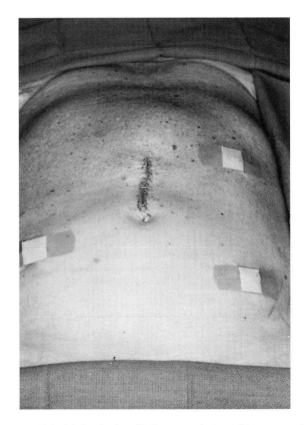

FIGURE 48.3. Abdominal wall after completion of laparoscopic-assisted ileocolic resection.

TABLE 48.2. Summary of published studies.

Author	n	Morbidity (%)	Length of stay (mean days)	Conversion (%)
Milsom et al. 1992[12]	9	0	7	0
Reissman et al. 1996[15]	30	10	5.2	10
Liu et al. 1995[21]	3	20	7	10
Bauer et al. 1995[2]	18	6.2	6.6	22
Reissman et al. 1996[15]	32	14	5.1	14
Alabaz et al. 1997[18]	26	15.3	7	11

quickly shifted to looking for benefits in terms of length of stay, decreasing morbidity, and pushing the limitations of what was initially believed to be feasible. During the past 8 years, we have learned more about results of surgery that have led us to reevaluate our traditional standards of management and better define the criteria to compare outcomes. As a result of these advances, we now do not routinely use postoperative nasogastric tubes, and the oral diet is advanced as tolerated without waiting for flatus or the passage of stool after both laparotomic and laparoscopic ileocolic resections. The focus, which initially concentrated on the ability to safely complete a laparoscopic case, has now expanded to looking for advantages in length of stay. Even more recently, evaluation of laparoscopic ileocolic resection has expanded to compare postoperative pain, adhesion formation, and cosmesis in the quest to provide safe, cost-effective surgery with maximal patient satisfaction. A summary of published studies is presented in Table 48.2.

One of the initial series describing laparoscopic ileocolic resection in 1993 described good results in highly selected patients. All patients in this early series were treated without the need for conversion and without complications. Eight of the nine patients had not had prior abdominal surgery and the mean length of stay was 7 days, not significantly different from the authors' experience with laparotomic resection.[12]

During the past 8 years, we have advanced our techniques and better described our results. Although initial reports frequently describe an entirely intracorporeal technique for ileocolic resection, this was found to be expensive, time consuming, and did not avoid an incision because the specimen would ultimately have to be removed. Furthermore, data have failed to show any significant difference with respect to length of hospital stay and duration of postoperative ileus when intracorporeal and extracorporeal mesenteric division and anastomosis were compared. Thus, the completely laparoscopic procedure has generally fallen out of favor.[13] Similarly, increased experience has supported the routine use of prophylactic bilateral ureteral stents in all patients with Crohn's disease undergoing laparoscopic ileocolic resec-

tion. In one series of elective laparoscopic and laparotomic procedures, the average time for catheter insertion was 17 min and bilateral catheterization was possible in 95% of the patients with no significant complications. In general, ureteric catheters expedite and possibly increase the safety of laparoscopic surgery for Crohn's disease by facilitating initial and subsequent identification of the ureters.[8]

Further work, with increased operative experience and larger, better-controlled studies, has supported a significant reduction in length of hospital stay and decreased postoperative pain management requirement. Length of stay after surgery has varied from 5 to 8 days; this has been shown to be significantly shorter in comparison with laparotomy.[2,13] Many retrospective comparisons have been made to laparotomy; results generally demonstrate statistically significantly shorter recovery periods after laparoscopy. This difference is particularly evident with more complicated Crohn's disease involving fistula, abscess, and strictures when compared with case-matched controls.[2,13] This issue will certainly be clarified by randomized controlled studies currently underway.[14] Evidence for a less painful surgery with more expeditious recovery is also supported by approximately half the preoperative utilization of morphine equivalents and by a significantly better surgical recovery index.[15]

The presence of a fistula was initially thought to be a contraindication to laparoscopic surgery; however, this belief has since been proven otherwise. Although it is associated with a more difficult and longer procedure and therefore requires more experience, success has been demonstrated in patients with ileovesical, ileorectal, gastrocolonic, and ileoileal fistula without complications.[13]

Theoretically, it seemed plausible that less intraperitoneal trauma via a laparoscopic approach would result in fewer adhesions. Initial experiments with a porcine model supported these findings.[15–17] Alabaz et al. retrospectively surveyed 100 patients having undergone laparoscopic and laparotomic colorectal operations using a questionnaire to obtain long-term follow-up extending out to 6 years.[18] They found that laparotomy was associated with a higher incidence of symptomatic small bowel obstruction necessitating hospital admission (31% versus 8%). However, the need for reexploration in symptomatic small bowel obstruction was not significantly different (8% for laparotomy versus 4% for laparoscopy).

Further reviews in the form of well-matched cohort analysis quantify and compare results in terms of postoperative pain, cosmesis, and self-image. One such study demonstrated a 50% reduction in narcotics used after ileocolic resection when performed laparoscopically and documented an improved patient perception of postoperative results. This perception was associated with enhanced social interaction and a quicker return to normal activity.[19] Further substantiating these results, a different review used a patient questionnaire and documented a strong preference for laparoscopy, based on perceived cosmetic benefit. This preference remained strong even when patients were given hypothetical statistics for increased risk for ureteral injury and increased medical costs.[20]

Conclusion

Early interest in laparoscopic ileocolic resection for Crohn's disease was driven by case reports of success in completing the procedure with hope of few complications and expeditious recovery. Further evidence-based data continue to support the initial enthusiasm for this procedure. A range of studies varying from retrospective review to prospective randomized trials have documented reduced postoperative pain, reduced postoperative ileus, decreased hospitalization time, enhanced cosmesis, less disability, and decreased symptoms attributable to adhesion formation. These results support the benefit of laparoscopic ileocolic resection for Crohn's disease when performed with prudent patient selection by experienced personnel.

References

1. Bauer JJ, Harris MT, Grumbach NM, Gorfine SR. Laparoscopic-assisted intestinal resection for Crohn's disease. Which patients are good candidates? J Clin Gastroenterol 1996;23(1):44–46.
2. Bauer JJ, Harris MT, Grumbach NM, Gorfine SR. Laparoscopic-assisted intestinal resection for Crohn's disease. Dis Colon Rectum 1995;38(7):712–715.
3. Bauer JJ, Harris MT, Grumbach NM, Gorfine SR. Laparoscopic-assisted intestinal resection for Crohn's disease. Surg Endosc 1994;8:232–235.
4. Fleshman JW, Fry RD, Birnbaum EH, Kodner IJ. Laparoscopic-assisted and minilaparotomy approaches to colorectal diseases are similar in early outcome. Dis Colon Rectum 1996;39(1):15–22.
5. Watanabe M, Oghami M, Teramoto T, Hibi N, Kitajima M. Laparoscopically assisted surgery for Crohn's disease [abstract]. Nippon Geka Gakkai Zasshi 1997;98:4.
6. Joo JS, Agachan F, Wexner SD. Laparoscopic surgery for lower gastrointestinal fistulas. Surg Endosc 1997;11(12):116–118.
7. Wexner SD. Diagnostic laparoscopy. Editorial comment. II. In: Jager RM, Wexner SD (eds) Laparoscopic Colorected Surgery. New York: Churchill Livingstone, 1996:139–141.
8. Chen WT, Parameswaren S, Gilliland R, et al. The role of elective intraoperative ureteric catheterization in colorectal surgery. Dis Colon Rectum (in press).
9. Reissman P, Salky BA, Edye M, Wexner SD. Laparoscopic surgery in Crohn's disease. Surg Endosc 1996;10:1201–1204.
10. Bernstein MA, Dawson JW, Reissman P, Weiss EG, Nogueras JJ, Wexner SD. Is a complete laparoscopic colectomy superior to laparoscopic assisted colectomy? Surgery 1996;62:507–511.
11. Wexner SD. Laparoscopic colectomy. In: Keighley RBM, Williams NS (eds) Surgery of the Anus, Rectum and Colon, vol 2. Philadelphia: Saunders 1997;2:2434–2448.
12. Milsom JW, Lavery IC, Bohm B, Fazio VW. Laparoscopically assisted ileostomy in Crohn's disease. Surg Laparosc Endosc 1993;3:77–80.
13. Talamini MA, Moesinger RC, Kaufman H, Kutka M, Harris M, Bayless T. Laparoscopically assisted bowel resection for Crohn's disease: the best of both worlds. Presented at Digestive Disease Week, Washington, DC, May 1997.
14. Bessler M, Whelan RL, Halverston A, et al. Controlled trial of laparoscopic assisted versus open colon resection in a porcine model. Surg Endosc 1996;10:732–745.
15. Reissman P, Teoh TA, Skinner K, Nogueras JJ, Wexner SD. Adhesion formation after laparoscopic anterior resection in a porcine model: a pilot study. Surg Laparosc Endosc 1996;2:136–139.
16. Schafer M, Krahenbahl L, Buchler MW. Comparison of adhesion formation in open and laparoscopic surgery. Dis Surg 1998;15:145–147.
17. Schippers E, Tittle IA, Ottinger A, Schumpelick V. Laparoscopy versus laparotomy: a comparison of adhesion formation after bowel resection in a canine model. Dis Surg 1998;15:145–147.
18. Alabaz O, Iroatulam AJN, Nessim A, Weiss EG, Nogueras JJ, Wexner SD. Comparison of laparoscopic assisted and conventional ileocolic resection for Crohn's disease. Int J Colorect Dis 1997;12:182–185.
19. Chen HH, Wexner SD, Weiss EG, et al. Laparoscopic colectomy for benign colorectal disease is associated with a significant reduction in disability as compared with laparotomy. Surg Endosc 1998;12:1397–1400.
20. Dunker MS, Stiggelbaout AM, van Hogezand RA, Ringers J, Bemelman WA. Cosmesis and body image after laparoscopic assisted and open ileocolic resection for Crohn's disease. Surg Endosc 1998;12:1334–1340.
21. Liu CD, Rolandelli R, Ashley SW, Evans B, Shin M, Mcfadden DW. Laparoscopic surgery for inflammatory bowel disease. Am Surg 1995;61:1054–1056.

49
Restorative Proctocolectomy

Jonathan E. Efron and Juan J. Nogueras

Laparoscopic surgery has seen tremendous growth over the past decade.[1,2] These technological advances have extended to coloproctology where many colorectal procedures are now being successfully accomplished with the use of the laparoscope.[3–5] Restorative proctocolectomy with ileoanal reservoir reconstruction is currently the surgical procedure of choice for the treatment of either mucosal ulcerative colitis or familial adenomatous polyposis.[6–8] In 1992, Wexner et al. first noted the technical feasibility of this procedure with the aid of the laparoscope.[9] In 1994, Schmitt et al. reported on 22 patients who underwent laparoscopic-assisted total proctocolectomy with ileal pouch anal anastomosis.[10] A cohort group of 20 patients who underwent the standard procedure by laparotomy were matched for age and gender. No significant differences were found in hospital length of stay or resolution of ileus between the groups, but the laparoscopic group had increased morbidity and operative time. In 1995, Thibault and Poulin published their preliminary results on complete intracorporeal laparoscopic total proctocolectomy.[11] Mean operative time was 7 h and 18 min, with an average blood loss of 500 to 800 ml and a mean hospital stay of 10 days. Given these initial results, the authors modified their operative technique to a laparoscopically assisted approach, which resulted in a decrease in their operative time to 4 h. They also noted a decrease in the postoperative stay to 8.3 days.[12] Thus, they ultimately adopted the technique and recommendations of Wexner et al. and Schmitt et al.[9,10] The debate regarding the indications for performing this extensive laparoscopic procedure persists; however, the potential benefits of improved cosmetic results and decreased postoperative disability as compared to laparotomy are sufficient motivating factors to pursue and improve the laparoscopic techniques. Several authors have experience with laparoscopic-assisted restorative total proctocolectomy (Table 49.1).

Young, thin, cosmetically conscious, and physically active patients who wish to try to minimize the disability period are ideal candidates for the procedure.[15] All patients should undergo the same preoperative evaluation regardless of whether the procedure is planned by laparoscopy or laparotomy. In patients with colitis, pathological confirmation of the diagnosis of mucosal ulcerative colitis, as opposed to Crohn's disease, must be established by colonoscopy with multiple biopsies and small bowel radiographic contrast studies. Anal sphincter function should be assessed by manometry and possibly anal ultrasonography before performing any ileal pouch anal procedure.[16–18] The advisability of laparoscopic colon surgery for cancer is still being studied by a prospective randomized multi-institutional trial sponsored by the National Cancer Institute. For the present, patients with cancer and either colitis or polyposis, including perianal Crohn's disease, should not be considered for laparoscopic-assisted total proctocolectomy. Finally, all patients should have preoperative enterostomal evaluation for stomal marking and preoperative stomal education.

Preoperative bowel preparation includes a mechanical purgative and both oral and parenteral perioperative antibiotics.[19,20] Heparin or low molecular weight heparin and sequential compression stockings are also utilized to help limit the possibility of venous thrombosis. A nasogastric or orogastric tube is placed to empty the stomach, and the bladder is decompressed with a catheter. Cystoscopy and placement of bilateral ureteral catheters may be useful to facilitate recognition of the ureters. The patient is positioned in the supine, modified lithotomy position using Allen stirrups (Allen Medical, Bedford Heights, OH, USA). Minimal flexion of the hips and knees (no more than 15° flexion in each knee and hip) prevents interference with instrumentation during the procedure. Care must be taken to appropriately pad and protect all areas of the body from potential injury, specifically because of the lengthy procedure. The ulnar and perineal nerves are particularly vulnerable to pressure. Moreover, the patient should be firmly secured to the table to permit table tilt-facilitated retraction.

TABLE 49.1. Results of laparoscopic-assisted restorative total proctocolectomy.

Author	Operation	Number of cases	Mean operative time (min)	Conversion rate (%)	Mean days to oral intake	Mean length of stay (days)
Wexner et al.[9]	TPC + IAR	Open, 5	150	0	4.7	8
		Laparoscopic, 5	230		5.3	9.2
Schmitt et al.[10]	TPC + IAR	Open, 20	120	0	4.3	8.9
		Laparoscopic, 22	240		3.6	8.7
Tucker et al.[12]	TPC + IAR	11	327	NR	4.8	6
Thibault and Poulin[11]	TPC + ileostomy	4	438	0	4	10
Rhodes et al.[13]	TPC + IAR	5	310	0	NR	10
Liu et al.[14]	TPC + IAR	5	480	NR	NR	—

TPC, total proctocolectomy; IAR, ileoanal reservoir.

After prepping the skin and draping the patient, a 1-cm, supra- or infraumbilical incision is made; pneumoperitoneum is established by either insertion of a Veress needle or placement of a Hasson trocar. Placement of the Veress needle is accomplished by lifting the abdominal wall with two towel clips placed at the edges of the skin incision, and then by inserting the needle through the abdominal fascia. The passage of the needle through the fascia is felt as a sudden release of pressure. The correct placement of the needle is confirmed by aspirating and then flushing the needle with normal saline. Furthermore, the pressure increase during insufflation should be gradual. Once an adequate pneumoperitoneum is achieved, if the Veress needle was used, it is removed and a 10- or 12-mm trocar is inserted into the peritoneal cavity. The Hasson trocar is placed under direct vision into the peritoneal cavity by incising the fascia and peritoneum and then securing the trocar into position with two 2-0 vicryl or proline sutures. Carbon dioxide is insufflated to a pressure of 15 mmHg to create the pneumoperitoneum.

After insertion of the 0° or 30° camera into the abdominal cavity, inspection is undertaken. Generally, four additional 10-mm ports are required for the procedure, each of which is placed under direct vision. The precise placement of the ports is essential to provide maximal traction and exposure and is dependent on the patient's body habitus. The standard port locations are demonstrated in Figure 49.1. The superior ports are usually placed approximately a hand's breadth above the inferior ports, thus providing adequate room for the manipulation of the instruments. When placing the inferior ports, attention should be given to the possible location of pelvic drains or ileostomies, as these port sites may be used for either purpose if they prove to be necessary during the operation. The lower port incisions may also be incorporated into the Pfannenstiel incision through which the colon will be delivered for ligation and resection. Finally, transillumination of the abdominal wall with the laparoscope is essential during lateral port placement to verify the positions of the inferior epigastric vessels.

After successful port placement, any adhesiolysis should be performed, and the small bowel should be closely examined. This examination is best facilitated by beginning at the ileocecal valve and using two laparoscopic Babcock clamps gently and carefully to inspect the small intestine to ligament of Treitz for evidence of Crohn's disease. Although there is loss of the traditional tactile sense, an adequate bowel inspection is possible with the laparoscopic instruments. The experienced laparoscopic surgeon develops an instrument-facilitated tactile sensation. Findings suggestive of Crohn's disease of the small intestine include thickened mesentery with fat wrapping and strictures. In patients with familial adenomatous polyposis, large small bowel polyps may be appreciated during inspection and mesenteric desmoids may be discovered.

Mobilization of the colon begins at the ileocecal valve and ascending colon. During mobilization, the operation surgeon stands either on the opposite side of the colon being mobilized or between the patient's legs; positioning of the table is very important. Maintaining the table

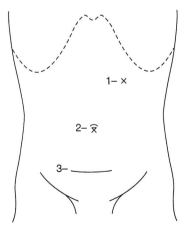

FIGURE 49.1. Standard port site placements for restorative proctocolectomy. *1*, left upper quadrant incision; *2*, paraumbilical incision; *3*, Pfannenstiel incision.

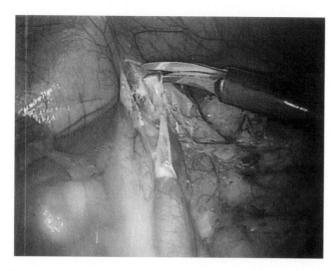

FIGURE 49.2. Electrocautery scissors used in restorative proctoscolectomy.

in the reverse Trendelenburg position with the right side up assists in keeping the right paracolic gutter and hepatic flexure free from small intestine, thereby facilitating mobilization of the cecum and ascending colon along the white line of Toldt. Mobilization is continued by medial and superior retraction of the colon. An electrocautery scissors (Fig. 49.2) or the ultrasonic scalpel (10-mm or 5-mm scalpel) (Fig. 49.3) combined with blunt dissection are used to dissect the colon free from its retroperitoneal attachments. Advantages of the harmonic scalpel over the electrocautery are twofold: a minimal amount of smoke is generated, and significantly larger blood vessels can be safely coagulated and divided. The right ureter and gonadal vessels are identified and protected as the dissection is continued along the superior mesenteric artery to the pancreas and duodenum. Full mobilization of the small bowel mesentery should occur during the laparoscopic phase because further mobilization through the lower abdominal incision is difficult and hampered by the location and site of the Pfanenstiel incision.

The transverse colon should be freed from the greater omentum by dissecting through the avascular plane formed by the fusion of the omentum and colonic mesentery. Difficulty may be encountered when attempting this dissection because the surgeon may not be able to obtain adequate tension between the colon and omentum to clearly define the avascular plane. Alternately, the omentum may be resected with the colon specimen by ligating the omentum's vascular supply below the gastroepiploic arcade with the harmonic scalpel, blunt dissection and placement of endoclips, or an endoscopic linear cutter, or with sutures.

Mobilization of the sigmoid and descending colon is best performed with the patient in the Trendelenburg position with the right side down. The small intestine is displaced to the right upper quadrant, allowing visualization of the left paracolic gutter. Dissection along the white line of Toldt with the harmonic scalpel is again facilitated by medial and superior traction of the colon, and the left ureter and gonadal vessels are identified as the colonic mesentery is dissected free from the retroperitoneum.

Exposure of the splenic flexure is attained with the patient in the reverse Trendelenburg position with the right side down. Gentle medial traction is undertaken while the colon is freed from the lienocolic ligament. Splenic lacerations are usually caused by excessive tension placed on the omentum, and not the colon; hence, excessive traction on the omentum should be avoided. Approaching the splenic flexure from two directions, progressing superiorly along the left paracolic gutter and separating the omentum from the transverse colon as it approaches the splenic flexure, may also avoid injury to the spleen. Generally, visualization of the splenic flexure is better with a laparascope than through a midline incision, and may be further enhanced by the use of a 30° laparoscopic camera and reverse Trendelenburg (head-up) position.

After complete mobilization of the colon and small bowel mesentery has been performed, a Pfannenstiel incision is made incorporating the lower port sites. The mobilized colon can then be eviscerated and its mesentery ligated. The proctectomy is performed under direct vision and completed with either mucosectomy or stapling with a 30-mm linear stapler. The ileal pouch is created under direct vision, and either a handsewn or double-stapled anastomosis is performed depending on the surgeon's preference. If required, a loop ileostomy is

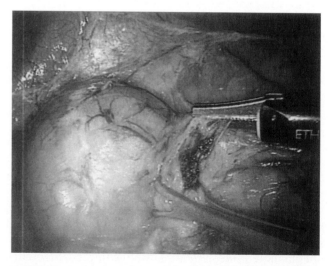

FIGURE 49.3. Ultrasonic scalpel used in restorative proctocolectomy.

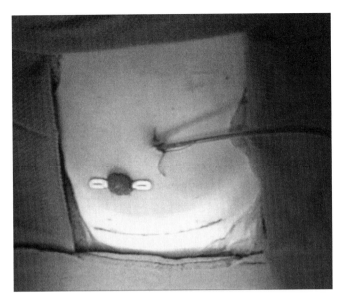

FIGURE 49.4. Pfannenstiel incision used in laparoscopic colorectal surgery.

effected through the right superior trocar incision,[21] and the pelvic drains may exit the abdomen through the left superior or inferior trocar sites.[22] All other fascial defects are then closed with suture material of the surgeon's choice. It is easiest to close the fascial port site defects under direct vision through the abdominal incision. The Pfannenstiel fascial defect can be closed with a running suture, and all skin incisions are closed with running subcuticular sutures. At the conclusion of the procedure, the patient will have a left upper quadrant incision, the paraumbilical incision (possibly used as a drain site), and the Pfannenstiel incision (Fig. 49.4). Alternatively, all the vessels may be ligated in an intracorporeal fashion, followed by creation of a small incision for pouch construction and anastomosis. The added time and expense do not seem justifiable given that an incision is still required for specimen extirpation.

Wishner et al. described a significant learning curve for surgeons performing laparoscopic-assisted colectomies, which varied from 30 to 70 cases depending on the procedure being performed.[23] Similarly, Larach et al. reported a higher morbidity for the cases performed earlier in the learning curve of laparoscopic colorectal surgeons.[24] Considering all the laparoscopic-assisted procedures performed in the specialty of colon and rectal surgery, none is more daunting than restorative proctocolectomy. Given the high morbidity associated with laparoscopic colorectal surgery, only the most experienced laparoscopic colorectal surgeons should attempt this procedure. The debate on the efficacy of laparoscopic-assisted restorative proctocolectomy will continue; however, technological advances and the

improved laparoscopic skills of colorectal surgeons may prove clear benefits. The benefits may include reduced adhesion formation,[25] decreased disability,[26] less immune system trauma,[27] diminished pain,[28] expedited recovery, and lower morbidity[29] as compared to laparotomy. However, at the present time the only clearly proven benefit is superior cosmesis.

References

1. Jager RM, Wexner SD (eds) Laparoscopic Colorectal Surgery. New York: Churchill Livingstone, 1996.
2. Sackier J, Wexner SD (eds) Protocols in General Surgery: Laparoscopic Colorectal Surgery. New York: Wiley, 1999.
3. Chen HH, Wexner SD, Weiss EG, et al. Laparoscopic colectomy for benign colorectal disease is associated with a significant reduction in disability as compared with laparotomy. Surg Endosc 1998;12(12):1397–1400.
4. Wexner SD, Latulippe JF. Laparoscopic colorectal surgery and cancer. Swiss Surg 1997;3(6):266–273.
5. Reissman P, Cohen S, Weiss EG, Wexner SD. Laparoscopic colorectal surgery: ascending the learning curve. World J Surg 1996;20(3):277–281.
6. Kelly KA. Anal sphincter saving operations for chronic ulcerative colitis. Am J Surg 1992;163:5.
7. Wexner SD, Alabaz O. Anastomotic integrity and function: role of the colonic J-pouch. Semin Surg Oncol 1998; 15(2):91–100.
8. Haray PN, Amarnath B, Weiss EG, Nogueras JJ, Wexner SD. Low malignant potential of the double-stapled ileal pouch-anal anastomosis. Br J Surg 1996;83(10):1406.
9. Wexner SD, Johansen OB, Nogueras JJ, Jagelman DG. Laparoscopic total abdominal colectomy. A prospective trial. Dis Colon Rectum 1992;35(7):651–655.
10. Schmitt SL, Cohen SM, Wexner SD, Nogueras JJ, Jagelman DG. Does laparascopic-assisted ileal pouch anal anastomosis reduce the length of hospitalization? Int J Colorect Dis 1994;9:134–137.
11. Thilbault C, Poulin EC. Total laparoscopic proctocolectomy and laparoscopy-assisted proctocolectomy for inflammatory bowel disease: operative technique and preliminary report. Surg Laparosc Endosc 1995;5:472–476.
12. Tucker JG, Ambroze WL, Orangio GR, Duncan TD, Mason EM, Lucas GW. Laparoscopically assisted bowel surgery. Analysis of 114 cases. Surg Endosc 1995;9(3):297–300.
13. Rhodes M, Stitz RW. Laparoscopic subtotal colectomy. Semin Colon Rectal Surg 1994;5:267–270.
14. Liu CD, Rolandelli R, Ashley SW, Evans B, Shin M, McFadden DW. Laparoscopic surgery for inflammatory bowel disease. Am Surg 1995;61(12):1054–1056.
15. Wexner SD. Total Laparoscopic proctocolectomy and laparoscopic-assisted proctocolectomy for inflammatory bowel disease: operative technique and preliminary report. Surg Lap Endosc 1997;1:79–80.
16. Takao Y, Weiss EG, Nogueras JJ, Wexner SD. Should ileoanal pouch surgery be denied to patients with low resting pressures? Am Surg 1997;63(8):726–731.
17. Morgado PJ Jr, Wexner SD, James K, Nogueras JJ, Jagelman DG. Ileal pouch-anal anastomosis: is preoperative anal

manometry predictive of postoperative functional outcome? Dis Colon Rectum 1994;37(3):224–228.

18. Joo JS, Latulippe JF, Alabaz O, Weiss EG, Nogueras JJ, Wexner SD. Long-term functional evaluation of straight coloanal anastomosis and colonic J-pouch: is the functional superiority of colonic J-pouch sustained? Dis Colon Rectum 1998;41(6):740–746.

19. Cohen SM, Wexner SD, Binderow SR, et al. Prospective, randomized, endoscopic-blinded trial comparing pre-colonoscopy bowel cleansing methods. Dis Colon Rectum 1994;37(7):689–696.

20. Oliverira L, Wexner SD, Daniel N, et al. Mechanical bowel preparation for elective colorectal surgery. A prospective, randomized, surgeon-blinded trial comparing sodium phosphate and polyethylene glycol-based oral lavage solutions. Dis Colon Rectum 1997;40(5):585–591.

21. Wexner SD, Taranow DA, Johansen OB, et al. Loop ileostomy is a safe option for fecal diversion. Dis Colon Rectum 1993;36(4):349–354.

22. Reissman P, Cohen SM, Weiss EG, Wexner SD. Simple technique for pelvic drain placement in laparoscopic abdominoperineal resection. Dis Colon Rectum 1994; 37(4):381–382.

23. Wishner SD, Baker JW Jr, Hoffman GC, et al. Laparo-scopic-assisted colectomy: the learning curve. Surg Endosc 1995;9:1179–1183.

24. Larach SW, Patankar SK, Ferrara A, Williamson PR, Perozus, Lord AS. Complications of laparascopic colorectal surgery. Analysis and comparison of early versus latter experience. Dis Colon Rectum 1997;40:592–596.

25. Sardinha TC, Wexner SD. Laparoscopy for inflammatory bowel disease: pros and cons. World J Surg 1998; 22(4):370–374.

26. Chen HH, Wexner SD, Weiss EG, et al. Laparoscopic colectomy for benign colorectal disease is associated with a significant reduction in disability as compared with laparotomy. Surg Endosc 1998;12(12):1397–1400.

27. Allendorf JD, Bessler M, Horvath KD, Marvin MR, Laird DA, Whelan RL. Increased tumor establishment and growth after open vs laparoscopic bowel resection in mice. Surg Endosc 1998:12(8):1035–1058.

28. Franklin ME Jr, Rosenthal D, Abrego-Medina D, et al. Prospective comparison of open vs. laparoscopic colon surgery for carcinoma. Five-year results. Dis Colon Rectum 1996;39(suppl 10):S35–S46.

29. Jerby BL, Milsom JW. Role of laparoscopy in the staging of gastrointestinal cancer. Oncology (Huntingt) 1998; 12(9):1353–1360.

50
Surgery for Rectal Prolapse

Yik-Hong Ho and Francis Seow-Choen

The common indications and contraindications for rectal prolapse surgery are shown in Table 50.1. Preoperative preparations include bowel preparation, prophylactic antibiotics (the authors prefer cephtriaxone and metronidazole), and bladder catheterization. The operation is performed under general anesthesia, without the use of nitrous oxide during laparoscopy to limit bowel distension.

Surgical Technique

Positioning and Setup

The patient is placed in a supine modified lithotomy position with the legs supported in Allen stirrups (Allen Medical, Bedford Heights, OH, USA). The head is supported by a rubber head ring and the shoulders are supported for steep Trendelenburg tilt. Both arms are kept straight alongside the body and protected in towel wraps. The surgeon, camera assistant, and scrub nurse stand on the patient's right side. The camera assistant stands on the surgeon's left and the scrub nurse on the surgeon's right. The first assistant stands on the patient's left side. Monitors are placed on the left and right sides where they can be conveniently viewed by the operative team (Fig. 50.1).

Cannula Port Placements

A Hasson cannula is placed infraumbilically by an open technique to accommodate the camera and carbon dioxide (CO_2) insufflation. Under direct camera vision guidance, 10- to 12-mm ports are inserted into the right and left lower abdomen; 5-mm ports are inserted into the right and left upper abdomen, with the right port intentionally inserted medially to facilitate pelvic dissection (Fig. 50.2).

Following cannula insertion and suture anchorage, the patient is tilted 25° to 30° head down and 15° to 20° left side up laterally. This positioning assists in gravitating the small bowel and omentum away from the operating field.

Procedure

After general abdominal exploration, any residual small bowel in the operative field is gently placed into the right upper quadrant with endoscopic graspers.

Isolation of Inferior Mesenteric Arteries

The first assistant places two endoscopic graspers upon the medial side of the sigmoid mesentery, which is tented up by retraction toward the anterior abdominal wall and to the left. This maneuver allows identification of the inferior mesenteric artery on this aspect of the sigmoid mesentery. The peritoneal layer of the latter is divided with electrocautery just inferior to and along the length of the inferior mesenteric artery.

The first assistant then grasps the incised peritoneum near the upper edge, which will display the plane between the retroperitoneal structures and the sigmoid mesentery. This plane is developed by the surgeon with a judicious combination of sharp electrocautery and blunt sweeping dissection to identify and displace the left ureter to a posterolateral position. Similarly, the left gonadal vessels and preaortic hypogastric nerve plexus are left intact upon the retroperitoneum. The dissection is continued proximally to the origin of the inferior mesenteric artery and laterally to reach the lateral attachments of the sigmoid (Fig. 50.3).

Ligation of Inferior Mesenteric Artery

The sigmoid mesentery proximal to the inferior mesenteric artery pedicle is incised. Through this window, the jaws of an endoscopic vascular 30-mm linear stapler are opened to include the vascular pedicle (including the inferior mesenteric vein if both safe and feasible). Having ensured that no other structures are inadvertently included in the jaws, the staples are fired and the vascular pedicle is transected. This particular step is done in preparation for subsequent resection of the sigmoid colon

TABLE 50.1. Indications and contraindications for rectal prolapse surgery.

Indications
  Full-thickness rectal prolapse
  Significant circumferential rectal intussusception clearly causing obstructed defaecation
  Solitary rectal ulcer syndrome or colitis cystica profunda refractory to conservative management
Contraindications
  Previous abdominal rectopexy, especially with large bowel resection or pelvic mesh
  Extensive adhesions
  Sexually active male patient
  Morbid obesity

(resection rectopexy), which is not obligatory unless constipation is a significant complaint and colonic transit time test is normal. If colonic transit time test is abnormal, an ileoproctostomy may be more appropriate.

Lateral Detachment of the Sigmoid Colon

The sigmoid colon is retracted with triangulation toward the right. Lateral attachments of the sigmoid colon to the abdominal wall that are thus displayed can be safely cut

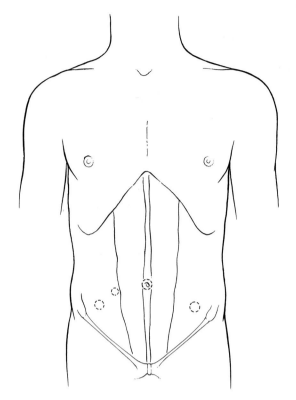

FIGURE 50.2. Cannula placement. *A*, Hasson port (10mm); *B*, 10- or 12-mm ports; *C*, 5-mm port.

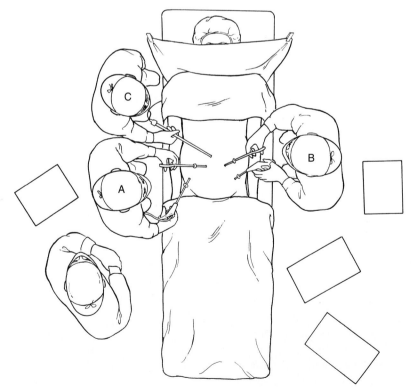

FIGURE 50.1. Positions of patient, operative team, and equipment. *A*, Surgeon; *B*, first assistant; *C*, camera assistant; *D*, scrub nurse; *E*, monitor, light source, and camera system; *F*, monitor; *G*, CO$_2$ insufflator; *H*, electrocautery unit.

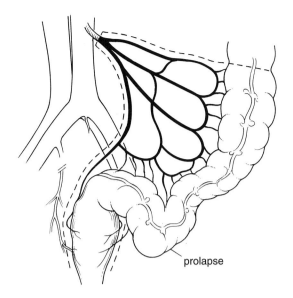

FIGURE 50.3. Dissection of sigmoid mesentery continued to (A) origin of inferior mesenteric artery. The (B) left ureter and (C) gonadal vessels are identified and preserved.

when the ureter and gonadal vessels have been cleared away by the previous retroperitoneal dissection.

Pelvic Dissection

Dissection of the lateral sigmoid attachments is continued distally down the left base of the mesorectum, to the level of the anterior peritoneal reflection. The rectum is then retracted ventrally and to the left while the peritoneum of the right mesorectal base is similarly incised with electrocautery. Subsequently, when the rectum is drawn proximally and lifted anteriorly, the plane between the mesorectum and the presacral fascia (including hypogastric nerves) can be identified. This plane is developed by sharp dissection, with preservation of the nerves, distally to the anorectal junction on the pelvic floor (Fig. 50.4). The lateral rectal stalks are preserved to avoid undue postoperative constipation symptoms.[1] The distal extent of the dissection is confirmed by rectal digital palpation of the tip of the instrument at the posterior anorectal junction.

Resection of the Sigmoid Colon

The distal end of the sigmoid colon and its mesentery are stapled and transected with an endoscopic linear stapler. The sigmoid colon is then delivered from the abdomen through a 4-mm-long suprapubic Pfannenstiel incision. A suitable length of the sigmoid colon is resected, and the distal end is closed around the detached anvil of an intraluminal circular stapling instrument. The proximal end, including the stapler anvil, is then returned into the abdomen, the incision closed, and pneumoperitoneum reconstituted. Reanastomosis is accomplished by intra-anal introduction of the intraluminal circular stapling instrument (Fig. 50.5).

Sutured Rectopexy

The rectum is gently retracted to the left, and an endoscopic suturing device (Endostitch; United States Surgi-

FIGURE 50.4. Retraction of the rectum proximally and forward displays the plane to be developed between the mesorectum and presacral fascia. The pelvic hypogastric nerves are carefully preserved upon the presacral fascia.

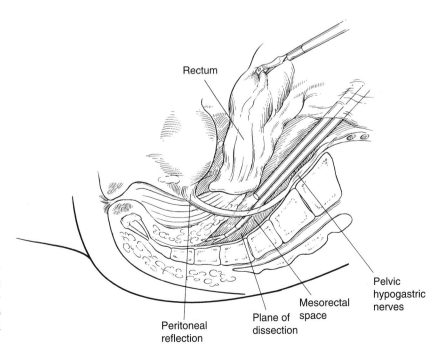

Rectum

Peritoneal reflection

Plane of dissection

Mesorectal space

Pelvic hypogastric nerves

cal, Norwalk, CT, USA) is employed to insert a 2-0 vicryl stitch into the presacral fascia at the level of the sacral promontory (Fig. 50.6), on the right side of the midline. This instrument has a special needle (with two sharp ends) that can be passed securely from each of its two jaws. A suture can thus be expediently inserted into tissue grasped between the jaws of the instrument; care is taken to avoid the ureters and pelvic nerves.

The rectum is then drawn proximally out of the pelvis; at the place where it approximates the sacral promontory stitch, the other end of the suture is passed though the mesorectal edge. The suture is then tied down by an intracorporeal knotting technique and the suture ends cut and extracted (see Fig. 50.6). This suturing procedure is repeated on the left side of the rectum, resulting in the rectum being held straight out of the pelvis, under mild tension. Alternative laparoscopic rectopexy techniques that have been described include the use of polypropylene mesh and a laparoscopic hernia stapler,[2–4] as well as anterior resection alone.[5]

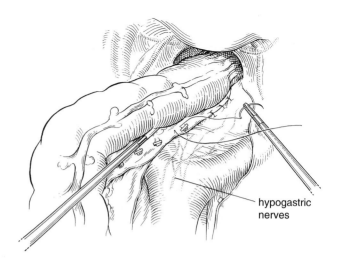

FIGURE 50.6. As the rectum is retracted away, a stitch is placed into the presacral fascia using an Endostitch endoscopic suturing device. After the suture is continued through an appropriate mesorectal edge of the proximally drawn colon, it is tied down by an intracorporeal knotting technique.

Closure of Wounds

The surgical field is checked for hemostasis. The cannulas are removed and the wounds sutured. A rectal tube is routinely inserted.

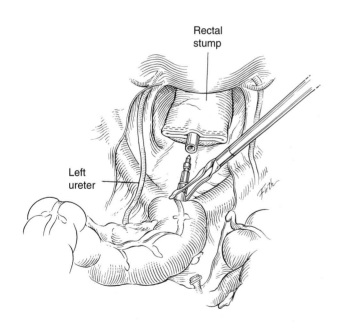

FIGURE 50.5. Reanastomosis of the colon end closed over a detached anvil to the stapled-off rectal stump, with intraluminal circular stapler introduced transanally.

Conclusion

There are many methods of performing surgery for rectal prolapse, including abdominal nonlaparoscopic, abdominal laparoscopic, and perineal approaches. The laparoscopic approaches appeared to offer significant benefits in terms of cosmesis, return of bowel function, decrease in morbidity, length of hospital stay, and length of time to return of bowel function. Only with longer follow-up will function results and recurrence rates become known.

References

1. Speakman CT, Madden MV, Nicholls RJ, Kamm MA. Lateral ligament division during rectopexy causes constipation but prevents recurrence: results of a prospective randomized study. Br J Surg 1991;78:1431–1433.
2. Cuesta MA, Borgstein PJ, De Jong D, Meijer S. Laparoscopic rectopexy. Surg Laparosc Endosc 1993;3:456–458.
3. Darzi AW, Lewis C, Guillou P, Monson J. Stapled laparoscopic rectopexy for rectal prolapse. Surg Endosc 1994;8:233.
4. Cuschieri A, Shimi SM, Vander Velpen G, Banting S, Wood RAB. Laparoscopic prosthesis fixation rectopexy for complete rectal prolapse. Br J Surg 1994;81:138–139.
5. Ballantyne GH. Laparoscopic assisted anterior resection for rectal prolapse. Surg Laparosc Endosc 1992;2:230–236.

51
Laparoscopic Management of Bowel Obstruction

Alon J. Pikarsky and Petachia Reissman

Although some progress in laboratory and imaging studies has been made, the management of intestinal obstruction is still a challenge for the surgeon. Depending on the etiology, intestinal obstruction may be treated conservatively or surgically. As adhesions from previous abdominal surgery are the leading cause of intestinal obstruction,[1] conservative treatment is always attempted first, but any signs or symptoms of bowel ischemia require immediate surgical intervention. In many ways, the wisdom of the adage "never let the sun set on a bowel obstruction" remains the safest guideline whenever any uncertainty exists. Prompt recognition of the need for operative intervention when indicated remains the key to successful management of bowel obstruction.

During the past two decades, few major advances have been made in the management of bowel obstruction, and most surgeons continue to rely on clinical criteria as well as laboratory and radiographic findings to determine if and when to operate on these patients. The most common causes for most cases of small bowel obstruction (SBO) eventually requiring operative intervention are adhesions, followed by hernias and neoplasms.[2] Combined, these etiologies account for 70% to 80% of all cases. When discussing large bowel obstruction (LBO), one must also consider volvulus of the sigmoid and colonic pseudoobstruction, Ogilvie's syndrome.[3] At least 50% of surgical cases are directly related to postoperative adhesions. In these cases, initial nonoperative management is acceptable, with success rates ranging from 50% to 85%. Aggressive, early surgical intervention to avoid ischemic bowel must be balanced against the significant morbidity (30%) and even mortality of such an undertaking. Specifically, previous abdominal surgery and suspected intestinal adhesions along with dilated bowel were initially considered a contraindication to laparoscopy because of the risk of bowel injury and limited visualization.[4] However, both increased surgical experience and improved surgical instrumentation have facilitated a change in opinion to include bowel obstruction as a potential indication for laparoscopic surgery.[5]

Diagnostic laparoscopy can help avoid laparotomy and allow therapeutic laparoscopy in suitable cases. Laparoscopy in the setting of bowel obstruction does, however, pose certain hazards to the patient. The dilated bowel increases the risk of bowel injury at the entry site, especially at the first entry port. Manipulating friable, edematous bowel may cause bowel injury and perforation. Manipulation of gangrenous bowel without rapid vascular control may lead to endotoxic sepsis. These problems can be limited by using an open-first trocar insertion technique and by handling the bowel loops gently.

Another concern related to the laparoscopic technique is the effect of pneumoperitoneum on mesenteric blood flow. Kleinhaus[6] studied the effect of CO_2 insufflation at different intraperitoneal pressures on mesenteric blood flow in dogs. Mesenteric blood flow was reduced to 70% of baseline when the intraperitoneal pressure was 20mmHg. When this pressure was increased to 40mmHg, mesenteric flow was further reduced to 50% of baseline values. When a second group of dogs was subjected to partial balloon occlusion of the superior mesenteric artery, mesenteric blood flow was 50% of baseline at intraperitoneal pressures of 20mmHg and 40% at 40mmHg.

The effect of intraperitoneal pressure on femoral artery flow was even more pronounced. It seems that gas insufflation exerts its hemodynamic effect by two mechanisms. The first is a decrease in cardiac output, as venous return from the lower half of the body is reduced. Additionally, the impact on femoral blood flow suggests either a direct effect on the abdominal aorta and its branches, or a differential response in peripheral resistance in various vascular beds. It is therefore prudent to perform laparoscopy in a patient with acute intestinal obstruction when the intraperitoneal pressure does not exceed 10 to 15mmHg.

TABLE 51.1. Criteria for laparoscopic small bowel obstruction management.

1. Mild abdominal distension[a]
2. Proximal obstruction[a]
3. Partial obstruction[a]
4. Anticipated simple "single band" obstruction[a]
5. Localized radiographic distension
6. No signs of systemic sepsis
7. No history of prior enterolysis
8. Prepare for a laparotomy if necessary

[a] Adapted from Duh.[7]

Because of the many pitfalls and suspected difficulties, even the experienced surgeon must have a low threshold to conversion where there is suspected bowel compromise or extremely dense adhesions. To reduce the chances of accidental enterotomies, an open technique for placement of the initial cannula is advocated. Manipulating the thin-walled, friable, and dilated bowel may result in damage with spillage of large amounts of contaminated succus entericus into the abdominal cavity, which in turn may lead to intra-abdominal abscess or generalized sepsis. Therefore, only atraumatic instruments should be used. Due to these potential complications, Duh[7] has outlined a number of criteria to select patients for laparoscopic management of SBO; we have added several other criteria (Table 51.1).

Obviously, the aim of surgery for intestinal adhesions is relief of the obstruction, if possible, with prevention of recurrent obstruction. Therefore, the indications for laparoscopic adhesiolysis include patients who had previous abdominal surgery and present with transient recurrent episodes or an acute progressive onset of intestinal obstruction. The criteria for laparoscopic surgical treatment of an acute intestinal obstruction are identical to those for a laparotomy and include failure of conservative treatment with increasing pain, progressive dilatation of bowel loops on repeated radiographs, leukocytosis, fever, and development of localized tenderness with peritoneal signs. In chronic recurrent intestinal obstruction, additional findings may include weight loss, postprandial bloating, and alternating diarrhea and constipation.

Technique

In preparation for laparoscopy, the stomach and bladder are drained by catheters. Additionally, in cases of previous pelvic surgery, radiation, prior pelvic sepsis, or multiple lower abdominal surgeries, bilateral ureteric catheters are extremely useful for rapid and safe intraoperative identification of the ureters. For cases in which preoperative evaluation was inconclusive for intraluminal obstruction, intraoperative colonoscopy or enteroscopy should be considered. Therefore, placement of the patient in a modified lithotomy position may be helpful. The operating room setup should include at least two video monitors to enable comfortable inspection for both the surgeon and assistants. All patients should be aware of the potential for a laparotomy, a bowel resection, and a stoma, contingent upon intraoperative findings; routine preoperative enterostomal therapy consultation is helpful.

The initial creation of the pneumoperitoneum should be carefully planned and executed. When choosing the site for placement of the first trocar, previous incisions, including scars from previous laparoscopy should be avoided if possible, because bowel or omentum may be adherent. After the site is chosen, an open technique is used to insert a blunt-tip Hasson trocar or a 10-mm port with video capability. For the Hasson technique, an incision of 10 mm or larger is made followed by incision of the fascia and peritoneum under direct vision. If the site is away from the midline, careful muscle splitting is performed to avoid injury to the epigastric vessels. Once the peritoneal cavity is entered, either a pursestring suture or two stay sutures of the fascia are placed. The blunt-tip trocar or the 10-mm port is now introduced, and the fascial sutures are snugly secured. Therefore, even if a longer skin incision is made, no air leakage will occur. If the initial site is amid multiple adhesions, an effort should be made to close the fascia to prevent air leakage and an alternative site should be chosen. Direct visualization of the peritoneal cavity permits lysis of adhesions in the subumbilical area sufficient to allow placement of a 10-mm trocar under direct visual control. A 0° laparoscope is initially used. Recently, small miniscopes have been introduced for diagnosis as well as surgical purposes. These scopes, which range in diameter between 1.7 and 3.5 mm, can be connected to ordinary laparoscopic cameras. Although the concept is appealing, the technology is still under development, as the resolution of most of these cameras is suboptimal. The second port is used for lysis of adhesions to the abdominal wall, using a 5- or 10-mm scissors with cautery or the harmonic scalpel (Ethicon Endosurgery, Cincinnati, OH, USA) as needed for hemostasis. As the adhesions are lysed and more of the peritoneal cavity can be inspected, additional ports are placed for traction, exposure, and suction-irrigation. Repositioning of the camera and instruments in different ports is usually required when adhesions of omentum and bowel to the abdominal wall are divided. External manual compression often allows delivery of the adhesions into the operative field without requiring an additional port. Once the abdominal wall is cleared of adhesions, careful inspection of the bowel is undertaken.

With the first trocar in place, pneumoperitoneum not exceeding 15 mmHg is established during which there is careful observation of the hemodynamic status of the patient. With any change in the patient's stability, the intra-abdominal pressure should be decreased. Once the scope is in the peritoneal cavity, an initial general inspection is performed for detection of obvious bowel ischemia or gangrene, perforation, or fecal content in the peritoneal cavity, all of which require prompt laparotomy. Other findings that may account for the patient's symptoms but are unrelated to bowel obstruction, such as diverticulitis or pancreatitis, should be treated as appropriate. If the distended bowel loops appear massively dilated, very thin walled, and are anticipated to be very friable and difficult to manipulate safely, one should consider a laparotomy. If no obvious findings are noted during the initial inspection, two more 5- or 10-mm ports are placed on each side below the midline port. The inspection is performed using a two-hand (hand-over-hand) technique with an atraumatic ring clamp and frequent shifting of the operating table position according to the area inspected. Peritoneal fluid, usually present in these cases, is aspirated and can be sent for gram stain, amylase, bilirubin, and culture.

Small Bowel Obstruction

Small Bowel Obstruction Related to Adhesions

In cases of SBO, the small bowel is inspected in a retrograde fashion commencing at the cecum, gently grasping it with the atraumatic graspers using the hand-over-hand technique. The distal small bowel is decompressed and can be evaluated until it enters an area of adhesions where a transitional zone with dilated obstructed bowel is noted. After localizing the point of transition, the underlying pathology can be clarified. In cases where a single adhesive band is causing the obstruction, it can be grasped and divided using scissors, the harmonic scalpel, or electrocautery. When using electrocautery one has to be extremely careful not to injure the adjacent bowel. In other cases where a conglomerate of bowel is captured between a network of adhesive bands, careful sharp dissection of the adhesions should be carried out until the bowel is completely mobilized. Gentle pushing rather than grasping is a safer means of providing traction to facilitate dissection. Similarly, table tilt can help facilitate exposure. After full enterolysis, care must be taken to carefully inspect the entire small bowel. Once again, the bowel should be gently manipulated by pushing with closed instruments rather than by grasping with open ones. Individual areas, especially those sites from which adhesions were divided, need to be inspected. In any questionable areas, myotomy and certainly any enterotomies should be repaired. These maneuvers can be

effected by either intracorporeal or extracorporeal suture techniques. Alternatively, hernia staplers may be suitable for this maneuver.

If any doubts exist, extracorporeal inspection is safest. However, a number of adjunct techniques may be included. Oral or transanal endoscopy with the colonoscope, submersion of the loop in question under water, may follow. More proximal gentle occlusion and endoscopic air insufflation can confirm any injured areas. An alternative technique includes instillation of carbon dioxide through the nasogastric tube with distal gentle occlusion of the bowel, again carefully inspecting any areas in question. One of the major dangers in laparoscopic enterolysis is failure to detect injured areas, mandating subsequent reoperation or potentially leading to enterocutaneous fistulas. Indeed, of the 35 patients treated laparoscopically, as reported by Bailey,[8] 5 required early reoperation (14%) compared with 4 of 88 patients (4.6%) treated by laparotomy. Of the 5 patients, 2 had reobstruction, possibly due to missed obstructing bands, and 3 were operated for perforation due to missed injuries during the procedure. If a loop of bowel needs to be resected, general principles of laparoscopic colorectal surgery should be applied. The anastomosis is best performed extracorporeally after the bowel is exteriorized through a small, protected incision such as during laparoscopic-assisted colectomy.

Chronic Abdominal Pain

Unfortunately, it is difficult to judge the results of laparoscopic enterolysis for bowel obstruction as it is obfuscated in many series by the inclusion of patients with chronic abdominal pain. Although gynecologists consider adhesions as a major cause of abdominal pain, this theory is less accepted by colorectal and general surgeons. Nonetheless, there may be certain patients in whom chronic pain is a feature in addition to chronic intermittent or acute relapsing SBO. Many of the series in the literature include patients admitted for *elective* enterolysis for chronic abdominal pain. Although some of these patients may be candidates, care should be taken to communicate to patients that reoperation will allow division of adhesions, may allow relief of obstruction, but may do nothing to address any preexisting pain. Appropriate preoperative evaluations in these patients include not only extensive review of all prior hospitalization records for bouts of obstruction but also review of prior plane radiographs, small bowel series, enteroclysis studies, and other gastrointestinal investigations.

Tumors

Tumors are a much less common cause of SBO than are postoperative adhesions. However, an older patient or a patient who has not had prior abdominal surgery is at a higher risk of presenting with this cause of SBO. Initial exploration is undertaken in the same fashion as in SBO related to adhesions. After inspecting the collapsed distal bowel, the tumor is identified as the obstructing mass. When resecting a tumor, one is obliged also to resect the nodal basin, including a wide resection margin in the mesentery. Although technically feasible as an intracorporeal procedure, the time commitment, cost, potential for contamination, need for a subsequent incision for specimen delivery, and lack of any demonstrable benefit militate against its use. Instead, the bowel containing the tumor should be exteriorized through an appropriately placed and protected incision. The tumor should then be resected with a wide mesenteric margin, and ultimately intestinal continuity should be restored. A thorough inspection of the abdominal cavity including all surfaces of the liver should be undertaken to exclude metastatic disease. If the tumor is fixed to surrounding organs, causing a conglomerate of bowel loops or associated with severe shortening of the mesentery, as in cases of carcinoid tumors, the safest approach may be conversion to a laparotomy. Judgement and critical appraisal of one's skill and available instrumentation must supercede the desire for a technical triumph.

Ischemic or Gangrenous Bowel

Ischemic and gangrenous bowel in the setting of SBO are related to a closed-loop obstruction, usually caused by an adhesive band. Because venous occlusion precedes the arterial occlusions, the ischemic loop appears congested with dilated veins, despite visible arterial pulsation. Subsequently, secondary arterial thrombosis occurs. Newly developed Doppler probes may help determine arterial mesenteric pulsation during the laparoscopic inspection. Whether by laparotomy or laparoscopy, dividing the obstructive band in these circumstances requires extreme caution. The compromised loop of bowel should be manipulated as minimally as possible; attempts should be made instead to grasp the band itself. After freeing the obstructed loop, it should be left in situ for 15 to 20 min while the rest of the bowel is inspected. Because the loop might revert to a viable state, it may be difficult to later recognize. Accordingly, clips should be carefully applied to the mesentery at the bowel junction at both the proximal and distal limits of the ischemia. Normal color, peristalsis, and reversal of the venous congestion are positive signs, indicating that the obstruction was relieved and the loop is viable. If the bowel is gangrenous and mandates resection, the procedure is completed as a laparoscopically assisted small bowel resection with extracorporeal anastomosis. Before completion of either procedure, extensive normal saline irrigation should be undertaken.

Large Bowel Obstruction

The most common etiology for LBO necessitating immediate intervention is an obstructing tumor.[9] To date, the precise role of laparoscopic surgery for the curative treatment of carcinoma of the colon is not yet established. We therefore do not recommend a laparoscopic approach for obstructing colonic carcinomas at this stage. If a carcinoma is suspected, intraoperative colonoscopic verification should be undertaken. The procedure may then be converted to a laparotomy. However, if metastatic disease is present, a palliative resection may be laparoscopically appropriate. Appropriate preoperative investigation including such methods as endoscopy, flat and upright x-ray, endoscopy, water-soluble contrast enema, and CT scan should allow appropriate diagnosis of LBO. It should be relatively infrequent that a LBO is not preoperatively detected and becomes an intraoperative laparoscopic diagnosis. Efforts should be made to distinguish between these entities before surgery because of the vastly different methods of treatment. Specifically, the patient with a complete left-sided colonic obstruction may require a stoma (which may be permanent) or a subtotal colectomy, which may necessitate a laparotomy and significantly alter bowel habits. Diverticulitis and inflammatory bowel disease may sometimes present as colonic obstruction. Techniques to treat these entities are discussed separately in other chapters.

Volvulus

Volvulus of the sigmoid colon is initially treated by decompression of the colon. Suboptimal decompression or recurrence of the volvulus is an indication for resection.[10] Opinions differ regarding the extent of the resection, and although some authors advocate subtotal colectomy, many surgeons consider sigmoid colectomy the procedure of choice. Laparoscopic sigmoid resection can be preceded by "on table" lavage, using the appendix as the inflow tract. The appendix is exteriorized through the right lower quadrant port, and the terminal ileum is clamped through the other working channel. The sigmoid colon, after being divided with an endo-GIA stapler at the rectosigmoid junction, is exteriorized through a small incision in the left lower quadrant that serves as the outflow tract for the lavage. Using a 0° camera inserted in the umbilicus and two working ports along the right anterior axillary lines, the sigmoid colon is freed from its lateral attachments. The colon is transected at the rectosigmoid junction with a linear endo-stapler, taking care not to open the peritoneal reflection. A 5-cm incision is made in the left iliac fossa through which the sigmoid colon can be exteriorized. Control of the sigmoidal arteries can be extracorporeally undertaken, followed by resection. The detachable anvil of a 33-mm circular stapler is secured to the colon by a pursestring suture. The colon is returned to the abdominal cavity, after which a 33-mm working port is inserted through the incision and pneumoperitoneum is reestablished. The circular stapler is introduced through the rectum, and an end-to-end colorectal anastomosis is constructed. Alternatively, intracorporeal vascular ligation can be undertaken as for any standard sigmoid colectomy. However, the redundancy and mobility of the sigmoid provide a unique opportunity to expedite and decrease cost by performaning a laparoscopic-assisted procedure.

Ogilvie's Syndrome

Colonic pseudoobstruction (Ogilvie's syndrome) is part of the differential diagnosis of colonic obstruction. Common in eldery, debilitated patients following surgery, trauma, or sepsis, the syndrome is manifested by marked gaseous dilatation of the colon.[11] Both diagnosis and treatment include colonoscopy to exclude mechanical obstruction and allow decompression. Colonic decompression as an adjunct to treatment of the underlying condition is mandated when the cecal diameter on a plain radiograph increases (>9–12 cm). Colonoscopic decompression is successful in 85% of cases, although a second or third attempt may be required. Alternatives to colonoscopic decompression include epidural morphine instillation. The success rate of any of these procedures, including colonoscopic decompression, is generally contingent upon correction of the underlying abnormalities. In most cases, protein, albumin, and electrolyte abnormalities need to be reversed to prevent recurrence of Ogilvie's syndrome. In some recalcitrant cases, either because the underlying etiology cannot be corrected or because recurrent Ogilvie's syndrome is noted even after correction, surgery is necessary.

If the cecum shows signs of ischemia or perforation, resection is required. Otherwise, if the cecum is viable, a cecostomy can be created. Laparoscopy offers excellent exploration in these moribund patients. The cecum is gently grasped through a right anterior axillary line port, at the level of the umbilicus. This grasper is used to manipulate the cecum from side to side to evaluate its viability and to exclude perforation. Four T-fasteners (Flexico Introducer Gastrostomy Kit; Ross Laboratories, Columbus, OH, USA) are introduced through the abdominal wall into the cecum, under direct laparoscopic control. Pneumoperitoneum is reduced to 8 mmHg, and the fasteners are retracted to attach the cecum to the abdominal wall. Using the Seldinger technique, a 16F bladder catheter (stiffened by a stylet introducer) is inserted into the cecum. The presence of leak is radiographically ruled out by injecting soluble contrast material into the bladder catheter. The bladder catheter can now be connected to a bag for gravity drainage. The fasteners may be cut close to the skin 14 days after placement, and the metal bars will pass in the stool. This method avoids laparotomy in the absence of bowel infarction in these high-risk patients.

Cecostomies can be difficult to manage. Alternatively, a Thurbolt "blowhole" transverse colostomy can be performed. This technique entails maturation of only the antemesenteric border of the sigmoid colon rather than its full thickness of both walls. The maturation can be undertaken either laparoscopically or as a trephine procedure. The advantage of laparoscopy is that it allows complete abdominal inspection as opposed to the trephine procedure, which only allows maturation of the stoma.

Contraindications

The absolute contraindications for laparoscopic treatment of intestinal obstruction in chronic, recurrent, or acute episodes are similar to those in other laparoscopic procedures and include coagulopathies and inability to tolerate general anesthesia. Relative contraindications include the following.

Severe abdominal distension with massively dilated small bowel: this condition may be associated with higher risk of bowel injury during the insufflation and dissection as well as limited exposure and visualization.

Peritonitis: in cases of localized or diffuse peritonitis, perforated or gangrenous bowel may already be present; if compromised bowel is found, it may increase the risk of septic complications following surgery; laparotomy with prompt resection and rapid completion of the procedure is desired.

The final contraindication and perhaps the most important relates to the surgeon's sound judgment concerning safety during the procedure: in the presence of extremely dense adhesions and fused loops of bowel, the risk of enterotomy is increased. In such cases, laparotomy will help ensure the patient's safe outcome.

Results

Clinical experience with laparoscopy as a primary diagnostic and therapeutic tool in patients with SBO is gradually increasing (Table 51.2). Since the case reported by Bastug et al. in 1991,[12] other reports with more patients have appeared. Keating in 1992[14] was successful in laparoscopic adhesiolysis in 5 patients with SBO. Two years later, Franklin[15] reported 23 patients treated over a period of 2 years. As seen in Table 51.2, 20 of these patients were suc-

TABLE 51.2. Resutls of laparoscopic small bowel obstruction (SBO) management.

Author	Number of patients	Morbidity	Mortality	Correct diagnosis	Laparoscopy treatment	Conversion
Bastug[12]	1	0	0	1	1	0
Adams[13]	3	0	0	3	3	0
Keating[14]	5	0	0	5	5	0
Franklin[15]	23	4	0	23	20	3
Ibrahim[16]	33	1	1	28	22	5 (6 assisted)
Bailey[8]	55	4	1	50	31	9 (15 assisted)

cessfully treated laparoscopically. Ibrahim[16] and Bailey[8] in two more recent reports have treated larger numbers of patients, and it seems from these reports that the conversion rate is overall approximately 10% to 20%, with morbidity and mortality comparable to that achieved with conventional open treatment of SBO. All these reports lack long-term follow-up, and the impact of laparoscopy on recurrence of adhesions and bowel obstruction requires such long-term follow-up. Indeed, one of the potential advantages of laparoscopy, particularly in the setting of SBO, is a decreased rate of adhesion formation. Several animal models have shown a decreased rate of adhesion formation. Using a model of anterior resection in pigs, we have shown reduction of both rate and severity of adhesion formation when comparing laparoscopy to conventional laparotomy.[17] In at least one report,[8] the patients who were laparoscopically managed were discharged earlier than those managed by laparotomy. However, the laparoscopically treated patients did show a trend to less severe disease. Overall, 27 patients treated laparoscopically left the hospital within 3 days.

Laparoscopy also has a potential role for treating chronic pain caused by adhesions. Several reports addressed the use of laparoscopy for the evaluation and treatment of chronic abdominal and pelvic pain caused by postoperative adhesions. In a retrospective study by Lavonius et al.,[18] 46 patients underwent laparoscopy for chronic abdominal pain, having an average duration of symptoms of 3.5 years. Of these 46 patients, 72% had had previous surgery. In 29 patients, adhesions were found to be the cause of the pain, 24 of whom underwent concomitant adhesiolysis with resultant resolution of the symptoms. Fayez and Clark[19] had the same results in 156 patients presenting with chronic abdominal pain following surgery, and several other retrospective studies concur with these findings.[20,21]

New Directions

Until recently, adhesion-related research has focused upon defining the incidence, causes, and treatment of adhesive disease. However, within the past few years, significant progress has been made in potentially limiting the development of adhesions. Several animal studies have shown the efficacy of hyaluronic acid-carboxymethylcellulose (HA/CMC) in decreasing the rate of adhesion formation. Hadaegh et al.[22] used 60 rabbits to show that HA/CMC significantly reduces adhesion formation when complete anastomoses are constructed. Importantly, HA/CMC did not affect the wound healing process when an incomplete anastomosis was constructed. In these cases, however, HA/CMC did not affect adhesion formation. The application of HA/CMC was also found to decrease adhesions in a uterine horn injury in rabbits[23] and in the presence of foreign bodies (mesh application) in rats. Again, neither of these studies reported adverse effects on wound healing.[24]

Human studies have also demonstrated a significant reduction in adhesion formation using HA/CMC. Specifically, Becker et al.[25] described their prospective randomized surgeon-blinded study of 183 patients in whom Seprafilm™ (Genzyme Corp., Cambridge MA, USA) was placed. A significant decrease in adhesion formation to the site of application was noted in patients who received Seprafilm™ after restorative proctocolectomy, as compared to a control group. Subsequently, Wexner et al.[26] (one of the original investigators in the study by Becker et al.[25]) documented a 75% rate of successful relief of chronic bowel obstruction in 15 patients in a compassionate use application.[26] Last, Salum et al.[27] compared 259 consecutive patients in whom Seprafilm™ was placed during colorectal surgery to a group of 179 patients who underwent a procedure and diagnosis-matched surgery without the application of Seprafilm™. There was more than a 50% reduction in the need for laparotomy for bowel obstruction in the Seprafilm™ group during a mean follow-up of 65 months; the same reduction was not noted in the non-Seprafilm™ group at a mean follow-up of 81 months.

Although it is very exciting to consider that there may be potential to actually reduce the formation of adhesions or at least the need for laparotomy for treatment for those adhesions, to date there is no means of easy laparoscopic application. However, during laparoscopic-assisted procedures, the 12 × 8 cm sheets of Seprafilm™ can be cut into smaller pieces and placed through the 3-

to 5-cm-long laparoscopic-assisted incisions. This method has become our routine practice since U.S. Food and Drug Administration approval of Seprafilm™ in August 1996.

The other concern in routine placement of Seprafilm™ is its use in the "high-risk" setting. Specifically, the patient in whom it may be most efficacious is the patient with the most tenacious adhesions who has undergone enterolysis for obstruction. This is the very patient in whom an enterotomy or myotomy may have been created. To answer this question, Moreira et al.[28] prospectively randomized 160 injured sites of bowel in a rabbit model. The randomization groups included repaired enterotomies, repaired and unrepaired myotomies, and a control group. Seprafilm™ was associated with a statistically significant decrease in the incidence of adhesions to these sites without causing any increase in septic sequelae such as abscess, phlegmon, or anastomotic leak.

Conclusion

The role of laparoscopy in the diagnosis and treatment of bowel obstruction is not yet fully established. The recent increase in the number of publications on this topic reflects greater experience with this modality and presumably more enthusiasm for it. It seems that laparoscopy has a definite role in establishing an early diagnosis in patients with SBO. Whether the long-term effect of laparoscopic adhesiolysis on the formation of adhesions will prove to be more favorable compared with conventional laparotomy has yet to be proven in long-term studies. So far, based on animal studies, this hypothesis seems to be true. As with any new approach, it is crucial to be aware of the limitations and potential disadvantages of this procedure to limit any adverse outcome. Judgment, rather than any instrument or technique, remains the best tool that the surgeon possesses.

References

1. Bastug DF. Laparoscopic adhesiolysis for small bowel obstruction. Surg Laparosc Endosc 1991;4:259–62.
2. Mucha P. Small bowel obstruction. Surg Clin N Am 1983; 67:597–620.
3. Anuras S. Colonic pseudoobstruction. Am J Gastroenterol 1984;79:525–532.
4. Reissman P. Laparoscopic colorectal surgery: ascending the learning curve. World J Surg 1996;20:277–282.
5. Sackier J, Wexner SD (eds) Protocols in General Surgery. Laparoscopic Colorectal Surgery. New York: Wiley, 1999.
6. Kleinhaus S. Effects of laparoscopy on mesenteric blood flow. Arch Surg 1978;113:867–869.
7. Duh QY. Small bowel obstruction. In: Toouli J, Gossot D, Hunter JG (eds) Endosurgery. New York: Churchill Livingstone, 1996:425–431.
8. Bailey IS. Laparoscopic management of acute small bowel obstruction. Br J Surg 1998;85:84–87.
9. Serpell JW. Obstructing carcinoma of the colon. Br J Surg 1989;76:965–969.
10. Mellor SG. The aetiology and management of sigmoid volvulus in the UK: how much colon need to be excised? Ann R Coll Surg Engl 1990;72:193–195.
11. Geelhoed GW. Colonic pseudo-obstruction in surgical patients. Am J Surg 1985;149:258–265.
12. Bastug DF, Trammell SW, Boland JP, Mantz EP, Tiley EH III. Laparoscopic adesiolysis for small bowel obstruction. Surg Laparosc Endosc 1991;1(4):259–262.
13. Adams S. Laparoscopic management of acute small bowel obstruction. Aust N Z J Surg 1993;63:39–41.
14. Keating J. Laparoscopy in the diagnosis and treatment of acute small bowel obstruction. J Laparosc Endosc Surg 1992; 2:239–244.
15. Franklin ME. Laparoscopic surgery in acute small bowel obstruction. Surg Laparosc Endosc 1994;4:289–296.
16. Ibrahim IM. Laparoscopic management of acute small-bowel obstruction. Surg Endosc 1996;10:1012–1015.
17. Reissman P, Teoh TA, Skinner K, Burns JW, Wexner SD. Adhesion formation after laparoscopic anterior resection in a porcine model: a pilot study. Surg Laparosc Endosc 1996; 6:136–139.
18. Lavonius M, Gulichsen R, Laine S, Ovaska J. Laparoscopy for chronic abdominal pain. Surg Laparosc Endosc 1999; 9:42–44.
19. Fayez JA, Clark RR. Operative laparoscopy for the treatment of localized chronic pelvic pain caused by postoperative adhesions. J Gynecol Surg 1994;10:79–83.
20. Klingensmith ME, Soybel DI, Brooks DC. Laparoscopy for chronic abdominal pain. Surg Endosc 1996;10: 1085–1087.
21. Miller K, Mayer E, Moritz E. The role of laparoscopy in cronic and recurrent abdominal pain. Am J Surg 1996;172: 353–356.
22. Hadaegh A, Bruns J, Burgess L, Rose R, Rowe E, Lamarte WW, Becker JM. Effects of hyaluronic acid/carboxymethylcellulose gel on bowel anastomoses in the New Zealand white rabbit. J Gastrointest Surg 1997;1: 569–578.
23. Leach RE, Burns JW, Dawe EJ, SmithBarbour MD, Diamond MP. Reduction of postsurgical adhesion formation in the rabbit uterine horn model with use of hyaluronate/carboxymeth-cellulose gel. Fertil Steril 1998;69:415–418.
24. Alponat A, Lakshminarasappa SR, Yavuz N, Goh PM. Prevention of adhesions by Seprafilm™, an absorbable adhesion barrier: an incisional hernia model in rats. Am Surg 1997;63:818–819.
25. Becker JM, Dayton MT, Fazio VW. Prevention of postoperative abdominal adhesions by a sodium hyaluronate-based bioresorbable membrane: a prospective, randomized, double-blind multicenter study. J Am Coll Surg 1996;183: 297–306.

26. Wexner S, Beck D, Seprafilm™ Compassionate Study Group. Clinical resolution of life threatening recurrent adhesive disease by Seprafilm™: a compassionate use treatment series [abstract]. Dis Colon Rectum 1998;41:A58.

27. Salum M, Lam DTY, Wexner SD, et al. Does bioresorbable membrane of modified sodium hyaluronate and car-

boxymethylcellulose (Seprafilm™) have possible short term beneficial impact. Dis Colon Rectum 2001;44:706–712.

28. Moreira H Jr, Wexner S, Yamaguchi T, et al. Use of bioresorbable membrane (sodium hyaluronate and carboxyme + hylcellulose) after controlled bowel injuries in a rabbit model. Dis Colon Rectum 2000;43:182–187.

52
The Role of Transanal Endoscopic Microsurgery and Intraoperative Colonoscopy

Luca A. Vricella and Bruce A. Orkin

Transanal Endoscopic Microsurgery

The principles of laparoscopic surgery can be utilized in the management of lesions that involve the mid- and upper rectum. Using constant insufflation and specifically designed instruments, transanal endoscopic microsurgery (TEM), provides improved visualization of the rectum and allows surgical endoscopic manipulation and resection of lesions previously thought to be inaccessible by a transanal approach.[1] Extirpation of superficial rectal carcinomas, large sessile villous adenomas, or disc excision of the base of an incompletely excised polyp can now be safely accomplished in selected patients with the use of TEM. This chapter focuses on the technical aspects of this new therapeutic modality[2-6] as well as on those of intraoperative colonoscopy.

Patient Selection and Preoperative Evaluation

Careful patient selection is of foremost importance in TEM. Because of instrumentation length, lesions localized beyond 20 cm from the anal verge are not candidates for transanal endoscopic resection. The normal narrowing of the sigmoid colon as opposed to the rectum and the angulation of the rectosigmoid junction may further reduce this limit. The distance from the anus must also allow for a 1-cm margin proximal and distal to the lesion. Tumors located in the lower third of the rectum (within 8 cm of the anal verge) may be safely and efficiently excised by conventional transanal techniques. Also, lesions in the distal rectum may not be suitable for TEM because the beveled end of the operating proctoscope may not remain completely within the lumen, making it difficult to maintain insufflation. Also, bleeding may be more profuse because of proximity to the hemorrhoidal vessels.[7] Furthermore, these lesions are often easily removed by standard transanal technique. Small, pedunculated neoplasms of the mid and upper rectum are candidates for endoscopic excision by means of flexible or rigid sigmoidoscopy. For large or even circumferential tumors located 8 cm cephalad, TEM is a much more elegant and complete form of excision, as opposed to piecemeal endoscopic removal by other techniques. Lesions of the middle third of the rectum may be excised transanally with other types of retractors or by transsphincteric or parasacral approaches such as the York-- Mason or Kraske methods, respectively. Nevertheless, these procedures are laborious and associated with substantial morbidity.[8,9]

Malignant lesions may be excised using TEM, but the depth of penetration and pathological features of the lesion limit the indications for local excision. Local excision of rectal malignancies is predicated on selection of lesions with low risk for lymphatic or distant spread and, thus, a high likelihood of cure. Classically, mobile neoplasms (suggesting superficial invasion) with a diameter smaller than 3 cm, exophytic morphology, and involvement of less than one-third of the rectal circumference are candidates for transanal excision. Preoperative staging is limited because lymph node status cannot be directly assessed until pathological examination. Currently, the risk of lymphatic or distant spread seems to correlate best with depth of invasion into the rectal wall. Lymphatic metastasis are present in less than 5% of patients with T1 carcinomas or those limited to the submucosa. Infiltration into or through the muscularis propria (T2 and T3 lesions) is associated with higher incidences of nodal involvement (15% and up to 50%, respectively) as well as disseminated disease and higher local recurrence rates.[9-11] These statistics may be analyzed together. Because less than 50% of patients with lymphatic involvement will be cured by radical surgery, even with adjuvant therapy, and only 5% or less of patients with T1 lesions will have lymph node metastases, less than 2% of these patients would benefit from radical resection. Furthermore, no statistically significant difference in local recurrence and 5 year mortality has been noted when comparing outcomes for matched groups with T1 lesions.[12,13] Therefore, TEM excision may be recommended for patients with T1 lesions of the proximal and midrectum.

Endorectal ultrasound (EUS) has become a major determinant of local resectability, having played a pivotal role in the preoperative staging of patients with lesions of the middle and upper rectum for more than a decade.[14] Specificity and sensitivity in detecting depth of wall penetration have been reported to be as high as 96% and 89%, respectively, in experienced hands. Sensitivity in detecting lymphatic disease is, however, well under 80% because lymphatic involvement is often microscopic and EUS only detects grossly enlarged nodes.[15] EUS is also of practical value in the follow-up of patients who have undergone TEM as early local recurrence may be found before the development of other signs or symptoms. Some authors have advocated preoperative staging with magnetic resonance imaging (MRI) or computerized tomography (CT). We have not found CT to accurately stage the local disease although liver involvement may be seen, and, even though MRI with an endoluminal coil is reasonably accurate, it is more expensive and no more accurate than EUS.

Once the patient is selected for TEM, a colonoscopy is performed to exclude the presence of synchronous pathology. Preoperative CT of the abdomen may be obtained to detect hepatic metastases in patients with a malignancy. If the liver is extensively involved, TEM may still be considered an option for local control and palliation.[16] Transanal endoscopic microsurgery (EM) may also be selectively considered in rare high-risk patients with T2 and T3 rectal carcinomas, following a detailed discussion of the increased risk of local recurrence and lymphatic spread.

Tumor differentiation and lymphovascular invasion are often discussed as separate prognostic factors. Poorly differentiated lesions and those tumors with involvement of the submucosal lymphatics and vessels are more likely to have spread to the lymph nodes. Therefore, conventional surgical resection is generally a more appropriate approach for these patients.

Although TEM is primarily used for transanal local excision of rectal polyps and early carcinomas, other indications have been explored. The technique has been applied to the treatment of rectal prolapse, solitary rectal ulcers, and rectal stenosis.[7,10] We have found that other approaches are much more fruitful when treating patients with prolapse. Excision of symptomatic solitary rectal ulcers is reasonable in the occasional patient without prolapse. Benign stenoses of the mid and upper rectum may be treated by transanal stricturoplasty with the assistance of the TEM apparatus. Malignant stenoses are best treated by proctectomy, but palliative transanal treatments such as laser recanulation, stents, and even circumferential transanal excision with anastomosis may be used in selected cases. For the purpose of this chapter, we describe the technical aspects of TEM as they apply to the curative resection of rectal neoplasms because this diagnosis is by far the most frequent indication for the procedure.

Instrumentation and Preoperative Preparation

The basic instrumentation for TEM consists of (1) an operating proctoscope attached to the "basic element," (2) the optical system, (3) the insufflation apparatus, and (4) the TEM instruments. In addition, a standard electrocautery unit, a rigid sigmoidoscope, and a wall suction are needed.

The basic element consists of a metal ring or collar with a handle. The operating proctoscope is docked to one side of the basic element, and a faceplate is attached to the other. Each element is locked into place to make the system airtight. The unit is anchored to the operating table using a Martin arm with a universal double-ball-and-socket joint system. This arm is easily adjusted during the course of the procedure to allow for the frequent repositioning of the TEM unit needed to keep the operating field within the usable area of the scope. The operating proctoscopes provided with the set are 12 and 20 cm long and have an external diameter of 40 mm; two faceplates are supplied to close the system. The first has a simple window and an attachment for a fiberoptic light source. This type is used for initial insertion and positioning of the operating proctoscope. An insufflation port is mounted on the basic unit whereas the second faceplate is the working unit. The older version has five large ports, four of which are raised and lipped. The first port is for the visual system, and the other three are used for instruments (Fig. 52.1); the newer units have four ports,

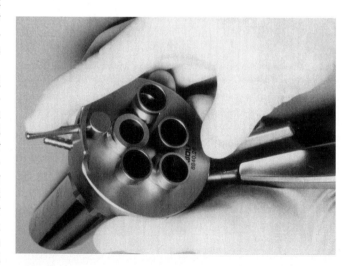

FIGURE 52.1. Proctoscope with working insert (faceplate) in place.

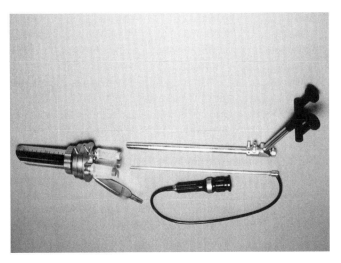

FIGURE 52.2. Basic element, optical system, and side-viewing optical port.

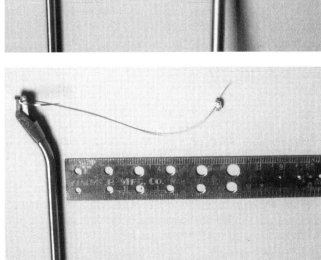

as the fifth was unnecessary. Plastic sleeves and caps are mounted on each of the four ports to provide a gas-tight seal.

The visual system provides a binocular, three-dimensional, direct view of the operative field including approximately sixfold magnification, depending on how close to the lesion it is placed. An additional monocular view is provided for the assistant, which is generally attached to a standard video camera so that the entire team may view the procedure on a monitor (Fig. 52.2). The shaft of the visual system is advanced through the working faceplate and down the superior side of the proctoscope. The tip is beveled to view the field at a 45° downward angle, mirroring the bevel of the operating scope.

FIGURE 52.4. A. The suture is pulled taught with the needle holder (left hand), and the silver clip is applied with the right-handed instrument. B. The silver clip is then released.

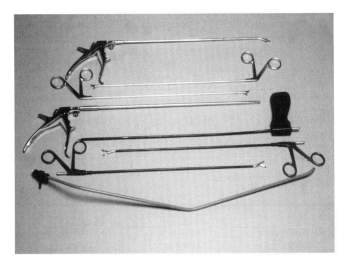

FIGURE 52.3. Typical instrument set for transanal endoscopic microsurgery (TEM).

To support the endosurgical unit that provides insufflation, irrigation, and suction, a bundle of tubes runs from the unit to the operating system. The unit distends the rectum with carbon dioxide (CO_2) with flow rates up to 6 liters/min, maintaining and monitoring intracavitary pressures through a separate line at 12 to 15 mmHg. The unit also supplies low-pressure suction using a roller-pump mechanism and low-pressure irrigation to clear the view.

The instruments used for TEM are angulated downward, paralleling the 45° viewing angle. Included in the typical set are straight and angulated, locking needle drivers, right- and left-angled forceps, right and left curved scissors, suture clip appliers, and a high-frequency electrocautery knife (Fig. 52.3). The clip appliers facilitate placement of a silver clip to anchor the proximal and distal end of the running suture in place of tying a suture (Fig. 52.4A,B). A sliver clip is placed on a 3-0 polydioxanone suture (PDS II; Ethicon Endosurgery, Sommerville, NJ, USA) at 6cm from the needle. The suture is trimmed and is subsequently used to reapproximate the rectal defect following tumor excision.

Preoperative bowel preparation includes a mechanical cleansing with either 4 liters oral polyethylene glycol solution or 90ml sodium phosphate, followed by oral antibiotics; systemic antibiotics are administered on the induction of anesthesia. The risks of the procedure are discussed at length with the patient and family, with particular emphasis placed on the possibility of conversion to laparotomy, as well as the possibility of local recurrence of carcinoma and of undetected lymphatic disease. Other complications specific to TEM are discussed, including bleeding, pelvic infection, suture line dehiscence, incontinence, urinary retention, rectovaginal fistula, and rectal stenosis.

Intraoperative Technique

The procedure is usually undertaken under general endotracheal anesthesia, although regional anesthesia has been used in selected patients. A urinary catheter is inserted, after which the patient is appropriately positioned to ensure that the lesion is in the dependent aspect of the operating field. The exact location of the lesion within the rectum is determined by preoperative rigid proctoscopy and is confirmed with proctoscopy at the beginning of the procedure. The later examination is concluded with intraluminal lavage with povidone-iodine (Betadine). For posterior lesions, the easiest to approach, the patient is placed in the lithotomy position. Anterior rectal lesions require the patient to be in the prone jack-knife position. The surgeon must sit between the patient's legs, so the patient's thighs are flexed at 90° at the hips and knees, and stirrups support the legs. For lateral tumor locations, the patient is placed in the lateral decubitus position with the legs flexed and placed on an arm board to the left or right; accordingly, the perineum is positioned well beyond the edge of the operating table. Pressure points are padded with foam, and intravenous fluid administration is minimized during the procedure to decrease the risk of postoperative urinary retention.

On completion of positioning, rigid proctoscopy is performed to again confirm the location of the tumor and to irrigate the field. The perineum and, if necessary, the vagina are prepped and draped in a sterile fashion. After digital dilatation of the anal canal, the operating proctoscope attached to the basic unit is inserted into the rectum, and the obturator is removed. The window faceplate is attached to the basic unit and the rectum is manually insufflated. The operating proctoscope is positioned with the right portion of the lesion in the lower middle of the field. The window faceplate is exchanged for the working faceplate. The optic system is inserted and posi-

tioned to view the entire field. Each of the instrument ports is occluded with a sleeve and cap that are squeezed when exchanging instruments to minimize CO_2 loss. The tubing lines from the endosurgical unit are attached to the appropriate sites for CO_2 insufflation, pressure monitoring, irrigation, and suction. The electrocautery and fiberoptic light cords are attached to the cautery knife and optical system, respectively. Insufflation is begun, and the field is examined for optimal positioning. A forceps is inserted through the left port in the faceplate, the cautery knife through the right port, and the angled suction instrument through the inferior port (Fig. 52.5). Escape of CO_2 into the proximal colon has not been a significant problem as it is rapidly absorbed and exhaled.

Manipulation of the operating instruments during TEM is severely limited by the diameter of the operating proctoscope and the fact that they must be used in parallel. This technical limitation must be overcome during TEM training because most new practitioners of the technique are used to working at right or acute angles during laparotomy or laparoscopy; this feature contributes to the significant learning curve associated with this procedure.

The margins of resection are demarcated with spot electrocauterization. This step is essential because it becomes very difficult to determine the correct line of dissection once the excision is begun. Some surgeons infiltrate the submucosal plane along the margins with dilute epinephrine to minimize bleeding, although we have not found this step to be necessary. The dissection begins at the right edge of the lesion and proceeds to the left. The extreme right margin is divided with the cautery knife, held in the right hand, and then the edge on the

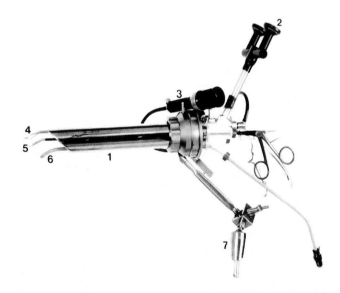

FIGURE 52.5. Fully assembled transanal endoscopic microsurgical unit: *1*, proctoscope; *2*, optic system; *3*, side-viewing port; *4*, needle holder; *5*, forceps; *6*, suction catheter; *7*, Martin arm.

lesion side is grasped with the forceps, held in the left hand. The lesion can then be pulled to the left, maintaining traction on the plane of dissection, while the cautery knife in the right hand continues the resection. All vessels are cauterized and immediately controlled upon visualization because any bleeding will rapidly obscure the field. Most bleeding is controlled by direct cauterization; occasionally a vessel may need to be grasped with the forceps and cauterized by transferring the cord to the post on the handle of the forceps.

Typically, the lesion is removed by full-thickness excision of the wall into the pericolic fat at right angles to the plane of the mucosa. Less frequently, tumors that are of benign appearance on exam, EUS, and biopsy may be excised in the submucosal plane. This method may be helpful for anterior lesions in women because of concerns regarding entry into the vagina or cul-de-sac. However, larger adenomas have up to a 30% to 50% risk of harboring a focus of occult cancer. If a focus of invasive carcinoma is identified on postoperative pathological examination, this submucosal excision may be deemed inadequate. Some authors have even advocated deeper excision of perirectal fat to attempt to include mesorectal lymph nodes;[3] however we do not believe that this approach is justified. In addition, the defect left after mucosectomy and partial wall excision may be more difficult to close than a full-thickness excision because of undue tension on the suture line.[17] Some surgeons choose to leave these wounds open to heal secondarily. Our usual practice is to performed full-thickness excisions, except in occasional cases.

It is crucial to manipulate only the normal tissue around the margin of the lesion rather than the lesion itself, to avoid tearing, bleeding, or seeding into the excision bed. The operating proctoscope must be frequently repositioned to optimize the exposure necessary for such a technique. Following complete excision, the specimen is firmly grasped with the forceps and removed as a unit with the faceplate, taking care to maintain its orientation. The specimen is carefully pinned onto a corkboard that is labeled to orient the pathologist. Insufflation is discontinued, and a gauze pad is placed into the excision bed. Should there be any question of tumor-free margins, frozen-section examination may be indicated to guide further resection of the appropriate area.

The gauze sponge is removed, and the site is irrigated through the open scope. The working faceplate is reattached to the basic element and insufflation is resumed. The defect is usually closed in a transverse fashion from right to left with a running 3-0 polydioxanone suture placed through the full thickness of the rectal wall. Smaller defects may be longitudinally reapproximated from proximal to distal if the diameter of the lumen will not be compromised. A sliver clip is placed 6 cm from the needle, and the excess suture is removed. The extreme right side of the defect is grasped and required to facilitate the suture being placed through this corner, pulling it through until the silver clip secures it in place. The needle driver is manipulated by the right hand and the needle always points to the left. Rather than using the needle driver to rotate and force the needle through the tissue, the forceps held in the left hand brings the full thickness of the rectal wall over the needle. The suture is run over and over starting within the defect and taking the upper edge and then below from the lower mucosal surface and back into the defect. After each upper bite the suture is pulled tight by withdrawing the needle driver distally into the operating scope. Once the closure is complete, a second silver clip is applied to the far left end of the taut suture and the suture is cut. Because all sutures are 6 cm in length, closure of large defects may require more than one suture. If the peritoneal cavity has been entered either intentionally or inadvertently, the defect may still be primarily closed; however, it may be difficult to maintain a good view. Once closure is satisfactory, insufflation is discontinued and the operating proctoscope is removed. Rigid proctoscopy is performed again to examine the suture line for hemostasis and completeness and to ensure patency of the rectal lumen.

Postoperative Care

Patients in good health with smaller lesions are discharged home on the day of the procedure. Patients with large lesions, a long procedure, or significant comorbidity are admitted for 1 to 3 days and may receive additional doses of antibiotics. The diet is advanced as tolerated, and the patients are discharged on a bowel management program consisting of a high-fiber diet, a fiber supplement, stool softeners, and increased fluid intake. Selected patients with very large lesions are kept in the hospital for 3 days and are constipated with codeine and loperamide for 48 h. At the time of discharge, printed instructions regarding signs and symptoms of complications are given to the patient and discussed in detail. Patients are seen for follow-up in the clinic initially in 6 weeks and then for proctoscopy at 3 months and regularly thereafter for 1 year. Colonoscopy is repeated after 1 year and regularly thereafter as dictated by findings. Follow-up in patients with an invasive malignancy includes EUS and carcinoembryonic antigen (CEA) levels every 3 months. Imaging of the liver and chest is performed 1 year postoperatively and as indicated thereafter.

Results of TEM

The technique of TEM was developed by Professor Gerhart Buess and his coworkers in Germany and has been clinically applied in a large series since 1983.[18-21]

Because of the extensive training and significant learning curve required to be proficient with TEM and the costs inherent to the equipment, few centers are routinely performing TEM.[22–26] In a recent review,[27] we reported the results of 153 patients who underwent TEM at five U.S. institutions. The lesions removed were primarily adenomas ($n = 82$, 53.6%) and carcinomas ($n = 54$, 35.3%). Other indications for the procedure ($n = 17$, 11.1%) were less common (5 carcinoids, 1 solitary rectal ulcer, 3 rectal strictures, 1 rectal stump excision in two stages, 3 endometriosis, 1 rectal prolapse, 2 enterovaginal fistulas). Neoplasms were equally divided into mid- and proximal rectal lesions, and a full-thickness excision was performed in all cases. Intraoperative difficulties were encountered in 14 patients (9.1%) and required conversion to a laparotomy in 9 cases (5.8%). Only 1 conversion was necessitated due to entry into the peritoneal cavity, whereas 8 were converted because of the lack of proximal exposure. Minor postoperative complications (fever, *Clostridium difficile* diarrhea, and urinary retention) occurred in 18 patients (11.7%). Three patients experienced rectal bleeding but none of them required reoperation; 1 developed pneumonia; and 1 patient had a significant suture line disruption. Major late complications included 3 cases of mild incontinence, 2 of which were transient and 2 of rectal stenosis. The mean operative time was slightly longer for adenomas than for carcinomas, probably because of their large size (116 versus 109 min). Average hospital stay was also longer for patients with adenomas (3.2 versus 2.2 days); there was no perioperative mortality. Our current protocol includes more aggressive discharge on the day of surgery.

During long-term follow-up, local recurrence occurred in 10%, 40%, and 66% for T1, T2, and T3 lesions, respectively. All six T2 patients with recurrence underwent salvage abdominoperineal resection. Recurrence rates for adenomas were 11%. In case of incomplete resection or local recurrence, a secondary procedure can be performed with curative intent.[28]

Similar results have been reported in other larger series. In 236 patients undergoing TEM, Mentges et al. reported a morbidity and mortality of 5.5% and 0.3%, respectively. After 24 months follow-up, 2 patients with T1 lesions (3.6%) experienced local recurrence.[29] In a multi-institutional retrospective study, 1900 cases from 57 German institutions were reviewed.[30] On pathological evaluation, 1411 adenomas and 433 carcinomas were excised. The conversion rate to a laparotomy was between 1.2% and 11.6%, with 3 deaths (0.2%) and 120 complications (6.3%).

Kreis and colleagues investigated long-term functional results after TEM, reporting superior results in comparison to low anterior resection. In particular, no difference between preoperative and postoperative minor fecal incontinence was observed (6 of 42 patients; 14.2%).[31]

Banerjee et al. prospectively studied 36 patients undergoing TEM with proctography and manometry, reaching similar conclusions.[32] In their series, no differences in maximal squeeze pressures were found; however, lower resting pressures and loss of the rectoanal inhibitory reflex in 7 patients were observed. Nevertheless, there were no changes in clinical function 12 months postoperatively.

Given this experience, it is reasonable to support transanal excision of rectal neoplasms for benign adenomas and for T1 carcinomas. Clearly, patients with T3 lesions are not adequately treated with local approaches, and adjuvant chemotherapy and radiation have not proven to be reasonable alternatives to radical surgery. T2 lesions are also not well treated with local excision alone, and whether adjuvant therapy is a reasonable alternative to radical extirpation remains to be seen.

Intraoperative Colonoscopy

The intraoperative use of colonoscopy is a very useful and important technique in selected cases. This discussion focuses on the indications and technique of intraoperative colonoscopy (IOC). Intraoperative colonoscopy is seldom required if the preoperative evaluation has been thorough. The most common indications for intraoperative endoscopy are summarized in Table 52.1. There are no absolute contraindications to the use of IOC; however, the surgeon must balance the benefits of intraoperative colonic evaluation with the inherent risk of prolonging the procedure. This decision is really only a consideration in patients who are poor operative candidates or become unstable during the procedure. Nevertheless, IOC can be successfully undertaken in up to 97% of cases and, in skilled hands, does not add more than 15 min to the total operative time.[33]

TABLE 52.1. Indications for intraoperative endoscopy.

1. Gastrointestinal bleeding
     Massive
     Occult
2. Localization of nonpalpable lesions
     Small colon cancer
     Polyps
     Incomplete polypectomy sites
3. Search for synchronous lesions
4. Evaluation of incidental lesions
5. Miscellaneous
     Retrieval of foreign bodies
     Traumatic injuries
     Inflammatory bowel disease
     Laparotomy/laparoscopic-assisted colonoscopic polypectomy

Gastrointestinal (GI) Bleeding

In cases of intermittent or chronic bleeding without precise preoperative localization, IOC may help to identify the source of bleeding and guide the extent of resection. Routine evaluation of GI bleeding should localize more than 95% of bleeding sites. However, occasionally patients present with intermittent bleeding requiring transfusions in whom preoperative localization has failed. Panendoscopy may be intraoperatively performed using the colonoscope to first perform an upper endoscopy and complete enteroscopy followed by colonoscopy. IOC enables the surgeon to identify vascular ectasias, which will characteristically appear as tortuous vessels on transillumination of the bowel wall.[34] In the uncommon setting of acute, massive GI hemorrhage, IOC may play a crucial role if the patient is taken to the operating suite without prior localization studies (colonoscopy, bleeding scan, or angiography). Preoperative colonoscopy is in fact notoriously inaccurate in finding the source of bleeding in instances of severe active hemorrhage. IOC can be greatly facilitated in this setting by the use of on-table colonic lavage.[35]

Localization of Nonpalpable Lesions

Intraoperative colonoscopy is invaluable in localizing nonpalpable lesions, such as benign neoplasms, small carcinomas, and polypectomy sites. Preoperative colonoscopy is often inaccurate in precisely defining the distance of the lesion from the anal verge. Small lesions may also be difficult to palpate if located on the mesenteric surface or if there is abundant adipose tissue surrounding the colon. Localization of lesions during laparoscopic colectomy is becoming a common indication for IOC. Because many lesions are not visible from the serosal aspect of the bowel and palpation is not an option, IOC may rapidly and accurately identify the location of the lesion to be excised.

Perhaps one of the most frequent indications for IOC is to localize the site of a recent polypectomy of a lesion requiring further resective therapy. The surgeon should not remove a segment of the colon without being sure of the location of the polypectomy site. Cecal localization is generally fairly accurate but preoperative colonoscopic identification of any site from the upper ascending colon to the rectum can be unreliable. When indicated, operative resection should be performed within 2 to 3 weeks from the time of the polypectomy. IOC is commonly used to localize the polypectomy site because they are rarely palpable, and this approach is very successful if the mucosal defect has not completely healed. If there is going to be a longer period until surgery or if IOC is not available in the operating room, prompt repeat colonoscopy should be performed with marking of the site with a dye, such as indocyanine green, India ink, or methylene blue. The marking should be at four positions, specifically at 90° intervals around the bowel circumference rather than at 90° intervals around the lesion. The reason for this preference is because the possibility that all four marks in the latter setting could be on the mesenteric border. In this situation, the marking may be invisible during laparoscopy and even during laparotomy. Circumferential marking helps ensure that at least one ink spot will be antimesenteric and more readily visualized at the time of surgery.

Colonic Evaluation

Before operating on a patient with a colonic neoplasm, the entire colon should be examined, as there is a high rate of synchronous polyps (27%–75%) and colorectal cancers (1.7%–7.6%), which can alter the operative plan.[33,36] Colonic evaluation is usually preoperatively achieved by either colonoscopy or air-contrast barium enema and sigmoidoscopy. Therefore, intraoperative colonic evaluation for this reason is rarely necessary. However, in the case of partial or complete obstruction, preoperative exclusion of synchronous lesions may not be possible. On-table lavage with IOC and primary anastomosis is a viable option for many of these patients. In practice, most surgeons intraoperatively palpate the remaining colon and defer endoscopic examination, preferring elective colonoscopy approximately 6 months later. IOC is to be encouraged in this setting because of its efficiency and to obviate a second operative procedure in case a synchronous lesion is present.

Incidental Lesions and Other Indications

Intraoperative colonoscopy may be useful in better evaluating lesions incidentally found at the time of laparotomy. This approach avoids enterotomies and unnecessary contamination. IOC may also be useful in addressing mucosal extent of inflammatory bowel disease and strictures. The expanding list of indications for IOC also includes retrieval of foreign bodies and, arguably, laparoscopically assisted colonoscopic polypectomy.

Intraoperative Technique

The instrumentation used for IOC is the same as that used for conventional colonoscopy. A standard 160-cm flexible scope is employed, and most systems now use a three-color video chip rather than a fiberoptic bundle. The patient is placed in the modified lithotomy position for access to both the abdomen and the perineum. We generally perform a rigid sigmoidoscopic exam with irrigation of the rectum with povidone-iodine solution to assess the adequacy of the bowel preparation and to facilitate the colonoscopy; minimal gas is insufflated at that time. The abdomen and perineum are prepped and the patient is draped. The abdomen is entered by either laparotomy or laparoscopy. Should the need for IOC be discovered during laparoscopy or laparotomy when the patient is positioned supine, the colonoscope may be inserted into the anus by flexing the right leg and maneuvering beneath the drapes.[37] However, it is preferable to have all patients scheduled for abdominal intestinal procedures to be positioned in the modified lithotomy position. A noncrushing bowel clamp or umbilical tape is used to occlude the terminal ileum. The endoscopist maintains the tip of the colonoscope centered in the bowel lumen and advances or withdraws the scope as the operative team gently assists with advancement and pulling the bowel onto the scope (accordioning). Communication between the endoscopist and the operating team is critical to avoid injury to the bowel. Excessive insufflation should be avoided, and the bowel should not be stretched. The sigmoid colon should be accordioned and may be kept this way by having an assistant manually compress it into the pelvis and left iliac fossa. The splenic flexure may be supported with a hand placed laterally and superiorly. Rarely, mobilization of the splenic or hepatic flexures may be necessary to facilitate the endoscopy. A bowel clamp may be temporarily placed on the transverse colon to avoid proximal dilation early in the procedure. The mucosa is viewed as the endoscope is advanced, rather than during withdrawal of the instrument; this method avoids mistaking iatrogenic injury of the mucosa for intrinsic pathology. Evaluation is completed with transillumination of the wall, while dimming the operating theater lights to facilitate marking any lesions with a suture. The endoscope may often be advanced into the terminal ileum for examination and transillumination of any vascular ectasias. During removal of the scope, as much of the insufflated air as possible should be removed to ease the subsequent operation and closure of the abdomen.

The findings of IOC can frequently alter the extent of resection at the time of surgery. In a report,[38] IOC changed the planned procedure in up to 16.4% of cases. Although complications such as injuries due to manipulation of the splenic flexure, bleeding after biopsy or polypectomy, and perforation can occur, rates in larger series appear to be similar to those of conventional colonoscopy.[38–40]

Conclusion

Transanal endoscopic microsurgery is an innovative procedure that allows excision of lesions in the mid- and upper rectum, with curative intent, short hospitalization, and few perioperative complications. However, it demands acquisition of specific technical skills and requires a well-orchestrated surgical team and very expensive equipment. Nonetheless, for a very few caudally selected patients, TEM allows a minimally invasive approach with achievement of long-term results quite comparable to conventional radical procedures. Because of the training, expense, and limited number of patients in whom it may be used, TEM is likely to remain in the hands of a limited number of surgeons.

Intraoperative colonoscopy has rapidly expanded in its potential applications during colorectal procedures and is often instrumental in changing the planned procedure. In experienced hands, it allows precise localization of intraluminal or vascular pathology with minimal impact on operative time; this technique should be available to all surgeons.

Acknowledgments. The authors thank the Richard Wolf Medical Instruments Corporation for providing photographs of the TEM instruments.

References

1. Orkin BA. Transanal endoscopic microsurgical excision. In: Shirmer BD, Rattner DW (eds) Ambulatory Surgery. Philadelphia: Saunders, 1998:435–445.
2. Buess G, Hutterer F, Theiss J, et al. Das System fur die transanale endoskopische rectumoperation. Chirurg 1984; 55:667–680.
3. Buess G, Theiss R, Gunther M, et al. Endoscopic surgery in the rectum. Endoscopy 1985;17:31–35.
4. Buess G, Kipfmuller K, Ibald R, et al. Clinical results of transanal endoscopic microsurgery. Surg Endosc 1988;2: 245–250.
5. Buess G, Theib R, Gunther M, et al. Endoscopic operative procedure for the removal of rectal polyps. Colo-Proctology 1984;6:254–261.
6. Buess G, Kipfmuller K, Theib R, et al. Clinical results of transanal endoscopic microsurgery. Surg Endosc 1988;2: 245–250.
7. Saclarides TJ, Smith L, Ko ST, Orkin BA, Buess G. Transanal endoscopic microsurgery. Dis Colon Rectum 1992;35: 1183–1191.
8. Allgower M, Durig M, Hochstetter A von, Huber A. The parasacral sphincter-splitting approach to the rectum. World J Surg 1982;6:539–548.
9. Orkin BA. Local treatment of rectal neoplasms. In: Mazier WP, Levien DH, Luchtefeld MA, Senagore A (eds) Surgery of the Colon, Rectum and Anus. Philadelphia: Saunders, 1995:470–489.
10. Smith LE. Transanal endoscopic microsurgery for rectal neoplasms. Gastroint Clin N Am 1993;3:329–341.
11. Saclarides TJ, Bhattacharya AK, Britton-Kuzel C, et al. Predicting lymph node metastases in rectal cancer. Dis Colon Rectum 1994;37:52–57.

12. Winde G, Nottberg H, Keller R, et al. Surgical cure for early rectal carcinomas (T1). Transanal endoscopic microsurgery versus anterior resection. Dis Colon Rectum 1996;39(9): 969–976.

13. Hildebrandt U, Feifel G. Preoperative staging of colorectal cancer by intrarectal ultrasound. Dis Colon Rectum 1985: 28(1):42–46.

14. Hildebrandt U, Schuder G, Feifel G. Preoperative staging of rectal and colonic cancer. Endoscopy 1994;26(9):810–812.

15. Turler A, Shafer H, Pichlmaier H. Role of transanal endoscopic microsurgery in the palliative treatment of rectal cancer. Scand J Gastroenterol 1197;32(1):58–61.

16. Said S, Stippel D. Ten years experience with transanal endoscopic microsurgery. Histopathologic and clinical analysis. Chirurg 1996;67(2):139–144.

17. Lezoche E, Guerrieri M, Paganini A, et al. Is transanal microsurgery (TEM) a valid treatment for rectal tumors? Surg Endosc 1996;10:736–741.

18. Buess G, Mentges B, Manncke K, et al. Technique and results of transanal endoscopic microsurgery in early rectal cancer. Am J Surg 1992;163:63–70.

19. Buess G, Mentges B, Manncke K, Stanlinger M, Becker HD. Minimal invasive surgery in the local treatment of rectal cancer. Int J Colorect Dis 1991;6:77–81.

20. Mentges B, Buess G, Effinger S, et al. Indications and results of local treatment of rectal cancer. Br J Surg 1997;84: 348–351.

21. Said S, Stippel D. Transanal endoscopic microsurgery in large sessile adenomas of the rectum. A 10-year experience. Surg Endosc 1995;9(10):1106–1112.

22. Saclarides TJ. Transanal endoscopic microsurgery. Surg Clin N Am 1997;77(1):229–238.

23. Saclarides TJ. Transanal endoscopic microsurgery. A single surgeon's experience. Arch Surg 1988;133:595–599.

24. Smith LE, Orkin BA. Transanal microscopic excision of rectal neoplasms [abstract]. Surg Endosc 1994;8:468.

25. Steele RJ, Hershman MJ, Mortensen NJ, et al. Transanal endoscopic microsurgery. Initial experience from three centers in the United Kingdom. Br J Surg 1996; 83(2):207–210.

26. Stipa S, Lucandri G, Stipa F, et al. Local excision of rectal tumors with transanal endoscopic microsurgery. Tumori 1995;81(suppl 3):50–56.

27. Smith LE, Ko ST, Saclarides T, et al. Transanal endoscopic microsurgery. Initial Registry results. Dis Colon Rectum 1996;39:S79–S84.

28. Mentges B, Buess G, Effinger G, et al. Local therapy of rectum carcinoma. Chirurg 1996;67(2)133-138.

29. Mentges B, Buess G, Shafer D, et al. Local therapy of rectal tumors. Dis Colon Rectum 1996;39(8):886–892.

30. Salm R, Lampe H, Bustos A, et al. Experience with TEM in Germany. Endosc Surg Allied Technol 1994;2(5): 251–254.

31. Kreis ME, Jehle EC, Haug V, et al. Functional results after transanal endoscopic microsurgery. Dis Colon Rectum 1996;39(10):1116–1121.

32. Banerjee AK, Jehle EC, Kreis ME, et al. Prospective study of the proctographic and functional consequences of transanal endoscopic microsurgery. Br J Surg 1996;83(2): 211–213.

33. Brullet E, Montane JM, Bombardo J, et al. Intraoperative colonoscopy in patients with colorectal cancer. Br J Surg 1992;79(12):1376–1378.

34. Orkin BA, Fazio VW. Vascular ectasias of the colon. In: Fazio VF (ed) Current Therapy in Colon and Rectal Surgery. Philadelphia: Dekker, 1989:238–245.

35. Whelan RL, Buls JG, Goldberg SM, et al. Intraoperative endoscopy: University of Minnesota experience. Am Surg 1989;55:281–286.

36. Orkin BA. Treatment of rectal cancer. In: Beck DE, Wexner SD (eds) Fundamentals of Anorectal Surgery. New York: McGraw-Hill, 1992:279.

37. Orkin BA. Intraoperative colonoscopy. Semin Colon Rectal Surg 1992;3(1):35–41.

38. Sakanoue Y, Nakao K, Shoji Y, et al. Intraoperative colonoscopy. Surg Endosc 1993;7(2):84–87.

39. Saclarides TJ, Wolff BG, Pemberton JH, et al. Clean sweep of the colon. The use of intraoperative colonoscopy. Dis Col Rectum 1989;32(10):864–866.

40. Cohen JL, Forde KA. Intraoperative colonoscopy. Ann Surg 1988;207(3):231–233.

53
Laparoscopic Ultrasound in Minimally Invasive Procedures in the Abdomen and Pelvis

Anthony J. Senagore and Peter W. Marcello

The rapid application of minimally invasive techniques to increasingly complex intraabdominal and pelvic surgical procedures has demanded an increased ability to visualize pathology. Increased ability to "see" the pathology is required because of the current limitations of the traditional tactile evaluation of the intraabdominal viscera and associated pathology. This discussion reviews the current state of the art for applications of ultrasound visualization during laparoscopic procedures.

The majority of the probes used for laparoscopic ultrasound (LUS) employ compact linear array transducers fixed on rigid or flexible shafts that can negotiate standard abdominal wall ports.[1,2] The laparoscopic transducer frequencies parallel the traditional general use counterparts, ranging from 5.0 to 10.0MHz.[3] An additional benefit can be derived by using probes with Doppler ultrasound, spectral analysis, or color imaging, which may improve the clinical assessment. It is important to select the appropriate probe frequency to visualize the intended structure, recalling that the higher the frequency, the less the depth of penetration, and therefore the closer the field of resolution. Generally, probes with frequencies of 6.5 to 7.5MHz are optimal for LUS.

Laparoscopic Ultrasound of the Pancreas

Laparoscopic ultrasound has become an important component of the staging process for pancreatic neoplasms.[4-6] Laparoscopic evaluation of the peritoneal surfaces allows the identification of metastatic disease, which avoids unnecessary laparotomy in patients without duodenal obstruction. The recent addition of LUS for evaluation of the liver and pancreas adds further information that can help select patients for curative resection. Features of potential nonresectability based on LUS of the gland itself include tumors larger than 5cm, vascular invasion, and regional lymphadenopathy (>10mm).[7] Obviously, any abnormal lesions can be biopsied under LUS guidance to direct clinical decision making. Incorporation of LUS for staging pancreatic cancer increases the specificity from 50% to 88% and the positive predictive value from 65% to 89%.[7] There is also some evidence that LUS of the pancreas may be useful for identifying pancreatic islet cell tumors, which allows for laparoscopic resection.[8,9]

Laparoscopic Ultrasound of the Biliary Tract

Laparoscopic cholecystectomy has become the standard approach to symptomatic cholelithiasis and has led to additional maneuvers to study the biliary tree to avoid leaving untreated choledocholithiasis. A recent National Institutes of Health consensus statement advocated preoperative endoscopic retrograde cholangiography with or without papillotomy for this problem. However, this approach is invasive with a predictable morbidity and mortality.[10] LUS can obtain the same information without invading the common bile duct; the technique of LUS of the biliary tree has been described elsewhere but is briefly reviewed here.[11-13] The LUS probe is inserted via the epigastric port to allow the transducer to be placed in direct contact with the duct, which provides a transverse image of the duct lumen. The entire length of the duct must be examined from the bifurcation of the right and left ducts to the duodenal entrance. The classic "mouse head" is demonstrated by the simultaneous imaging of the adjacent hepatic artery and portal vein.[14] LUS imaging of the biliary tree has demonstrated excellent sensitivity (72%–100%) and accuracy (97%–100%) in a number of studies, which compares favorably to cholangiography.[15-19]

Laparoscopic Ultrasound in Pelvic Surgery

Laparoscopic ultrasound offers the potential for evaluating lymph node pathology in association with pelvic malignancies, where current clinical staging modalities are limited.[20] Even clinical evaluation of metastatic lymph nodes via palpation is limited to 44% accuracy.[21] Pelvic lymph node dissection via either open or laparoscopic approach is the most accurate staging modality for uterine and cervical malignancies.[22–24] However, these procedures include the risk of subsequent bowel adhesions, increased toxicity with postoperative radiotherapy, and lymphedema.[22–24]

LUS potentially confirms nodal status without extensive dissection, reducing both operative complications and the sequelae of lymph node dissection. A recent report of 11 patients with metastatic lymph nodes from pelvic malignancies demonstrated a 91% sensitivity and a 100% specificity.[24] A longitudinal to transverse diameter ratio of 2 or less confirmed the presence of metastatic involvement and avoided the need for complex ultrasonic or waveform analysis of lymph node architecture.[25,26] Although this modality may limit the need for extensive pelvic lymph node dissection as well as specify the use of perioperative radiotherapy, further experience is required.

Laparoscopic Hepatic Ultrasound

Laparoscopic resection of colorectal cancer has been proposed as an alternative to conventional resection. The benefits of a minimally invasive approach, as demonstrated in colonic resection of benign diseases, have been shown in the early results of several small independently managed prospective randomized clinical trials of laparoscopic resection for colorectal cancer.[27–31] Earlier return of gastrointestinal function, earlier resumption of diet, reduced postoperative pain, and improved pulmonary function have led to a reduction in hospital length of stay. However, early reports of minimally invasive resection of colorectal malignancy identified the issues of port site metastases and resection margins and staging difficulties. Adherence to accepted principles of oncologic resection including proximal vessel ligation, wide mesenteric resection, appropriate tumor-free resection margins, and evaluation of the liver parenchyma is mandatory if laparoscopic resection is to offer the same opportunity for cancer cure as do conventional procedures.

Because manual liver palpation is not laparoscopically feasible, other modalities must be utilized to assess the liver at the time of resection. Preoperative liver ultrasound or contrast-enhanced computerized tomography (CT) is commonly employed to assess the liver for synchronous metastases. However, during conventional surgery, intraoperative liver ultrasound has been shown to be one of the most sensitive methods of detecting hepatic lesions.[32,33] Intraoperative ultrasound also offers the ability to perform guided biopsy of small lesions. With the development of LUS probes, intraoperative LUS may be utilized in a similar fashion as in laparotomy. LUS has been evaluated not only in the assessment of synchronous colorectal malignancies but also in staging of upper gastrointestinal malignancies and in determining the feasibility of hepatic resection in both primary and metastatic disease without the morbidity of a laparotomy.[34]

There are several reports describing the technique of laparoscopic liver ultrasound for colorectal cancer screening.[35–38] At our institution, a standardized approach is undertaken with the assistance of an experienced radiologist.[35,36] After creation of the pneumoperitoneum, two 10- or 12-mm cannulas are placed, one below the umbilicus and the other in the right lower quadrant (Fig. 53.1). Following diagnostic laparoscopy, the patient is tilted into the reverse Trendelenberg position. A flexible-tip, multifrequency (5–6.5–7.5 MHz) convex array transducer probe is inserted through the right lower quadrant cannula and is guided to the liver surface with the operator standing between the patient's legs (Fig. 53.2). The ultrasound image is simultaneously observed with the

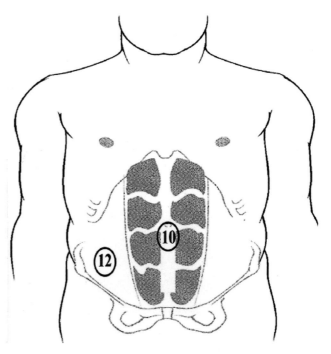

FIGURE 53.1. Port placement for laparoscopic ultrasound (LUS). The camera is placed through the umbilical trocar. Following diagnostic laparoscopy, the LUS probe is passed through the right lower quadrant trocar. *10*, 10-mm port; *12*, 12-mm port.

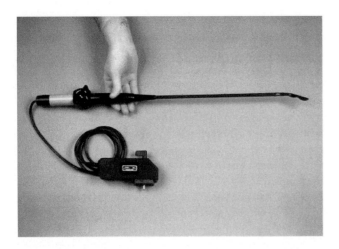

FIGURE 53.2. A flexible tip, multifrequency (5–6.5–7.5 MHz) convex array transducer probe (Bruel & Kjaer, Marlborough, MA).

laparoscopic camera image on a monitor placed above the patient's right shoulder. The liver is systematically evaluated by a standardized sequence to ensure a complete evaluation (Fig. 53.3). Focal abnormalities identified by ultrasound are typically characterized as cysts, hemangiomas, metastases, or indeterminate lesions. Needle biopsy of suspicious lesions is feasible under ultrasound guidance through a separate puncture site in the right upper quadrant.

Although there are numerous reports demonstrating the efficacy and feasibility of laparoscopy and LUS in the staging of upper gastrointestinal malignancies, few studies have evaluated the role of intraoperative laparoscopic liver ultrasound in the staging of colorectal malignancies (Table 53.1). In an earlier report from our institution, the results of 22 patients who underwent laparoscopic palliative and curative resection of colorectal cancer combined with laparoscopic liver ultrasound were reported;[35] all patients underwent preoperative CT scan. A complete and expeditious evaluation of all liver segments was successfully performed by LUS in all patients. The median duration of the procedure was 10 (range, 5–15) min. Sixteen focal abnormalities were identified by LUS in 7 patients compared with 10 lesions by preoperative CT scan. Seven of the lesions were deemed metastatic by preoperative CT scan. LUS correctly identified all these lesions and found one additional metastasis that was not identified by CT scan. This finding led to the conversion from laparoscopy to a laparotomy procedure, with subsequent hepatic biopsy confirmation of a metastatic adenocarcinoma. The patient underwent a simultaneous wedge liver resection and rectal resection.

Based on the positive results of this initial series, laparoscopic liver ultrasound was incorporated into the

prospective randomized trial comparing laparotomy and laparoscopy and resection of colorectal cancer at Cleveland Clinic (Ohio).[27] We have recently presented a larger prospective blinded comparison of LUS versus contrast-enhanced CT scan in patients entered into the laparoscopic cancer trial.[36] Fifty-four consecutive patients underwent preoperative CT scan, diagnostic laparoscopy, and laparoscopic liver ultrasound. At the time of surgery, the radiologist was blinded to the results of the preoperative CT scan. Patients randomized to laparotomy also underwent liver ultrasound and bimanual liver palpation. The median time to complete the LUS remained at 10 min. There was, however, one capsular tear in the liver related to the LUS that required conversion and suture repair, resulting in a morbidity rate of 1.9%. The yield was calculated using the number of lesions identified by each imaging modality divided by the total number of lesions identified by any modality (see Table 53.1). Conventional intraoperative ultrasound did not identify any additional abnormalities when compared to LUS. The yield for metastatic lesions was 93% for LUS and 89% for CT scan. Combining benign and metastatic lesions the yield was significantly higher for LUS (91%) when compared to preoperative CT scan (68%). After a median follow-up of 17 months, no additional liver metastases have been identified.

The results of this larger series have been confirmed by several other groups.[37,38] In a review of 33 patients with colorectal cancer by Goletti et al.,[38] laparoscopic liver ultrasound had a sensitivity of 100% compared with

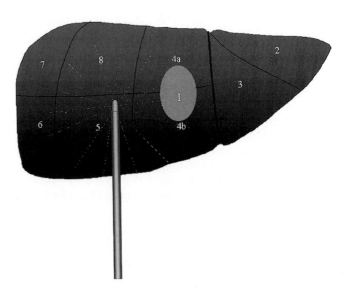

FIGURE 53.3. Systematic evaluation of the liver with a laparoscopic probe commences with examination of segments 6 and 7 and moves medially. After examination of the liver anteriorly, the probe may be passed under the liver to allow evaluation of the caudate lobe (segment 1) if necessary.

Table 53.1. Results of laparoscopic liver ultrasound for colorectal cancer.

Author	Year	n'	Preoperative evaluation	Metastases		Benign	
				Sensitivity (%)	Specificity (%)	Sensitivity (%)	Specificity (%)
Marchesa et al.[35]	1996	22	CT scan	100	100	100	100
Jerby et al.[36]	1998	54	CT scan	93	—	90	—
Goletti et al.[38]	1998	33	US, CT scan	100	—	—	—
Kumar et al.[37]	1998	76	US, MRI	90	100	—	100

US, ultrasound; MRI, magnetic resonance imaging.

62.5% for preoperative ultrasound and CT scan. Combining the results of the initial laparoscopy and laparoscopic liver ultrasound, the therapeutic plan was altered in 11 cases (33%); 4 cases (12%) were altered by the results of the LUS alone.

Laparoscopic liver ultrasound has been utilized not only in the screening of colorectal liver metastasis but also in the therapeutic management of these lesions. An alternative to liver resection, cryoablation of liver metastasis requires "real-time" ultrasound to assess the zone of freezing. A minimally invasive approach to cryoablation may reduce the morbidity associated with conventional techniques. A recent study from our institution has reported the successful completion of laparoscopic cryoablation of liver metastases in seven patients.[39] In four of the patients, laparoscopic liver ultrasound identified additional treatable lesions that were previously unrecognized. This early report demonstrates the potential application of laparoscopic ultrasonography in the management of liver metastasis.

With the increasing application of minimally invasive techniques to the management of intra-abdominal malignancies, laparoscopic liver ultrasound is an integral component of the evaluation of metastatic spread. In patients with colorectal malignancy who undergo a laparoscopic resection, LUS allows a safe and expeditious evaluation of the liver parenchyma. When compared to preoperative CT scan, the yield for metastatic lesions is comparable and the overall yield is superior. LUS also allows intraoperative biopsy and subsequent alteration in therapy, which cannot be afforded by other preoperative modalities. In addition, laparoscopic liver ultrasound may play a role in the treatment of hepatic metastases when combined with laparoscopic cryoablation.

Conclusion

Laparoscopic ultrasound offers an easy-to-use, minimally invasive technique to augment intraoperative evaluation. Although it does not completely replace the tactile sensation upon which surgeons often rely, LUS can in many cases provide visual documentation of the anatomic and pathological features essential to safe surgery. Moreover, the technique itself appears safe. It is important that laparoscopic surgeons master the skills of this rapidly developing technology to allow continued advancement of minimally invasive procedures. Unresolved issues include interobserver and intraobserver variability and the volume of cases needed to achieve proficiency at both the technique and image interpretation (the learning curve).

References

1. Jakimowicz JJ. Technical and clinical aspects of intra-operative ultrasound applicable to laparoscopic ultrasound. Endosc Surg Allied Technol 1994;2:119–126.
2. John TG, Banting SW, Pye S, et al. Preliminary experience with intracorporeal laparoscopic ultrasonography using a sector scanning probe. A prospective comparison with intraoperative cholangiography in the detection of choledocholithiasis. Surg Endosc 1994;8:1176–1180.
3. John TG, Garden OJ. Clinical experience with sector scan and linear array ultrasound probes in laparoscopic surgery. Endosc Surg Allied Technol 1994;2:134–142.
4. Catheline JM, Turner R, Rizk N, Barrat C, Champault G. The use of diagnostic laparoscopy supported by laparoscopic ultrasonography in the assessment of pancreatic cancer. Surg Endosc 1999;13:239–245.
5. Palazzo L, Roseau G, Gayet B, et al. Endoscopic ultrasonography in the diagnosis and staging of pancreatic adenocarcinoma. Results of a prospective study with comparison to ultrasonography and CT scan. Endoscopy 1993;25:143–150.
6. Irving AD, Cuschieri A. Laparoscopic assessment of the jaundiced patient: a review of 53 patients. Br J Surg 1978;65:678–680.
7. Murughiah M, Paterson-Brown S, Windsor JA, Miles WFA, Garden OJ. Early experience of laparoscopic ultrasonography in the management of pancreatic carcinoma. Surg Endosc 1993;7:177–181.
8. Gagner M, Pomp A, Herrera MF. Early experience with laparoscopic resections of islet cell tumors. Surgery (St. Louis) 1996;120:1051–1054.
9. Sussman LA, Christie R, Whittle DE. Laparoscopic excision of distal pancreas including insulinoma. Aust NZ J Surg 1996;66:414–416.

10. King CMP, Reznek RH, Dacie JE, Wass JAH. Review. Imaging islet cell tumours. Clin Radiol 1994;49:295–303.

11. Bezzi M, Merlino P, Orsi F, et al. Laparoscopic sonography during abdominal laparoscopic surgery: technique and imaging findings. AJR Am J Roentgenol 1995;165:1193–1198.

12. Lirici MM, Caratozzolo M, Urbano V, et al. Laparoscopic ultrasonography: limits and potential of present technologies. Endosc Surg Allied Technol 1994;2:127–133.

13. Yamamoto M, Stiegmann GV, Durham J, et al. Laparoscopy-guided intracorporeal ultrasound accurately delineates hepatobiliary anatomy. Surg Endosc 1993;7:325–330.

14. Machi J, Sigel B, Zaren HA, et al. Technique of ultrasound examination during laparoscopic cholecystectomy. Surg Endosc 1993;7:544–549.

15. Cavina E, Goletti O, Buccianti P. Echolaparoscopy: an indispensable procedure for laparoscopic surgery. Endosc Surg 1994;2:143–148.

16. Rothlin MA, Schlumpf R, Largiarder F. Laparoscopic sonography. An alternative to routine intraoperative cholangiography? Arch Surg 1994;129:694–700.

17. John TG, Banting SW, Pye S, Paterson-Brown S, Garden OJ. Preliminary experience with intracorporeal laparoscopic ultrasonography using a sector scanning probe. A prospective comparison with intraoperative cholangiography in the detection of choledocholithiasis. Surg Endosc 1994;8:1176–1181.

18. Stiegmann GV, Soper NJ, Filipi CJ, McIntyre RC, Callery MP, Cordova JF. Laparoscopic ultrasonography as compared with static or dynamic cholangiography at laparoscopic cholecystectomy. A prospective multicenter trial. Surg Endosc 1995;9:1269–1273.

19. Santambrogio R, Bianchi P, Opocher E, et al. Intraoperative ultrasonography (IOUS) during laparoscopic cholecystectomy. Surg Endosc 1996;10:622–627.

20. LaPolla JP, Schlaerth JB, Gaddis O, Morrow CP. The influence of surgical staging on the evaluation and treatment of patients with cervical carcinoma. Gynecol Oncol 1986;24:194–206.

21. Kinney WK, Hodge DO, Egorshin EV, Ballard DJ, Oodratz KC. Surgical treatment of patients with stage IB and IIA carcinoma of the cervix and palpably positive pelvic lymph nodes. Gynecol Oncol 1995;57:145–149.

22. Recio FO, Piver MS, Hempling RE. Pretreatment transperitoneal laparoscopic staging pelvic and paraaortic lymphadenectomy in larg (>5 cm) stage 1b2 cervical carcinoma. Report of a pilot study. Gynecol Oncol 1996;63:333–336.

23. Querleu D, Leblanc E, Castelain B. Laparoscopic pelvic lymphadecetomy in the staging of early carcinoma of the cervix. Am J Obstet Gynecol 1991;164:579–581.

24. Childers JM, Hatch KD, Tran AN, Surwit EA. Laparoscopic para-aortic lymphadenectomy in gynecologic malignancies. Obstet Gynecol 1993;82:741–747.

25. Vassallo P, Wernecke K, Roos N, Peters PE. Differentiation of benign from malignant superficial lymphadenopathy: the role of high resolution. US Radiol 1992;183:215–220.

26. Choi MY, Lee JW, Kyung JJ. Distinction between benign and malignant causes of cervical, axillary and inguinal lymphadenopathy: value of Doppler spectral waveform analysis. AJR 1995;165:981–984.

27. Milsom JW, Bohm B, Hammerhofer KA, et al. A prospective, randomized trial comparing laparoscopic versus conventional techniques in colorectal cancer surgery: a preliminary report. J Am Coll Surg 1998;187:46–54.

28. Lacy AM, Garcia-Valdecasas JC, Pique JM, et al. Short-term outcome analysis of a randomized study comparing laparoscopic vs open colectomy for colon cancer. Surg Endosc 1995;9:1101–1105.

29. Stage JG, Schulze S, Moller P, et al. Prospective randomized study of laparoscopic versus open colonic resection for adenocarcinoma. Br J Surg 1997;84:391–396.

30. Schwenk W, Bohm B, Witt C, et al. Pulmonary function following laparoscopic or conventional colorectal resection. Arch Surg 1999;134:6–12.

31. Stocchi L, Nelson H. Laparoscopic colectomy for colon cancer: trial update. J Surg Oncol 1998;68:255–267.

32. Stone MD, Kane R, Bothe A Jr, Jessup JM, Cady B, Steele GD. Intraoperative ultrasound imaging at the time of colorectal cancer resection. Arch Surg 1994;129:431–435.

33. Rafeaelson SR, Kronborg O, Larsen C, Fenger C. Intraoperative ultrasonography in detection of hepatic metastases from colorectal cancer. Dis Colon Rectum 1995;38:355–360.

34. John TG, Greig JD, Crosbie JL, Miles WF, Garden OJ. Superior staging of liver tumors with laparoscopy and laparoscopic ultrasound. Ann Surg 1994;220:711–719.

35. Marchesa P, Milsom JW, Hale JC, O'Malley CM, Fazio VW. Intraoperative laparoscopic liver ultrasonography for staging of colorectal cancer: initial experience. Dis Colon Rectum 1996;39:S73–S78.

36. Jerby B, Milsom J, Hale J, Herts B, O'Malley C. A prospective blinded comparison of laparoscopic ultrasonography and computed tomography (CT) for liver assessment in patients with colorectal cancer. Dis Colon Rectum 1998;41:A23–A24.

37. Kumar H, Hartley J, Heer K, Duthie G, Avery G, Monson J. Efficacy of laparoscopic ultrasound scanning (USS) in detection of colorectal liver metastases during surgery. Dis Colon Rectum 1998;41:A24.

38. Goletti O, Celona G, Galatioto C, et al. Is laparoscopic sonography a reliable and sensitive procedure for staging of colorectal cancer? A comparative study. Surg Endosc 1998;12:1236–1241.

39. Iannitti DA, Heniford T, Hale J, Grundfest-Broniatowski S, Gagner M. Laparoscopic cryoablation of hepatic metastases. Arch Surg 1998;133:1011–1015.

54
Avoiding Complications

Marc E. Sher and T. Cristina Sardinha

Despite the many potential benefits of laparoscopic colorectal surgery, as has been reported for ileoanal reservoir surgery and other advanced colorectal surgical procedures, complications are also inevitable. Complications may be related to the laparoscopist's experience. The learning curve specific to colorectal surgery is both steep and lengthy.[1-5] Moreover, the consequences of an anastomotic leak are potentially catastrophic; hence requirements for avoidance of complications include technical precision, advanced skills, and extensive training.

Many surgeons have adapted this new technology without the benefit of formal training such as within a traditional surgical residency program or fellowship. The lack of organized progressive experience coupled with the complexity of the procedure increased and intensified the resultant morbidity attributed to the laparoscopic approach.[2,3] Proper case selection and prudent judgment advocating timely conversion have become inherent and exaggerated necessities for a successful outcome.[6,7] Different and unusual complications such as port site recurrences[8,9] and hernias have mandated a reevaluation of this approach, not only within local quality assurance surgical forums but also by the enrollment of patients in multi-institutional prospective randomized trials.[8,9] This novel procedure is associated with immense theoretical benefits in the treatment of colorectal pathology. However, extensive training, supervision, and credentialing of surgeons keen to adapt this technology are essential to surpass the difficult learning curve.[10-13]

Complications of laparoscopic colorectal surgery can be categorized as:

1. a result of the steep and lengthy learning curve
2. Attributed directly and specifically to the laparoscopic approach
3. resulting from errors in judgment and case selection

Complications attributed to the learning curve are not surprising. Laparoscopic colectomy challenges even the most adept instrumentalist who also has an innate gift of transforming three-dimensional anatomy to the two-dimensional video screen. Laparoscopic colectomy requires extensive mobilization of a large hollow organ in multiple quadrants of the abdomen. In addition, extensive vascular control of a fat-laden mesentery requires costly instrumentation to ensure safety. Finally, a well-vascularized, tension-free circumferentially intact anastomosis must be constructed, often in a narrow pelvis. The potential for complications is undoubtedly increased as each and every new and unfamiliar step is taken.[14,15]

Complications specific to the laparoscopic approach include port site hernias, port site recurrences, and pneumoperitoneum-related problems. Direct trocar-related injuries to bowel and vascular structures are not uncommon, yet are possibly avoidable. Faulty positioning, difficult exposure, and the loss of tactile sensation may predispose to complications specific to laparoscopic technology. The list includes ureteral, vascular injury, and contamination and sepsis from bowel injury.

Complications resulting from poor surgical judgment are often due to inadequate case selection and the inappropriate application of this technology to treat all pathology regardless of patient outcome. No single surgical tool, procedure, or approach is universally applicable. Laparoscopy is no different; there still remains an important role for the traditional laparotomy. Other complications resulting from poor judgment stem from inappropriately prolonged operating times and reluctance to convert to a laparotomy when indicated.

The Steep and Lengthy Learning Curve

Complications are in part reflective of the operating surgeon's experience. Agachan and associates[4] reported a progressive decrease in the complication rate at the Cleveland Clinic Florida from 29% to 11% and then 7%

during the years 1991, 1993, and 1995, respectively. The learning curve appeared to have required 55 laparoscopic colorectal procedures to stabilize the complication rate; 70 cases were required to significantly reduce the mean operative time. Nevertheless, the learning curve in this series could have been a reflection of case selection, because total abdominal colectomies were abandoned early in the series in favor of segmental colectomies and other less formidable procedures.

Simons et al.[3] used operative time only as an indication of learning and reported a need for about 11 to 15 cases. Falk et al.[13] noted a 50% reduction in operating room time during a 10-month span. Other authors[14–16] have corroborated experience in the operating room and careful case selection as the most critical variables in avoiding morbidity.

The definition of the learning curve is arbitrary and difficult to assess. Some authors[2–5,14] have used operating time while others have used morbidity. Furthermore, procedures differ with respect to complexity, the patient's body habitus, and the underlying pathology. Some patients may have had multiple prior procedures, harbor a large phlegmonous mass, or have dense severe adhesions. The role of complexity has been demonstrated, as Reissman et al.[1] reported an overall complication rate of 42% for total abdominal colectomies, significantly higher than the 9% reported for segmental colectomies.

Senagore et al.[2] analyzed 60 consecutive patients who underwent a laparoscopic colectomy and divided them into three groups of 20 patients based on surgeon's experience. The 30% incidence of pulmonary complications in the first group decreased to 5% in the next two groups. They emphasized the mastery of technical skills in enterolysis as being of paramount importance, paralleling the learning curve. After this education, inadvertent enterotomies and other complications were minimized, as was the conversion rate. Agachan et al.[5] concurred, documenting adhesions resulting from prior laparotomy or inflammation that made dissection tedious and prolonged operative time. Conversely, despite the increased complexity inherent in procedures performed on patients with abscesses, fistulae, and dense adhesions, operating times were shortened, reflecting improved skills and operator learning with more experience.

Sher et al.[17] compared laparoscopic resection versus traditional resection for patients with acute diverticulitis stratified by severity of disease. More than 85% of the conversions were directly related to the intense inflammatory process. After the first four cases, patients with Hinchey II diverticular disease had a morbidity rate of 14.3%, approximately half the rate noted in patients with Hinchey II disease treated by laparotomy. Thus, after ascending the learning curve, even patients with Hinchey II diverticular disease should be considered for the laparoscopic approach.

Pandaya et al.[18] reviewed the indications for conversion among 200 consecutive patients. Their conversion rate was 23.5% (47 patients). They noted a change in the reasons for conversion from the initial technical problems (reflecting the learning curve) to patient-related limitations such as a large phlegmon, dense adhesions, bulky tumors, and fixed pathology. They recommended laparotomy if any of these features were preoperatively identified and early conversion when and if such were laparoscopically encountered. Their conversion rate of 36% was statistically greater in the first 50 patients (first quarter) than the 16% of subsequent quarters (51–200 patients). Thus, as did Agachan et al.,[5] they noted a learning curve of 50 patients. They emphasized the importance of case selection and recommended avoiding procedures such as reversal of Hartmann's and surgery on the distal rectum.

The Laparoscopic Approach

Complications specific to the laparoscopic approach can be separated into those problems attributed to the use of pneumoperitoneum, trocar-related difficulties, and direct laparoscopic limitations such as faulty positioning, difficult exposure, and loss of tactile sensation.

Pneumoperitoneum-Associated Complications

Intraperitoneal insufflation of carbon dioxide can elevate the arterial content of carbon dioxide (CO_2) by transperitoneal and subcutaneous absorption.[14] Therefore, continuous capnometry is mandatory, as are blood gas measurements in prolonged cases. The CO_2 gas used should be warmed to help prevent hypothermia; most healthy patients will develop only minimal hypercarbia. Patients with cardiopulmonary dysfunction can develop severe hypercarbia and acidemia, provoking numerous complications.[12]

Extensive subcutaneous emphysema sequesters large amounts of CO_2, which can overwhelm the endogenous clearance mechanism and further exacerbate the respiratory acidosis.[12] This occurrence is typical in thin-skinned, frail elderly patients with cardiopulmonary disease. This problem can be avoided by carefully anchoring the ports and having an assistant ensure port stability during the introduction and extraction of instruments through the ports. The intraabdominal pressure should be kept at 15 mmHg because higher pressures can decrease venous return. This level is especially important in volume-depleted patients, particularly after a bowel preparation. Furthermore, increased intraabdominal pressure may alter pulmonary mechanics, decreasing compliance and forcing the diaphragm cephalad. Ventilating the lower lobes for patients with obstructive pulmonary disease may be difficult and require increasing the ventilator's inflation pressure.

Trocar-Associated Complications

The major risk with trocars is related to the initial blind insertion. Adherent organs and vessels within or deep to the abdominal wall may be injured. The Hasson technique eliminates the complications of blind Veress needle and the initial trocar insertion; the Hasson technique is not without morbidity, as avulsion of adhesions or even enterotomy can occur. Nevertheless, the complication rate appears to be both lower and less consequential than with the closed technique. Regardless of technique of initial port placement, all subsequent trocars should be placed under direct vision, specifically avoiding the epigastric vessels. This positioning can be difficult in obese patients in whom the epigastric vessels cannot be easily transilluminated. To help decrease the chance of epigastric vessel injury, subsequent ports are placed lateral to the vessels. This position also facilitates mobilization of the right or left colon, allowing maximum distance between ports. The skin incision should be large enough and the abdomen should be fully distended, so that excessive force is not required to place the trocar.

The incidence of port site hernias is probably increased secondary to frequent manipulation and dissection that is required through larger, atypically placed trocars. Thus, all defects made by trocars 10mm or larger should be carefully sutured closed, a maneuver that can be difficult and frustrating in obese patients. Sometimes the skin incision must be enlarged, obviating one of the benefits of laparoscopic surgery. A few sophisticated devices (Endo-Judge, UR-6 needle; Ethicon Endosurgery, Cincinnati, OH, USA) have been developed to assist in this tedious but essential task.

Procedure-Associated Complications

The patient should be positioned to allow padding of all areas of potential bodily injury. In addition, because of the various positions needed to effect the surgery, the patient should be safely secured to the table to prevent slippage when in extreme positions.[19] The risk of thromboembolic complications is higher in lengthier operative cases and also with the use of pneumoperitoneum; venous blood return from the lower limbs is reduced. Intermittent sequential compressive stockings have been shown to lower the risk of postoperative deep venous thrombosis during laparoscopic colorectal procedures.[19] Lengthy procedures carry the risk of hypothermia and increased wound infections. Therefore, any obstacle that prevents timely progression of the procedure should dictate early conversion to laparotomy to avoid significant complications.

Exposure and visualization of the ureter in every case will minimize potential for injury. A preoperative CT scan or intravenous pyelogram (IVP) may confirm the location and identify any deviation associated with a large neoplasm or inflammatory mass. Ureteric catheterization should be considered in these cases, just as when approached via laparotomy. Furthermore, ureteral catheters should be preoperatively placed in all cases of acute diverticulitis where an inflammatory mass may obscure anatomy. The ureters must be identified before vessel or bowel transection (Fig. 54.1).

Injury to the bowel can be minimized by the use of atraumatic bowel clamps when manipulating and mobilizing the intestine. The clamp should never be locked and should always be kept within the visual field on grasping, opening, inserting, and extracting. In this way, inadvertent injury may be avoided. Also, this suggested guideline should help to avoid entrapment injury whereby the omentum or epiploica catches on extraction of the instrument. Trocars, electrocautery, and direct trauma from instruments can cause enterotomies. Thermal injury is often unrecognized; thus, precision, insulation, and visual field awareness are of paramount importance.

Complete dissection and visualization of the mesenteric vascular pedicle is essential before clipping, stapling, and transecting (Fig 54.2). Proper dissection will help decrease the bulk of tissue in the staples and secure hemostasis. The Harmonic scalpel (Ethicon Endosurgery) may be helpful, particularly with a bulky inflamed mesentery, to secure a passageway in the mesorectum for the stapling of the rectal stump (Fig. 54.3).

Last, of particular concern is the potential for metastatic tumor recurrences at the port sites.[8,9,20,21] Thus far, reports are anecdotal and the true incidence uncon-

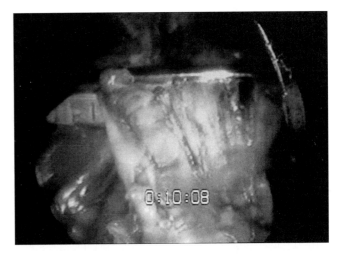

FIGURE 54.1. Complete dissection and visualization of the mesenteric pedicle.

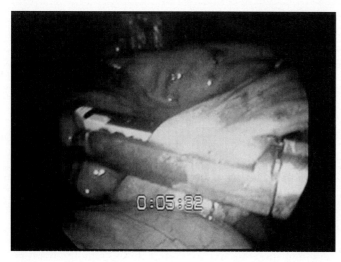

FIGURE 54.2. Identification of ureters before vessel or bowel transection.

firmed. Nevertheless, specimens should always be placed in a protective bag or delivered through an impervious wound protector before extraction. Careful handling of the tumor specimen to prevent disruption, aerosolization, and implantation is mandatory. Until results of prospective randomized trials are published, this approach for cancer should be limited to patients enrolled in prospective randomized, externally monitored, peer-reviewed trials.

Errors in Judgment and Case Selection

Early conversion to laparotomy should be regarded as sound and appropriate judgment. It is the key to avoiding complications and the best way to ensure a successful outcome. Conversion should never be thought of as an indication of failure. Prolonged laparoscopy before conversion adversely increases the overall morbidity and cost.[18,22,23] Early conversions may still allow therapeutic benefits and cost savings to be realized.

Sher et al.[15] found no differences in either the hospital stay or the morbidity type or incidence for patients who required conversion compared to patients treated by laparotomy for acute diverticulitis. In a review of 200 cases, excessive tumor bulk, dense adhesions, fixed pathology, and phlegmonous disease secondary to diverticulitis were defined as the technical limitations of the laparoscopic approach. The authors also warned against laparoscopy for the reversal of a Hartmann procedure after pelvic sepsis and for distal rectal surgery.

Larach et al.[22] favored early conversion for patients with unclear anatomy secondary to adhesions, obesity, or any other prohibitive obstacle. If the ureter was not visualized, a laparotomy was mandatory. They were able to

reduce the iatrogenic complications related to inexperience with technique from 7.3% to 1.4%. If any of the principles or criteria set was not accomplished, timely abandonment was regarded as sound judgment. This approach explains why the overall conversion rate was unchanged in their later experience.

Kockerling et al.[23] reviewed one year's experience in Germany and Austria, which included 500 patients from 18 centers; the overall conversion rate was 7%. Most conversions were undertaken early in the procedure for anatomic reasons and tumor size or location. The zero intraoperative complication rate was attributed to timely conversion.

Case selection is probably the most important factor in avoiding complications. As with any other tool, selected application gained by experience will offer the best outcome. Hence, random application of the laparoscope to all colorectal pathology even when technically feasible should be discouraged. One must identify a subset of patients who will truly benefit from a laparoscopic approach and discourage the use of the laparoscope for other reasons.

Kockerling et al.[23] and other authors[24–27] have identified differences in complication rates specific to intestinal pathology. For instance, introperative complications such as bleeding and enterotomy were common with low anterior resections; these procedures also had the highest conversion rate. Resection for acute diverticulitis was also associated with bleeding complications due to the thick, inflamed, friable mesentery. In contrast, laparoscopic sigmoid colectomies for cancer, abdominal perineal resections, stomas, and rectopexies carrier less morbidit intraoperative complications and deemed more suitable for a laparoscopic approach. Lumley et al.[6] also noted technical difficulty with low anterior resections and total

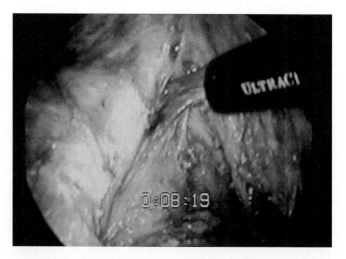

FIGURE 54.3. Dissection of the mesentery using the Harmonic scalpel (Ethicon Endosurgery, Cincinnati, OH).

colectomies because of the lack of a linear cutter to allow for precise laparoscopic-assisted low rectal division in the confines of a narrow pelvis with pneumoperitoneum; they advocated a laparotomy. Sher et al.[17] noted an increased morbidity and conversion rate with Hinchey II as compared to Hinchey I diverticular disease and recommended operating for the latter indication first. Molenaar et al.[7] and Kohler et al.[24] also documented the limitations associated with inflammatory disease and excluded all patients with a preoperatively fixed mass. The exact method to identify patients with diverticulitis and freely mobile bowel not firmly adhered to the left gutter or contingent organs was unclear, however. The goal should be to the avoidance of complications, not of conversions.

Conclusion

Avoiding complications associated with the application of minimally invasive technology to colorectal disorders can be achieved in the same way that any other unfamiliar innovative technology is adapted to the surgical forum. Progressive technical experience, careful and thoughtful case selection, early conversion to laparotomy, and advances in technology will all help ensure the desired outcome.

References

1. Reissman P, Cohen S, Weiss E, et al. Laparoscopic colorectal surgery: ascending the learning curve. World J Surg 1996;20:277–282.
2. Senagore AJ, Luchtefeld MA, Mackeigan JM. What is the learning curve for laparoscopic colectomy? Am Surg 1995; 61:681–685.
3. Simons AJ, Anthone GJ, Ortega AE. Laparoscopic-assisted colectomy learning curve. Dis Colon Rectum 1995;38: 600–603.
4. Agachan F, Joo JS, Weiss EG, et al. Intraoperative laparoscopic complications; are we getting better? Dis Colon Rectum 1996;39:S14–S19.
5. Agachan F, Joo JS, Sher M, et al. Laparoscopic colorectal surgery: do we get faster? Surg Endosc 1997;11:331–335.
6. Lumley JW, Fielding GA, Rhodes M, et al. Laparoscopic-assisted colorectal surgery: lessons learned from 240 consecutive patients. Dis Colon Rectum 1996;39:155–159.
7. Molenaar CBH, Bijnen AB, De Ruiter P. Indications for laparoscopic colorectal surgery: results from the Medical Centre Alkmaar, The Netherlands. Surg Endosc 1998;12: 42–45.
8. Pahlman L. The problem of port-site metastases after laparoscopic cancer surgery. Ann Med 1997;29:477–481.
9. Schaeff B, Paolucci V, Thomopoulos J. Port site recurrences after laparoscopic surgery. Dig Surg 1998;15:124–134.
10. Weiss EG, Wexner SD. Training and preparing for laparoscopic colectomy. Semin Colon Rectal Surg 1994;5:224–227.
11. See WA, Cooper CS, Fisher RJ. Predictors of laparoscopic complications after formal training in laparoscopic surgery. JAMA 1993;270:2689–2692.
12. Beck DE. Laparoscopic surgery. In: Hicks TC, Beck DE, Opelka FG, Timmcke AE (eds) Complications of Colon and Rectal Surgery. Baltimore: Williams & Wilkins, 1996: 153–162.
13. Falk PM, Beart RW Jr, Wexner SD, et al. Laparoscopic colectomy: a critical appraisal. Dis Colon Rectum 1993;36: 28–34.
14. Beck DE, Opelka FG. Laparoscopic complications. In Jager R, Wexner SD (eds) Laparoscopic Colorectal Surgery. New York: Churchill Livingstone, 1996:267–276.
15. Sher ME. United States. In: Wexner SD (ed). Laparoscopic Colorectal Surgery. New York: Wiley-Liss, 1999:541–550.
16. Larach SW, Patankar SK, Ferrara A, et al. Complications of laparoscopic colorectal surgery. Dis Colon Rectum 1997;40: 592–596.
17. Sher ME, Agachan F, Bortul M, et al. Laparoscopic surgery for diverticulitis. Surg Endosc 1998;11:264–267.
18. Pandaya S, Murray JJ, Coller JA, et al. Laparoscopic colectomy: indications for conversion to laparotomy. Arch Surg 1999;134:471–476.
19. Schwenk W, Bohm B, Junghans T, et al. Intermittent sequential compression of the lower limbs prevents venous stasis in laparoscopic and conventional colorectal surgery. Dis Colon Rectum 1997;40:1056–1062.
20. Milsom JW, Bohm B, Hammerhoffer K, et al. A prospective randomized trial comparing laparoscopic versus conventional techniques in colorectal cancer surgery: a preliminary report. J Am Coll Surg 1998;187:46–57.
21. Stage JG, Schulze S, Moller P, et al. Prospective randomized study of laparoscopic versus open colonic resection for adenocarcinoma. Br J Surg 1997;894:391–396.
22. Larach SW, Gallagher J, Ferrar J. Lessons learned from laparoscopic colectomy. Semin Colon Rectal Surg 1999; 10:59–63.
23. Kockerling F, Schneider C, Reymond MA. Early results of a prospective multi-center study on 500 consecutive cases of laparoscopic colorectal surgery. Surg Endosc 1998;12: 37–41.
24. Kohler L, Rixen D, Troidl H. Laparoscopic colorectal resection for diverticulitis. Int J Colorect Dis 1998;13:43–47.
25. Sardinha TC, Wexner SD. Laparoscopy for inflammatory bowel disease: pros and cons. World J Surg 1998;22:37.
26. Bouillot JL, Aouad K, Badaway A, et al. Elective laparoscopic-assisted colectomy for diverticular disease. Surg Endosc 1998;12:1393–1396.
27. Lacy AM, Garcia-Valdecasas JC, Delgado S, et al. Postoperative complications of laparoscopic-assisted colectomy. Surg Endosc 1997;11:119–122.

55
Cost Considerations

Johann Pfeifer and Selman Uranüs

The revolution in laparoscopic minimally invasive surgical technology and techniques has introduced a constellation of new issues, not the least of which are economic outcomes and cost. These considerations have become an especially important topic due to the steady increase in health care costs in Western countries. Insurance companies, health maintenance organizations, managed care directors, governmental legislative bodies, surgeons, and even patients today contend with health care resource management. While studies on the clinical aspects of laparoscopy have been widely published, the few economic outcome studies have lead to more confusion than resolution of important questions as a consequence of the varied inconsistent and conflicting results. The other major problem is that the majority of studies to date have reported "charges" and not costs; these charges are artificial and may not accurately depict true costs. The aim of this chapter is to highlight the problems of cost calculations in general and of cost studies in laparoscopic colorectal surgery in detail.

What to Measure?

The goals of health care have been defined by Lohr in 1988 as "to limit mortality, disease, disability, and discomfort, and optimize satisfaction."[1] Quality-adjusted life years (QUALYs) and costs per QUALY are research efforts aimed at answering questions that previously seemed irrelevant. However, society is confronted with rising costs and limited resources, and the public demands value for money.[2] To analyze all aspects of cost calculations in laparoscopic surgery, many considerations must be taken into account (Fig. 55.1). The total economic impact of a surgical procedure includes the direct medical expenses charged to the payor, the patient's lost salary, and the employer's lost revenues and/or incremental costs incurred due to the patient/employee's absence. Thus, there are two main cost categories: (1) direct

medical costs, which include the initial operation with the costs of treatment of any complications, and (2) the indirect costs. This latter group includes all expenses related to the fact that the patient is absent from normal activity.

Direct Medical Costs

Direct medical costs are directly related to the surgical procedure (Fig. 55.2); they can be divided into short-term costs and follow-on direct costs.

Short-term costs are those expenses that occur between the time of initial presentation and evaluation through hospital admission until discharge. These costs can be further divided into labor, supplies, diagnostic tests, and capital items.

Labor. Labor includes the number of hours required and cost per hour for the surgeon, the anesthesiologist, and other staff to evaluate and treat the problem.
Supplies. Measurement of supply input should focus on the quantity used as well as the cost for each item. Supplies consist of medical instruments and other supplies. Billing for medical supplies varies from hospital to hospital. Furthermore, the quantity of a given product used in a given hospital is important for price calculations. For reusable instruments, maintenance of instruments must also be calculated as an expense. The problem is that objective data are seldom available; often one must decide between actual costs or charges (to the patient's bill). Other supplies are charges for tapes, dressings, intravenous fluids, medications, and all other ancillary requirements.
Diagnostic tests. Some evaluations may be necessary to make the diagnosis. The personnel, equipment, and the time necessary to arrive at the diagnosis and prepare for treatment should be taken into account when calculating costs for individual procedures.

FIGURE 55.1. Direct and indirect costs that should be considered in calculating the cost of a laparoscopic procedure.

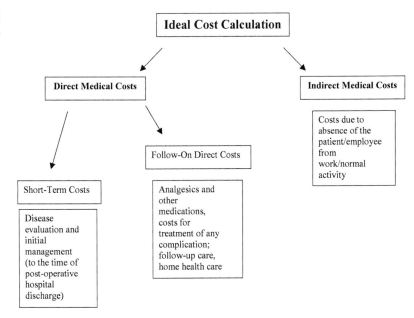

Capital items. The most expensive items are the charges for the operating theater, the intensive care unit, and the hospital bed. Other items may be costs for administration, utilities, and nursing.

Follow-on direct costs are those expenses that must be paid after the initial procedure (even if not reimbursed by payors), such as analgesics and other medications, as well as follow-up visits and management of any complications.

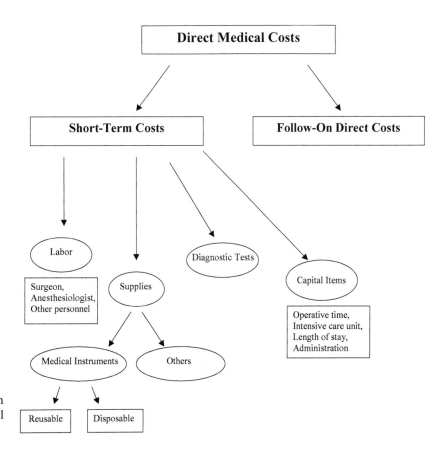

FIGURE 55.2. Short-term and follow-on direct costs that add up to the direct medical cost of a laparoscopic procedure.

Indirect Medical Costs

Indirect costs should include all expenses that can arise from the absence of the patient from work and normal activity. This loss is usually very difficult to estimate. However, true cost and outcome studies should include all the expenses until the patient returns to normal activity.

- For employers, indirect costs may include substitute workers, lost revenues, and disability costs.
- For payors of workers' compensation and disability, indirect costs may include dispensation made to a recovering worker.
- For workers having no disability compensation coverage, indirect costs may be lost salaries.

Special Consideration for Costs

In the calculations for cost studies, it is of immense importance to know the level of expertise of the surgeon performing the operation. There has been much discussion (especially when laparoscopic surgery was in the developmental stage) about the increased time required for surgery as compared to laparotomy. The learning curve had costs that were difficult to justify compared to laparotomy.[3] However, as surgeons' skills and instrumentation improved, costs for operative time and equipment decreased, making laparoscopic operations less expensive. Cuschieri et al. suggested that the new laparoscopic operating methods should be reported in steps. After 20 to 50 procedures (constituting the learning curve), comparison with laparotomy may be valid.[4] Furthermore, instrument preferences are often highly individual and should be a part of each cost analysis.

Another important cost effectiveness factor is length of hospital stay. Patients can be routinely and safely discharged much earlier than previously thought possible.[5-9] However, hospital stay has a major impact on costs as a fixed capital item. Therefore, many studies that compared laparoscopy with "historical controls" were based upon potentially erroneous assumptions.[10-12]

Disposable Versus Reusable Instruments

Since the introduction of laparoscopy, one debate has centered on reusable versus disposable instruments. Costs, safety, and hygiene are cited considerations.

1. Costs. If disposable instruments are used, it is of tremendous importance not only to calculate the actual price of (or charge for) the instrument but also to include costs for instrument disposal (hazardous waste handling or sterilization). Reusable instrument calculations should include initial purchase price, costs for maintaining the instrument, replacement charges, as well as costs for cleaning, repair, repacking, and sterilization. It is often very difficult to calculate prices, especially if "semi-reusable instruments" are used. In this group some parts of instruments are reusable and other parts are disposable. For example, a clip applicator is reusable, whereas a clip magazine is disposable.

2. Safety. There is no difference in safety between reusable and disposable instruments.[13,14]

3. Hygiene. Several studies have addressed the issue of hygiene with reusable instruments.[15,16] However, no study has proven that any complications are due to unsanitary reusable instruments.[13,14]

TABLE 55.1. Costs of colon resection: laparoscopy versus open procedure.

Author	Year	Laparoscopy ($)	Open ($)	Net	Converted ($)
Falk[10]	1993	12,000	12,500	−500	15,000
Vayer[19]	1993	26,662	22,938	+3,724	13,956
Senagore[20]	1993	12,131	14,496	−2,365	17,583
Musser[21]	1994	9,811	Not stated		11,207
Reiver[22]	1994	23,294	19,384	+3,910	Not stated
Hoffmann[23]	1994	12,464	10,213	+2,250	13,956
Pfeifer[5]	1995	29,626	22,938	+6,688	13,954
Bokey[24]	1996	6,021	5,235	+786	Not stated
Liberman[25]	1996	Costs, 11,528	13,426	−1,898	Not stated
		Charges, 36,745	29,981	+6,764	Not stated
Bruce[26]	1996	10,230	7,068	+3,162	Not stated
Bergamaschi[27]	1997	10,929	9,944	+985	Not stated
Psaila[28]	1998	4,712	5,362	−650	Not stated
Mean cost ($)		15,953	14,506	+1,905	14,276

All prices in U.S. dollars.

TABLE 55.2. Costs of appendectomy: laparoscopy versus open procedure.

Author	Year	Laparoscopy ($)	Open ($)	Net
Cohen[29]	1993	9,656	8,384	+1,272
Williams[30]	1994	7,500	5,700	+1,800
Buckley[31]	1994	7,238	5,343	+1,895
Martin[32]	1995	6,077	7,227	−1,150
Richards[33]	1996	4,900	4,950	−50
McCahill[34]	1996	7,760	5,064	+2,696
Heikkinen[35]	1998	4,557	6,039	−1,482
Johnson[36]	1998	Normal, 6,430	Normal, 6,669	−239
		Perforated, 7,506	Perforated, 10,504	−2,998
Mean cost ($)		6,847	6,653	193

All prices in U.S. dollars

To achieve an appropriate balance among costs, safety, and hygiene, most studies indicate that the effectiveness of a combination of disposable (first trocar) and reusable instruments (further trocars) is preferred.[6,17,18]

Cost Studies

Cost considerations expressed in outcome studies can only assess part of the actual costs. Each surgeon has to discuss the economic impact of laparoscopic surgery in his or her department or hospital. Calculations for costs vary greatly among hospitals, regions, and countries. Furthermore, cost considerations must always be evaluated in view of the operative caseload for each department. Some recent publications of cost and outcome studies are shown in Tables 55.1 and 55.2.

Laparoscopy-Related Cost Considerations

From the aforementioned cost studies up to now the following trends can be recognized. First, in almost all series the cost of a converted procedure was more than that of either laparoscopy or laparotomy. Second, there is a trend toward higher costs for the laparoscopic procedure. These data result from the longer operative time and more sophisticated equipment used. However, as mentioned, true economic impact has not yet been calculated.

Conclusion

Cost considerations can be calculated only for a given laparoscopic procedure in a given hospital with given staff surgeons and a given frequency of operations performed, as cost calculations are a dynamic process. For surgeons, however, quality for the patient is the most important point. To solve the problem of increasing costs in health care, all parties involved in this system must work collectively together to manage this issue.

References

1. Lohr KN. Outcome measurements: concepts and questions. Inquiry 1988;25:37–50.
2. Kievit J. Decision analysis, cost-benefits analysis and cost-effectiveness analysis in surgical research. In: Troidl H, McKneally MF, Mulder DS, Wechsler AS, McPeek B, Spitzer WO (eds) Surgical Research. New York: Springer, 1998:555–570.
3. Reissman P, Cohen S, Weiss EG, et al. Laparoscopic colorectal surgery: ascending the learning curve. World J Surg 1996;20:277–281.
4. Cuschieri A, Ferreira E, Goh P, et al. Guidelines for conducting economic outcomes studies for endoscopic procedures. Surg Endosc 1997;11:308–311.
5. Pfeifer J, Wexner SD, Reissman P, et al. Laparoscopic vs open colon surgery. Costs and outcome. Surg Endosc 1995;9: 1322–1326.
6. Wexner SD, Reissman P, Pfeifer J, et al. Laparoscopic colorectal surgery: analysis of 140 cases. Surg Endosc 1996; 10:133–136.
7. Rajagopal AS, Thorson AG, Sentovich T, et al. Decade trends in length of postoperative stay following abdominal colectomy [abstract]. Dis Colon Rectum 1994;37:26.
8. Reissman P, Teoh TA, Cohen SM, et al. Is early oral feeding safe after elective colorectal surgery? A prospective randomized trial. Ann Surg 1995;222:73–77.
9. Schoetz DJ Jr, Bockler M, Rosenblatt MS, et al. "Ideal" length of stay after colectomy: whose ideal? Dis Colon Rectum 1997;40(7):806–810.
10. Falk PM, Beart RW, Wexner SD, et al. Laparoscopic colectomy: a critical appraisal. Dis Colon Rectum 1993;36:28–34.
11. Monson JRT, Darzi A, Carey PD, et al. Prospective evaluation of laparoscopic-assisted colectomy in an unselected group of patients. Lancet 1992;340:831–833.

12. Phillips EH, Franklin M, Carroll BJ, et al. Laparoscopic colectomy. Ann Surg 1992;212:703–707.

13. Lefering R, Troidl H, Ure B. Entscheiden die Kosten? Einweg oder wiederverwertbare Instrumente bei der laparoskopischen Cholecystektomie? Chirurg 1994;65: 317–325.

14. Paolucci V, Schaeff B, Gutt C, et al. Einmal versus wiederverwendbare Instrumente in der laparoskopischen Chirurgie eine kontrollierte Untersuchung. Zentralbl Chir 1995;120:47–52.

15. Des Coteaux J, Poulin E, Julien M, et al. Residual organic debris on processed surgical instruments. J Assoc Oper Room Nurses 1995;62:23–29.

16. Fengler TZ, Pahlke H, Kraas E. Five-year-experience with laparoscopic instruments and accessories. Minim Invasive Med 1995;4:153–158.

17. MacFadyen BV, Lenz S. The economic considerations in laparoscopic surgery. Surg Endosc 1994;8:748–752.

18. Kriwanek S, Armbruster C, Dittrich K, et al. Einmal versus wiederverwendbare Instrumente in der laparoskopischen Cholecystektomie Kostenkalkulation und Nutzwertbestimmung. Acta Chir Austriaca 1997;29:42–49.

19. Vayer AJ, Larach SW, Williamson PR, et al. Cost effectiveness of laparoscopic assisted colectomy. Coloproctology 1994; 16:190–195.

20. Senagore AJ, Luchtefeld MA, MacKeigan JM, et al. Open colectomy versus laparoscopic colectomy: are there differences? Am Surg 1993;59:549–554.

21. Musser DJ, Boorse RC, Madera F, et al. Laparoscopic colectomy: at what cost? Surg Laparosc Endosc 1994;4:1–5.

22. Reiver D, Kmiot WA, Cohen SM, et al. A prospective assessment of laparoscopic versus open procedures in colorectal surgery [abstract]. Dis Colon Rectum 1994;37:22.

23. Hoffmann GC, Baketr JW, Fitchett CW, et al. Laparoscopic assisted colectomy: initial experience. Ann Surg 1994;219: 732–743.

24. Bokey EL, Moore WE, Chapuis PH, et al. Morbidity and mortality following laparoscopic-assisted right hemicolectomy for cancer. Dis Colon Rectum 1996;39:S24–S28.

25. Liberman MA, Phillips EH, Carroll BJ, et al. Laparoscopic colectomy vs traditional colectomy for diverticulitis. Outcome and costs. Surg Endosc 1996;10:15–18.

26. Bruce CJ, Coller JA, Murray JJ, et al. Laparoscopic resection for diverticular disease. Dis Colon Rectum 1996;39: S1–S6.

27. Bergamaschi R, Arnaud JP. Immediately recognizable benefits and drawbacks after laparoscopic colon resection for benign disease. Surg Endosc 1997;11:802–804.

28. Psaila J, Bulley SH, Ewings P, et al. Outcome following laparoscopic resection for colorectal cancer. Br J Surg 1998; 85:662–664.

29. Cohen M, Dangleis K. The cost-effectiveness of laparoscopic appendectomy. J Laparosc Endosc 1993;3:93–97.

30. Williams MD, Miller D, Graves E, et al. Laparoscopic appendectomy: is it worth it? South Med J 1994;87:592–598.

31. Buckley R, Hall T, Muakkassa F, et al. Laparoscopic appendectomy: is it worth it? Am Surg 1994;60:30–34.

32. Martin LC, Puente I, Sosa JL, et al. Open versus laparoscopic appendectomy. A prospective randomized comparison. Ann Surg 1995;222:256–261.

33. Richards K, Fisher K, Flores J, et al. Laparoscopic appendectomy: comparison with open appendectomy in 720 patients. Surg Laparosc Endosc 1996;6:205–209.

34. McCahill LE, Pellegrini CA, Wiggins T, et al. A clinical outcome and cost analysis of laparoscopic versus open appendectomy. Am J Surg 1996;171:533–537.

35. Heikkinen TJ, Haukipuro K, Hulkko A. Cost effective appendectomy: open or laparoscopic? A prospective randomized study. Surg Endosc 1998;12:1204–1208.

36. Johnson AB, Peetz ME. Laparoscopic appendectomy is an acceptable alternative for the treatment of perforated appendicitis. Surg Endosc 1998;12:940–943.

56
Avoidance and Treatment of Urological Complications

Roland N. Chen

The incidence of ureteral injury during open colorectal surgery has been reported to be 0.71% for colorectal procedures[1] and as high as 3.7% for abdominoperineal resections.[2] Laparoscopic surgery poses additional challenges for the colorectal surgeon because of the lack of tactile feedback and potential difficulties with exposure. A 0.6% to 1.6%[3,4] incidence of ureteral injuries has been reported for laparoscopic gynecological procedures. Clearly, the incidence of iatrogenic urologic injury varies depending on patient selection factors such as history of radiation or the likelihood of retroperitoneal or pelvic fibrosis. The risk of iatrogenic urological injury also depends on the location of the pathology and the extent of dissection required to complete the laparoscopic procedure.

Ureteral Anatomy

Because the ascending and descending colon are, in part, within the retroperitoneal space, the ureters must be considered during their surgical dissection. The ureters course medially in the retroperitoneum posterior to the colon mesentery (Fig. 56.1). The proximal to midureters are immediately lateral to the great vessels and anterior to the psoas muscle. The ureters cross the iliac vessels at their bifurcation and travel posterolaterally along the pelvic sidewall (Fig. 56.2). The ureters then cross under the vas deferens, in men, and the infundibulopelvic ligament, in women, before passing under the obliterated umbilical artery and into the posterolateral aspect of the bladder where they enter via a muscular sheath (Figs. 56.3, 56.4). Because of the proximity of the distal ureters to the gynecological organs and rectum, most iatrogenic ureteral injuries occur to the distal one-third of the ureters,[5] particularly in the region of the pelvic brim.

Avoidance of Ureteral Injury

The most important aspect of avoiding ureteral injury is to be aware of its possibility. Patients who are particularly susceptible to ureteral injury include those with significant retroperitoneal inflammation, such as patients with inflammatory bowel disease or pelvic abscess. Patients with infiltrative cancer or a history of abdominal or pelvic radiation are also at increased risk for iatrogenic ureteral injury.

Ureteral catheters may be placed before colon surgery to aid in identifying the ureters via palpation during difficult cases. Because the ureteral catheters can be difficult to palpate laparoscopically, intraoperative manipulation of the ureteral catheters via the urethra as the retroperitoneum is inspected for motion may aid in the identification of the ureters. If a ureter cannot be identified in the region of large bowel pathology and the risk of ureteral involvement is high, it would be prudent to identify the ureter away from the pathology and trace it into the region of involvement. Illuminated ureteral catheters may facilitate their identification[6] but are expensive and should be reserved for particularly difficult cases. Ureteral catheters that emit infrared light are also available with an infrared laparoscopic camera system (Fig. 56.5).

Recognition and Treatment of Urinary Tract Injuries

Discovering an iatrogenic urinary tract injury intraoperatively is far preferable to discovering the problem in the postoperative period. Most clues that the urinary tract has been injured are relatively obvious, such as the sudden intraoperative onset of hematuria or insufflation of the bladder catheter drainage bag with CO_2. Preoperative placement of ureteral catheters facilitates the intra-

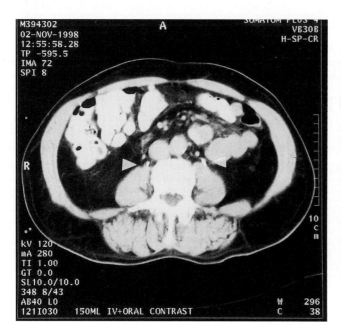

FIGURE 56.1. In the upper retroperitoneum, the ureters (*arrowheads*) are anterior to the psoas muscles and posterior to the ascending and descending colon mesentery.

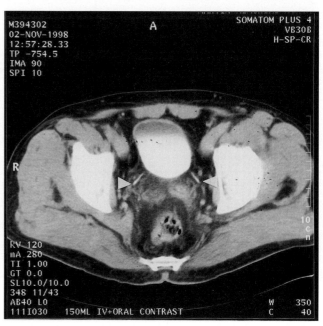

FIGURE 56.3. In men, the most distal ureters (*arrowheads*) are anterior to the seminal vesicles and distant to the rectum.

operative recognition of a ureteral injury[1] by the surgeon's direct visualization of the catheter during dissection. In the absence of a ureteral catheter, a ureteral injury could much more easily be missed. If suspicion for a ureteral injury exists, a ureteral catheter can be placed cystoscopically at any point during the procedure and then irrigated with methylene blue or saline solution.

Extravasation of irrigant should be evident. If there is any suspicion for bladder injury, the bladder catheter should be similarly irrigated with methylene blue or saline solution.

If a urinary tract injury is recognized intraoperatively, steps can be taken immediately to repair the injury. If a very small ureterotomy (<1–2mm) has been made,

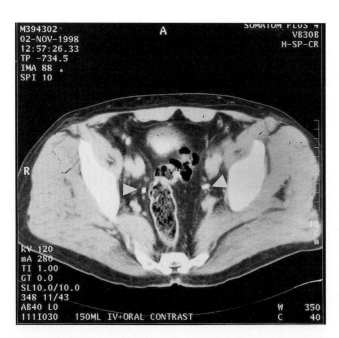

FIGURE 56.2. In the pelvis, the ureters (*arrowheads*) are lateral to the sigmoid colon along the pelvic sidewall.

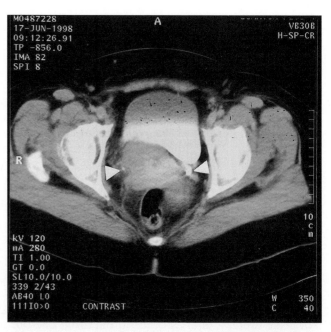

FIGURE 56.4. In women, the most distal ureters (*arrowheads*) are lateral to the uterus and considerably anterior to the rectum.

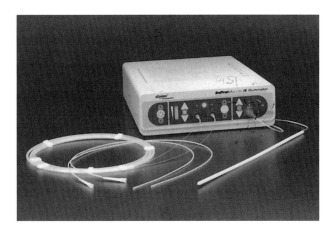

FIGURE 56.5. Infrared ureteral catheter system. (Courtesy of Stryker Endoscopy, San Jose, CA.)

placement of an indwelling ureteral stent and a retroperitoneal drain should suffice. Larger lacerations may require the additional placement of a few small (4-0 or smaller) interrupted absorbable sutures. The closure should be transversely performed if possible so as not to compromise the diameter of the ureter. If a significant injury occurs or if the ureter is completely transected, however, reconstruction will be necessary via open or laparoscopic ureterotomy or ureteral reimplantation, depending on the site and extent of injury. The end(s) of the ureter should be debrided and spatulated, but mobilized no more than necessary. The goal of any such procedure is to create a watertight, tension-free anastomosis with a good blood supply to each end of the ureter. If the ureteral injury involves inadvertent ligation, the ligated segment usually should be excised and a ureteroureterotomy performed. Placement of a drain adjacent to the anastomosis is generally recommended following such procedures. In extreme circumstances when a significant length of ureter is lost and when there is insufficient length to perform a ureteral reimplant, options include complex open reconstructive procedures such as the construction of an ileal ureter, transureteroureterostomy, autotransplantation, or nephrectomy. Such complex procedures should probably not be undertaken at the time of initial ureteral injury.

If a bladder injury has occurred, the bladder may be repaired in one or two layers via an open or laparoscopic approach using absorbable sutures. Care should be taken not to injure or obstruct the urethra and bladder neck or the ureters and their orifices during bladder repair. A large bladder catheter ($\geq 20F$) should be placed for 1 to 2 weeks, depending on the size of the injury. A gravity cystogram may be performed to confirm absence of extravasation before bladder catheter removal.

Patients with an initially unrecognized urinary tract injury may present with flank or abdominal pain, fever, leukocytosis, or prolonged ileus. Although unusual, postoperative oliguria or anuria could be noted if both ureters are injured. CT is a valuable tool for identifying urinary tract injury. If extravasation of contrast or a collection is seen on CT, a drain should be placed and the fluid sent for creatinine level. Other diagnostic procedures that may be performed to locate or characterize urinary tract injury include intravenous pyelography, cystography, cystoscopy, and retrograde pyelography.

Conclusion

Urinary tract injuries are uncommon during laparoscopic or open colon surgery. However, the ureters and bladder may be injured if significant inflammation and fibrosis are present. Awareness of the possibility of urinary tract injury and steps to prevent injury, such as preoperative placement of ureteral catheters, can further reduce the incidence of such events. Intraoperative recognition is far preferable to postoperative diagnosis of a urinary tract injury. Fortunately, the urinary tract is relatively forgiving so long as the urine is diverted with an indwelling ureteral stent or a large bladder catheter during the healing process.

References

1. Bothwell WN, Bleicher RJ, Dent TL. Prophylactic ureteral catheterization in colon surgery. Dis Colon Rectum 1994;37: 330–334.
2. Andersson A, Bergdahl L. Urologic complications following abdominoperineal resection of the rectum. Arch Surg 1976; 111:969–973.
3. Harkki-Siren P, Kurki T. A nationwide analysis of laparoscopic complications. Obstet Gynecol 1997;89:108–112.
4. Saidi MH, Sadler RK, Vancaillie TG, et al. Diagnosis and management of serious urinary complications after major operative laparoscopy. Obstet Gynecol 1996;87:272–276.
5. Selzman AA, Spirnak JP. Iatrogenic ureteral injuries: a 20-year experience in treating 165 injuries. J Urol 1996;155: 878–881.
6. Low RG, Moran ME. Laparoscopic use of the ureteral illuminator. Urology 1993;42:455–457.

57
Avoidance and Treatment of Vascular Complications

Mark K. Grove and Mark E. Sesto

Vascular complications are uncommon but potentially catastrophic sequelae of laparoscopic surgery. Although the term vascular injury connotes an iatrogenic breech in a vessel wall, equally significant vascular complications can result from the hemodynamic effects of pneumoperitoneum or the inadvertent introduction of gas into the circulation. The avoidance of vascular complications during laparoscopic surgery is based on both an appreciation of vascular anatomy and a sound understanding of physiological principles related to pneumoperitoneum.

Complications Related to Venous Stasis

Risk factors for venous thromboembolism are well characterized and thus, measures to prevent perioperative deep venous thrombosis (DVT) have become standard.[1,2] The creation of pneumoperitoneum in conjunction with laparoscopic procedures has specific implications with respect to venous stasis and the potential for thromboembolic events. Studies have demonstrated that lower extremity venous stasis occurs when intra-abdominal pressure exceeds 14 mmHg.[3] Furthermore, a tendency toward hypercoagulability is seen in patients following pneumoperitoneum. Despite these factors which, in aggregate, would be anticipated to increase the likelihood of venous thromboembolism following laparoscopy, the incidence of clinical venous thromboembolism may, in fact, be lower than with comparable procedures performed by laparotomy.

In this regard, in one series of more than 500 laparoscopic colorectal procedures, no instances of DVT or pulmonary embolism were observed.[4] Although speculative, the low incidence of venous thromboembolic events following laparoscopic colorectal surgery may relate to the placement of the patient in the Trendelenburg position during many such procedures. It is currently recommended that prophylactic measures be employed in patients at risk for DVT in whom laparoscopic surgery is being performed.[5] Prophylaxis should include mechanical measures (pneumatic compression) supplemented by anticoagulation with heparin or low molecular weight heparin, as indicated. The use of pneumatic compression has been shown to improve venous hemodynamics during laparoscopic surgery.[6,7]

Effects of Pneumoperitoneum on the Mesenteric Circulation

Experimentally, the increased abdominal pressure associated with induction of pneumoperitoneum has been shown to decrease splanchnic perfusion.[8] The clinical implications of relative mesenteric hypoperfusion, however, are unclear as visceral ischemic manifestations are exceedingly uncommon following routine laparoscopic procedures. Richmond et al. have reported a collected series of five cases of mesenteric ischemia attributed to laparoscopy.[9]

Gas Embolism

Gas embolism may appropriately be considered a vascular complication of laparoscopy. The rare incidence of this potentially lethal complication may be attributed to the rapid dissolution of carbon dioxide (CO_2) in the blood. The introduction of large volumes of CO_2 into the circulation, however, can result in precipitous cardiovascular collapse. A high index of suspicion regarding CO_2 embolism must be maintained when a patient develops hemodynamic instability or collapse during laparoscopy, particularly in association with bradycardia and cyanosis. Monitoring end-tidal CO_2 may help confirm the diagnosis, although an increased end-tidal CO_2 reflecting hypercapnia is not invariably observed. In nearly two-thirds of

FIGURE 57.1. A. Location of abdominal wall and retroperitoneal vessels relative to the umbilicus and rectus muscles. B. The retroperitoneal mesenteric attachments of the colon. The superior mesenteric and left iliac vessels are particularly vulnerable to injury during division of the transverse mesocolon and sigmoid mesocolon, respectively.

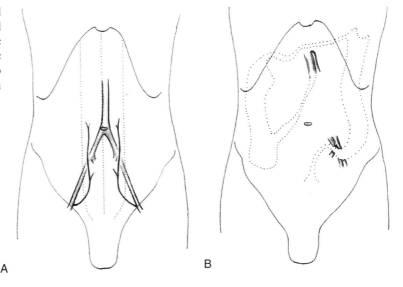

A   B

reported cases of CO_2 embolism, cardiovascular colla- pase occurred during or immediately following insuffla- tion.[10] In most cases inadvertent vascular cannulation with a Veress needle was suspected.

In cases of gas embolism, management is directed toward immediate cessation of insufflation and release of pneumoperitoneum. The patient should be placed in the steep Trendelenburg and left lateral decubitus posi- tion. Aspiration of gas from the right atrium by central venous cannulation can be a lifesaving maneuver in such cases.

Vascular Injury Related to Veress Needle Placement and Cannulation

The potential for direct vascular injury begins with peri- toneal cannulation (Fig. 57.1). Often, pneumoperitoneum is established by introduction of a Veress needle through a periumbilical incision. Injury to the aortic bifurcation or iliac vessels can occur with blind introduction of the Veress needle into the peritoneal cavity. In anatomic studies, the aortic bifurcation has been demonstrated to lie within 5 cm above the umbilicus in approximately two- thirds of patients in the supine position and at or below the umbilical level in the remainder.[11] It is important to note that although positioning the patient in the 'head- down' position during cannulation has been advocated to reduce the likelihood of visceral injury, this maneuver can displace the umbilicus in a cephalad direction. However, in this position the aortic bifurcation lies at or below the umbilicus in 60% of patients, predisposing to major vas- cular injury with blind cannulation. The dorsal lithotomy position can further alter the position of the retroperi- toneal vessels referable to the umbilicus.[12]

The proximity of the aorta, inferior vena cava, and iliac vessels to the abdominal wall also varies greatly with the body habitus of the patient.[13] In thin patients, the aorta can lie just a few centimeters deep to the umbilicus (Fig. 57.2). If a closed cannulation technique is employed, the potential for vascular injury must be minimized by introducing the Veress needle or trocar with proper ele- vation of the abdominal wall and by ensuring adequate pneumoperitoneum.

Large series suggest that up to 90% of major vascular injuries have resulted from blind introduction of a peri- toneal needle or cannula.[14–16] Veress needle injuries accounted for the preponderance of these. Injuries sus- tained during initial trocar placement are thought to

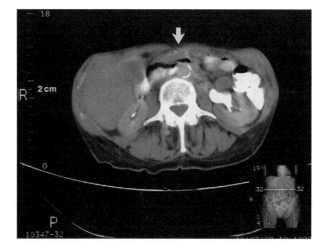

FIGURE 57.2. The retroperitoneal vessels can be located just a few centimeters below the anterior abdominal wall, rendering them vulnerable to injury during peritoneal cannulation.

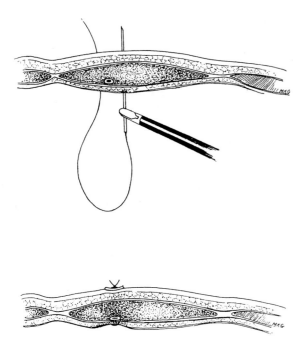

FIGURE 57.3. Cross-sectional representation of rectus sheath demonstrates transabdominal mattress suture compressing the epigastric artery. The suture is removed several days after the procedure.

result from inadequate pneumoperitoneum. These observations have led some authorities to advocate open cannulation, as originally described by Hasson, in preference to closed cannulation.[17–21] The data comparing these techniques, although uncontrolled, support the superiority of the former method, limiting major and potentially lethal vascular injury.

Undoubtedly, the vessel most commonly injured in laparoscopic procedures is the epigastric artery. This vessel may be particularly vulnerable in laparoscopic colorectal procedures because of the proximate sites of trocar insertion used in such procedures. Injuries to the inferior epigastric artery may go unrecognized due to temporary tamponade by both the cannulae and the pneumoperitoneum. The importance of direct laparoscopic inspection of the port site on withdrawl of the cannulae and decompression of the pneumoperitoneum to ensure proper hemostasis bears emphasis in this regard. Significant bleeding may occur in such cases into the peritoneal cavity, the preperitoneal space, or the rectus sheath. Temporary hemostasis is usually not problematic, being effected by reintroduction of a cannula. Suture control is achieved by transmural introduction of a monofilament mattress suture on a straight needle above and below the port site (Fig. 57.3).

In contrast to the burgeoning experience and literature relating to laparoscopic gastrointestinal and solid organ

procedures, intracorporeal vascular surgical techniques are largely undeveloped. Although anecdotal reports of aortofemoral bypass performed laparoscopically have been described,[22] vascular techniques in laparoscopic surgery cannot be viewed as standardized. As such, it must be emphasized that, in cases of injury to major vas-

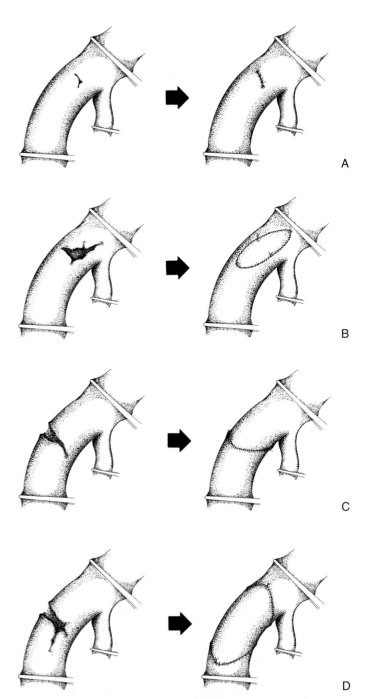

FIGURE 57.4. Techniques of vascular repair. A. Debridement and suture repair. B. Debridement with patch angioplasty. C. Segmental resection with end-to-end anastamosis. D. Segmental resection with interposition graft.

cular structures incurred during laparoscopy, conversion to laparotomy with direct vascular control and repair is imperative in all but the most exceptional circumstances.

Laparotomy will afford optimal vascular exposure and permit repair using standard techniques. In most cases, this resolution will involve direct suture repair using fine monofilament suture (Fig. 57.4A). In those unusual cases in which extensive disruption of the arterial or venous wall occurs, more elaborate reconstructive tehniques may be required, such as debridement and patch angioplasty (Fig. 57.4B) or segmental resection with end-to-end anastamosis or interposition grafting (Fig. 57.4C,D). Should the latter technique be required, autogenous grafting using the greater saphenous vein or, less commonly, the hypogastric artery should be employed if the reconstruction is being performed in a contaminated field.

The iliac vessels are at risk both during cannulation and during pelvic dissection. Acute compromise of the common or external iliac arteries in the absence of pre-existing atherosclerotic disease typically leads to severe limb ischemia; prompt and accurate repair of such injuries, using anatomic or extra-anatomic techniques, is essential. In contrast, prolonged attempts to salvage an injured hypogastric artery may not be justified, particularly if the contralateral internal iliac artery is intact or if proctosigmoidectomy has been performed. In such cases ligation can usually be performed without sequelae. Similarly, although repair of iliac venous injuries is preferable, if circumstances dictate, ligation is well tolerated. Swelling can be anticipated following iliac vein ligation, and the use of compression stockings can be helpful.

Injury to the superior mesenteric vessels, vulnerable during mobilization and resection of the transverse colon, can have devastating consequences (Fig. 57.1B). This portion of the procedure may be particularly difficult when the transverse colon is foreshortened by malignant or inflammatory disease. Should injury to either the superior mesenteric artery or vein occur, precise repair with preservation of patency is imperative to prevent extensive mesenteric infarction. In contrast to spontaneous mesenteric venous thrombosis, thrombectomy should be attempted in iatrogenic superior mesenteric vein thrombosis in an attempt to restore venous patency.

References

1. Clagett GP, Anderson FA, Geerts W, et al. Prevention of venous thromboembolism. Chest 1998;114(suppl):531–560.
2. Collins R, Scrimgeour A, Yusuf S, et al. Reduction in fatal pulmonary embolism and venous thrombosis by perioperative administration of subcutaneous heparin. N Engl J Med 1988;318:1162–1173.
3. Reymond MA, Christen Y, Morel P, et al. Pneumoperitoneum-related circulatory changes of the lower extremities. In: Rosenthal RJ, Friedman RL, Phillips EH (eds) The Pathophysiology of Pneumoperitoneum. Berlin: Springer-Verlag, 1998:28–41.
4. Kockerling F, Schneider C, Reymond MA, et al. Early results of a prospective multicenter study on 500 consecutive cases of laparoscopic colorectal surgery. Laparoscopic Colorectal Surgery Study Group (LGSSG). Surg Endosc 1998;12:37–41.
5. Society of American Gastrointestinal Endoscopic Surgeons. Global statement on deep venous thrombosis prophylaxis during laparoscopic surgery. Surg Endosc 1999;13:200.
6. Christen Y, Reymond MA, Vogel JJ, et al. Hemodynamic effects of intermittent compression of the lower limbs during laparoscopic cholecystectomy. Am J Surg 1995;170:395–398.
7. Schwenk W, Bohm B, Junghans T, et al. Intermittent sequential compression of the lower limbs prevents venous stasis in laparoscopic and conventional colorectal surgery. Dis Colon Rectum 1997;40:1956–1962.
8. Ishizaki Y, Bandai Y, Shimomura K, et al. Changes in splanchic blood flow and cardiovascular effects following peritoneal insufflation of carbon dioxide. Surg Endosc 1993;7:420–423.
9. Richmond BK, Lucente FC, Boland JP. Laparoscopy-associated mesenteric vascular events: description of an evolving clinical syndrome. J Laparoendosc Adv Surg Tech A 1997;7:363–367.
10. Lowham AS, Filipi CJ, Tomonaga T. Pneumoperitoneum-related complications: diagnosis and treatment. In: Rosenthal RJ, Friedman RL, Phillips EH (eds) The Pathophysiology of Pneumoperitoneum. Berlin: Springer-Verlag, 1998:28–41.
11. Nezhat F, Brill AI, Nezhat CH, et al. Laparoscopic appraisal of the anatomic relationship of the umbilicus to the aortic bifurcation. J Am Assoc Gynecol Laparosc 1998;5:135–140.
12. Hurd WW, Bude RO, DeLancey JOL, et al. Abdominal wall characterization with magnetic resonance imaging and computed tomography: the effect of obesity on the laparoscopic approach. J Reprod Med 1991;36:373–376.
13. Hurd WW, Burd RO, DeLancey, et al. The relationship of the umbilicus to the aortic bifurcation: implications for laparoscopic technique. Obstet Gynecol 1992;80:48–51.
14. Usai H, Sayad P, Hayek N, et al. Major vascular injuries during laparoscopic cholecystectomy: an institutional experience with 2589 procedures and literature review. Surg Endosc 1998;12:960–962.
15. Hanney RM, Alle KM, Cregan PC. Major vascular injury and laparoscopy. Aust NZ J Surg 1995;65:533–535.
16. Seville LE, Woods MS. Laparoscopy and major retroperitoneal vascular injuries (MRVI). Surg Endosc 1995;9:1096–1100.
17. Hasson HM. A modified instrument: method for laparoscopy. Am J Obstet Gynecol 1971;110:886–887.
18. Witz M, Lehman JM. Major vascular injury during laparoscopy. Br J Surg 1997;84:800.
19. McKernan JB, Champion JK. Access techniques: Veress needle-initial blind trocar insertion versus open laparo-

scopy with the Hasson trocar. Endosc Surg Allied Technol 1995;3:35–38.

20. Sigman HH, Fried GM, Garzon J, et al. Risks of blind versus open approach to celiotomy for laparoscopic surgery. Surg Laparosc Endosc 1993;3:296–299.

21. Bonjer HJ, Hazebroek EJ, Kazmier G, et al. Open versus closed establishment of pneumoperitoneum in laparoscopic surgery. Br J Surg 1997;84:599;602.

22. Berens ES, Herde JR. Laparoscopic vascular surgery: four case reports. J Vasc Surg 1995;22:73–79.

Section VII
Diagnostic Laparoscopy and Acute Abdomen

Steve Eubanks, MD
Section Editor

58
Principles of Diagnostic Laparoscopy

Ross L. McMahon

In 1901 Kelling, a surgeon from Dresden, performed the first successful laparoscopy in a dog[1-4] before the Seventy-third Congress of German Naturalists and Physicians. He anesthetized an area of the abdominal wall and introduced a puncture needle through which room air (filtered by sterile cotton) was injected into the peritoneal cavity to produce a pneumoperitoneum. He then introduced a larger trocar and introduced a Nitze cystoscope through it. Through a second trocar site, he inserted a probe to manipulate the contents of the abdominal cavity. A more detailed report was to follow but was never published.[4]

Later, in 1910, Jacobaeus described the technique in humans afflicted with ascites. After experimenting on 20 cadavers with a trocar he invented, he performed laparoscopy on 17 patients with ascites and thoracoscopy on 2 patients with empyema. He did not introduce air through a separate needle, as did Kelling, instead insufflating air through the original trocar.[4] He advocated the technique as an "early" diagnostic tool for malignancy.[3,5]

The first laparoscopy in the United States was performed in 1911 by Bertram Bernheim, a surgeon at Johns Hopkins. He was apparently unaware of the work of Kelling and Jacobaeus. He utilized a 0.5-in.-diameter proctoscope through a epigastric incision. No pneumoperitoneum was used; however, he reported visualizing stomach, gallbladder, liver, and peritoneum.[4]

The first large-scale series of diagnostic laparoscopy in humans was presented in the United States in 1920 by Orndoff. He described 42 cases of "peritoneoscopy" in the *Journal of Radiology*.[4] He described the then novel pyramidal trocar blade and utilized fluoroscopy to decrease visceral injury during trocar insertion. In 1928, Kalk and Bruhl[3,6] described one of the first large-scale reports of laparoscopy. Ruddock, in 1937, demonstrated the efficacy and safety of diagnostic laparoscopy with a report of 500 patients without a single mortality.[1,7] Since the founding work of these and other pioneers, diagnostic laparoscopy has slowly evolved into an invaluable

tool for the diagnosis of intra-abdominal and pelvic disease.

Diagnostic laparoscopy has been in the armamentarium of the gynecological surgeon for many years. Recognized more than 30 years ago by gynecologists as a useful technique for evaluating pelvic pathology, diagnostic laparoscopy now is one of the most frequently performed gynecological procedures. However, diagnostic laparoscopy has only recently been embraced by the general surgeon. Before the laparoscopic cholecystectomy, which caused a revolution in general surgery, few general surgeons utilized the technique. Increasingly, general surgeons are using laparoscopic techniques for the diagnosis of a wide range of abdominal diseases. The application of the laparoscopic technique to the treatment of many of these diseases has accelerated the use of laparoscopy as a diagnostic tool.

The use of laparoscopy in the diagnosis of abdominal diseases has rapidly expanded over the last few years. Surgeons are now expanding the role of the laparoscope to include preoperative staging of a wide range of cancers, posttreatment or second-look laparoscopy for numerous malignancies, liver disease, and ascites. The number of treatment options available through the laparoscope are also increasing rapidly.

Indications

The indications for laparoscopy are numerous and still expanding. However, there are several widely accepted indications for diagnostic laparoscopy, which are described here and listed in Table 58.1.[8]

Acute Right Lower Quadrant Abdominal Pain

Although not traditionally considered an indication for laparoscopy, the increasing use of laparoscopic appen-

TABLE 58.1. Current indications for diagnostic laparoscopy.

1. Acute right lower quadrant pain
2. Chronic abdominal/pelvic pain
3. Infertility
4. Evaluation of an abdominal mass
5. Liver disease
6. Liver tumors
7. Ascites
8. Tumor staging
9. Second-look posttreatment evaluation

dectomy has liberalized the laparoscopic evaluation of right lower quadrant pain. Laparoscopy helps diagnose the problem and, in most instances, the treatment can be carried out using the laparoscopic technique. The situation of the female with right lower quadrant (RLQ) pain is especially well suited to differentiation and treatment through the laparoscope. The wide differential diagnosis and high negative appendectomy rate have led many to adopt diagnostic appendectomy in virtually all females with RLQ pain who would otherwise undergo appendectomy.

Chronic Abdominal or Pelvic pain

One of the most frustrating problems in gastrointestinal and gynecological medicine for both patient and physician is chronic abdominal pain. In some cases, a barrage of tests leaves both physician and patient with no understanding of the etiology. Admittedly, a large number of these patients will ultimately not have any identifiable organic disease; however, when all noninvasive tests have failed to detect any disease process, diagnostic laparoscopy should be considered as a final step to rule out organic disease. In one prospective study by Wood and Cuschieri, 30% of patients with unexplained abdominal pain had significant pathology, including unsuspected malignancy. This topic is further explored in Chapter 63.

Liver Disease

Diagnostic laparoscopy with laparoscopic biopsy is indicated for cirrhotic patients when a standard biopsy is not diagnostic or is undesirable (e.g., small liver, large-volume ascites).[8,9] Patients with advanced liver disease may be more prone to hemorrhage following biopsy. However, during laparoscopy, directed hemostasis can be applied to any bleeding biopsy site using electrocautery or other hemostatic technique.

Liver Tumors

Evaluation of primary or secondary hepatic malignancies may be improved with laparoscopy[8,10,11] as 80% to 90%

of these lesions are at the surface of the liver and two-thirds of the liver's surface can be visualized with the laparoscope. Laparoscopic biopsy is particularly helpful when hepatic neoplasm is suspected and blind percutaneous biopsy is negative. When surgical resection is a therapeutic option, laparoscopy may reveal small (less than 2 cm) satellite lesions that might not be detected using other modalities.

Ascites

When the etiology of ascites remains elusive, laparoscopy may prove helpful, especially when the ascites are secondary to tuberculosis or carcinomatosis.[8]

Infertility

A standard part of the workup for infertility has included diagnostic laparoscopy. The fimbria, tubes, uterus, and ovaries can be evaluated and the presence of scarring or other abnormalities that might increase infertility documented. This examination is usually combined with chromotubation, often using indigo-carmine dye to assess patency of the fallopian tubes. The failure of dye to pass freely may indicate intratubal pathology, which may contribute to a patient's inability to conceive.[12]

Tumor Staging

Laparoscopy can be useful in helping to stage several malignancies, including lymphoma, pancreatic,[8,13] gastric, and esophageal cancer.[8,14] A thorough discussion of laparoscopy for malignancy is addressed in Chapter 63.

Second Look: Posttreatment

Several authors have espoused the utility of laparoscopy to detect occult disease posttreatment with chemotherapy or radiotherapy.[8] This added information has allowed clinicians to alter a patient's treatment protocol in attempts to eradicate the residual disease.

Palpable Mass

The presence of an abdominal mass that cannot be adequately characterized by noninvasive and semi-invasive methods (e.g., US, CT, MRI, flexible endoscopy) may be readily visualized and identified by diagnostic laparoscopy and biopsy.[8] Not only can the diagnosis with histology be made using this technique, but the true extent, including involvement of adjacent structures, of the mass can also be established.

Miscellaneous

Other indications in which laparoscopy may prove useful include fever of unknown origin, critically ill patients with suspected abdominal pathology, obscure gastrointestinal bleeding, trauma, and second look after reconstruction/resection for mesenteric ischemia.[8]

Contraindications

Contraindications, both relative and absolute, are described here and listed in Table 58.2.[8]

Absolute Contraindications

Known Ruptured Diaphragm[8]

Patient with known ruptured diaphragm should not undergo pneumoperitoneum.[8] Insufflation of the abdomen of patients with diaphragmatic ruptures may lead to tension pneumothorax and consequent hemodynamic and respiratory deterioration. These adverse effects can be eliminated by utilizing alternatives to pneumoperitoneum.

Hemodynamic Instability[8]

A patient who is so severely sick or injured that hemodynamic reserves are exhausted should not undergo laparoscopy to find the source of the problem. The added hemodynamic changes induced by pneumoperitoneum along with the increased delay invoked by laparoscopy are unacceptable in a hemodynamically compromised patient.[8] Few treatment options are viable through the laparoscope in a patient this ill. An expeditious laparotomy and correction of the problem should be performed without delay.

Relative Contraindications

Mechanical or Paralytic Ileus

A patient with highly distended air- or air/fluid-filled loops of bowel should probably not undergo laparoscopy

TABLE 58.2. Contraindications to diagnostic laparoscopy.

Absolute	Relative
Known diaphragmatic hernia	Mechanical or paralytic ileus
Hemodynamic instability	Uncorrected coagulopathy
	Generalized peritonitis
	Severe cardiopulmonary disease
	Large hiatus hernia
	Irreducible external hernia
	Abdominal wall infection

because the risk of perforating bowel is markedly increased.[8] If such a patient required laparoscopy, the Hasson technique could be considered, using great care. Also, the intra-abdominal pressure, already elevated by the distended bowel, should be carefully monitored to avoid abdominal compartment syndrome during evaluation.

Uncorrected Coagulopathy

If coagulopathies can be corrected, laparoscopy can be performed with little risk of bleeding. However, uncorrected coagulopathies increase the risk of bleeding,[8] and as a result the success rate of laparoscopy is lowered and the complication rate increased. Clinical judgment must prevail on a case-by-case basis.

Generalized Peritonitis

Generalized peritonitis is usually an indication for a laparotomy,[8] and many consider laparoscopy as unnecessary and time-consuming foreplay. However, in certain instances, the cause of generalized peritonitis (e.g., perforated duodenal or gastric ulcer) can be dealt with laparoscopically. Again, clinical judgment and insight as to the surgeon's abilities are required.

Severe Cardiopulmonary Disease

Patients suffering from severe cardiac disease should receive a careful workup before undergoing laparoscopy.[8] Stable angina is not a contraindication, but close communication with the anesthesiologist regarding intraoperative hemodynamic changes is important. Severe obstructive lung disease may lead to hypercarbia from the CO_2 pneumoperitoneum, and a resultant acidosis may develop. There are many alternatives to CO_2 pneumoperitoneum that should be considered in patients at risk of severe hypercarbia.

Large Hiatal Hernia

Large hiatal hernias can cause a pneumomediastinum upon induction of pneumoperitoneum.[8] The determination of the size of hiatus hernia where this poses a danger to the patient has yet to be determined scientifically. Removal of the hernia sac during repair of paraesophageal and large hiatal hernias may result in the appearance of pneumomediastinum on postoperative chest x-ray.

Abdominal Wall Infection

Abdominal wall infection is considered by the Society of American Gastrointestinal Endoscopic Surgeons (SAGES) as a relative contraindication for laparoscopy.[8]

Some of the concerns include dissemination of infection, induction of bacteremia, decreased oxygenation of the affected tissue secondary to increased intra-abdominal pressure, and CO_2 diffusion.

Instruments

The instrumentation of diagnostic laparoscopy does not vary much from the instrumentation required for any laparoscopic procedure. A 0° laparoscope may be sufficient for most examinations; however, the surgeon should have a 30° or even a 45° scope on hand should visualization be problematic. A standard light source, fiberoptic cable, and insufflator, all commonly used for laparoscopic cholecystectomies, will suffice. The table should be adjustable for both the headup and headdown position. Side-to-side adjustment is also very helpful, as is a method of securing the patient to the table. A standard 10-mm trocar, disposable or reusable, for the laparoscope is essential as is at least one 5-mm trocar or smaller. Instruments such as a blunt probe, suction-irrigation, a traumatic graspers, as well as a good pair of laparoscopic scissors should be readily available (Fig. 58.1). Mini-laparoscopic instrumentation may be used, which is discussed in another chapter. Clip appliers, stapler, and needle driver should also be available. A uterine manipulator, such as the Hulka tenaculum, is very useful if the patient has been placed in the lithotomy position. A coagulation device is also required.

Differential Diagnosis

The differential diagnosis of a patient undergoing a diagnostic laparoscopy depends on the indication for the laparoscopy. However, the most common findings in a patient with acute abdominal pain are appendicitis, pelvic inflammatory disease, ruptured ovarian cyst, adnexal torsion, and ectopic pregnancy. Many of these diagnoses can be inferred or suspected on the bases of preoperative history, physical examination, and laboratory or radiologic investigations.

Approach to Diagnostic Laparoscopy

After induction of general anesthesia, the patient can be placed either flat or in a modified lithotomy position. The former position is preferred for male patients and when the diagnosis is very unlikely to be of pelvic origin whereas the latter is preferred in a female patient when the diagnosis is less clear. The bladder should be emptied. A pelvic examination in the female is advisable. A tenaculum such as the Hulka tenaculum is also a very useful and easily applied instrument.

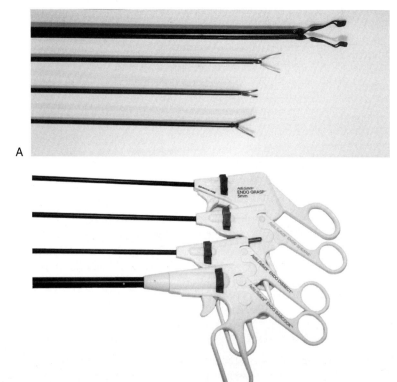

A

B

FIGURE 58.1. Selection of instruments for use during diagnostic laparoscopy. A. Graspers and Babcock clamp. B. Disposable grasper handles. (Courtesy of United States Surgical, Norwalk, CT, USA.)

Port Site Placement

The umbilicus is usually chosen for the site of a Veress needle insertion and ultimately laparoscope location because it represents the thinnest accessible portion of the anterior abdominal wall, whereby the deeper tissue planes are tethered to the layers above. Variations of insertion technique at this position have been described.[15] If potential complications (e.g., adhesions) are thought to exist, alternative sites for Veress needle insertion include a position 2 to 3 cm below the midpoint or the left costal margin or the left ninth intercostal space. From these positions, both a gas-distended stomach and an enlarged spleen can be hazardous. Insertion of the Veress needle in the left lower quadrant and at the supraumbilical point has also been described (Fig. 58.2).

Port site placement will vary somewhat with the indications for laparoscopy; however, a few generalizations can be made. In most circumstances, an umbilical port (usually 10 mm) is used for the scope. If the diagnosis is not obvious, a second port to allow manipulation of the intrabdominal organs is required.

If RLQ pain is the indication, a second port should be considered, either in the midline just above the symphysis pubis or in the left lower quadrant (LLQ); this allows good manipulation of the bowel, appendix, and pelvic organs. If the patient is in stirrups and a tenaculum is placed on the cervix, then excellent visualization of the lower abdomen and pelvis can be expected.

If upper abdominal pain is the presenting problem, then a left upper quadrant port with possible addition of an epigastric port should be considered to allow manipulation of the upper abdominal organs.

Operator Placement

Alignment of the surgeon's visual axis and hands should focus on the area of interest. The surgeon should be placed opposite the area being exposed and work across the midline of the abdomen. If the RLQ is being explored for possible appendicitis, then the surgeon should be standing on the patient's left side. If the LUQ is being explored, the surgeon should be on the patient's right. Conversely, the assistant (in most instances) is best suited on the opposite side to the surgeon. Monitors should be placed directly in front of both surgeon and assistant to aid in keeping the visual/hand alignment.

Procedure

If the pelvic organs are to be assessed, it is strongly encouraged to place the patient in the modified lithotomy position. A complete pelvic exam can be performed under general anesthesia. A tenaculum can be placed on the cervix. The 10-mm trocar should be placed in the sub-

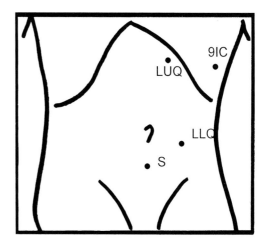

FIGURE 58.2. Alternate sites for Veress needle insertion: left upper quadrant (LUQ); 9th intercostal space (9IC); suprapubic (S); left lower quadrant (LLQ).

umbilical position. A Hasson technique is becoming the preferred method; however, the Veress technique is still acceptable. A CO_2 pneumoperitoneum of approximately 12 mmHg should be achieved. A 0° or 30° laparoscope should be placed in the abdominal cavity. A thorough examination of the upper and lower abdomen should be carried out in a systematic fashion. If this does not reveal the diagnosis, a 5-mm trocar or minilaparoscopy port can be placed in the lower abdomen. The midline suprapubic position is an excellent choice. An instrument to move the bowel, pelvic organs, and appendix around is necessary; this can be accomplished by using a blunt probe, a nontraumatic grasper, or a Babcock clamp. The pelvis and lower abdomen should then be carefully explored in a systematic fashion.

All adhesions should be carefully taken down to expose the area of interest; this should be done in nonvascular tissue planes and bleeding should be kept to an absolute minimum as blood may severely limit visualization and thus the ability to complete the diagnostic evaluation. A routine order of areas to be explored will ensure all areas are explored and none are missed. The tenaculum, if present, will aid in examining the pouch of Douglas and the tubes and ovaries. An example of a routine order for examination would be as follows: first, retrovert the uterus and examine the peritoneum of the anterior cul-de-sac for endometriosis. Anterior, then posterior uterine surfaces are then examined noting the size, shape, and color of the uterus. Next, the uterus is anteverted and the posterior cul-de-sac, uterosacral ligaments, and anterior sigmoid colon are examined, again noting any findings. The adnexa are then examined from left to right. Manipulation of the uterus during this step will aid in ovary exposure. Characteristics of the ovary in terms of size, color, and texture as well as the

TABLE 58.3. Differential diagnosis.

1. Acute right lower quadrant abdominal pain
   a. Appendicitis
   b. Pelvic inflammatory disease
   c. Ruptured ovarian cyst
   d. Adnexal torsion
   e. Ectopic pregnancy
2. Chronic pelvic pain
   a. Endometriosis
   b. Fitz–Hugh–Curtis syndrome
   c. Adhesions
   d. Malignancy

presence of any cysts should be noted. Attention is then directed at the appendix, right colon and finally the ileocecal valve and the terminal ileum. The order of this examination is variable depending on both surgeon and the patient's presenting symptoms; it is provided as an example only.

Specific Findings

The results of the diagnostic laparoscopy can be quite numerous and depend on the indications for the procedure. However, the most common scenarios are listed in Table 58.3. Broadly speaking, in the scenario of acute abdominal pain in the female, the results are likely to be one of the following: normal, appendicitis, pelvic inflammatory disease, ruptured ovarian cyst, or adnexal torsion. An ectopic pregnancy should be diagnosed preoperatively with a high β-hCG and an ultrasound that shows no fetus within the uterus.

Appendicitis

The specifics of treating acute appendicitis are discussed in Chapter 61. Briefly, in the majority of patients, the appendix can be safely removed using the laparoscope, which usually involves the addition of a second large-caliber trocar (10 or 12 mm) (Table 58.4). Both stapled and endoloop techniques have been described; the choice of operation depends on many factors such as surgeon preference, appendiceal thickness/condition, and cost.

Pelvic Inflammatory Disease

Pelvic inflammatory disease (PID) is confirmed by the presence of inflammatory exudates in the pelvis, erythemia of the fallopian tubes, and occasionally tubal abscess. It is wise at this point to obtain gynecological advice, but general principles hold: drainage, irrigation, and antibiotics.

Ruptured/Hemorrhagic Corpus Luteum Cyst

Evidence of a ruptured ovarian cyst includes the absence of other pathology, presence of fluid in the pelvis and cul-de-sac, and remnants of the cyst wall on the ovary. A hemorrhagic cyst will show evidence of hemorrhage on the ovary. It is important to ensure that a complete evaluation of the pelvis and abdomen has been done. When cyst pathology is the only finding, irrigation of the pelvis is all that is necessary.

Torted Adnexa

In some cases, the diagnosis of a torted ovary is not made preoperatively. Indeed, some cases of ovarian tortion mimic appendicitis. The presence of a ovary twisted on its mesentery is easily documented at laparoscopy. The options for treatment include simple detortion and oophorectomy. The decision on which option to perform depends on the degree of ischemia, presence of infarction, and the patient's wishes for future fertility.

Ectopic Pregnancy

In the unfortunate event of a patient at diagnostic laparoscopy without a preoperative diagnosis of ectopic pregnancy, the diagnosis can be made during laparoscopy. A tubal pregnancy often appears as a bulge in the tube with a bluish hue.[12] The choice of procedure (either salpingectomy or salpingostomy) should be based a number of factors: the patient's condition; the patient's desire to maintain fertility; the size of the ectopic pregnancy; the condition of the tube; and finally the skill of the surgeon. If at all possible, a gynecologist should be consulted.

Conversion

Reasons to convert to an open procedure are varied and too numerous to list here. However, the basic logic behind the decision to convert can indeed be explained. The basic premise in converting to an open procedure is

TABLE 58.4. Approach based on operative findings.

Operative findings	Approach
Acute appendicitis	Add additional trocars: total 3 (1, 10-mm; 1, 12-mm; 1, 5-mm)
Evidence of ruptured ovarian cyst	Irrigation and closure
Adnexal torsion	Gynecology consult—detortion ± oopherectomy
Ruptured ectopic pregnancy	Gynecology consult— ±salpingotomy
Pelvic inflammatory disease	Irrigation, ensure adequate drainage, postoperative antibiotics

TABLE 58.5. Indications for conversion to open procedure.

1. Complication not amenable to laparoscopic control/repair
   a. Massive bleeding
   b. Complex enterotomies
   c. Cystotomy
   d. Ureter injury
   e. Other organ injury that cannot be assessed adequately

2. Lack of visualization
   a. Bloody field
   b. Anatomic details unclear
   c. Retraction problems
   d. Exposure difficulties

3. Instrumentation problems
   a. Obese patient presenting trocar and instrument length
      problems
   b. Instrument angle

that one cannot perform the necessary procedure laparoscopically. Although that may seem basic and an oversimplification, this premise is often overlooked or unappreciated. A list of factors affecting the decision to convert can be found in Table 58.5. The reason that a procedure cannot be finished laparoscopically is often a result of one of several factors: visualization, instrumentation, or complication.

A lack of visualization, or unclear anatomy, is one of the most frequent reasons for conversion to an open procedure. Visualization can often be enhanced by the addition of a scope of 30°, 45°, or greater degree. The ability to expose the area of interest to complete the exam is paramount. Several techniques have been advocated to improve laparoscopic exposure including tilting the table headup, or headdown, and lateral angulations. Having the patient in stirrups with a tenaculum attached to the cervix will facilitate visualization of the pelvis; this allows mobilization of the uterus and can be very helpful in improving visualization of pelvic structures. However, the anatomy can still be difficult to identify and, depending on the patient's symptoms and the surgeon's judgment, this is an indication to convert to an open procedure.

Instrumentation can also be a limiting factor during laparoscopic surgery. Instrument problems include exposure problems, inability to reach the area of concern (due to instrument length, patient girth, or instrument angle), and inability to perform the function needed. Addition of ports and advanced instrumentation alleviates some of these problems, but if one is unable to perform the necessary procedure with the instruments available, an indication for conversion to open exists.

Complications leading to conversion to an open procedure include any complications that cannot be handled in a safe fashion laparoscopically, of course depending on the surgeon's abilities. Well-accepted indications for conversion to an open procedure are massive bleeding, complex enterotomies, or inability to fully determine the nature of the complication.

The three broad categories leading one to convert the laparoscopic procedure to an open one overlap and rarely exist in isolation, nor do these factors occur in isolation from the surgeon. The abilities and judgment of the surgeon play a key role. It is paramount to remember that the decision to convert a laparoscopic procedure to an open one is not a failure but rather sound surgical judgment.

Complications

Complications of laparoscopy are described here and listed in Table 58.6. Complications can be broadly defined as general (often caused by any operation or anesthesia) or specific (caused by the nature of the procedure itself). Specific complications can be further grouped by when they are encountered during the operation. Complications can be encountered during many stages of the operation: during insertion of the Veress needle; upon obtaining access for Hasson trocar; during trocar insertion; during the performance of the procedure itself; or as a result of the pneumoperitoneum. The rates of vascular and visceral injury in several large studies of Veress

TABLE 58.6. Complications of diagnostic laparoscopy.

Technique	Study	Year	Number of laparoscopies	Vascular injury	Visceral injury	Rate per 1000 cases
Veress	Loffer and Pent[16]	1975	32,719	NR	22	0.67
	Mintz[17]	1977	99,204	30 Veress	5 Veress	0.35
				18 trocar	26 trocar	0.44
	Bergqvist[18]	1987	75,035	4 Veress	NR	0.07
				1 trocar		
	Querleu et al.[19]	1993	17,521	4	7	0.63
Hasson	Hasson[20]	1980	200	0	0	0
	Lafullarde[21]	1999	803	0	0	0

NR, not reported.

needle, trocar insertion, and Hasson insertion are listed in Table 58.6 and discussed here.

Veress Needle Insertion

During Veress needle insertion, damage to vessels may occur. A report of more than 99,000 laparoscopies in 1977 by Mintz showed a rate of major vascular injury by the Veress needle alone of 0.3 in 1,000.[17] In contrast, Bergqvist and Bergqvist reported, in 1987, 4 vascular injuries secondary to Veress needle insertion in more than 75,000 laparoscopies, giving a rate of 0.07 in 1,000.[18] Querleu et al. reported a rate of vascular injury specifically due to the Veress needle of 0.2 per 1,000 with the only death in their study occurring secondary to major hemorrhage from a Veress needle insertion.[19]

The viscera that is most likely to be injured during Veress needle insertion is the small bowel. The incidence of bowel injury is suspected to be greater than that reported. Due to the small needle size and the proximity of any injury to the eventual camera site, these injuries may not be noticed intraoperatively. Indeed, because of the small size of the needle, some of these injuries may resolve without need for repair. Delay in recognition, however, increases the morbidity considerably. Loffer and Pent reported a rate of visceral perforation at 0.67 in 1000,[16] and Mintz reported a rate of perforations specifically associated with Veress needle insertion of 0.05 in 1000.[17] Querleu et al. quoted a rate of 0.4 per 1000 cases of visceral injury,[19] and roughly half of visceral injuries were diagnosed during the laparoscopic procedure.[17,19]

Trocar Injuries

Devastating complications of trocar (i.e., major vessel or visceral injury) should only occur with blind insertion either directly or after creation of pneumoperitoneum with a Veress needle. The rates of vessel injury directly related to trocar insertion were reported by Mintz at 0.18 per 1000, and Bergqvist and Bergqvist reported a rate of 0.01 per 1000. Bowel injuries are also a problem with trocar insertion. The rates of visceral injury caused specifically by the trocar were reported by Mintz at 0.26.

Nuzzo et al. reported that the highest rate of complications is associated with the insertion of the Veress needle and trocar.[22] They presented data from nine major studies of laparoscopic cholecystectomy between 1991 and 1996 involving more than 160,000 patients. They concluded that the 0.05% to 0.2% mortality rate was due to Veress needle or trocar insertion. At least half of the visceral injuries (0.1%–0.4% total) were also related to the Veress needle or trocar. Overall, the incidence of bowel

and vascular complications due to the Veress needle technique is between 0.63 and 0.8 per 1000.[17,19]

Hasson Insertion

Although considered by many surgeons as considerably more safe than Veress needle insertion, the Hasson technique, published by Hasson in 1971,[23] may also cause specific complications. Hasson described his method for open insertion of the trocar, thereby (1) guaranteeing pneumoperitoneum and (2) avoiding the dangers described of blind trocar insertion. By dissecting down to and suturing to the fascia, the peritoneum is exposed, and safe placement of a blunt trocar is facilitated. Perone confirmed the usefulness of this technique in 585 patients, of whom 173 (29.5%) had undergone previous abdominal surgery and, therefore, had the potential of viscera adjacent to the anterior abdominal wall.[24,25] No major complications (major vascular injury or bowel injury) were reported. Lafullarde et al. also reported their experience with the Hasson technique.[21] In 802 laparoscopies, they reported no major vascular or visceral injuries.

Procedural Injuries

Injuries during the procedure are varied and numerous. Injuries to the vascular, alimentary, and urinary systems are the most common and occur from a number of mechanisms: direct cut or puncture; thermal injury secondary to cautery; crush injury from graspers; and traction injuries. Injury to solid organs can also occur from similar mechanisms. Much attention has been placed on potential cautery injury, both primary and secondary from arcing or poor instrument insulation. However, according to Levy et al. many of the injuries formerly ascribed to cautery burn may be related to the insertion of trocars.[26]

Pneumoperitoneum Complications

Carbon dioxide (CO_2) is the gas most commonly used to establish pneumoperitoneum. Pneumoperitoneum with CO_2 induces several well-characterized physiological responses.

CO_2 Absorption

As the rate of absorption of CO_2 across the peritoneum overcomes the ability of the repiratory and the buffer systems to compensate, the patient's $PaCO_2$ rises; this is reflected in the end-tidal CO_2, which should be measured in every patient. In patients with limited repiratory reserve, the $PaCO_2$ may be measured directly with arterial blood gas measurements intraoperatively.

Arrhythmia

Up to 20% of patients experience cardiac arrhythmias from the CO_2 pneumoperitoneum.[27] The most common dysrhythmias are tachycardia, premature ventricular contraction, and bradycardia; most are transient and do not lead to clinical instability.

Cardiac Output

Stroke volume, and subsequently cardiac output, may be diminished by severe hypercarbia, particularly with high intrabdominal pressures or high altitudes. The high intrabdominal pressures may result from insufflator malfunction or incomplete muscular paralysis.

Hypotension is thought to result from a combination of myocardial depression from acidosis and decreased venous return secondary to vensous compression.

Gas Embolism

Carbon dioxide is a diffusible gas. As a result, when small amounts of CO_2 enter the bloodstream either from absorption from the peritoneal surface or from direct injection into the circulation, minimal physiological consequences result. However, when larger amounts of CO_2 enter the vasculature, a gas embolism syndrome and potential fatality result. Fortunately, the incidence of gas embolism during laparoscopy is rare, between 1 and 4 per 65,000 laparoscopies.[27] Unexplained hypotension, change in cardiac rhythm, new heart murmur, and increased endtidal CO_2 suggest CO_2 embolism. Hypoxia, pulmonary hypertension, and right ventricle obstruction may result, which may lead to right ventricular failure. Treatment consists of immediate release of pneumoperitoneum, positioning the patient in the headdown, left-sidedown position, aspirating the right ventricle through a central line, and increasing FiO_2 to 100%.

Pulmonary Complications

During laparoscopy, several respiratory changes result, most of which are caused by either the absorption of carbon dioxide or pressure from the pneumoperitoneum. Both functional residual capacity (FRC) and forced expiratory volume (FEV) decrease as much as 23%.[27] Atelectasis is present postlaparoscopy in as many as 50% of patients. Pressure and stretching of the diaphragm causing diaphragmatic dysfunction is now implicated as a possible cause.[27]

In the hand of the experienced laparoscopic surgeon, the complication rate and the mortality rate should be quite low. One review of more than 46,000 cases reported a mortality rate of 0.054%, which compares favorably with the mortality rate of other invasive interventions.

The application of laparoscopic technique has revolutionized the role of the laparoscope in general surgery and led to the rapid application of laparoscopic techniques to a wide range of general surgical problems. The result is that diagnostic laparoscopy is quickly replacing diagnostic laparotomy for many disease processes and patient presentations.

References

1. Berci G. Elective and emergent laparoscopy. World J Surg 1993;17(1):8–15.
2. Kelling G. Ueber Oesophagoskopie, Gastroskopie und Kolioskopie. Munch Med Wochenschr 1902;1:21–24.
3. Khaitan L, et al. Diagnostic laparoscopy outside of the operating room. Semin Laparosc Surg 1999;6(1):32–40.
4. Davis CJ, Filipi CJ. A history of endoscopic surgery. In: Arregui ME, et al. (eds) Principles of Laparoscopic Surgery: Basic and Advanced Techniques. New York: Spinger-Verlag, 1995.
5. Jacobaeus H. Uber die moglichkeit, die zystskopie bei untersuchung seroser hohlunger anzuwenden. Munch Med Wochenshcr 1910;57:2090–2092.
6. Kalk H, Bruhl W. Leitfaden der Laparoscopie und Gastroskopie. Stuttgart: Thieme, 1951:1–158.
7. Ruddock C. Peritoneoscopy. Surg Gynecol Obstet 1937;65:523.
8. Guidelines for diagnostic laparoscopy. Society of American Gastrointestinal Endoscopic Surgeons (SAGES). Surg Endosc 1993;7(4):367–368.
9. Bruguera M, et al. A comparison of the accuracy of peritoneoscopy and liver biopsy in the diangosis of cirrhosis. Gut 1974;15(10):799–800.
10. Brady PG, et al. A comparison of biopsy techniques in suspected focal liver disease. Gastrointest Endosc 1987;33(4):289–292.
11. Coupland GA, Townend DM, Martin CJ. Peritoneoscopy—use in assessment of intraabdominal malignancy. Surgery 1981;89(6):645–649.
12. Diamond MP. A Manual of Clinical Laparoscopy. New York: Parthenon, 1998.
13. Andren-Sandberg A, et al. Computed tomography and laparoscopy in the assessment of the patient with pancreatic cancer. J Am Coll Surg 1998;186(1):35–40.
14. Bogen GL, Mancino AT, Scott-Conner CE. Laparoscopy for staging and palliation of gastrointestinal malignancy. Surg Clin N Am 1996;76(3):557–569.
15. Toth A, Graf M. The center of the umbilicus as the Veress needle's entry site for laparoscopy. J Reprod Med 1984;29(2):126–128.
16. Loffer FD, Pent D. Indications, contraindications and complications of laparoscopy. Obstet Gynecol Surv 1975;30(7):407–427.
17. Mintz M. Risks and prophylaxis in laparoscopy: a survey of 100,000 cases. J Reprod Med 1977;18(5):269–272.
18. Bergqvist D, Bergqvist A. Vascular injuries during gynecologic surgery. Acta Obstet Gynecol Scand 1987;66(1):19–23.
19. Querleu D, et al. Complications of gynecologic laparoscopic surgery—a French multicenter collaborative study [letter]. N Engl J Med 1993;328(18):1355.

20. Hasson HM. Window for open laparoscopy [letter]. Am J Obstet Gynecol 1980;137(7):869–870.
21. Lafullarde T, Van Hee R, Gys T. A safe and simple method for routine open access in laparoscopic procedures. Surg Endosc 1999;13(8):769–772.
22. Nuzzo G, et al. Routine use of open technique in laparoscopic operations [see comments]. J Am Coll Surg 1997; 184(1):58–62.
23. Hasson HM. A modified instrument and method for laparoscopy. Am J Obstet Gynecol 1971;110(6):886–887.
24. Rosen DM, et al. Methods of creating pneumoperitoneum: a review of techniques and complications. Obstet Gynecol Surv 1998;53(3):167–174.
25. Perone N. Laparoscopy using a simplified open technique. A review of 585 cases. J Reprod Med 1992;37(11):921–924.
26. Levy BS, Soderstrom RM, Dail DH. Bowel injuries during laparoscopy. Gross anatomy and histology. J Reprod Med 1985;30(3):168–172.
27. Cooperman AM. Complications of laparoscopic surgery. In: Arregui ME, et al. (eds) Principles of Laparoscopic Surgery—Basic and Advanced Techniques. New York: Springer-Verlag, 1995.

59
Bedside Laparoscopy

Leena Khaitan

The first diagnostic laparoscopy (DL) was performed in 1901 by Kelling in the dog.[1] This technique was extended to humans by Jacobaeus in 1910 by inflating the abdominal cavity with air, permitting the evaluation of the abdominal cavity under direct visualization.[2] The first large-scale series of diagnostic laparoscopy in humans was presented in 1928 by Kalk and Bruhl.[3] Since that time, laparoscopic techniques have been applied to an increasing number of abdominal procedures. Laparoscopy has become another tool in the surgeon's armamentarium of diagnostic and therapeutic techniques.

Increasingly, surgeons are using laparoscopic techniques outside the operating room to help evaluate the patient with an unknown intraperitoneal process. Diagnostic laparoscopy has been used in the trauma bay, emergency room, intensive care unit, and even the office. Therapeutic laparoscopy is also becoming more commonplace in these settings as surgeons become more versatile with its use. In this chapter, laparoscopy is taken out of the operating room to the patient's bedside.

Indications for Bedside Laparoscopy

Bedside laparoscopy is a skill reserved primarily for diagnostic purposes. Currently, there are a variety of diagnostic techniques available to the surgeon that include ultrasound, computed tomography, MRI, diagnostic peritoneal lavage, and, ultimately, exploratory laparotomy. Although the radiographic techniques are noninvasive, they offer varying degrees of diagnostic efficacy. Additionally, it is quite difficult to transport the patient from the intensive care unit (ICU) to the radiology suite. The risks of endotracheal tube dislodgment, IV infiltration, and monitor dysfunction are common, as previously reported.[4] Outpatients may face difficulties in obtaining the necessary diagnostic studies. The studies can be troublesome to schedule due to lack of availability, limitations by the insurance company, or difficulty with transport.

DL provides a method to effectively evaluate the peritoneum under direct visualization with minimal associated morbidity and mortality in whatever setting the patient may present to the surgeon. DL can be used in most patients with an unknown intraperitoneal process. It is particularly helpful in very ill patients in whom the surgeon wishes to avoid a negative laparotomy or if a surgeon wishes to achieve the most accurate diagnosis with the least morbidity to the patient.

Bedside laparoscopy is applicable in many settings throughout the hospital. A patient may come to the emergency room with abdominal pain with a vague history. Diagnostic laparoscopy can be performed using small instruments under local anesthesia to determine possible causes for the pain. DL is especially useful in this setting when a young woman is evaluated for lower abdominal pain, as it may distinguish gynecological from nongynecological etiologies. It may provide more information than one would obtain from physical examination or computed tomography alone. In the trauma bay, the use of laparoscopy is controversial, and studies reflecting the efficacy of DL in the trauma setting are reviewed later in this chapter. One place where bedside laparoscopy has become markedly useful to the general surgeon is in the intensive care unit. DL can allow one to determine the presence of multiple intra-abdominal conditions. It can also allow one to avoid a negative laparotomy in these already critically ill patients. In the office, laparoscopy is used mostly by the gynecologists to evaluate pelvic disorders, as is discussed in another chapter. These indications are disucssed in more detail later (Table 59.1).

Contraindications to Diagnostic Laparoscopy

There are relatively few contraindications to DL. Awareness of existing contraindications allows avoidance of unnecessary patient harm. Relative contraindications

481

TABLE 59.1. Indications for bedside laparoscopy in the emergency room, the trauma bay, and the intensive care unit.

Abdominal pain of unknown etiology
Sepsis
Unexplained acidosis
Clinical, laboratory, or radiologic suspicion for an intra-abdominal
    process without a clear diagnosis
Confirming an intra-abdominal process
Fever and/or leukocytosis in an obtunded or sedated patient not
    explained by another identifiable problem such as pneumonia, line
    sepsis, urosepsis
Unexplained abdominal distension
Right lower quadrant pain in a young woman in the emergency room
Equivocal evidence of fascial penetration on local stab wound
    exploration
Questionably tangential gunshot wound and with potential fascial
    penetration

include: coagulopathy, previous abdominal surgery, morbid obesity, irreducible external hernia, cardiorespiratory insufficiency, lack of technical or staffing support, or a patient who is immediately postoperative. Also, one may not be able to technically perform the diagnostic laparoscopy in a patient with a tense, distended abdomen. None of these indications is absolute, so the clinician must use his own clinical accumen in determining the risks and benefits to the patient. Absolute contraindications remain subjective.

Preparation for Bedside Laparoscopy

One can easily be prepared to do bedside laparoscopy by stocking a cart with the following equipment and sterile drapes (Fig. 59.1). This cart can be kept in the intensive care unit (ICU) for ready availability, or in the emergency department, or if such a cart exists in the operating room, it should be a mobile unit that can be easily moved. Staff trained in the use of this equipment should be available at all times. In today's financial climate, this may not always be possible, so the surgeon should be familiar with setup and troubleshooting of the equipment.[5,6] Bedside laparoscopy provides the surgeon the versatility to take the procedure to the patient and to avoid the inconvenience or risks of transporting the patient.

Instrumentation

Diagnostic laparoscopy outside of the operating room requires few instruments. It is important for the surgeon to be familiar with these instruments and their availability. For safe DL, the basic instruments include a 0° or angled laparoscope, monitor, two trocars, manipulating instruments, a light source and cord, insufflator with appropriate tubing, and often a syringe or suction setup.

These instruments should be stored on one portable cart that can be easily accessed and transported to the location where it is needed (see Fig. 59.1).

More recently, minilaparoscopic instruments have become increasingly popular, especially in the office or trauma bay. These instruments are 1 to 2mm in size, fit through specialized miniports, and can even be placed under local anesthesia. An additional advantage of the mini-instruments is that the trocars can easily be repositioned multiple times with minimal morbidity to the patient (Fig. 59.2).

Telescope

The quality of the visual image is of utmost importance to the laproscopic surgeon. The Hopkin's rod lens system, which allows light to be transmitted through a series of glass rods with a series of lenses on the ends, has revolutionized the optics in laparoscopic surgery. These scopes are available in 0°, 30°, and 45° lenses. The 45° scope provides the most versatility as it allows one to see around corners and underneath structures. Diagnostic laparo-

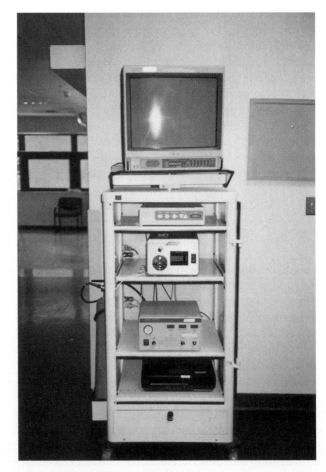

FIGURE 59.1. Portable laparoscopy cart with monitor, light source, insufflator, and sterile drapes.

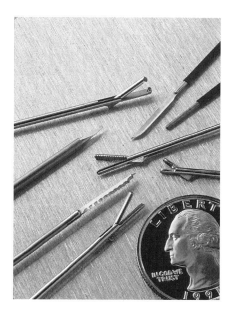

FIGURE 59.2. Microlaparoscopy instruments.

scopists must be familiar with its use and manipulation. A 0° scope is sufficient to provide the surgeon with adequate information pertaining to further care of the patient.

In addition to having different angles, the scopes now come in different sizes. The most commonly used scope is the 10-mm scope; 5-mm and 2-mm scopes are available that provide an image that is similar but not equal to that of a 10-mm scope. Smaller instruments allow for less anesthesia and less discomfort to the patient. As optics move toward digitalization, the images from the smaller scopes will improve. The gallbladder pictured in Figure 59.3 is seen through a 2-mm scope. Note see that the resolution is quite clear.

Camera

The camera is as important as the telescope. Three-chip cameras are recommended, although a single-chip camera can be used at the loss of significant resolution. The cameras are designed to fit with the different size scopes. The cameras are also improving in resolution as digital technology advances.

Monitor

The monitor screen allows a two-dimensional projection of the image so that all who are involved in the procedure can see what the surgeon is seeing. The monitor is the third piece in the image circuit following the scope and camera. All three components must provide adequate resolution so the surgeon can effectively operate under clear visualization. The monitors come in different sizes

and with different resolutions. The screen must be at least 10 in. in diameter so that it can be observed comfortably from a distance of 3 to 4 feet. A high-resolution monitor is preferred to make the image as accurate as possible. The quality of the picture on the screen is important, particularly when assessing patients for intestinal ischemia. A slight aberrance in the quality or coloring of the picture can lead to a misdiagnosis. In Figure 59.3, a gangrenous gallbladder is pictured as seen on a high-resolution screen through a 2-mm scope. If one altered the coloring of the picture, or if the resolution of the monitor was poor, the surgeon might have difficulty interpreting the picture on the screen. Additionally, the monitor allows for teaching and can be used to videotape the case or capture still photos for documentation on the chart.

There are headsets available that allow three-dimensional visualization of the peritoneum. This technology is in its infancy, remains expensive, and has not yet been popularized. Also, visualization of the procedure is limited to those who are wearing the special headsets designed to provide a three-dimensional picture.

Trocars

For DL, generally only two trocars are required. One 2-, 5-, 10-, or 12-mm port is used for introduction of the scope, depending on its diameter. Another 2- or 5-mm trocar is used as a blunt-tipped manipulating instrument.

Light Source

Traditionally, a bright light source such as a xenon 300-V light is necessary to transmit light through the camera to provide adequate visualization in the abdomen. One must also have a light cord to connect the source to the scope.

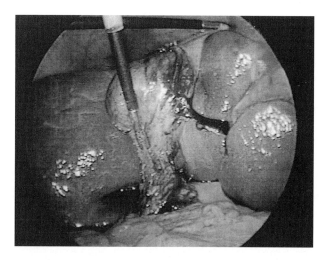

FIGURE 59.3. Gangrenous gallbladder as seen through a 2-mm scope.

Insufflator

One can use the Veress needle (in the virgin abdomen) or the Hasson trocar (surgeon's preference, or in patients who have undergone previous surgery) to provide access to the abdominal cavity for peritoneal insufflation. CO_2 insufflation is the gas of choice for DL. Virtually any system can be used to obtain a intra-abdominal pressure of 12 to 15 mmHg. However, lower pressures of 8 to 10 mmHg are better tolerated by patients who are awake during the procedure and usually provides adequate visualization.

Laparoscopic Instruments

A limited number of laparoscopic instruments are desirabe but not all are necessary; these can be 5-mm or 2-mm instruments. The instruments one might need include blunt-tipped, atraumatic grasping forceps, blunt probes, biopsy forceps, "peanuts" or Kittners, and biopsy needles. It also may be helpful to have an instrument for suction, In general, instrumentation that is disposable may be easier to maintain and stock.

Anesthesia

General or local anesthesia can be used. In critically ill patients, general anesthesia may consist of only a benzodiazapine (midazolam) and a shor-acting paralytic (cis-atracurum, diprivan). Less insufflation combined with local anesthesia can be used in patients with a contraindication to general anesthesia or if the procedure is being performed as an outpatient.

"Is an anesthesiologist needed to perform this procedure?" In most cases, no. In the intensive care unit, medications can be administered by the ICU team, especially for the patient who is intubated and even paralyzed. Procedures that would be performed in the office, emergency department, or trauma bay are usually be done under local anesthesia.[6-8] If the patient receives conscious sedation along with local anesthesia, monitoring is recommended. Depending on the depth of sedation, an anesthesiologist may be needed if deemed necessary by the surgeon performing the procedure.

Laparoscopic Technique

The preferred initial entry site into the penitoneal cavity is the umbilicus. The Veress needle or Hasson technique can be used, depending on the history of previous surgery or the preference of the surgeon.

Once the abdomen is insufflated, the scope is inserted. Inspection of the abdomen is carried out in an orderly fashion. All four quadrants are inspected to look for any gross abnormalities. The presence of fluid is sought in the pelvis and in the right and left paracolic gutters. If fluid is found, it is aspirated and sent for Gram stain and culture. A second trocar is ideally placed below the right costal margin (or in an area free of intrapenitoneal adhesions) under direct visualization lateral to the rectus sheath for careful manipulation of intra-abdominal structures.

It is helpful if the patient bed used for the procedure can be placed in Trendelenburg or reverse Trendelenburg and rotated from side to side to use gravity so one can easily see all organs; this can be difficult in the outpatient setting where the beds are not as mobile. The ICU beds usually have Trendelenburg and reverse Trendelenburg capabilities. If the patient is awake, the surgeon can ask the patient to move from side to side to further visualize the right and left paracolic gutters.

It does not matter where in the abdomen one begins exploration as long as inspection is done systematically. One of the most common causes of intra-abdominal pathology in the intensive care patient is acalculous cholecystitis.[9] The gallbladder should be carefully inspected and lifted by placing a blunt instrument under the gallbladder or gingerly grasping it with atraumatic graspers so as not to injure the organ; this allows some tactile sense to determine if the gallbladder is distended or edematous. Additionally, one should inspect the liver, a portion of the duodenum, and the stomach.

Next, the right lower quadrant, the appendix, and the cecum are visualized. It is sometimes helpful to rotate the patient to the left to more adequately view these structures. The patient can then be flattened and placed in Trendelenburg position to view the pelvic structures. If one is evaluating the pelvis, it is helpful for the patient to have an empty bladder, especially at the time of trocar placement, which can be achieved by having the patient void prior to the procedure or by placing a Foley catheter. The camera is slowly moved around the peritoneal cavity to allow thorough inspection of all quadrants. The small bowel, colon, spleen, and stomach should be visualized. If necessary to run the small bowel, a third trocar is placed. The ileocecal valve is identified and the small bowel is inspected carefully by progressing proximally to the ligament of Treitz. Using this technique, the retroperitoneal structures cannot be inspected completely; one should keep this in mind.

At the end of the procedure, the abdomen should be completely desufflated to minimize postoperative shoulder pain. The trocars are removed, and the scope site and any incisions greater than 5 mm should be closed at the level of the fascia. The skin can be approximated using staples or sutures.

Laparoscopy in the Trauma Patient

The use of diagnostic lapascopy in the trauma population is controversial. Concern regarding the use of laparoscopy in trauma revolves around the equipment costs, availability, setup time, and potential complications of pneumoperitoneum including gas embolus and pneumothorax. Initially, laparoscopy required general anesthesia and the use of an operating room. With the advent of minilaparoscopic instruments, this procedure can be performed in the trauma bay under local anesthesia by a skilled operator. Thus, the procedure is not much more invasive than a diagnostic peritoneal lavage.[10]

Diagnostic peritoneal lavage (DPL) is the gold standard diagnostic modality for intra-abdominal trauma, although computed tomography (CI) scan and ultrasound are becoming increasingly popular. DPL is limited, however, because it is nonspecific and cannot identify the type of injury or degree of injury to organs. The indications for diagnostic laparoscopy in trauma are similar to the indications for a DPL, including Glasgow Coma score of 13 or less neurological deficit, equivocal abdominal examination, unexplained episodic hypotension (systolic BP < 90), factors precluding reliable and timely follow-up examination, or equivocal fascial penetrance in penetrating trauma.[11] A nontherapeutic laparotomy rate as high as 20% has been reported following a positive DPL.[12,13] If a patient has a positive DPL, laparoscopy can be used as an adjunct to define the injury as one that is minor and can be managed nonoperatively versus one that requires exploratory laparotomy. Thus, the number of nontherapeutic laparotomies can be reduced. The same holds true for the patient who has positive or equivocal findings on a CT. Laparoscopy can detect a diaphragmatic injury that would not be seen on CT scan or by DPL.[14] One may be able to identify a hollow viscus injury that may not have been clearly recognized on CT or by DPL. The utility of DL applies to both blunt and penetrating trauma. A word of caution: one must recognize the limitations of laparoscopy in evaluating the retroperitoneum. Another diagnostic modality is necessary to evaluate this space. Computed abdominal and pelvic tomogram is the gold standard.

DL is helpful but cannot replace laparotomy in the trauma situation. However, it may aid in identifying those patients who have positive findings on CT, ultrasound (US), or DPL but can be spared a nontherapeutic laparotomy. Gazzaniga et al. published a series of 37 trauma patients who underwent emergency diagnostic laparoscopy. Nontherapeutic laparotomy was avoided in 10 (42%) of 24 patients with blunt trauma.[15] In a prospective analysis of 182 diagnostic laparoscopies performed in hemodynamically stable trauma patients with equivocal abdominal exams, negative laparotomies were avoided in a large group of patients with stab wounds, gunshot wounds, and blunt trauma on the basis of laparoscopic findings.[16] A large retrospective multicenter series on the use of laparoscopy in penetrating trauma reported avoidance of laparotomy in 54.3% of patients based on laparoscopic findings; 26 patients also had therapeutic procedures performed laparoscopically. The avoidance of laparotomy in a patient may lead to a quicker recovery.[17]

Laparoscopy in the Emergency Room

Diagnostic laparoscopy can be helpful in the emergency room setting for a young woman with right lower quadrant pain, to rule out appendicitis in an equivocal exam, to rule out intestinal ischemia, and sometimes to evaluate an acute abdomen. This procedure can be diagnostic and therapeutic.

A limiting factor in the use of DL in the emergency department is that DL can be performed only by surgeons, and a surgeon is not always available in the emergency department. The quality of the equipment and the experience of the operator can vary greatly. Ultimately, exploratory laparotomy remains the gold standard.

The literature on the use of laparoscopy for the outpatient with the acute abdomen is sparse. One interesting paper worthy of note reviews the use of laparoscopy in the pregnant patient with an acute abdomen at a single institution. Laparoscopy identified 34 patients with symptomatic biliary disease, 5 with appendicitis, and the rest with bowel obstruction or pelvic mass. Twenty-three patients required surgical intervention during their pregnancy, of which 15 were done laparoscopically. Women were operated during all trimesters with no morbidity.[18] DL can also be helpful in the nonpregnant patient in diagnosing appendicitis versus a gynecological process.

Laparoscopy in the Intensive Care Unit

The critically ill patient can be a diagnostic challenge to the surgeon when called upon to rule out an intra-abdominal process. Intra-abdominal complications in the critically ill are not very common, but when they do occur, they are associated with high morbidity and mortality. There are very few reports describing the use of diagnostic laparoscopy in this population. Those who have used DL in the ICU have found it to be very useful in terms of high diagnostic value with minimal morbidity. Often these are patients with multisystem organ failure, and little help is provided by history and physical examination. Open exploration provides high risk with unknown gain to the patient. The scenario is often the following: A patient is admitted to the intensive care unit after coronary artery bypass grafting or myocardial infarction with a rocky hospital course. Then, the patient develops fever of unknown origin, abdominal distension of unknown etiology, or unexplained acidosis. They

TABLE 59.2. Differential diagnosis of abdominal process in critically ill patients necessitating diagnostic laparoscopy.

Acalculous/calculous cholecystitis
Gangrenous bowel
Bowel/mesenteric ischemia
Perforate diverticulitis
Perforated peptic ulcer
Other perforated viscus
Acute appendicitis
Pancreatitis
Bowel obstruction
Intra-abdominal hemorrhage

appear to have slight abdominal tenderness on physical exam; however, due to sedation or their illness, they are depressed neurologically and are unable to provide one with a reliable exam. The differential diagnosis includes cholecystitis, appendicitis, and intestinal ischemia (Table 59.2). The key to helping these patients who are so critically ill is to make the diagnosis of an intra-abdominal process as early as possible in its course. In the ICU population, there is usually a delay in the decision to operate for several reasons, including reluctance to operate in the abscence of a definite diagnosis, fear of the harmful physiological effects of a negative laparotomy, unrealistic faith in antimicrobial therapy, and a delay in carrying out special diagnostic investigations.[19] DL provides one with a minimally invasive way to accurately and quickly diagnose or rule out an intra-abdominal process. Because DL is minimally invasive, it allows one to avoid all delays and proceed with treating the patient in a timely fashion.

A thorough review of the literature reveals very little published experience with diagnostic laparoscopy in critically ill patients. The groups that have evaluated DL in critically ill patients have found it to be a useful diagnostic technique which the patients tolerated well.

Brandt et al. have presented two studies on this topic. One reviews 9 trauma patients who are in the ICU setting and are suspected of having acalculous cholecystitis. Four patients had positive studies, and 5 patients had negative studies, which spared them a nontherapeutic laparotomy.[20] In the study of medical/surgical patients in the ICU, 25 patients underwent DL with 12 positive and 13 negative laparoscopic explorations. In this study, laparoscopic findings led to a change in management in 9 patients, earlier exploration in 4 patients, and avoidance of laparotomy in 5 patients. DL led to a change in therapy 40% of the time.[21] Bender and Talamini also evaluated the role of DL in ICU patients, noting that DL provided a surgeon the ability to accurately make a diagnosis without any unnecessary diagnostic delays.[22] The results of these studies are presented in Table 59.3.[20-23] Another article regarding the use of laparoscopy in the intensive care unit compares DL with diagnostic peritoneal lavage. The overall result was that causative findings were made apparent by DL in 5 of 12 patients.[24]

Thus, DL can be useful in diagnosing intra-abdominal processes in critically ill patients. However, one must realize the limitations of this diagnostic modality. The benefits of DL are that a definitive diagnosis can be established at the bedside and that some patients are spared a nontherapeutic laparotomy and its associated sequelae.

Laparoscopy in the Office

In the office setting, laparoscopy is currently primarily performed by gynecologists. The procedure is usually performed using minilaparoscopic instruments under local anesthesia. Patients tolerate the procedure well, and, in cases of undiagnosed abdominal pain, the patient can direct the surgeon to the point of maximal pain or tenderness.[6,25] Office DL has been described as useful in evaluating patients for carcinomatosis, endometriosis, chronic pelvic pain, and ovarian cancer. Some groups have shown this to be very helpful in diagnosis of various pelvic processes outside the operating room setting. Office-based sterilization has become commonplace. Schnepper reported 810 sterilizations attempted in the office under local anesthesia with 808 successes. The only complication was wound infection in 3 patients.[26]

Another application of office laparoscopy is to diagnose and potentially treat chronic pelvic pain. Twenty-two women underwent microlaparoscopy under local anesthesia with successful diagnosis in all patients. Patients were able to direct the surgeon to the location

TABLE 59.3. Review of Reports in Literature to Date on Diagnostic Laparoscopy in the ICU.

Author	Number of patients	Age (years)	Positive laparoscopy	Operative time (min)	Change in clinical management
Brandt et al. (1994)[20]	9		4		5 (55%)
Brandt et al. (1993)[21]	25		12	51	9 (36%)
Bender et al. (1992)[22]	7	64.3	5		2 (29%)
Forde et al. (1992)[23]	10		4		6 (60%)

of the pain because they were awake during the procedure. Nine of 14 patients with endometriosis had fulguration of their lesions in the office, and 7 of 8 patients with pelvic adhesions underwent adhesiolysis in the offices.[6,7] Additionally, office laparoscopy for pelvic pain has been shown to have an 80% reduction in cost when compared with traditional laparoscopy.[25]

Runowicz described office laparoscopy as a screening tool for ovarian cancer with the adjunctive use of microultrasound to image the internal structures of the ovary. This method cannot be used to screen the population at large but can be useful as a secondary test in working up a patient suspected of having ovarian cancer.[27]

Comparison of Diagnostic Laparoscopy to Other Diagnostic Modalities

Brandt et al. retrospectively reviewed the accuracy of DL compared to CT scan, ultrasound, and MRI (Table 59.4). Not all patients had all the diagnostic studies. Results by DL were compared to findings at exploratory laparotomy or autopsy. Overall, DL is 96% sensitive, according to this review.[20] In Table 59.5, the advantages of DL are compared to the other diagnostic modalities.[28] The gold standard remains laparotomy, but because DL appears to be equally effective in a trained person's hands, the minimally invasive technique is the less morbid diagnostic test for the patient.

Walsh et al. prospectively compared DL to DPL in accuracy of diagnosis and time of procedure. In comparison to diagnostic peritoneal lavage, DL was superior in providing a diagnosis and defining the need for further exploration. Laparoscopy required an average of 19 min and DPL took 14 min. Therefore, in experienced hands, laparoscopy can provide an accurate diagnosis in a timely fashion.[24]

Potential Complications and Management

Bedside laparoscopy is a versatile and useful technique to diagnose intra-abdominal processes. However, there are several potential complications. Awareness of these complications will allow the surgeon to avoid these potential complications and recognize them if they should occur. First, on introduction of the Veress needle, one can injure the bowel, which may necessitate a laparotomy in a patient who may not have needed one; this can be avoided by using meticulous surgical technique with placement of the Veress needle and trocars. After the first trocar is placed, the others should be inserted under direct visualization. If a patient has had a prior procedure, one may wish to insert the first trocar in the lateral abdomen away from the incision. One may also utilize the Hasson technique of trocar placement. Thus, even the first trocar can be placed under direct visualization with minimal risk to intraperitoneal contents.

Another potential complication and disadvantage of bedside laparscopy is a missed lesion. Bedside laparoscopy is limited to pathology that can be identified by viewing surface anatomy alone. Therefore, retroperitoneal lesions or pathology in hidden loops of bowel may be missed. Inadequacy of equipment may also hinder one from effectively interpreting the condition of the bowel, resulting in a missed pathological condition. These potential complications can be avoided by being aware of the limitations of laparoscopy. If retroperitoneal pathology is suspected clinically, then laparoscopy may not be the best diagnostic approach. To avoid missed bowel conditions, one should have well-maintained equipment, the surgical skills to manipulate the bowel laparoscopically, the ability to rotate the bed to be able to inspect all quadrants thoroughly, and a 45° scope that allows one to see around all structures well. Despite all these precautions, one may

TABLE 59.4. Comparison of diagnostic laparoscopy with other techniques of diagnosing intrabdominal processes.

Study	Computed tomography	Ultrasound of the abdomen	Exploratory laparotomy	Diagnostic laparoscopy
Brandt et al. (1994)[19]	1 true −	2 true −	5 true −	5 true −
	1 true +	2 true +	4 true +	4 true +
	1 false −	1 false −		
	0 false +	2 false +		
Number of patients in study	3/9	7/9	9/9	9/9
Brandt et al. (1993)[20]	5 true −	5 true −	13 true −	0 true −
	3 true +	3 true +	12 true +	25 true +
	1 false −	2 false −		
	0 false +	1 false +		
Number of patients in study	9/25	11/25	25/25	25/25

TABLE 59.5. Different diagnostic modalities to evaluate the abdomen.

Investigations	Advantages	Disadvantages
Diagnostic peritoneal lavage	Inexpensive Easy to perform Expeditious Transportable Few complications Sensitivity >95% Determines character of fluid	Invasive Nonspecific Cannot identify type of injury Cannot identify severity of injury Not reliable for diphragm or retroperitoneal injuries High false-positive rate High nontherapeutic laparotomy rate
Computed tomography	Noninvasive Localizes site of injury Best for solid organ injuries Best for retroperitoneal injuries	Expensive Need skilled technician Time consuming Availability May miss bowel injuries
Ultrasonography	Noninvasive Easy to perform Expeditious Transportable	Less sensitive than CT Large learning curve Availability May miss bowel injuries Cannot localize injury Unreliable in obese patients
Diagnostic laparsocopy	Accurately localizes injury Demonstrates active bleeding Localizes source of bleeding Best for diaphragm injuries Can be therapeutic Decreases nontherapeutic laparotomies (about 25%)	Expensive Invasive Time consuming May miss retroperitoneal injuries May need anesthesia Gas embolism Tension pneumothorax if diaphragm injury present Difficult to quantify blood volume

Source: From Runowicz.[27]

still miss some pathology. In this instance, one must rely on clinical judgement and treat the patient appropriately.

Finally, the bowel or any other structure can be injured during this procedure. One must use good surgical technique and be able to recognize injury. At the end of the procedure, be sure to close all fascial defects that are greater than 5 mm. Otherwise, one may create a chronic ascites leak that may be difficult to contain.

Conclusion

When called upon to evaluate a critically ill patient, a patient with abdominal pain in the office, patients with equivocal abdominal findings in the emergency department, or patients suffering abdominal trauma, a surgeon must appropriately select from the diagnostic tools available to quickly and accurately evaluate the patient. Diagnostic laparoscopy provides a minimally invasive method to determine the presence of an intra-abdominal process effectively and accurately. The patient is subjected to minimal morbidity with a precise diagnosis in most cases.

As technology advances, imaging is improving, and 2-mm scopes have resolution approaching that of 10-mm scopes. Placing a minilaparoscope is similar to a needle biopsy through the abdominal wall. DL with the standard-size laparoscopic instruments currently available is minimally invasive when compared to the alternative of exploratory laparotomy. DL allows avoidance of multiple diagnostic tests that can be expensive, lack sensitivity, and are not therapeutic. Furthermore, this procedure can be performed at the bedside in the trauma bay, emergency department, intensive care unit, or office.

Another advantage of DL is that it is very cost effective. DL is performed efficiently provided one has the proper equipment and well-trained personnel. DL allows the avoidance of several less sensitive but more expensive radiologic tests. DL can be shown to be cost-effective when considering the ability to make a rapid and accurate diagnosis that allows early intervention while avoiding other diagnostic studies and unnecessary laparotomy. Additionally, it is well known that hospital stay after laparoscopy is often shorter than after laparotomy.

Unfortunately, there are also some disadvantages to this diagnostic modality, particularly in the intensive care unit. These patients are already very sick and often expected to have poor outcomes regardless of the intervention. Nontherapeutic laparotomies can be avoided in this population with DL. DL is accurate, but thus far has not been shown to improve the overall survival or outcome of these patients. Additionally, not all institutions have the resources available to evaluate the patient with DL. Furthermore, DL is an invasive procedure with inherent potentially serious complications.

In conclusion, laparoscopy can be used in several settings outside the operating room. The procedure is most often diagnostic and occasionally can be therapeutic. In the diagnostic capacity, laparoscopy can be very helpful when the findings are positive. One should always interpret negative findings with caution even though DL is quite specific. As laparoscopic instruments become smaller and technology more portable, these procedures may become increasingly applicable. Laparoscopy should be used whenever indicated with the expectation of having accurate results in a timely fashion.

References

1. Kelling G. Ueber oesophagoskopie, gastroskopie, und kolioslopie. Munch Med Wochenschr 1902;49:21.
2. Jacobaeus HC. Uber die moglichkeit, die zystskopie bei untersuchung seroser hohlunger anzuwenden. Munch Med Wochenschr 1910;57:2090–2092.
3. Kalk H, Bruhl W. Leitfaden der Laparoscopie und Gastroskopie. Stuttgart: Thieme, 1951:1–58.
4. Indeck M, Peterson S, Smith J, Brotman S. Risk, cost, and benefit of transporting ICU patients for special studies. J Trauma 1988;28(l):1020–1025.
5. Brooks DC. Bedside laparoscopy in the critically ill ICU patient. In: SAGES Course Hand Book. Society of American Gastrointestinal Endoscopic Surgeons. 1997:8–12.
6. Demco LA. Patient-assisted laparoscopy. J Am Assoc Gynecol Laparosc 1996;3(suppl 4):S8.
7. Almeida OD Jr, Val Gallas JM. Office microlaparoscopy under local anesthesia in the diagnosis and treatment of chronic pelvic pain. J Am Assoc Gynecol Laparosc 1998;5(4):407–410.
8. Hall TJ, Donaldson R, Brennan TG. The value of laparoscopy under local anaesthesia in 250 medical and surgical patients. Br J Surg 1980;67:751–753.
9. Brandt CP, Priebe PP, Jacobs DG. Value of laparoscopy in trauma ICU patients with suspected acute acalculous cholecystitis. Surg Endosc 1994;8(5):361–364; discussion 364–365.
10. Berci G. Elective and emergent laparoscopy. World J Surg 1993;17:8–15.
11. Salvino CK, Esposito TJ, Marshall WJ, et al. The role of diagnostic laparoscopy in the management of trauma patients: a proliminary assessment. J Trauma 1993;34(4):506–513.
12. Soderstrom CA, Du Pries RW, Cowley RA. Pitfalls of peritoneal lavage in blunt abdominal trauma. Surg Gynecol Obstet 1980;151:513.
13. Peterson SR, Sheldon GF. Morbidity of negative finding at laparotomy in abdominal trauma. Surg Gynecol Obstet 1979;148:23.
14. Leppaniemi AK, Elliot DC. The role of laparoscopy in blunt abdominal trauma. Ann Med 1996;28(6):483–489.
15. Gazzaniga AB, Stanton WW, Bartlett RH. Laparoscopy in the diagnosis of blunt and penetrating injuries to the abdomen, Am J Surg 1976;131:315–318.
16. Fabian TC, Croce MA, Stewart RM, et al. A prospective analysis of diagnostic laparoscopy in trauma. Ann Surg 1993;217:557–564.
17. Zantut LF, Ivatury RR, Smith RS, et al. Diagnostic and therapeutic laparoscopy for penetrating abdominal trauma: a multicenter experience. J Trauma Injury Infect Crit Care 1997;42(5):825–831.
18. Gurbuz AT, Peetz ME. The acute abdomen in the pregnant patient. Is there a role for laparoscopy? Surg Endosc 1997;11(2):98–102.
19. Nel CJC, Pretorius DJ, De Vaal JB. Re-operation for suspected intra-abdominal sepsis in the critically ill patient. South Afr J Surg 1986;24:60–62.
20. Brandt CP, Priebe PP, Jacobs DG. Potential of laparoscopy to reduce non-therapeutic trauma laparotomies. Am Surg 1994;60:416–420.
21. Brandt CP, Priebe PP, Eckhauser ML. Diagnostic laparoscopy in the intensive care patient. Avoiding the non-therapeutic laparotomy. Surg Endosc 1993;7:168–172.
22. Bender JS, Talamini MA. Diagnostic laparoscopy in critically ill intensive-care-unit patients. Surg Endosc 1992;6:302–304.
23. Forde KA, Treat MR. The role of peritoneoscopy (laparoscopy) in the evaluation of the acute abdomen in critically ill patients. Surg Endosc 1992;6:219–221.
24. Walsh RM, Popovich MJ, Hoadley J. Bedside diagnostic laparoscopy and peritoneal lavage in the intensive care unit. Surg Endosc 1998;12(12):1405–1409.
25. Palter SF, Olive DL. Utility, acceptance and cost-benefit analysis of office laparoscopy under local anesthesia for chronic pelvic pain. J Am Assoc Gynecol Laparosc 1995;2(suppl 4):S39–S40.
26. Schnepper FW. Office-based sterilization by open laparoscopy. J Am Assoc Gynecol Laparosc 1996;3(suppl 4):S45.
27. Runowicz CD. Office laparoscopy as a screening tool for early detection of ovarian cancer. J Cell Biochem (Suppl) 1995;23:238–242.
28. Memon MA, Fitzgibbons RJ Jr. The role of minimal access surgery in the acute abdomen. Surg Clin N Am 1997;77(6):1333–1353.

60
Diagnostic Laparoscopy for Pelvic Pain

Linda Fetko

Pelvic pain is a common presenting complaint of women, accounting for more than 25% of all gynecological office visits and more than 40% of all laparoscopic procedures.[1] Pelvic pain is traditionally thought of as either acute or chronic, with pain of more than 6 months duration defining chronic pelvic pain. In clinical practice, however, acute presentations or exacerbations of chronic pelvic pain are also common.

Acute pelvic pain, by its very nature, frequently demands prompt diagnosis and treatment. Laparoscopy is often ideally suited for both. Chronic pelvic pain demands thorough evaluation to arrive at a diagnosis and appropriate therapy; again, laparoscopy often is a useful adjunct.

Initial Evaluation of the Patient with Pelvic Pain

Initial evaluation of the patient with pelvic pain includes a detailed history, including gynecological and obstetrical histories, and physical examination. The physical examination should include a pelvic exam. Laboratory tests and radiologic studies should be added as indicated.

Immediate goals should be to determine the need for supportive measures, the presence or absence of pregnancy, and the most likely cause of the pain. If the patient is pregnant, it will be necessary to determine whether the pregnancy is intrauterine or ectopic and whether the source of the pain is the pregnancy or another cause.

History

Any history of pelvic pain should include a detailed history of the characteristics of the pain[2] and a complete gynecological and obstetrical history. The nature of the pain may be intermittent or constant, sharp or dull. A distended hollow viscus, such as from a ureteral or bowel obstruction, is often associated with intermittent pain of a colicky nature. Peritoneal irritation, as from appendicitis, pelvic inflammatory disease, or a ruptured ovarian cyst, often causes constant acute pain.

The severity of the pain should be assessed. Pain scales are helpful in assessing changes in severity over time. Sudden versus gradual onset can be an important diagnostic clue. Sudden onset or exacerbation of pain suggests rupture or perforation of a pelvic organ, whether fallopian tube, bowel, or ovarian cyst. Gradual onset suggests a more indolent etiology, such as infection associated with pelvic inflammatory disease. Duration and change over time may provide insight into the cause of the pain if matched with the natural history of the condition.

Relationship to menstrual cycle provides important diagnostic clues. Pain at midcycle may be due to ovulation and a ruptured ovarian cyst. Pain during menstruation may be caused by endometriosis or dysmenorrhea. Pain after amenorrhea may signal an early pregnancy complication.

Associated symptoms may also provide insight into the etiology of the pain. Symptoms such as nausea, vomiting, diarrhea, or anorexia may point to a gastrointestinal source. Urinary tract involvement may be signaled by frequency, urgency, and dysuria.

A gynecological and obstetrical history is crucial in identifying risk factors for certain conditions that may present with pelvic pain. A full gynecological history includes last menstrual period, an assessment of the regularity of menses, sexual activity including new sexual partners, and birth control method. Obstetrical history includes prior miscarriages or ectopic pregnancies, both of which increase the risk of recurrence.

Physical Examination

A general physical examination, including heart rate, blood pressure, orthostatics, and temperature, aids in determining the acuity of the condition as well as possible etiologies.

Abdominal examination should include inspection, auscultation, palpation, and percussion. Pelvic examination should be performed. Inspection of the external female genitalia includes the Bartholin's glands, hymen, and urethra. Introduction of a vaginal speculum allows visualization of the uterine cervix, assessment for infections of the lower genital tract, and collection of samples for wet prep, cultures, and Papanicolau smear. Bimanual examination should include an assessment of the uterine cervix for cervical motion tenderness; the uterus for size, shape, mobility, and tenderness; and the pelvis for palpable masses and tenderness.

Laboratory Studies

White blood cell count, hemoglobin/hematocrit, and human chorionic gonadotropin-β subunit (β-hCG) may be helpful in determining the presence of infection, hemorrhage, and pregnancy, respectively. Cervical cultures, wet prep, urinalysis, urine culture, blood cultures, erythrocyte sedimentation rate, and tumor markers may also be useful. A type and screen or cross-matching of blood may be indicated preoperatively.

Radiologic studies, such as pelvic and abdominal ultrasounds, CT, or MRI, may assist with the diagnosis or improve planning of operative approach.

General Considerations for Pelvic Laparoscopy

Laparoscopy devoted to the pelvis and pelvic organs differs somewhat from laparoscopy when upper abdominal disease is suspected. Preoperative preparation, entry into the abdomen, and trocar placement may require accommodation by the surgeon when pelvic, rather than abdominal, pathology is expected.

Preoperative Preparation

Before sterilely preparing the abdomen, shaving or clipping of the pubic hair may be desirable, especially if a suprapubic port is planned. Shaving or clipping is not usually necessary at the umbilicus. Surgical prep generally includes the vagina and external genitalia. Either in-and-out catheterization or continuous drainage of the bladder should be obtained, depending on the anticipated length of the surgical case.

Uterine manipulation is often desirable and may be facilitated by placing the patient in a modified lithotomy position with the thighs in the same plane as the abdomen, using adjustable stirrups. Uterine manipulation may then be obtained by applying one of several instruments currently available. A Hulka uterine manipulator is generally the standard choice, but in women who

may have an intrauterine pregnancy, a simple spongestick in the vagina is preferable. Numerous less traumatic alternative uterine manipulators are now available commercially and may be used instead of a Hulka manipulator.

Entry into the Peritoneal Cavity

Entry into the peritoneal cavity may be obtained through open laparoscopy, insufflation using a Veress needle, or direct trocar insertion. As the techniques of open laparoscopy are covered elsewhere in this volume, they are not addressed here.

As both Veress needle insertion and direct trocar insertion are essentially blind procedures, anatomic landmarks must be positively identified before insertion is performed. The umbilicus generally lies at the level of L4 and the aortic bifurcation, although in heavy women the umbilicus may be well caudal of this area. The sacral promontory may be easily palpated in thin women. The surgical table should remain horizontal during Veress needle and direct trocar insertion.

Veress needle insufflation is optimally performed in the periumbilical area because the fascia is nearest the skin surface at this point. A skin incision is made with the scalpel, and the Veress needle is pressed against the fascia. As the lower anterior abdominal wall is lifted, the Veress needle is inserted through the layers of the abdomen, directed in the midline toward the hollow of the sacrum, just below the sacral promontory. In thin women, approximately a 45° angle is appropriate; however, in progressively more obese women, the angle of insertion will gradually approach 90°.

Veress needle location within the peritoneal cavity may be confirmed by filling the needle hub with sterile saline, lifting the lower anterior abdominal wall, and observing the fall of the saline level. An alternative technique is to attach a syringe of sterile saline to the Veress hub, inject 2 to 3 ml saline into the peritoneal cavity, and then attempt to withdraw. The aspiration of the saline or the presence of urine, blood, or stool would indicate improper placement.

Insufflation with carbon dioxide (CO_2) is next performed. Observation of a filling pressure less than 15 mmHg, the presence of dullness over the liver on percussion of the abdominal wall, and symmetrical filling of the abdomen all indicate proper intraperitoneal placement. Improper placement between the fascia and peritoneum would be indicated by high filling pressures, asymmetry in the abdominal wall, and a lack of dullness over the liver. If these signs occur, a second Veress puncture can often be performed with success. After the desired pneumoperitoneum is obtained (generally between 2 and 3 liters), the Veress needle is removed. The trocar with its sleeve can then be inserted into the peritoneal cavity using the same angle and orientation as was used for Veress insertion.

Direct insertion of the trocar into the peritoneal cavity may also be performed, either with or without laparoscopic guidance. If direct insertion is to be performed without watching the advancement of the instrument through the layers of the anterior abdominal wall, the same angle of approach and orienting features should be used as for Veress needle insertion. Lifting upward on the lower anterior abdominal wall, either by hand or with towel clips, facilitates the opening of the potential space between the peritoneum and the pelvic organs. Once the trocar is in the peritoneal cavity, pneumoperitoneum is easily obtained.

Relative contraindications for Veress or direct trocar insertion include suspected pelvic adhesions, prior laparoscopy or laparotomy at the proposed site of entry, abdominal mass, and marked obesity. In these cases, open laparoscopy may be the safer choice.

Trocar Placement

For purely diagnostic pelvic laparoscopy, a suprapubic port is frequently the only additional port required. With the patient in Trendelenburg position, a point in the midline approximately 2 cm above the symphisis is incised transversely. The trocar may then be inserted into the abdomen under direct visualization. If difficulty with insertion is encountered, the trocar should be oriented either directly toward the uterus or into the camera trocar sleeve.

For cases in which operative laparoscopy is likely, ports in the right and left lower quadrants are useful. The side opposite that of the suspected pathology will allow greater maneuverability of the laparoscopic instruments. Care must be taken to avoid the inferior epigastric vessels, which course through this area.

Laparoscopy for Specific Causes of Pelvic Pain

Despite the best efforts of the clinician, the initial evaluation of the patient may not be diagnostic. Certain diagnostic dilemmas, such as pelvic inflammatory disease versus appendicitis or threatened abortion versus ectopic pregnancy, may elude definitive preoperative diagnosis. Fortunately, with the widespread availability of laparoscopy, such diagnoses may be definitively made with minimally invasive techniques. As diagnostic laparoscopy for appendicitis, intestinal disorders, and malignancy is covered in later chapters, the remainder of this chapter focuses on laparoscopy for gynecological causes of pelvic pain.

Ectopic Pregnancy

With both increasing use of assisted reproductive technologies and the increasing incidence of pelvic inflammatory disease, the incidence of ectopic pregnancy has increased more than fourfold over the past 20 years.[3] As undiagnosed and untreated ectopic pregnancies remain the leading cause of maternal death in the first trimester,[4] definitive diagnosis and treatment of this condition is critical.

Risk factors for ectopic pregnancy include prior ectopic pregnancy, history of tubal surgery including tubal ligation or tubal reanastomosis, use of assisted reproductive technologies, contraception with an intrauterine device, and history of pelvic inflammatory disease.

Pelvic (including endovaginal) ultrasound, in conjunction with highly sensitive assays for β-hCG, has become the primary modality for diagnosis of this potentially fatal condition. Endovaginal ultrasound is able to identify an intrauterine gestational sac as early as 35 days after the last menstrual period, when β-hCG levels reach approximately 1500 mIU/ml. Using serum levels of β-hCG in conjunction with ultrasound, patients presenting with pain and an early pregnancy can be determined to have a definite intrauterine pregnancy, a definite extrauterine (ectopic) pregnancy, a probable ectopic pregnancy, or be too early to determine.

It is important to mention that the simultaneous occurrence of an ectopic and an intrauterine pregnancy, once thought to occur in only 1:30,000 pregnancies,[5] is increasingly common due to assisted reproductive technologies and the increasing incidence of ectopic pregnancies. Heterotopic pregnancies now occur in 1 in 3889[6] to 1 in 6778[7] pregnancies. As a result, the presence of an intrauterine pregnancy does not preclude the simultaneous presence of an ectopic, extrauterine pregnancy.

For those patients in whom the diagnosis remains in doubt, diagnostic laparoscopy, either with or without concomitant dilation and curettage, should be considered. For patients with ectopic pregnancy, diagnosed either during or before laparoscopy, laparoscopy remains a hallmark of therapy. Although laparotomy may be preferable in cases of hemodynamic instability, the laparoscopic approach offers less adhesion formation, shorter hospitalizations, and shorter convalescence.[8]

Ectopic pregnancy is most often located in the fallopian tube and may be identified as a swollen, bluish, hyperemic segment of tube often accompanied by blood dripping from the ipsilateral fimbria and hemoperitoneum. The opposite tube should always be visualized laparoscopically, both for comparison and to evaluate for concurrent pathology.

For unruptured tubal pregnancies, especially those in the ampullary region of the tube, conservative treatment with linear salpingostomy may be performed laparoscopically. The tube is opened opposite the mesosalpinx over the area of distension. Scissors, point cautery, or hook cautery instruments work well for this task. The ectopic pregnancy may then be removed with hook cautery, forceps, or hydrodissection. Hemostasis is achieved through cautery. The pregnancy should then be removed from the abdomen using an endocatch bag, directly through the trocar sleeve, or via culdotomy.

For ruptured tubal pregnancies, or in cases of implantation in the isthmic region of the tube, salpingectomy may be the preferred approach. Salpingectomy may be distal, segmental, or total, depending on the location of the ectopic pregnancy, the degree of associated tissue damage, concurrent pathology, and the patient's wishes for future fertility. The tube may be isolated with monopolar cauterization, bipolar cauterization, or endoloops. The isolated segment is then excised with scissors, cautery, or a stapling device and removed from the abdomen.

Pelvic Inflammatory Disease

Pelvic inflammatory disease (PID) is an infection of the upper genital tract. The term encompasses salpingitis, oophoritis, parametritis, and even pelvic peritonitis. Sexually transmitted diseases such as those caused by *Neisseria gonorrheae* and *Chlamydia trachomatis* are the primary causative agents; however, the infection is often polymicrobial. PID occurs in 1% to 2% of young, sexually active women each year and accounts for 250,000 to 300,000 hospitalizations each year.[9] Women with multiple sexual partners are four to six times more likely to develop PID than monogamous women. Barrier contraceptives and oral contraceptives reduce the risk of acute PID.

Pain in the lower abdomen is the most common presenting symptom of acute PID and occurs in more than 90% of patients. A purulent vaginal discharge is present in 75% of patients with acute PID.[10] The triad of pelvic pain, fever, and leukocytosis is present in only 15% to 30%.[11]

Laparoscopy remains the gold standard for the diagnosis of pelvic inflammatory disease. Although most cases are diagnosed clinically, in cases of diagnostic dilemmas laparoscopy should be considered. Although laparoscopy may miss very early cases of PID, it is especially useful at excluding other diagnoses. In a study by Jacobson and Westrom of 814 women with clinically presumed acute PID, 65% had laparoscopic evidence of salpingitis, 23% had normal findings, and 12% had other pelvic pathology.[11]

The laparoscopic appearance of pus dripping from the inflamed fallopian tubes clinches the diagnosis. Findings may also include erythematous, indurated, edematous fallopian tubes, pockets of purulent material, or tuboovarian abscess. Aspirated fluid should be sent for culture. Pelvic adhesions are frequently present, and perihepatic adhesions (Fitz–Hugh–Curtis syndrome) may also be seen. Pelvic and abdominal irrigation with normal saline or lactated Ringer's to reduce colony count may be helpful. Treatment is by broad-spectrum antibiotics and should include all sexual partners.

Tuboovarian Abscess

Defined as an abscess with its wall composed of the fallopian tube and ovarian parenchyma, the tuboovarian abscess is a sequela of late or inadequately treated PID. Laparoscopy may be used to diagnose and drain unruptured tuboovarian abscesses. Henry-Suchet et al. reported a 90% cure rate in a series of 50 women whose tuboovarian abscesses were drained through the laparoscope.[12]

Rupture of a tuboovarian abscess may be life threatening. Pain, usually acute and severe, is the usual presenting complaint. Signs of generalized peritonitis are present, and a pelvic mass may be palpable. Although laparoscopy may be diagnostic, definitive therapy includes the removal of pus, abscess, uterus, tubes, and usually ovaries. Because of the acuity of the condition and the distortion of anatomy, laparotomy is the preferred approach.

Pelvic Tuberculosis

Pelvic tuberculosis is a rare disease in the United States but is a common cause of infertility and PID in other parts of the world. With the increasing incidence of tuberculosis and human immunodeficiency virus (HIV), as well as immigration from Asia, the Middle East, and South America, it is likely to become more common in the United States. *Mycobacterium tuberculosis* or *Mycobacterium bovis* are the causative agents, and venereal transmission has been reported although hematogenous spread from a pulmonary focus is more common.

The clinical presentation of pelvic tuberculosis is often confusing but may include pelvic pain or infertility or both. A doughy adnexal mass and ascites may also be present. Endometrial biopsy or dilation and curettage may be diagnostic, and hysterosalpingogram may be suggestive, but often the diagnosis requires visualization of the pelvis.

Laparoscopic findings of pelvic tuberculosis include widespread adhesions, miliary tubercles involving peritoneal surfaces, and matted adnexal masses.[13] Conclusive diagnosis requires a positive culture, which may be obtained laparoscopically. Because of the likelihood of extensive pelvic adhesions, trocar insertion must be performed with great care. Treatment is by various combinations of isoniazid, rifampin, streptomycin, ethambutol, and pyrazinamide. Surgical therapy is reserved for medication failure or noncompliance and consists of total abdominal hysterectomy and bilateral salpingo-oophorectomy.[14]

Ovarian Cysts and Adnexal Masses

Physiological ovarian cysts and other adnexal masses may occasionally present with pelvic pain. Bimanual exam is an essential element in diagnosis, and attempts should be made to characterize the mass in terms of location, size, consistency, shape, mobility, tenderness, bilaterality, and associated findings. Imaging studies such as ultrasonography, CT, and MRI are often useful in predicting malignancy. However, surgery may be necessary to determine the nature of the mass, and visualization with laparoscopy will frequently permit a diagnosis while avoiding the morbidity of laparotomy.

Established indications for surgical visualization of an adnexal mass include ovarian mass more than 6 cm in diameter, adnexal mass more than 10 cm in diameter, mass developing after menopause, failure to discover the nature of the mass with radiographic studies, or persistence of a presumed physiological cyst.

Laparoscopic management of adnexal masses and ovarian cysts requires attention to patient selection. The potential for malignancy must be considered and addressed at the time of laparoscopy to avoid a delay in diagnosis. If laparoscopic findings are at all suggestive of malignancy, the following steps should be performed:

1. Obtain peritoneal washings
2. Perform a thorough exploration of the abdomen
3. Perform a thorough exploration of the pelvis
4. Obtain intraoperative pathology consultation
5. Consider laparotomy[15]

The most common ovarian mass is the physiological ovarian cyst, which occurs after failure of follicular rupture or corpus luteum regression. Such cysts are usually smooth, mobile, cystic, and slightly tender to palpation. In general, physiological cysts regress spontaneously and may be managed conservatively with observation for two menstrual cycles. However, persistent cysts and those causing pain may require surgical management. Laparoscopy is often ideal for both confirmation of the diagnosis and therapy.

In the case of a benign ovarian cyst, laparoscopic ovarian cystectomy is often feasible. The ovary should first be stabilized with atraumatic forceps. An incision is then made through the thin ovarian cortex overlying the cyst wall. Endoshears or monopolar cautery may be used. The cyst is then shelled out of the ovarian parenchyma using sharp or blunt dissection, electrocautery, or hydrodissection as appropriate. Twisting the cyst wall may facilitate stripping the cyst from the normal ovarian tissue. Although every effort should be made to prevent spillage of cyst contents intraperitoneally, dissection and cyst removal may be aided by decompressing the cyst by evacuating its contents. In the case of a physiological cyst, this is easily accomplished by inserting a spinal needle through the abdominal wall into the cyst under laparoscopic visualization and aspirating cyst contents.

After hemostasis is obtained, the ovarian incision may be left open to heal by primary intention or may be reapproximated with sutures. The use of bipolar cautery to reapproximate the ovarian tissues has also been reported.

Adnexal Torsion

Torsion of the adnexa is an infrequent cause of pelvic pain, but it is the fifth most common gynecological surgical emergency.[15] The classic presentation is acute onset of abdominal pain with findings of adnexal mass and peritonitis. Adnexal torsion is uncommon in the setting of normal adnexa. However, when masses occur in the adnexa, as with hydrosalpinges or ovarian cysts, adnexal torsion increases in frequency. Adnexal torsion has also been reported in the setting of a tubal stump, as following tubal ligation or subtotal salpingectomy.

Adnexal torsion may be suspected with ultrasound findings of adnexal mass and decreased or absent flow on Doppler ultrasound examination. Definitive diagnosis may be made laparoscopically when the twisted adnexa is seen.

Despite earlier concerns regarding the release of venous thromboemboli, recent studies by Mage and colleagues,[16] as well as by Shalev and Peleg,[17] have confirmed the safety and utility of conservative management by untwisting the structure. Viability of the organ may be confirmed by observing color changes as blood flow returns. The underlying cause (usually an ovarian cyst) should then be treated. Routine oophoropexy is not recommended. If return of blood flow is not observed or in cases of recurrent torsion, oophorectomy may be performed laparoscopically.

Pelvic Adhesive Disease

Adhesions are among the most common findings noted at diagnostic laparoscopy for the evaluation of pelvic pain.[18] In a study by Kresch et al., adhesions were found in 89% of women undergoing laparoscopy for pelvic pain.[19] Adhesions may result from previous surgical procedures, pelvic inflammatory disease, ruptured cysts, postpartum infections, appendicitis, and endometriosis.

Nonsurgical diagnosis of pelvic adhesive disease remains elusive. Physical examination was shown to be a poor predictor of the presence and location of adhesions visualized during subsequent laparoscopy in a study by

Stovall et al.[20] Radiologic imaging studies are likewise unhelpful.

Laparoscopy may be very informative in the patient with pelvic adhesive disease and may allow more successful treatment than laparotomy. Sutton and MacDonald have reported 85% relief of chronic pelvic pain after laparoscopic adhesiolysis,[21] and Steege and Stout reported significant relief of pain in 67% of patients after laparoscopic lysis of adhesions.[22] After laparoscopic lysis of adhesions, the total adhesion score is reduced approximately 50%.[23]

Laparoscopic adhesiolysis may be performed by a number of surgical techniques. Blunt dissection may be performed with nearly any laparoscopic instrument by placing traction on the adhesion. Blunt dissection is most successful with filmy adhesions and should be abandoned if bleeding is encountered. Sharp dissection with scissors is useful for thick adhesive bands or adhesions involving bowel. Electrodissection with either unipolar or bipolar devices is useful for vascular adhesions but should be avoided in close proximity to bowel or ureters. Laser dissection can provide precise cutting and coagulation in a single step. Hydrodissection with hydraulic pressure can create cleavage planes quickly and safely. The surrounding tissue damage associated with these various modalities must be considered when selecting these techniques.[24]

Endometriosis

Endometriosis is the presence of implants of endometrial tissue outside the uterus. The ovaries, uterine ligaments, rectovaginal septum, parietal peritoneum, bowel serosa, and appendix are common places for implantation to occur. Endometriotic implants may appear as black, puckered lesions, red polypoid material, or clear vesicles. The classic black or blue "powder-burn" implant is a consequence of regression. Red polypoid lesions are thought to have the greatest metabolic activity. Endometriomas, with their characteristic chocolate-colored fluid, may also be present.

At laparoscopy, endometriosis was found in 41 of 126 (32.5%) of women with undiagnosed pelvic pain. It is widely accepted that there is no relationship between the extent or location of endometriotic lesions and the severity of pain; however, the depth of the lesion may be associated with pain. In particular, lesions greater than 1 cm in depth may be associated with severe discomfort.[25]

Laparoscopic assessment of the pelvis allows the definitive diagnosis of endometriosis to be made. Pain, infertility, and failure of medical management are indications for surgery. Biopsies, ablation of endometriotic implants, adhesiolysis, ovarian cystectomy, oophorectomy, and salpingectomy may all be accomplished through the laparoscopic approach. Laparotomy is most

valuable in cases of extensive, deep pelvic adhesions or large endometriomas.

At least two laparoscopic ports should be placed, even for purely diagnostic procedures, to permit mobilization of pelvic organs and allow a complete survey of the pelvis. Basic techniques for the laparoscopic ablation of endometriosis include excision, coagulation, and vaporization. Coagulation may be accomplished with monopolar or bipolar cautery, thermocoagulation, or laser. Deep lesions should be excised with a tissue margin of at least 2 to 4 mm; laparoscopic treatment of these lesions is often complicated by the proximity to vital structures, such as blood vessels or ureters.[26]

Venous Congestion

Pelvic venous congestion is a controversial cause of pelvic pain. Stimuli that increase intra-abdominal pressure, such as prolonged standing or lifting, are thought to exacerbate the pain, which is commonly described as dull and aching. Despite descriptions of pelvic vein varicosities dating back to Richet in 1857, the diversity and nonspecificity of symptoms and the difficulty establishing the diagnosis have contributed to a lack of consensus regarding this condition.

Laparoscopy is of limited use in establishing a positive diagnosis of pelvic venous congestion because the dilated veins are often not recognized because of their retroperitoneal position, increased abdominal pressure with pneumoperitoneum, and increased venous drainage with Trendelenburg positioning.[27] Venography remains the gold standard of diagnosis, and the value of laparoscopy lies in the association between a nondiagnostic laparoscopy and vascular congestion on venography. In a study by Beard et al., 91% of women with pelvic pain and no other pathology on laparoscopy had dilated veins in the broad ligament and ovarian plexus that were demonstrated on venography.[28]

Microlaparoscopy and Awake Laparoscopy

Along with the drive to improve laparoscopic technology there is a drive to reduce the invasiveness of surgical procedures, especially those performed primarily for diagnostic purposes. Microlaparoscopy, using instruments and trocars from 0.5 to 3 mm in diameter, provides fertile ground for the fusion of these two directions.

Microlaparoscopy allows for decreased discomfort to the patient, permitting procedures under conscious sedation and local anesthesia. One application is conscious pain mapping, which enables the patient to participate in the localization of painful foci.[29] With the ability to better correlate laparoscopic findings with the patient's experience of pain, our ability to diagnose the cause of pain and thereby tailor the treatment will likely improve.

Conclusion

Laparoscopy is now established as a useful, and sometimes essential, tool in the diagnosis and therapy of pelvic pain. The early use of laparoscopy for the evaluation of pelvic pain frequently leads to earlier diagnosis and definitive treatment using minimally invasive techniques.

References

1. Howard FM. The role of laparoscopy in the evaluation of chronic pelvic pain; promise and pitfall. Obstet Gynecol Surv 1993;48:117–118.
2. Porpora MG, Gomel V. The role of laparoscopy in the management of pelvic pain in women of reproductive age. Fertil Steril 1997;68:765–779.
3. Goldner TE, Lawson HW, Xia Z, Atrash HK. Surveillance for ectopic pregnancy—United States, 1970–1989. MMWR 1993;42:73–85.
4. Grimes DA. The morbidity and mortality of pregnancy: still risky business. Am J Obstet Gynecol 1995;170:1489–1494.
5. DeVoe RW, Pratt JH. Simultaneous intrauterine and extrauterine pregnancy. Am J Obstet Gynecol 1948;56:1119–1126.
6. Bello GV, Schonholz D, Moshirpur J, Jeng D-Y, Berkowitz RL. Combined pregnancy: the Mount Sinai experience. Obstet Gynecol Surv 1986;41:603–613.
7. Hann LE, Bachmann DM, McArdle C. Coexistent intrauterine and ectopic pregnancy: a reevaluation. Radiology 1984;152:151–154.
8. Zouves A, Urman B, Gomel V. Laparoscopic surgical treatment of tubal pregnancy. A safe, effective alternative to laparotomy. J Reprod Med 1992;37:205–209.
9. Droegemueller W. Infections of the upper genital tract. In: Mishell DR, Stenchever MA, Droegemueller W, et al. (eds) Comprehensive Gynecology. St. Louis: Mosby, 1997:662.
10. Martens MG. Pelvic inflammatory disease. In: Rock JA, Thompson JD (eds) Te Linde's Operative Gynecology, 8th Ed. Baltimore: Lippincott Williams & Wilkins, 1997:660.
11. Jacobson L, Westrom L. Objectivized diagnosis of acute pelvic inflammatory disease. Am J Obstet Gynecol 1969;105:1088.
12. Henry-Suchet, Soler A, Loffredo V. Laparoscopic treatment of tubo-ovarian abscesses. J Reprod Med 1984;29:579.
13. Sutherland AM. Laparoscopy in diagnosis of pelvic tuberculosis. Lancet 1979;2:95.
14. Martens MG. Pelvic inflammatory disease. In: Rock JA, Thompson JD (eds) Te Linde's Operative Gynecology, 8th Ed. Baltimore: Lippincott Williams & Wilkins, 1997:678–684.
15. Sanfilippo JS, Rock JA. Surgery for benign disease of the ovary. In: Rock JA, Thompson JD (eds) Te Linde's Operative Gynecology, 8th Ed. Philadelphia: Lippincott Williams & Wilkins, 1997:630–633.
16. Mage G, Canis M, Mandes H, et al. Laparoscopic management of adnexal torsion: a review of 35 cases. J Reprod Med 1989;34:520.
17. Shalev E, Peleg D. Laparoscopic treatment of adnexal torsion. Surg Obstet Gynecol 1993;176:448.
18. Stout AL, Steege JF, Dodson WC, et al. Relationship of laparoscopic findings to self-report of pelvic pain. Am J Obstet Gynecol 1991;164:73–79.
19. Kresch AJ, Seifer DB, Sachs LB, et al. Laparoscopy in the evaluation of pelvic pain. Obstet Gynecol 1973;64:672.
20. Stovall TG, Elder RF, Lind FW. Predictors of pelvic adhesions. J Reprod Med 1989;34:345.
21. Sutton C, MacDonald R. Laser laparoscopic adhesiolysis. J Gynecol Surg 1990;6:155.
22. Steege JF, Stout AL. Resolution of chronic pelvic pain after laparoscopic lysis of adhesions. Am J Obstet Gynecol 1991;165:278.
23. Operative Laparoscopy Study Group. Postoperative adhesion development after operative laparoscopy: evaluation at early second look procedures. Fertil Steril 1991;55:700.
24. Namnoum AB, Murphy AA. Diagnostic and operative laparoscopy. In: Rock JA, Thompson JD (eds) Te Linde's Operative Gynecology, 8th Ed. Lippincott Williams & Wilkins, 1997:401–402.
25. Koninckx PR, Mueleman C, Demeyere S, et al. Suggestive evidence that pelvic endometriosis is a progressive disease, whereas deeply infiltrating endometriosis is associated with pelvic pain. Fertil Steril 1991;55:759.
26. Hesla JS, Rock JA. Endometriosis. In: Rock JA, Thompson JD (eds) Te Linde's Operative Gynecology, 8th Ed. Baltimore: Lippincott Williams & Wilkins, 1997:599–602.
27. Metzger DA. Pelvic congestion. In: Steege JF, Metzger DA, Levy B (eds) Chronic Pelvic Pain: An Integrated Approach. Baltimore: Saunders Co., 1998:153.
28. Beard RW, Highman JH, Pearce S, Reginald PW. Diagnosis of pelvic varicosities in women with chronic pelvic pain. Lancet 1984;2:946.
29. Palter SF, Olive DL. Office microlaparoscopy under local anesthesia for chronic pelvic pain. J Am Assoc Gynecol Laparosc 1996;3:359–364.

61
Diagnostic Laparoscopy for Suspected Appendicitis

Aurora D. Pryor

Historical Perspective

The first clear description of a case of appendicitis was an autopsy by Heister in 1711, written in 1753. He described a small abscess next to a black appendix in an executed criminal. Amyand performed the first described appendectomy in 1735; however, it was not performed for appendicitis. He operated on an 11-year-old boy with a scrotal hernia and fecal fistula, stemming from a pin perforating the appendix.[1] The next reported case of appendicitis is from Mestivier, who in 1759 identified a pin in the appendix with gangrenous changes of the cecum at autopsy.

Descriptions of pathology in this region go back much further. The first written report of pus in the right lower quadrant, likely due to appendicitis, dates as far back as A.D. 30–39. At that time, Aretus described drainage of an abscess in this region. His patient survived. In 1812, Parkinson attributed a patient's death to appendiceal perforation. In 1827, Melier described appendiceal perforation due to the buildup of fecal matter, progressive dilation, rupture, and peritonitis. He also suggested that surgical intervention could treat the disease. However, Dupuytren was the most prominent surgeon at the time and he disagreed. He supported the prevalent theory that right lower quadrant inflammation, "typhlitis," was caused by cecal pathology, temporarily suppressing interest in the investigation of appendicitis. In the 1830s, Bright and Addison described the clinical presentation of appendicitis, with subsequent peritonitis and death or abscess formation and drainage. Williard Parker published a series of four appendiceal abscesses treated with operative drainage in 1867, making this an established procedure. However, it took until 1886 for Reginald Fitz to associate this condition with the appendix. He identified appendiceal perforation in the majority of patients with typhlitis studied at autopsy and suggested that surgery might be curative for this so-called appendicitis.[2]

It was during this time that the first appendectomy for a preoperative diagnosis of appendicitis was performed.

In 1889, McBurney published his classic description of the disease presentation, including pain at the point "between an inch and a half and two inches from the anterior spinous process of the ilium on a straight line drawn from that process to the umbilicus."[3] He went on, in 1894, to describe the now standard muscle-splitting incision for appendectomy.[4] Lewis McArthur, to whom McBurney actually conceded priority, concurrently described this approach. Rockey and Davis suggested a transverse skin incision in the early 1900s.[1] Operative management of appendicitis underwent little change over the next 100 years.

Laparoscopy was first described in the U.S. literature in 1911.[5] Until the last decade, the procedure was mostly limited to gynecology. The first laparoscopic appendectomy was described by Kurt Semm, a gynecologist, in 1982.[6] Since that time, the technique of laparoscopic appendectomy (LA) has become more accepted within general surgery. There have been many trials demonstrating the safety of the procedure, but its utility remains debated. Laparoscopy has also been considered as a diagnostic aid and has been used successfully to confirm the diagnosis of appendicitis.

Anatomy

The appendix is a blind tubelike extension of the cecum near the area of the ileocecal valve. It extends outward from the base of the taenia. The appendix ranges in length from approximately 5 to more than 20 cm. The blood supply comes from the ileocolic artery via the appendiceal artery. As in the remainder of the intestinal tract, the vasculature is located in a mesentery, named the mesoappendix. The appendiceal walls are filled with lymphatic tissue. The mucosa of the appendix contains

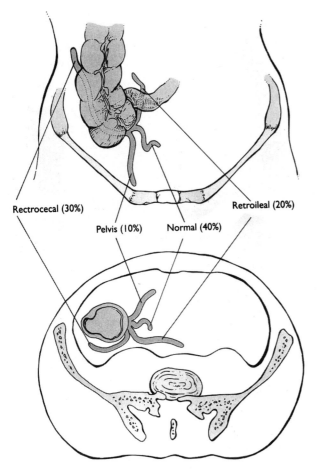

Rectrocecal (30%) Retroileal (20%)

Pelvis (10%) Normal (40%)

FIGURE 61.1. The variability of the appendiceal tip, with frequency in parentheses. (From DeMatos P, Ludwig KA. Laparoscopic appendectomy. In: Pappas TN, Chekan EG, Eubanks S (eds). Atlas of Laparoscopic Surgery, 2nd Ed. Philadelphia: Current Medicine, 1999:11.1–11.11.[8])

straight tubular glands, goblet cells, Paneth cells, and APUD cells. Absorptive cells are usually absent.[7]

The location of the appendix within the abdomen is variable. Figure 61.1 demonstrates the most common locations of the appendix and their relative frequencies.

Pathophysiology

Appendicitis is believed to begin with obstruction of the colonic orifice, with subsequent distention, followed by bacterial invasion of the wall leading to necrosis and eventually perforation. Foreign body, lymphatic proliferation, or tumor can cause obstruction of the appendiceal lumen. Typical foreign bodies can be ingested (seeds) or produced within the intestinal lumen (fecaliths). Lymphatic hyperplasia is most common in youths. Carcinoids and lymphomas are typical tumors leading to appendicitis. Within the obstructed appendix, mucosal cells con-

tinue to secrete fluid, causing the pressure to rise. When the intraluminal pressure exceeds venous pressure, venous stasis and ischemia result; this leads to mucosal ulceration and bacterial invasion. The infiltration of the wall with inflammatory cells leads to microabscess formation and arterial thrombosis. The wall becomes gangrenous and often perforates within 24 to 48h of the initial obstruction. Sequelae of appendicitis are related to perforation and include periappendiceal abscess, fistula, pylephlebitis, and hepatic abscess.[9]

Incidence

Appendicitis is the most frequent cause of abdominal emergency. Approximately 250,000 cases of appendicitis are treated in the United States each year. The highest incidence of appendicitis is in boys aged 10 to 19 years. Appendicitis is more common in men than women (1.4: 1) and in whites than nonwhites (1.5:1). The lifetime risk of appendicitis is 8.6% for males and 6.7% for females, but the risk of appendectomy is 12.0% for males and 23.1% for females, due to the higher rate of negative or incidental appendectomy in females (Fig. 61.2).[10]

Diagnosis

Clinical Presentation

The classic presentation of appendicitis begins with a history of gastrointestinal symptoms or discomfort for one to several hours before the actual onset of pain. Diarrhea or constipation may be present. Pain then usually begins as referred pain in the periumbilical region and shifts after several hours to the right iliac region once localized peritoneal irritation has progressed.

Nausea, vomiting, or anorexia typically develop after the onset of pain. If a patient is actually hungry, it can lead to doubt in the diagnosis. Tenderness over the area of the appendix, classically at McBurney's point, is usually progressive and may be absent early in the disease process. Tenderness on percussion, localized muscular rigidity, and hyperesthesia may also be present. A positive psoas sign, pain elicited during hip flexion against resistance, can also signify irritation in this area.

Over the course of the first 24h, low-grade fever usually develops, followed by a moderate leukocytosis. Tachycardia may also be an indication of peritoneal irritation. Gaseous distension from a reflex adynamic ileus, or referred pain in the testicle, may also occur.

The point of maximal tenderness is often over the area of McBurney's point, midway between the right anterior superior iliac spine and the umbilicus. However, if the appendix is not located in its usual intra-abdominal ori-

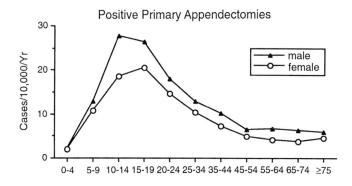

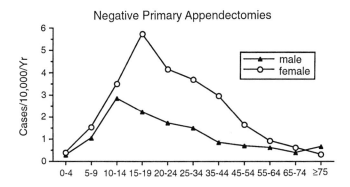

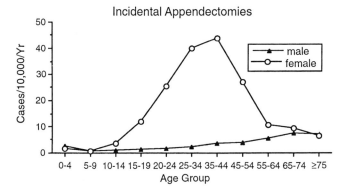

FIGURE 61.2. Annual incidence of appendectomy per 10,000 population in the United States, 1979–1984, divided by type of appendectomy, age, and sex. (From Addiss et al., with permission.[10])

Differential Diagnosis

There are many conditions that may mimic the presentation of acute appendicitis, and vice versa (Table 61.1). The presence or absence of systemic symptoms, which are more common with viral disease, can sometimes distinguish viral gastroenteritis. Bacterial gastrointestinal infection is usually associated with profound diarrhea. Rebound tenderness over the iliac region, or pain on slow deep palpation, can help differentiate appendicitis from pneumonia with abdominal symptoms. Chest x-ray and a careful chest examination are more definitive for the diagnosis of pneumonia. Acute hepatitis or diabetic ketoacidosis can also lead to confusing abdominal symptoms; these can be distinguished with appropriate laboratory data. One key feature of the history for a patient with possible appendicitis is previous abdominal surgery, particularly possible appendectomy.

Irritation or inflammation of the gallbladder, small intestine and kidney all can present like appendicitis. History, physical examination, and routine urinalysis should be carefully reviewed to exclude these alternatives. Rectus muscle hematomas usually present with a sudden onset following exertion. Bowel obstruction leads to abdominal distension early in the disease process. Diverticulitis may present similarly to appendicitis, but the pain usually localizes to the left iliac fossa.

Disease of the female reproductive organs can be especially difficult to distinguish from appendicitis. A pregnancy test can help to diagnose an ectopic pregnancy or threatened abortion. Pain and vomiting begin simultaneously with ovarian torsion. Timing at the midportion of the menstrual cycle is critical for diag-

TABLE 61.1. Some conditions that mimic appendicitis.

General conditions
  Duodenal ulcer
  Cholecystitis
  Perinephric abscess
  Pyelonephritis
  Kidney/ureteral stone
  Twisted omentum
  Crohn's disease
  Ileocecal carcinoma
  Intestinal obstruction
  Rectus muscle rupture
  Gastroenteritis
  Psoas abscess
  Meckel's diverticulum
Gynecologic conditions
  Ectopic pregnancy
  Ovarian torsion
  PID
  Ruptured luteal or follicular cyst (Mittelschmerz)

Source: Adapted from Cope's Early Diagnosis of the Acute Abdomen, 19th Ed.[12]

entation, the symptoms may vary. For instance, with a pelvic appendix, symptoms may include deep pelvic pain, bladder irritation or perirectal tenderness. Internal rotation of a flexed hip can elicit pain in this situation, the classic obturator sign.

If the diagnosis is missed in the first 24 to 48h, the appendix will perforate, leading to local or diffuse peritonitis. A mass can sometimes be palpated over the area of an abscess, or peritoneal signs may be present. Following perforation, fever and white count generally rise.[11]

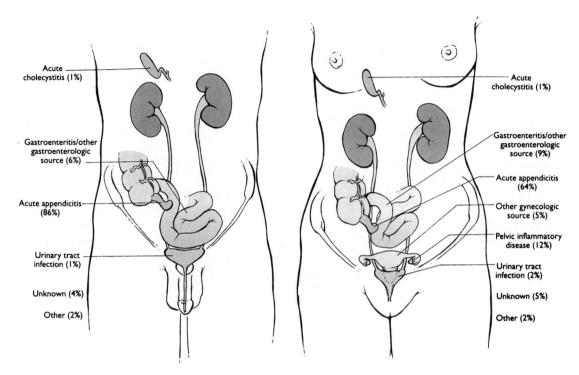

FIGURE 61.3. Final diagnosis for patients explored with a diagnosis of acute appendicitis, divided by sex. Incidence in parentheses. (From Lewis et al., with permission.[13])

nosing *Mittelschmerz*, pain due to a ruptured follicular cyst. Salpingitis is particularly difficult to differentiate from appendicitis, and the diagnosis is often made at operation.

Following perforation, if diffuse symptoms develop, the diagnosis of appendicitis becomes more difficult and the history more important. Primary or secondary peritonitis from any number of causes, including perforation of any viscera, becomes possible. Mesenteric vascular disaster or acute pancreatitis should also be considered.[12] The final diagnoses for 1000 patients treated for acute appendicitis are shown in Figure 61.3.

Adjunctive Testing

Many modalities have been suggested to confirm the diagnosis of presumed appendicitis. Plain films, ultrasound, and CT are often ordered in the emergency room for patients with abdominal pain. Although the classic plain film finding of a fecalith suggestive of appendicitis is well known, the diagnostic utility of these films for appendicitis has been debated. Based on plain films alone, radiologic suggestion of appendicitis is present in less than 10% of patients with pathologically proven appendicitis.[14] Ultrasound is widely used to aid in diagnosis of right lower quadrant pathology. However, accuracy ranges from 71% to 95%.[15–19] It is probably most helpful in women of reproductive age, where ovarian or uterine pathology can also be visualized.

Accuracy for diagnosing appendicitis with abdominal CT reportedly ranges from 93% to 98%. There has been some recent evidence that the use of preoperative CT can decrease the incidence of negative appendectomy. A report by Rao and colleagues demonstrated a change in the identification of a pathologically normal appendix following appendectomy from 20% (98/493) to 7% (15/209) after the instigation of a CT protocol. However, CT was performed in only 123 of these 209 patients. In addition, 206 patients who underwent appendiceal CT avoided operation based on the findings. CT was particularly helpful for diagnosis in adults and women.[20] Notwithstanding these excellent results, not all patients have access to high-quality radiologic equipment or analysis upon initial presentation. Some surgical papers report accuracy of CT or ultrasound diagnosis of appendicitis closer to 60%.[21]

Considering these findings, history and physical examination are the main tools used to diagnose appendicitis in the outpatient setting. Adjunctive testing is most commonly used for patients for whom the diagnosis is unclear or the operative risk is high. Delaying operation for additional testing could lead to an increased rate of perforation and therefore complication. An additional tool to aid in both diagnosis and management of appendicitis is laparoscopy, which prevents any therapeutic delay.

Surgical Management

Open Procedure

In the classic management of appendicitis, a patient is diagnosed with the disease by history and physical and taken to the operating room. Open appendectomy (OA) is typically performed through a right lower quadrant incision where only the appendix and local intestine are visualized. The outcome is generally excellent, with low morbidity. For unperforated appendicitis or a pathologically normal appendix removed at appendectomy, the complication rate is around 5% and mortality is less than 0.25%.[22] However, almost 20% of patients have perforated appendicitis.[10] In this group, morbidity jumps to 19% and mortality to 1.66%.[22] Because of the impressive increase in morbidity and mortality with perforation, a negative appendectomy rate of 10% 20% is still considered acceptable.[23]

Advent of Laparoscopy

During the past 20 years, the increased prevalence of laparoscopic surgery has led many surgeons to use diagnostic laparoscopy to reduce the negative appendectomy rate, without increasing the risk of perforation.[24] Laparoscopy also has the benefit of a more open-ended surgical procedure, in that other pathology identified during laparoscopic exploration can often be treated at the same time. This option is particularly helpful in patients in whom the diagnosis of appendicitis is more in doubt.

Diagnostic Laparoscopy

In early descriptions of diagnostic laparoscopy for suspected appendicitis, surgeons typically explored the abdomen through a laparoscope placed at the umbilicus. If the appendix was normal, the procedure terminated. If the appendix appeared inflamed, or was not visualized, the laparoscopic procedure was terminated and an open appendectomy performed.[25,26] This practice led to a reduction in the number of negative appendectomies, without serious complications. Other groups have suggested exploratory laparoscopy through the right lower quadrant appendectomy incision either before[27] or after appendectomy.[28] As surgical experience with laparoscopy has increased, laparoscopic appendectomy more frequently follows positive laparoscopic exploration.[29]

During diagnostic laparoscopy, extra-appendiceal pathology is occasionally identified. Many of these conditions can be treated laparoscopically, directly following laparoscopic exploration. In women of childbearing age, nonappendiceal pathology may be identified 25% of the time during exploration for suspected appendicitis.[30]

Ruptured tubo-ovarian abscess, ruptured dermoid cyst or endometrioma, adnexal torsion, and ectopic pregnancy are all potential causes of right lower quadrant pain in young women that can be managed with a minimally invasive approach.[31] Extra-appendiceal pathology is identified in only 5% on men less than 50 years old with a preoperative diagnosis of appendicitis. This rate increases to 20% for men (and women) more than 50 years of age.[30] The discharge diagnosis of "appendicitis" has been quoted as 64% in women and 86% in men (see Fig. 61.3). For this reason, diagnostic laparoscopy is more frequently recommended for women with a preoperative diagnosis of appendicitis.

The diagnosis of appendicitis becomes even more difficult in pregnant patients. As the uterus enlarges, the appendix is displaced out of its typical location toward the right upper quadrant. Acute cholecystitis and appendicitis are more difficult to differentiate in this situation, and operative management becomes more complex. Laparoscopic appendectomy has been successfully described in this situation and could be a helpful therapeutic strategy.[32,33]

Incidental Appendectomy

Incidental appendectomy is debated during laparoscopic surgery. When a right lower quadrant incision is made for open appendectomy, it is considered the standard of care to remove the appendix, regardless of the presence or absence of gross appendiceal pathology. One reason for this argument is that subsequent physicians who examine the patient will see the scar and expect that the appendix has been removed. With the more ambiguous placement of ports for the laparoscopic procedure, this is no longer the case.

There are advocates both for and against laparoscopic incidental appendectomy. Advocates of appendectomy argue that there is minimal added morbidity to the procedure, that occasionally (5%–26% of the time) the grossly normal appendix will show inflammation on pathological sectioning, and that appendectomy rules out the diagnosis of appendicitis during future attacks of right lower quadrant pain.[34,35] It can also be argued that one of the original tenets of laparoscopic surgery was to do the same procedure laparoscopically as you would do open, and this would include appendectomy. Opponents of incidental appendectomy cite the diagnostic utility of laparoscopy and support the lower rate of negative appendectomy that can be provided with this approach (1% versus 10%). However, these groups missed appendicitis based on gross findings at laparoscopy alone, requiring reoperation in up to 16% of patients initially spared appendectomy with this approach.[24,36] Strictly incidental appendectomy during surgery for another disease process is not indicated.

TABLE 61.2. Indications, benefits and contraindications for laparoscopic exploration in suspected appendicitis.

Indications/benefits
    Unclear diagnosis
    Young women
    Obese patients
    Decreased diagnostic delay

Contraindications (some relative)
    Young men
    Poor laparoscopic candidate
    Surgeon's technical ability

Based on these results, if a surgical disease is diagnosed at laparoscopy for appendicitis, it should be addressed at that time; this would include appendicitis, ectopic pregnancy, etc. To minimize the need for future intervention, the appendix should be removed regardless of obvious appendiceal pathology, unless a treatable nonrecurrent alternative for abdominal pain is identified (i.e., Meckel's diverticulum). Appendectomy is particularly important if an underlying recurrent disease process such as pelvic inflammatory disease or inflammatory bowel disease is identified. In these cases, it would be helpful to rule out the diagnosis of appendicitis for future bouts of right lower quadrant pain.

Indications for Appendectomy: Laparoscopic Versus Open

Many would argue that a diagnosis of probable appendicitis is all that is needed before proceeding with laparoscopic appendectomy. However, there are particular patient factors that support it more strongly. Young women, older patients of either sex, or immunocompromised patients in whom the diagnosis is less clear could arguably benefit from laparoscopic exploration before appendectomy. Obese patients, who often require a large incision for open appendectomy, could also profit from a laparoscopic approach.

Opponents of laparoscopy argue that the outcome of open appendectomy is not significantly different from the laparoscopic approach. It is argued that longer operative time and more expensive equipment outweigh any potential postoperative benefits. Patients with multiple prior abdominal operations or advanced pregnancy are generally considered to be poor laparoscopic candidates. The most controversial group of patients for diagnostic laparoscopy is young men with suspected appendicitis, who have a minimal rate of misdiagnosis.[37] Relative indications and contraindications are listed in Table 61.2.

Description of Procedure

Once the diagnosis of appendicitis is suspected and the decision to proceed with laparoscopic exploration is made, the patient is prepared for surgery. As diagnostic laparoscopy and appendectomy are fairly low-risk procedures, preoperative studies other than diagnostic ones should be tailored for the individual patient. A broad-spectrum antibiotic such as ampicillin sulbactam or cefotetan should be given within the hour before surgery, generally in the preoperative holding area.

In the operating room, the patient is placed in a supine position. General anesthesia is induced. The patient's left arm is tucked. A Foley catheter is usually placed to minimize the risk of bladder injury during the procedure. The surgeon stands on the patient's left. The assistant starts on the patient's right during port placement and exploration but moves to the left side if appendectomy is carried out. The monitors are placed at or just below the patient's umbilicus on either side of the table (Fig. 61.4).

A 10- to 12-mm port is placed at the umbilicus and the abdomen insufflated. The Hasson technique is advocated to prevent injury to intra-abdominal structures. However, blind placement of a Veress needle can also be used. Following placement of the laparoscope, visual exploration of the abdomen ensues. It is important to examine the entire abdomen to rule out pathology. An attempt is made to locate and visualize the appendix in the right lower quadrant. Trendelenburg positioning and rotating

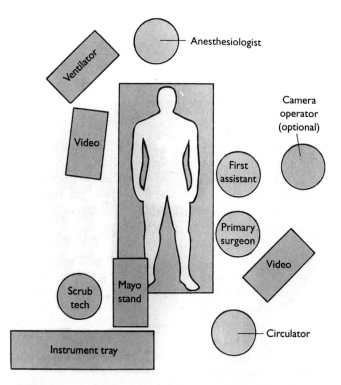

FIGURE 61.4. Operating room setup for diagnostic laparoscopy and anticipated laparoscopic appendectomy. (From DeMatos P, Ludwig KA. Laparoscopic appendectomy. In: Pappas TN, Chekan EG, Eubanks S (eds). Atlas of Laparoscopic Surgery, 2nd Ed. Philadelphia: Current Medicine, 1999:11.1–11.11.[8])

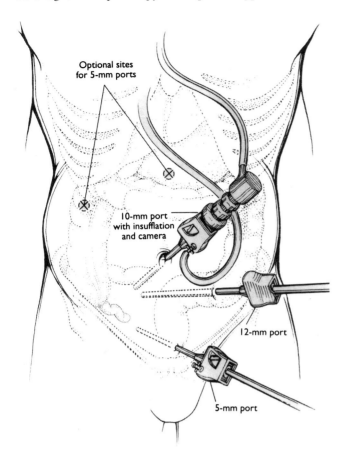

with identification of the appendix are running the small bowel to the ileocecal valve or following the taenia to the base of the cecum.

Once the appendix is identified, it is examined for signs of inflammation. In appendicitis the organ may be red or swollen, providing a relatively straightforward diagnosis. There may also be pus in the pericecal area with or without obvious appendiceal involvement; this can also be an indication of appendicitis. In this setting, other surrounding structures need to be carefully inspected for evidence of inflammation. If the appendix appears normal, the remainder of the abdomen is carefully and methodically inspected. If a finding other than appendicitis is identified, the procedure should be redirected accordingly.

To proceed with appendectomy, additional ports are placed as necessary. The appendix is then grasped and elevated. Care should be taken with inflamed or gangrenous tissues not to grasp the appendix itself. Holding the mesentery is preferable during mobilization. A suture loop can also be placed around the appendix to facilitate retraction. The mesentery is followed to the base of the appendix. A window is then created in the mesoappendix between the base of the appendix and the appendicular artery, using blunt dissection (Fig. 61.6). It is important to have this window adjacent to the cecum. The endoscopic stapler is then used to divide the appendix and the mesentery at this plane (Figs. 61.7, 61.8). The small bowel stapler should be used for the appendix and the vascular stapler for the artery. Either structure may be taken first.

The appendix is then removed through the 10- or 12-mm port. It can be brought out directly or with the use

FIGURE 61.5. Port placement for laparoscopic appendectomy. (From DeMatos P, Ludwig KA. Laparoscopic appendectomy. In: Pappas TN, Chekan EG, Eubanks S (eds). Atlas of Laparoscopic Surgery, 2nd Ed. Philadelphia: Current Medicine, 1999:11.1–11.11.[8])

the bed to the patient's left often aid in this step and the remainder of the procedure.

Additional ports can be placed to facilitate exploration (Fig. 61.5). It is best to place these extra ports where they will be most helpful for the subsequent procedure. To proceed with appendectomy, two additional ports are required; these include a 10- or 12-mm port to allow passage of the endoscopic stapler and a 5-mm port for a grasper. The 10- or 12-mm port is placed lateral to the epigastric vessels in the midportion of the left lower quadrant. The 5-mm port is placed in the suprapubic midline. An alternative is to place both operative ports in the midline, but this can provide less space for manipulation. Additional 5-mm ports are occasionally required to help with retraction during appendectomy.

Following port placement, attention is directed to identification of the appendix. Surrounding adhesions are divided sharply or with careful use of cautery, as necessary. A retrocecal appendix occasionally requires division of the peritoneum along the white line of Toldt; this can also be accomplished with a combination of blunt and sharp dissection plus electrocautery. Some tricks to aid

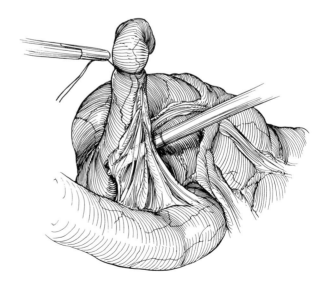

FIGURE 61.6. Elevating the appendix with the help of a suture loop and making the mesenteric window. (From Economou SG, Economou TS. Appendectomy. In: Atlas of Surgical Techniques. Philadelphia: Saunders, 1996:258–269.[38])

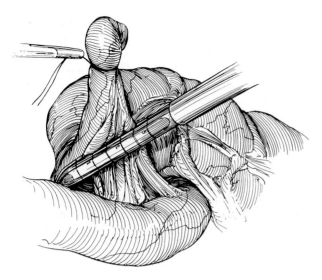

FIGURE 61.7. Dividing the mesentery. (From Economou SG, Economou TS. Appendectomy. In: Atlas of Surgical Techniques. Philadelphia: Saunders, 1996:258–269.[38])

of an endoscopic bag, depending on the degree of inflammation. Following removal of the appendix, the abdomen is irrigated and the appendiceal stump is visualized to ensure hemostasis. Small residual bleeding can be controlled with the electrocautery. A suture can be helpful if more control is needed. A final inspection of the abdomen is then performed.

The 10- to 12-mm operative port site is closed with an endoscopic closure device under laparoscopic visualization. The 5-mm port is removed and the site checked for hemostasis. Local anesthesia may be infiltrated at the port sites. The abdomen is then allowed to deflate. The fascia at the umbilical port site and the skin of all sites are then closed.

Following the procedure, the patient is started on a clear liquid diet. If the diet is well tolerated, regular food is generally started the next day and the patient is discharged.

Results

Expected Outcomes

During diagnostic laparoscopy, a diagnosis can be made in 84% to 100% of patients with suspected appendicitis.[21,29,39–43] Between 10% and 50% can avoid laparotomy or appendectomy based on another diagnosis made during exploration.[25,26,29,39,40,42,44,45] This number tends to be highest if only patients with a questionable diagnosis are explored. About 1% of all patients suspected to have appendicitis require an alternative surgical procedure, which may be performed by an open or laparoscopic

approach.[29] Laparoscopic exploration can help define this group.

The majority of published reports on laparoscopic appendectomy are limited to retrospective analyses. Recently there have been more prospective trials, some of which have been randomized. However, the numbers of patients included in these trials have been limited and the results varied. Within the past few years, there have been a limited number of authors compiling the results of these studies through meta-analyses. Meta-analyses do have limitations in the biases of the individual trials themselves. Items such as length of stay and operative time vary between centers. The skill level of the operating surgeon can also be variable. One additional major criticism of the individual studies is that patients who had to convert from the laparoscopic to open procedure were often excluded from analysis.[46] Despite these shortcomings, meta-analysis is an excellent tool for combining results from multiple trials. A 1999 meta-analysis covered 17 randomized controlled studies with a total of nearly 1800 patients. Laparoscopic appendectomy was associated with longer operating time (an extra 8 to 29 min; $p < 0.0001$), reduction in hospital stay (0.1–2.1 days; $p < 0.007$), and possibly an earlier return to normal activity. Wound infection was associated with open appendectomy.[46] Other analyses demonstrated a reduction in postoperative pain[47,48] and a trend towards increased intra-abdominal abscesses with laparoscopic appendectomy.[49]

Despite some variability in the conclusions of several meta-analyses, the statistically prominent outcomes are increased operative time, earlier return to normal activity, and possibly decreased postoperative pain with laparoscopic appendectomy. Other prominent trends that were significant in some analyses included decreased wound infection, earlier return to a regular diet, and faster hospital discharge with laparoscopic appendectomy. These results for one major study are shown in Table 61.3.

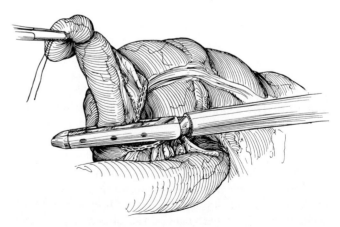

FIGURE 61.8. Dividing the base of the appendix. (From Economou SG, Economou TS. Appendectomy. In: Atlas of Surgical Techniques. Philadelphia: Saunders, 1996:258–269.[38])

TABLE 61.3. Summary of meta-analysis results.

Endpoint	Number of studies	Mean	p value
Postop stay, days	14	3.23 LA 3.84 OA	0.03
Days to solids	7	1.74 LA 1.96 OA	0.01
OR time, min	16	69.8 LA 51.5 OA	<0.0001
Days until normal activity	12	11.9 LA 19.0 OA	<0.0001
Postop pain	11		0.003
Wound infection	16	2.8% LA 7.1% OA	NS
Intra-abdominal abscess	15	2.02% LA 0.937% OA	NS

Means for laparoscopic (LA) and open appendectomy (OA) are listed, with the p value. NS, not significant.
Source: From Golub et al.,[49] with permission.

Pitfalls and Complications and Their Prevention and Management

Laparoscopic exploration is generally extremely well tolerated. Most studies report complication rates under 5%.[21,29,40] Laparoscopic appendectomy is also associated with low morbidity. The complication rate for both the laparoscopic and open procedures is around 8%, and the mortality rate is well under 1%. The major complications relate to the disease itself, and include intra-abdominal abscess, wound infection, and small bowel obstruction or ileus. Prophylactic antibiotics can minimize the infectious risk. Adequate, but localized, irrigation can help with abscess formation and motility issues. There are also complications inherent to laparoscopic surgery, such as needle, trocar, or cautery injury to bowel or vessels; these problems can be minimized with meticulous technique and open placement of the umbilical port.

If the appendiceal-cecal junction is not well defined during appendectomy, it is possible to amputate the appendix along its course and not at its base, which has led to a few cases of recurrent appendicitis following laparoscopic appendectomy.[50,51] However, this complication has also been reported from open appendectomy.[52] This complication can be avoided by adequate visualization of the pertinent anatomy, ensuring that the stapler is fired adjacent to the cecum. If necessary, a small portion of the cecum can be taken, without significant complication.

Conclusion

Laparoscopic exploration followed by possible appendectomy is a safe and straightforward approach to the management of appendicitis. Because of the ability to visualize the entire abdomen at operation, it has improved diagnostic utility over open appendectomy and

may therefore be advantageous for patients in whom the diagnosis is unclear. A significant percentage of this group can also avoid operative intervention beyond exploration. If the exploration is positive for appendicitis, proceeding to laparoscopic appendectomy has been shown to reduce postoperative hospital stay and decrease the time until a patient resumes normal diet and activity following surgery. Despite the reduction in wound infection with laparoscopic appendectomy, it has been associated with longer operative times and potentially higher rates of intra-abdominal abscess formation. The remaining complications from laparoscopic appendectomy are related to surgical error or diagnostic delay and can be minimized with careful technique and early intervention.

Diagnostic laparoscopy for suspected appendicitis is recommended for young women, the elderly, or other patients with unclear pathology because of its broader diagnostic ability and for obese patients because of its improved technical ease. Laparoscopic appendectomy can also be safely used for other patients with appendicitis, minimizing postoperative recovery time and potential pain.

References

1. Williams GR. A history of appendicitis with anecdotes illustrating its importance. Ann Surg 1983;197:495–506.
2. Royster HA. Appendicitis. New York: Appleton, 1927.
3. McBurney C. Experience with early operative interference in cases of disease of the vermiform appendix. NY Med J 1889;50:676–684.
4. McBurney C. The incision made in the abdominal wall in cases of appendicitis, with a description of a new method of operating. Ann Surg 1894;20:38–43.
5. Bernheim BM. Organoscopy: cystoscopy of the abdominal cavity. Ann Surg 1911;53:764–767.
6. Semm K. Advances in pelviscopic surgery. Curr Probl Obstet Gynecol 1982;5:1–42.
7. Ross MH, Reith EJ, Romrell LJ. Histology: A Text and Atlas, 2nd Ed. Baltimore: Williams & Wilkins, 1989:466.
8. DeMatos P, Ludwig KA. Laparoscopic appendectomy. In: Pappas TN, Chekan EG, Eubanks S (eds). Atlas of Laparoscopic Surgery, 2nd Ed. Philadelphia: Current Medicine, 1999:11.1–11.11.
9. Rubin E, Farber JL. Essential Pathology. Philadelphia: Lippincott, 1990:389–391.
10. Addiss DG, Shaffer N, Fowler BS, Tauxe RV. The epidemiology of appendicitis and appendectomy in the United States. Am J Epidemiol 1990;132:910–925.
11. Silen W. Appendicitis. In: Cope's Early Diagnosis of the Acute Abdomen, 19th Ed. New York: Oxford University Press, 1996:70–87.
12. Silen W. The differential diagnosis of appendicitis. In: Cope's Early Diagnosis of the Acute Abdomen, 19th Ed. New York: Oxford University Press, 1996:88–110.
13. Lewis FR, Holcroft JW, Boey J, Dunphy JD. Appendicitis: a critical review of diagnosis and treatment in 1000 cases. Arch Surg 1975;110:677–684.

14. Rao PM, Rhea JT, Rao JA. Plain abdominal radiography in clinically suspected appendicitis: diagnostic yield, resource use, and comparison with CT. Am J Emerg Med 1999;17: 325–328.

15. Yacoe ME, Jeffrey RB. Sonography of appendicitis and diverticulitis. Radiol Clin N Am 1994;32:899–912.

16. Puylaert JB. Imaging and intervention in patients with acute right lower quadrant disease. Baillieres Clin Gastroenterol 1995;9:37–51.

17. Incesu L, Coskun A, Selcuk MB, et al. Acute appendicitis: MR imaging and sonographic correlation. AJR Am J Roentgenol 1997;168:669–674.

18. Rioux M. Sonographic detection of the normal and abnormal appendix. AJR Am J Roentgenol 1992;158:773–778.

19. Balthazar EJ, Birnbaum BA, Yee J, et al. Acute appendicitis: CT and US correlation in 100 patients. Radiology 1994; 190:31–35.

20. Rao PM, Rhea JT, Rattner DW, Venus LG, Novelline RA. Introduction of appendiceal CT: impact on negative appendectomy and appendiceal perforation rates. Ann Surg 1999; 229:344–349.

21. Connor TJ, Garcha IS, Ramshaw BJ, et al. Diagnostic laparoscopy for suspected appendicitis. Am Surg 1995;61: 187–189.

22. Velanovich V, Satava R. Balancing the normal appendectomy rate with the perforated appendicitis rate: implications for quality assurance. Am Surg 1992;58:264–269.

23. Pappas TN, Gale F, Ross RP. Appendicitis can be treated safely with a negative appendectomy rate of 10%. Dig Surg 1989;6:74–77.

24. Leape LL, Ramenofsky ML. Laparoscopy for questionable appendicitis: can it reduce the negative appendectomy rate. Ann Surg 1980;191:410–413.

25. Kum CK, Sim EKW, Goh PMY, Ngoi SS, Rauff A. Diagnostic laparoscopy: reducing the number of normal appendectomies. Dis Colon Rectum 1993;36:763–766.

26. Tytgat SHAJ, Bakker XR, Butzelaar RMJM. Laparoscopic evaluation of patients with suspected acute appendicitis. Surg Endosc 1998;12:918–920.

27. Suh HH. A minimally invasive technique of appendectomy using a minimal skin incision and laparoscopic instruments. Surg Laparosc Endosc 1998;8:149–152.

28. Schrenk P, Rieger R, Shamiyeh A, Wayand W. Diagnostic laparoscopy through the right lower abdominal incision following open appendectomy. Surg Endosc 1999;13:133–135.

29. Moberg AC, Ahlberg G, Leijonmarck CE, et al. Diagnostic laparoscopy in 1043 patients with suspected appendicitis. Eur J Surg 1998;164:833–840.

30. Velanovich V, Harkabus MA, Tapia FV, Gusz JR, Vallance SR. When it's not appendicitis. Am Surg 1998;64:7–11.

31. Apelgren KN, Cowan BD, Metcalf AM, Scott-Conner CE. Laparoscopic appendectomy and the management of gynecologic pathologic conditions found at laparoscopy for presumed appendicitis. Surg Clin N Am 1996;76:469–482.

32. Gurbuz AT, Peetz ME. The acute abdomen in the pregnant patient: is there a role for laparoscopy? Surg Endosc 1997; 11:98–102.

33. Schreiber JH. Early experience with laparoscopic appendectomy in women. Surg Endosc 1987;1:211–216.

34. Greason KL, Rappold JF, Liberman MA. Incident al laparoscopic appendectomy for acute right lower quadrant abdominal pain: its time has come. Surg Endosc 1998;12: 223–225.

35. Grunewald B, Keating J. Should the "normal" appendix be removed at operation for appendicitis. J R Coll Surg Edinb 1993;38:158–160.

36. Thorell A, Grondal S, Schedvins K, Wallin G. Value of laparoscopy in fertile women with suspected appendicitis. Eur J Surg 1999;165:751–754.

37. Mutter D, Vix M, Bui A, et al. Laparoscopy not recommended for routine appendectomy in men: results of a prospective randomized study. Surgery 1996;120:71–74.

38. Economou SG, Economou TS. Appendectomy. In: Atlas of Surgical Techniques. Philadelphia: Saunders, 1996:258–269.

39. Cox MR, McCall JL, Padbury RTA, Wilson TG, Wattchow DA, Toouli J. Laparoscopic surgery in women with a clinical diagnosis of acute appendicitis. Med J Aust 1995;162: 130–132.

40. Jadallah FA, Abdul-Ghani AA, Tibblin S. Diagnostic laparoscopy reduces unnecessary appendicectomy in fertile women. Eur J Surg 1944;160:41–45.

41. Whitworth CM, Whitworth PW, Sanfillipo J, Polk HC. Value of diagnostic laparoscopy in young women with possible appendicitis. Surg Gynecol Obstet 1998;167:187–190.

42. Spirtos NM, Eisenkop SM, Spirtos TW, Poliakin RI, Hibbard LT. Laparoscopy—a diagnostic aid in cases of suspected appendicitis: its use in women of reproductive age. Am J Obstet Gynecol 1987;156:90–94.

43. Ure BM, Spangenberger W, Hebebrand D, Eypasch EP, Troidl H. Laparoscopic surgery in children and adolescents with suspected appendicitis: results of medical technology assessment. Eur J Pediatr Surg 1992;2:336–340.

44. Kuster GGR, Gilroy SBC. The role of laparoscopy in the diagnosis of acute appendicitis. Am Surg 1992;58:627–629.

45. Taylor EW, Kennedy CA, Dunham RH, Bloch JH. Diagnostic laparoscopy in women with acute abdominal pain. Surg Laparosc Endosc 1995;5:128–128.

46. Fingerhut A, Millat B, Borrie F. Laparoscopic versus open appendectomy: time to decide. World J Surg 1999;23:835–845.

47. Chung RS, Rowland DY, Li P, Diaz J. A meta-analysis of randomized controlled trials of laparoscopic versus conventional appendectomy. Am J Surg 1999;177:250–256.

48. Sauerland S, Lefering R, Holthausen U, Neugebauer EAM. Laparoscopic vs. conventional appendectomy—a meta-analysis of randomized controlled trials. Langenbecks Arch Surg 1999;383:289–295.

49. Golub R, Siddiqui F, Pohl D. Laparoscopic versus open appendectomy: a metaanalysis. J Am Coll Surg 1998;186: 545–553.

50. Greenberg JJ, Esposito TJ. Appendicitis after appendectomy: a warning. J Laparoendosc Surg 1996;6:185–187.

51. Devereaux DA, McDermott JP, Caushaj PF. Recurrent appendicitis following laparoscopic appendectomy: report of a case. Dis Colon Rectum 1994;37:719–720.

52. Demartines N, Largiader J. "Residual" appendicitis following incomplete appendectomy. Br J Surg 1996;83:1481.

62
Diagnostic Laparoscopy for Intestinal Disorders

James J. Gangemi and Edward G. Chekan

Intestinal disorders have long been within the realm of the general surgeon. More recently, several common intestinal disorders have been addressed laparoscopically. In this section, two major maladies of the small intestine are addressed: small bowel mesenteric ischemia and small bowel obstruction. Mesenteric ischemia can be subdivided into acute and chronic disease. Acute mesenteric ischemia is caused by thrombosis, embolism, or iatrogenic causes as is the case following abdominal aortic aneurysm repair. Chronic mesenteric ischemia is the result of severe atherosclerotic disease of the mesenteric arteries. Small bowel obstruction, on the other hand, can have a variety of etiologies, with the most common being adhesions, neoplastic disease, and hernia. Often, mesenteric ischemia and small bowel obstruction can occur together in that small bowel obstruction can lead to mesenteric ischemia.

This chapter provides a brief overview of small bowel mesenteric ischemia and obstruction along with a more in-depth discussion of the role for laparoscopy in diagnosing and treating these disease entities.

General Laparoscopic Issues

Laparoscopy can be used to diagnose a variety of intestinal disorders, and this evaluation can take place in a variety of settings ranging from a well-monitored bed, such as in the intensive care unit (ICU), to the operating suite. As a general rule, if the patient requires therapeutic intervention such as bowel resection, then the operation should be performed in the operating room. However, there are advantages to performing diagnostic studies in the ICU. For instance, intensive care unit laparoscopy obviates the need of transporting an unstable patient and unnecessary mobilization of expensive operating room resources.[1] In one report, a gangrenous small bowel segment was identified after an aortobifem

oral reconstruction for an abdominal aortic aneurysm using bedside laparoscopy.[2]

Irrespective of the location for diagnostic laparoscopy for evaluation of intestinal disease, it remains extremely important to continue to have access to the most advanced visualization equipment. Because operative decisions are largely based upon the optical image produced, laparoscopes and cameras should be chosen that produce high-quality images. Although miniscopes are available and are often tempting to employ in this circumstance, the image quality remains inferior to the more common 5- or 10-mm scope. Three-chip cameras or high-definition television can also be used to achieve high-quality reproduction of living tissues. Similarly, mini-instruments should not be used to manipulate distended bowel, as their inherently small gripping area can lead to intestinal perforation. Finally, during diagnostic or therapeutic laparoscopic procedures, equipment must always be readily available in the event that prompt laparotomy would become necessary.

Ischemic/Necrotic Bowel

Acute mesenteric ischemia was first described in the latter part of the fifteenth century.[3] In 1894, Councilman described the entity of chronic mesenteric ischemia.[4] In more modern times, Klass applied the general principles of vascular surgery and postulated a superior mesenteric artery (SMA) embolism as an etiology for acute mesenteric ischemia. The first clinically successful SMA embolectomy was credited to Shaw and Rutledge in 1957.[3]

An abrupt cutoff of mesenteric blood flow is typically the result of either acute vascular thrombosis or an embolism originating from the heart (i.e., myocardial infarction, ventricular aneurysm, atrial fibrillation, or mitral stenosis). Less common etiologies for acute mesenteric occlusion include either nonocclusive mesenteric ischemia (i.e., anaphylaxis, arterial vasospasm, or impaired capillary permeability)[3] or mesenteric venous thrombosis. Despite classical clinical descriptions, it is often challenging to discern acute from chronic mesenteric ischemia. The classic textbook presentation for acute mesenteric ischemia is an abrupt onset of intense abdominal pain that is "out of proportion to physical findings." The laboratory values are often nonspecific and may include metabolic acidosis, an elevated lactate level, and an elevated white blood cell count.[2] Although frequently discussed, mesenteric venous thrombosis is rare and is usually the result of a disruption in arterial blood flow or acute mechanical bowel obstruction. Occasionally, trauma, infectious diseases, neoplasms, portal hypertension, or acute fluid loss (i.e., diuretic use, polycythemia vera) are predisposing factors).[5] Not uncommonly, patients present with atypical abdominal pain and the possibility of ischemic bowel is raised. For instance, Serryn et al. reported a case of a young patient who underwent laparoscopy for suspected gynecological pathology but was found to have an infarcted intestine secondary to mesenteric thrombosis. This patient was treated with a laparoscopic bowel resection.[5]

Chronic mesenteric ischemia is the result of atherosclerotic occlusive disease that can manifest itself as intestinal gangrene, ischemic strictures, or colitis. By definition, the onset of symptoms in patients with chronic ischemia is insidious. Such patients may present with nonspecific abdominal pain (often beginning 30–90 min after ingesting a meal), diarrhea, or obstructive symptoms typical of intestinal stricture. A picture of acute ischemia can also be evident when a chronic vascular stricture becomes acutely thrombosed.

A challenging situation for clinicians often occurs when a patient presents with mesenteric ischemia in the early postoperative period. In such cases, incisional pain can be confused with ischemic pain. Also, the intubated or unresponsive patient can present clinical dilemmas. Following complicated coronary artery bypass, a patient is often intubated and sedated, requiring the diagnosis of intestinal ischemia to be based solely on objective criteria.

Angiography remains the gold standard for diagnosis of mesenteric ischemia. However, angiography is often precluded by the tenuous clinical status of the patient in that it is difficult to transport hemodynamically unstable patients or resuscitate them in the radiology department. Therefore, other interventions including endoscopy, laparotomy, and, most recently, laparoscopy have been used in managing such patients. Endoscopy has the advantage of being both safe as well as allowing for direct visualization of the gastric, duodenal, and colonic mucosa. In addition, its portability allows endoscopy to be an important diagnostic tool for postoperative intubated patients in the ICU. When laparotomy is the diag-

nostic modality of choice, special maneuvers (i.e., fluorescein injection) are sometimes necessary to discern viable versus nonviable segments of small intestine intraoperatively. Often, laparotomy is the only feasible diagnostic option despite concerns of exposing the patient to the risks of major abdominal surgery. However, when successful, the benefit of this approach is that it can be both diagnostic and therapeutic. Recently, laparoscopy has been successfully employed to help with both diagnostic and therapeutic interventions in the treatment of both acute and chronic mesenteric ischemia. Diagnostic laparoscopic intervention for mesenteric ischemia is best suited for patients who present a diagnostic dilemma, are clinically unstable, and so cannot be transported for fear of clinical decompensation. This group is the subgroup of patients in which laparotomy would be poorly tolerated. Whether performed in the ICU to avoid transportation or in the operating room to allow therapeutic intervention, laparoscopic interventions in these critically ill patients can help surgeons avoid unnecessary laparotomy and its associated morbidity.

Laparoscopy for Mesenteric Ischemia

The patient is placed supine and, occasionally, in the lithotomy position to allow for intraoperative colonoscopy. All patients undergoing diagnostic laparoscopy should have both a urinary catheter and nasogastric tube for decompression. Intestinal decompression creates more space within the abdominal cavity to allow intestinal manipulation, and decompression of the bladder is necessary to allow the operator clear visualization of the rectum. Before beginning any laparoscopic case, all the equipment should be tested to ensure proper functioning. It is most important to ensure that the camera is accurately white-balanced to control for "true color" representation on the monitor. The color of the intestine is frequently the determining factor when deciding on therapeutic maneuvers.

Access to the abdomen is gained by using the open (Hasson trocar) technique that allows the operator to directly visualize entrance into the peritoneal cavity and to most effectively avoid puncturing friable, ischemic, or distended bowel. The abdomen is insufflated with CO_2 to approximately 15 mmHg, and a laparoscope is inserted through an umbilical cannula into the abdomen to allow a systematic, circumferential review of the abdominal contents. Either a 30° or 0° scope can be used. However, the 30° scope offers the widest flexibility for complete intestinal visualization. Additional trocars (initially 5 mm) are placed laterally under direct visualization to help with peritoneal exploration. If more extensive bowel manipulation or resection become necessary, these trocars can be traded for 10- or 12-mm trocars. At least

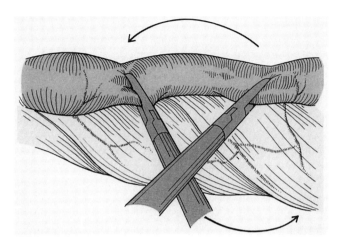

FIGURE 62.1. The entire small bowel is "run" from the ligament of Trietz to the terminal ileum to identify the area of concern. (From Figure 10.4 in *Atlas of Laparoscopic Surgery*. Pappas TN, Chekan EG, Eubanks WS, eds. 2E. 1999. Philadelphia: Current Medicine. Reproduced with permission.)

two trocars are necessary to allow two-handed, atraumatic handling of the bowel. Only large graspers or endobabcocks should be used for intestinal manipulation because small graspers or dissectors can cause perforation. An aspiration system should always be available for the aspiration and analysis of intraperitoneal fluid.

Once the trocars are in place, the omentum is gently retracted and the serosal surface of the bowel is inspected. Ischemic bowel can be represented by a wide range of colors, hence the importance of white-balancing the camera. Ischemic bowel can appear normal or pink if there is only mucosal ischemia, or black as in complete transmural necrosis. Therefore, it is very important to accurately note the color of the intestine. If there appears to be normal perfusion at first inspection, a methodical review of the entire small bowel should then be performed. This circumferential intestinal inspection begins at the ligament of Trietz, and the small bowel is then "run" using atraumatic bowel graspers and the hand-over-hand technique (Fig. 62.1). Care is taken to grab the bowel only with full-thickness large bites, as smaller bites have a tendency to tear the intestine, especially when intestinal integrity may already be tenuous as is the case with ischemia. If adhesions are encountered, they should be sharply divided with endoscopic scissors with minimal, if any, use of electrocautery to avoid energy conduction toward the intestine.

Whether the surgical approach is laparoscopic or open, identifying and grading intestinal ischemia can be the most challenging aspect of this operation. Although devices such as Doppler ultrasound, tissue oxygenation probes, and fluorescent dye have been used during laparoscopic exploration as in open procedures,[2] their dependability is equivocal, and often the margin of resec-

tion is based solely on visual judgement. For instance, dark-appearing bowel may be necrotic or may be normal and contain merely intraluminal blood or feces that cause it to appear black.[6]

Any segment of bowel that is obviously necrotic should be resected. Additional or larger trocars should be inserted if bowel resection is deemed appropriate. When performing a laparoscopic bowel resection, the ischemic area is first suspended between two graspers to allow clear visualization of the mesenteric arcade. Next, using sharp dissection, a window is created in the mesentery to define the proximal and distal extent of the bowel resection (Fig. 62.2). The bowel is then divided using an endoscopic stapling device. The mesentery is divided using either the endoshears and endoclips or, alternatively, by using the ultrasonic shears. After slight enlargement of one of the trocar sites, typically the umbilical port, the specimen is removed from the patient. The cut ends of the intestine are exteriorized through the same enlarged site to allow palpation and assessment of perfusion, as evidenced by bleeding, before extracorporeal anastamosis. The anastomosed bowel is then returned to the abdomen and the trocar sites are closed. Although multiple bowel segments can be resected by this method during a laparoscopic case, in the extreme cases of entire small bowel necrosis, the most prudent course of action may be to quit and close. In these unfortunate cases, any type of operative intervention would not be beneficial to the patient's care.

"Second-look" laparoscopy following primary laparotomy, laparoscopy, or interventional radiologic techniques in patients with mesenteric ischemia has been

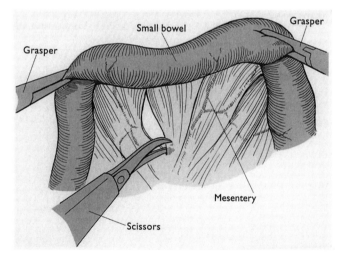

FIGURE 62.2. A window is created in the mesentery to mark the area of resection using both blunt and sharp dissection. (From Figure 10.6 in *Atlas of Laparoscopic Surgery*. Pappas TN, Chekan EG, Eubanks WS, eds. 2E. 1999. Philadelphia: Current Medicine. Reproduced with permission.)

reported as a useful approach. Slutzki et al. reported on five patients with acute ischemic bowel that initially underwent angiography followed by therapeutic laparotomy.[7] In this report, three patients underwent bowel resection and two were treated with an SMA embolectomy. Following these interventions, each patient underwent laparoscopic "second look" 48 to 72h later. In all patients, a second laparotomy was avoided. "Second-look" laparoscopy can be simplified by placing a trocar large enough to accommodate the laparoscope at the time of laparotomy. This trocar is then covered with a sterile dressing, such as a sterile towel held in place with a transparent adhesive covering.[7] At the time of the "second look," laparoscopy is used to assess bowel viability or to monitor recovery from the initial ischemic insult. Others have reported similar favorable results using this approach.[8–10]

Regan et al. used an alternative approach to avoid the primary laparotomy. These authors report one case of mesenteric ischemia in which the angiogram showed complete SMA occlusion. Instead of undergoing laparotomy, the patient was treated with intra-arterial infusion of thrombolytics until the embolus resolved and the angiogram returned to normal. On day 2, the patient was taken to the operating suite for diagnostic laparoscopy that revealed normal intestine, and the patient recovered uneventfully.[11]

There are some clear disadvantages to the laparoscopic approach for mesenteric ischemia. First, diagnostic laparoscopy does not always adequately evaluate the retroperitoneum (i.e., duodenum or rectum). Furthermore, as only the serosal surface of the bowel can be inspected, it may actually look normal in the early phases of intestinal ischemia. Using laparoscopic techniques, the operator is unable to palpate the small bowel mesentery to evaluate perfusion as is typically relied upon in judging intestinal viability in open cases. Finally, because the pneumoperitoneum used in laparoscopy can in and of itself depress mesenteric blood flow, high insufflation pressures should be avoided.

During any diagnostic laparoscopic procedure, open conversion is always a possibility. Conversion to an open approach should be considered in patients where bleeding is difficult to control, intestinal wall integrity has been violated, or poor image quality makes assessment of intestinal viability inconclusive.

Bowel Obstruction

Bowel obstructions are most commonly caused by adhesions (50%), hernias (15%), or neoplasms (15%).[12] Surgical history indicates that Praxagoras was the first to treat an intestinal obstruction in 350 B.C. by creating an intestinal fistula.[13] Since then, there has been debate as to whether surgical intervention or medical treatment with intravenous fluids and nasogastric decompression is the most appropriate treatment for patients with suspected bowel obstruction. Currently, scientific data support both surgical and medical modes of treatment.

Patients with small bowel obstruction can present with nonspecific signs or symptoms such as nausea, vomiting, and abdominal pain. On physical examination, the abdomen can be both tender and distended. The workup of such patients should include basic laboratory analysis to assess their level of hydration and to check for an elevated white blood cell count. Abdominal radiographs classically show evidence of distended loops of bowel, air–fluid levels, and an absence or paucity of air in the colon. The stasis of intraluminal intestinal contents may result in bacterial overgrowth, leading some patients to be toxic on presentation. Such patients require prompt surgical intervention.

For the majority of patients presenting in a less toxic manner, there are a variety of treatment options that range from conservative medical management to surgical intervention involving either laparotomy or laparoscopy. The patient's clinical status typically dictates the level and method of intervention.

In choosing between available surgical interventions for patients with bowel obstruction, the decision between laparotomy or laparoscopic management is based upon such patient factors as their level of acute distress, history of previous abdominal surgery, the availability of laparoscopic equipment, and the severity of bowel distension. In general terms, laparoscopic intervention should be reserved for hemodynamically stable patients without extensive intra-abdominal adhesions. Laparoscopic intervention for patients with small bowel obstruction should preferentially be performed in the operating room.

Laparoscopy for Small Bowel Obstruction

Because the majority of patients with bowel obstructions have distended loops of bowel, the open (Hasson trocar) technique is used to gain access to the abdomen. Laparoscopic exploration then proceeds in a fashion similar to that previously described for mesenteric ischemia.

Following general exploration, a transition point is sought between segments of distended loops of bowel and decompressed loops. If such a point is located, this confirms the diagnosis of bowel obstruction, which can usually be treated with simple lysis of adhesions. For a single adhesion, laparoscopic scissors with minimal use of electrocautery can be used to relieve the obstructed segment. However, while it is straightforward to apply laparoscopic techniques for lysis of a single offending band of adhesion, it is difficult to use laparoscopic tech-

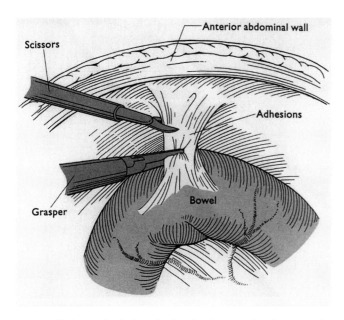

FIGURE 62.3. A single band of adhesion can be lysed under direct visualization using sharp dissection and minimal electrocautery. (From Figure 10.5 in *Atlas of Laparoscopic Surgery*. Pappas TN, Chekan EG, Eubanks WS, eds. 2E. 1999. Philadelphia: Current Medicine. Reproduced with permission.)

niques for extensive lysis of adhesions. Encountering extensive adhesions during laparoscopy is a relative indication for conversion to open laparotomy. Finally, if no such transition point between distended and decompressed loops is identified, the bowel is "run" along its entire length using the hand-over-hand technique. Care must be taken to avoid traumatic handling of these distended loops as they are often fragile, especially in patients with long-standing obstruction, and again excessive electrocautery should be avoided (Fig. 62.3).

Complications and Contraindications

Complications can occur during any operative procedure. During laparoscopic interventions for intestinal disorders, the majority of untoward events occur on entry into the abdomen. The dilated loops of intestine decrease the potential space of the peritoneal cavity, and as a result of the close proximity of these loops to the anterior abdominal wall, intestinal perforation can occur more often than during routine laparoscopic cases. Perforation can also result from either mishandling of the bowel or merely touching a distended or ischemic loop with compromised integrity. As long as the pneumoperitoneum pressure is kept at a minimum, complications resulting from increased intraperitoneal pressures are rare. However, it should be kept in mind that ischemic bowel, by definition, has a tenuous blood supply, and therefore overinflation

TABLE 62.1. Relative Contraindications for laparoscopy for intestinal disorders.

Dense adhesions
Inadequate or poorly functioning equipment
Prior abdominal surgery
Obesity

can decrease both venous and arterial blood flow to these segments. There are several relative contraindications for laparoscopic intervention in patients with ischemic bowel or bowel obstruction (Table 62.1).

Conclusion

Laparoscopic intervention is safe and effective for addressing patients with both small bowel ischemia and obstruction. However, patients should be carefully selected for these procedures. The laparoscopic evaluation of intraperitoneal contents is ultimately only as good as the equipment that is being used and the surgical experience of the person who is viewing the image. Laparoscopy is an effective tool for surgeons to keep in their surgical armamentarium when they are presented with the frequent, yet often confusing, clinical scenario of either bowel obstruction, mesenteric ischemia, or a combination of both.

References

1. Khaitan L, Chekan E, Brennan E, Eubanks W. Diagnostic laparoscopy outside of the operating room. Semin Laparosc Surg 1999;6:32–40.
2. Iberti T, Salky B, Onofrey D. Use of bedside laparoscopy to identify intestinal ischemia in postoperative cases of aortic reconstruction. Surgery 1989;105:686–689.
3. Boley S, Lawrence J, Sammartano R. History of mesenteric ischemia. Surg Clin N Am 1997;77:275–288.
4. Councilman W. Three cases of occlusion of the superior mesenteric artery. Boston Med Surg J 1894;130:410.
5. Serryn R, Schoofs P, Beatens P, Vanderkerkhove D. Laparoscopic diagnosis of mesenteric vein thrombosis. Endoscopy 1986;18:249–250.
6. Matern UP, Haberstroh JP, el Saman AP, Pauly EP, Salm RP, Farthmann EHP. Emergency laparoscopy. Technical support for the laparoscopic diagnosis of intestinal ischemia. Surg Endosc 1996;10:883–887.
7. Slutzki S, Hapern Z, Negri M, Kais H, Halevy A. The laparoscopic second look for ischemic bowel disease. Surg Endosc 1996;10:729–731.
8. Sackier J. "Second Look" laparoscopy in the management of acute mesenteric ischemia. Br J Surg 1994;81:1546.
9. Waclawiczek H, Holzinger J. Bedside laparoscopy instead of second-look operation bowel resection in scope of mesenteric infarction. Surg Endos 1996;10.

10. MacSweeny S, Postelthwaite J. "Second look" laparoscopy in the management of acute mesenteric ischemia. Br J Surg 1994;81:90.

11. Regan F, Karlstad R, Magnunson T. Minimally invasive management of acute superior mesenteric artery occlusion: combined urokinase and laparoscopic therapy. Am J Gastroenterol 1996;91:1019–1021.

12. Mucha P. Small bowel obstruction. Surg Clin N Am 1987; 67:597–620.

13. Jones RS. Intestinal obstruction. In: Sabiston D (ed) Textbook of Surgery: The Biologic Basis of Modern Surgical Practice. Philadelphia: Saunders, 1997:915–923.

63
Diagnostic Laparoscopy for Malignancy

Rebekah R. White and Douglas S. Tyler

As surgeons have become familiar with laparoscopic techniques for benign disease, the potential value of laparoscopy in the management of malignant disease has been increasingly recognized. Numerous studies have demonstrated the advantages of laparoscopic over open cholecystectomy in terms of length of hospital stay and recovery. The general acceptance of such benefits over laparotomy has resulted in the application of laparoscopic techniques to many other procedures, benign and malignant. Concerns over the adequacy of minimally invasive techniques for cancer operations initially limited their general practice to staging exploration before attempted resection of various malignancies. In the 1970s, several series demonstrated the ability of laparoscopy of diagnose occult metastases and to spare laparotomy.[1-3]

Meanwhile, fears of jeopardizing oncologic surgical principles with the laparoscopic approach have abated. Successful treatments of malignant colon,[4] stomach,[5] adrenal,[6] and pancreatic endocrine tumors[7] have all been described. Although associated with steeper learning curves than comparable open procedures, laparoscopic cancer resections—when performed by experienced surgeons—can provide adequate surgical margins and lymph node dissection with minimal tumor handling. Much attention has been paid to port site recurrence following laparoscopic colectomy, which has been reported to have an incidence as high as 1.6%.[8] This uncommon phenomenon has been attributed to spillage of tumor cells in the growth-conducive environment of CO_2 pneumoperitoneum[9] and may be minimized through avoidance of unnecessary manipulation of the tumor as well as improved specimen handling. Indeed, a more recent series reported the incidence of port site recurrence to be 0.8%[10]; in comparison, wound recurrence following open colectomy occurs in 0.6% of cases.[11] Animal studies have suggested that the preserved immune function after the less invasive laparoscopic approach may actually result in decreased propensity for tumors to spread.[12]

The increasing availability of preoperative therapies for certain localized tumors has made accurate diagnosis and staging more important than ever. The presence of metastatic disease is a contraindication for aggressive therapy in most patients. Computed tomography (CT) is the primary modality for staging of most gastrointestinal (GI) malignancies. Although continuously improving, CT cannot routinely detect liver lesions smaller than 0.5 cm and is notoriously insensitive for peritoneal disease. For certain tumors, angiography, endoscopic ultrasound (EUS), magnetic resonance imaging (MRI), and positron emission tomography (PET) may be valuable in combination with CT but, as individual imaging studies, remain inferior to CT scanning alone.

Laparoscopic staging may offer the opportunity to visualize small-volume metastatic deposits, detect cytological peritoneal spread, and, together with adjuncts such as laparoscopic ultrasound, accurately determine tumor resectability. Biopsies may safely be performed of indeterminate liver lesions, suspicious lymph nodes, and, in some situations, the primary tumor. When neoadjuvant therapy is intended, laparoscopic exploration may further allow for placement of enteral feeding access or performance of fertility-sparing procedures. In the event that metastatic disease is encountered, laparoscopic palliative procedures can potentially be performed.

Staging laparoscopy alone can be performed with very low morbidity, often with same-day discharge. At our institution, pneumoperitoneum is established using an open technique, and a 30° angled laparoscope is introduced. Two 5-mm trocars are placed in the right upper quadrant (Fig. 63.1); these may be exchanged for 10-mm trocars if a feeding jejunostomy or gastrojejunostomy is subsequently performed. A systematic, 360° inspection of the abdomen is performed, beginning with the liver and including the peritoneum, omentum, and entire bowel mesentery. A more extensive examination can be performed by entering the lesser sac by incising the gastrohepatic omentum. Biopsies are obtained of any

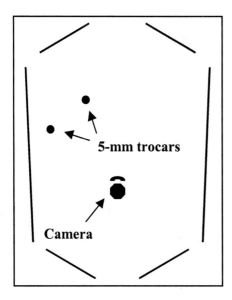

FIGURE 63.1. Placement of ports for laparoscopic staging.

suspicious lesions and sent for pathological examination. Biopsy of the primary tumor is generally avoided because of the theoretical risk of intraperitoneal dissemination. If no visible evidence of metastasis is present, 1 to 2 liters of saline are instilled, then collected for peritoneal cytology. Complications related to trocar placement and pneumoperitoneum are possible, as with any laparoscopic procedure, but the collective mortality for series in the literature approaches zero. Furthermore, although laparoscopy is usually done under general anesthesia, at least one center has reported successful performance of (one trocar) staging laparoscopy under local anesthesia.[13]

Laparoscopy in malignant disease has thus expanded from a laparotomy-sparing procedure for patients with advanced disease to a sensitive staging tool for patients with potentially curable disease. Like any staging modality, laparoscopic staging is most appropriately utilized when its outcome will affect management. The decision thus is affected by institutional factors such as the availability of neoadjuvant therapies and the quality of radiographic imaging. The need for operative palliation as well as the comfort level of the individual surgeon with laparoscopic palliative procedures may also enter into this equation. The potential roles of laparoscopic staging in the management of specific malignancies are discussed in the sections that follow.

Pancreatic Cancer

The potential value of laparoscopic staging is perhaps most appreciated for pancreatic cancer. More than 30% of patients with pancreatic cancer present with metastatic disease. Only 10% to 15% of patients with pancreatic cancer have tumors that are amenable to curative resection at the time of diagnosis. The remaining patients (approximately 50%) are considered unresectable because of local tumor invasion. Thus, despite improvement in the morbidity and mortality of pancreatic resection, the overall long-term survival for patients with pancreatic cancer remains less than 5%.[14] The appeal of avoiding unnecessary laparotomy, which is associated with increased morbidity and mortality and with decreased quality of life,[15,16] in patients with incurable disease is obvious.

Still, many patients are found to be unresectable on exploration following preoperative staging with state-of-the-art imaging modalities. Dynamic, contrast-enhanced CT is the most widely utilized technique, and numerous studies over the years have tracked its accuracy. In 1990, Warshaw et al. published a series in which CT predicted unresectablity with greater than 90% accuracy but correctly predicted resectability in only 45%.[17] CT failed to identify small liver metastases in 26% of patients and vascular invasion in 26%. In several subsequent studies, CT has predicted resectability with 57% to 88% accuracy.[18–21] Despite improvements in the technology, CT remains limited in its ability to detect and characterize small metastatic foci and in its sensitivity for vascular invasion. When performed in patients with resectable disease by CT, angiography improved the ability to predict resectability from 60% to 77% but was associated with a false-positive rate of 14%.[22] Endoscopic ultrasound marginally improved the ability to predict resectability but also has a tendency to overstage tumors, particularly those of large size.[23] MRI has not been shown to offer any additional staging information over CT.[17] PET has yet to find a role in the routine staging of pancreatic cancer.[24] In summary, angiography is used selectively at most centers, and endoscopic ultrasound has established a role mainly in the diagnosis of small pancreatic tumors.

Laparoscopic staging has been pursued as a means to visualize small-volume metastatic disease below the resolution of CT. Several series have addressed the value of laparoscopic staging in patients with radiographically localized disease before laparotomy for attempted resection. In two of the largest and most recent series, Fernandez-del Castillo et al.[25] and Conlon et al.[21] identified distant metastases in 24% and 19% of laparoscopically staged patients, respectively. These rates are somewhat lower than those of earlier series, perhaps because of interval improvements in CT resolution versus changes in the patient population. Subsequent resectability rates for patients with no evidence of unresectability by laparoscopy range from 37% to 91% (Table 63.1). In most of these series, laparoscopy was performed for the purposes of excluding extrapancreatic spread of disease. In two of these studies, negative laparoscopy was followed by laparoscopic ultrasound[26] or angiography[25] to evaluate for evidence of local tumor invasion, improving the actual resectability rate to 79% and 75%, respectively. The patients in the Duke series predominately showed locally advanced tumors on preoperative imaging studies with not unexpectedly higher rates of unresectability both on laparoscopy and on subsequent laparotomy.[27] In contrast, Conlon et al. at Memorial Sloan-Kettering (MSK) utilized a more extensive laparoscopic evaluation, including inspection of the lesser sac, which yielded an additional 9% of patients with vascular invasion as the sole reason for unresectability. The subsequent resectability rate in this series, which included some benign and malignant periampullary tumors other than pancreatic adenocarinoma, was 91%.

Standard laparoscopy lacks the tactile sensation and three-dimensional quality of open exploration. Laparoscopic ultrasound (LUS) has been proposed as an adjunct to standard laparoscopy to improve its capability to determine locoregional invasion, particularly retropancreatic vascular involvement. Early experience suggested that additional information could be obtained with LUS over laparoscopy alone.[28,29] John et al.[26] demonstrated that LUS had a positive predictive value for resectability of 79% as compared to 46% for standard laparoscopy. These results have been corroborated by subsequent series[30,31] as well as by a recent update of John et al.'s experience.[32] In the lattermost study, LUS was prospectively compared to transabdominal US, CT, and angiography; LUS was most reliable for determining overall resectability, with a positive predictive value of 68% and a negative predictive value of 97%. In all these series, the additional value of LUS over laparoscopy alone was greatest for assessment of local resectability although LUS detected intraparenchymal liver metastases missed by laparoscopy alone in up to 9% of patients.[30] In the MSK experience, LUS was most useful for the 14% of patients with "equivocal" findings, such as possible vascular or nodal involvement; LUS merely confirmed the findings of their standard "extended" laparoscopy in patients thought to be resectable or unresectable.[31] These studies, taken together, suggest that LUS may prove valuable in at least selected cases.

Another adjunct to laparoscopy worthy of mention is peritoneal lavage for cytology. The peritoneum is the second most common site of extranodal disease, following the liver. Laparoscopy alone can detect the almost 20% of patients with gross intra-abdominal spread. However, in the Massachusetts General Hospital experience, peritoneal cytology will be positive in another 8% of patients without other evidence of spread.[33] These patients have an outcome that is not significantly better than patients with visible metastases. Peritoneal lavage for cytology is a simple, inexpensive study that may be performed at the time of laparoscopy. As the results generally require more than a day for specimen preparation and pathological review, peritoneal lavage is optimally performed in situations in which the patient is not intended for immediate laparotomy.

A second domain of laparoscopic staging is in the screening of patients with radiographically localized disease for preoperative (neoadjuvant) therapy. It is generally accepted that complete surgical resection is necessary for long-term survival. In fact, patients with positive margins demonstrate survivals similar to those treated with chemoradiation alone.[34] High rates of positive margins, nodal metastases, and local recurrence underscore the locally aggressive nature of this disease.[35] Postoperative (adjuvant) chemoradiation following resection has been shown to increase survival from 11 to 12 months over resection alone and is considered standard of care at most centers.[36]

However, as many as 25% of patients do not receive intended postoperative therapy due to complications or prolonged recovery.[37] Therefore, in addition to the theoretical benefit of tumor downstaging, the advantages of preoperative (neoadjuvant) therapy include the assurance that chemoradiation will be received by all patients and at a time when oxygen delivery to the tumor is the greatest.

Series from several centers including our own have demonstrated that neoadjuvant therapy is feasible and is not associated with increased morbidity or mortality.[37-39] Although radiographic responses are modest compared to those for rectal and esophageal cancers, significant his-

TABLE 63.1. Results of staging laparoscopy for pancreatic cancer.

Author	Number of patients	Percent unresectable at laparoscopy	Percent resectable after negative laparoscopy	Percent unresectable after negative laparoscopy	
				Local	Distant
Warshaw et al. (1990)[17]	40	35	42	46	12
John et al. (1995)[26]	40	35	46	46	11
Fernandez-Del Castillo et al. (1995)[25]	114	24	37	61	2
Conlon et al. (1996)[21]	115	36	91	1.5	7.5
Holzman et al. (1997)[27]	28	54	38	54	8

tological responses have been seen. Complete pathological responses occur only rarely, but neoadjuvant therapy has been associated with lower rates of local recurrence and, in our experience, lower rates of positive margins and nodes (unpublished observations). Furthermore, commonly used neoadjuvant regimens—5-fluorouracil-(5-FU-) based chemotherapy combined with EBRT—are standard palliative regimens for unresectable patients that have been shown to increase survival in this group from 6 to 10 months over chemotherapy alone.[40] Combined chemotherapy and EBRT are not, however, standard therapy for patients with metastatic disease.

Proponents of neoadjuvant therapy, therefore, utilize staging laparoscopy not only to prevent patients with occult metastatic disease from undergoing unnecessary laparotomy but also to avoid the time, cost, and morbidity of unnecessarily aggressive chemoradiation. Many surgeons also routinely or selectively place feeding jejunostomy tubes at the time of laparoscopy in patients considered candidates for neoadjuvant therapy. Few studies have specifically examined the role of laparoscopy in the selection of patients for neoadjuvant therapy. The sensitivity of CT scanning for small-volume metastatic disease remains the critical factor for determining the value of laparoscopy. In our experience, more than 20% of patients with radiographically localized disease are determined to have gross or microscopic disease (liver 14%, peritoneal 5%, peritoneal cytology 5%) on laparoscopy that disqualifies them from receiving preoperative chemoradiation. This number, as would be expected, is comparable to those published for series in which laparoscopic staging was performed before laparotomy for attempted resection. LUS is not employed at our institution, as all patients with localized tumors are considered for neoadjuvant therapy, regardless of local resectability. Patients without evidence of metastatic disease on laparoscopy undergo Hickman catheter and feeding jejunostomy tube placement as well as peritoneal lavage for cytology in the same setting. Patients with localized disease following laparaoscopy receive preoperative chemoradiation, after which they are restaged by CT. Although the routine placement of enteral feeding access has not significantly influenced the subsequent morbidity or mortality of resection, the selective placement in nutritionally challenged patients may improve tolerance of neoadjuvant therapy.

Regardless of whether surgeons adopt preoperative or postoperative chemoradiation, most advocate staging laparoscopy before formal laparotomy. The laparotomy-sparing benefit of laparoscopic staging is diminished, however, if a patient requires subsequent laparotomy for palliation. Historically, staging was performed at the time of laparotomy. If the patient was found to be unresectable, prophylactic biliary and gastric bypass was performed. This practice was supported by reported incidences of biliary and gastroduodenal obstruction as high as 70% and 25% in patients with unresected pancreatic cancer.[41] With advanced laparoscopic techniques, laparoscopic gastrojejunostomy can be performed if necessary. In addition, although laparoscopic cholecystojejunostomy can be performed, endoscopic stenting can provide excellent biliary palliation with lower early morbidity, as has been shown in several randomized trials in the 1980s.[42–45] Metallic expandable stents can now offer longer patency[46] than their small, plastic, but easily removable predecessors. In addition, successful endoscopic palliation of malignant duodenal obstruction has been reported by several institutions.[47] Espat et al. reported a series of 155 patients with laparoscopically staged unresectable disease who did not undergo prophylactic surgical bypass.[48] Many of these patients underwent endoscopic biliary decompression, but only 2% of patients required subsequent laparotomy for palliation. The median survival of these patients was approximately 6 months; none received chemoradiation. Whether newer therapies will increase the demand for surgical palliation by increasing survival or decrease the demand by improving local tumor control is unclear.

Gastric Cancer

As is pancreatic cancer, gastric cancer in the United States is often advanced on presentation. At least 25% of patients have metastatic disease at the time of diagnosis, and more than 60% are stage III or IV.[49] Overall 5-year survival is only 14%, compared to 45% in Japan. Resection is necessary for long-term survival, and local recurrence is common, even after complete resection. Unlike pancreatic cancer, however, the treatment of gastric cancer has traditionally included surgical resection, even for patients with metastatic disease. Preoperative staging for the patient diagnosed with gastric cancer may have included at most a CT scan, followed by laparotomy for complete staging and subtotal or total gastrectomy.

However, the availability of multimodality therapies as well as laparoscopic approaches to palliation and even resection of gastric cancer have increased the importance of accurate preoperative staging. Although the best radiologic modality for hepatic metastases, CT scanning has serious limitations for tumor (T) and nodal (N) staging. CT understages a large percentage of primary tumors while overstaging others; CT is neither sensitive nor specific for nodal disease.[50] Endoscopic ultrasound has, therefore, emerged as the imaging study of choice for locoregional staging. EUS has an 86% concordance with pathologic T stage and is highly predictive of local recurrence, less than 20% for T1 or T2 and greater than 75% for T3 or T4 disease.[51] Although better than CT, the accuracy of EUS for nodal staging ranges from only 60% to

80%.[50,51] While the ability of current generation CT to detect hepatic lesions continues to improve, the accurate identification of small-volume metastatic disease and—important for gastric cancer—distant (N2) nodal disease remains elusive.

Although not as extensively studied as for pancreatic cancer, the ability of laparoscopy to identify occult metastatic disease not detected by high-quality CT scanning has been examined in a number of recent series (Table 63.2). Laparoscopic staging is most valuable for metastatic disease (M stage), which was identified in 24% to 37% of patients with radiographically localized disease (Table 63.2). The prevalence of liver metastases in these series is quite variable, in part because of the inclusion of patients with metastases on CT in one series[52] and to the restricted use of CT in another.[53] The sensitivity of laparoscopy in general is higher for peritoneal (69%–94%) than for hepatic metastases (33%–100%), although the prevalence of the liver as the sole site of metastasis is low compared to pancreatic cancer. The identification of nodal metastases by laparoscopic appearance alone was not very sensitive,[50,52] although nodal disease is not an absolute contraindication to resection at some centers. When therapeutically relevant, nodal stage sensitivity may be improved with laparoscopic lymph node sampling.[53]

Following from the success of EUS in predicting local recurrence and from experience with pancretic and hepatobiliary tumors, laparoscopic ultrasound has been proposed to further improve the detection of hepatic and nodal disease.[54] LUS may eventually even approach or surpass the accuracy of EUS for T staging. Published experience with LUS in gastric cancer is limited, but early series in the literature suggest that LUS provides excellent imaging of the primary tumor.[55,56]

More than 80% of patients without evidence of metastatic disease by laparoscopy proceeded to resection in these series. At least one-third were spared laparotomy. Futhermore, for all patients in these series with laparoscopically staged metastatic disease who did not undergo palliative resection, fewer than 1% required subsequent laparotomy for palliation. The majority of these patients can be adequately palliated through advances in nonsurgical therapies such as radiation, chemotherapy, enteral nutrition, and endoscopic laser and stenting. These patients, whose mean life expectancy is approximately 6 months, benefit from the avoidance of gastrectomy with significantly decreased length of hospital stay.[57]

Laparoscopic staging is thus recommended for patients in whom the presence of metastatic disease will affect either the surgical approach or the patient's candidacy for preoperative multimodality therapy. Where it is routinely used, EUS may occupy a key role in this algorithm. For patients with small tumors by EUS, the risk of metastasis is sufficiently low that the yield of laparoscopy is probably not high enough to warrant its routine use. Thus, for the majority of surgeons who perform open gastric resection, patients who are T1 or T2N0 by EUS may proceed directly to laparotomy. However, at centers where laparoscopic gastrectomy is practiced, patients with small tumors by EUS may be appropriate for laparoscopic exploration followed by resection. Although a number of groups have published experience with this procedure,[5,58] laparoscopic resection is less common than for other abdominal malignancies, perhaps due to the steep learning curve and low volume of cases.

Laparoscopic staging may have more widespread value for patients with large tumors. For the asymptomatic patient with locally advanced disease, the identification of metastatic disease may allow the patient to avoid laparotomy altogether. The symptomatic patient with metastatic disease may be a candidate for laparoscopic palliation, such as gastrojejunostomy of partial gastrectomy. Locally advanced patients without metastatic disease may be offered preoperative (neoadjuvant) chemotherapy with one of several multidrug regimens at many centers. Response rates of up to 70% have been demonstrated, leading to complete resectability in almost 50% of patients with previously unresectable tumors.[59] It is for this group that accurate staging is perhaps most important, as patients with occult metastatic disease may be subjected to the side effects of these often toxic chemotherapy regimens. Significant overstaging or understaging of patients within the context of experimental protocols will also falsely affect our assessment of treatment results.

The role of laparoscopy in the management of tumors of the esophagus and gastroesophageal (GE) junction

TABLE 63.2. Results of staging laparoscopy for gastric cancer.

Author	Number of patients	Prevalence of metastases detected by laparoscopy (%)			Prevalence of metastases missed by laparoscopy (%)		
		Liver	Peritoneum	Nodal	Liver	Peritoneum	Nodal
Lowy (1995)[**]	71	1	23	NS	3	1	NS
Stell et al. (1996)[52]	103	25	9	25	1	4	22
Burke et al. (1997)[57]	111	3	25	1	0	3	3
Asencio et al. (1997)[53]	76	16	21	39	0	3	24

deserves mention. Advances in nonsurgical palliation, such as endoscopic stenting, radiation, and photodynamic therapy, have diminished the need for palliative resection. In three recent series, laparoscopy detected distant metastases in fewer than 10% of patients with adenocarcinoma of the esophagus or GE junction and in no patients with squamous carcinoma of the esophagus.[56–61] The addition of laparoscopic ultrasound in two of these series improved sensitivity to between 70% and 90%, particularly improving the detection of celiac lymphoadenopathy.[56,60] The yield for occult metastases is still low compared to that for the other malignancies discussed in this chapter. For patients who are candidates for neoadjuvant therapies, however, staging laparoscopy may identify those patients with unsuspected metastases as well as provide an opportunity for obtaining enteral feeding access before multimodality therapy.

Colorectal Cancer

As the majority of patients with colorectal cancer will require resection for either cure or palliation, complete staging can generally be performed at the time of resection. For patients undergoing laparotomy, this is accomplished with nearly 100% sensitivity through direct visualization, palpation, and biopsy of suspicious lesions. Rectal cancer patients who are candidates for local procedures are reliant on nonoperative staging, utilizing EUS for regional nodal disease and CT for distant metastasis. The limitations of CT scanning for detecting liver metastases are generalizable. Therefore, staging laparoscopy will theoretically yield a significant percentage of patients with metastases not detected by CT. However, unless the patient is a candidate for neoadjuvant therapy of a locally advanced tumor, the presence of metastases is not going to affect the operative approach. The role of laparoscopy in the staging of patients with rectal cancer for neoadjuvant therapy has not been extensively studied. A recent paper from MSK reported a series of 14 patients with near-obstructing rectal cancer who underwent staging laparoscopy.[62] Four patients (29%) had unsuspected peritoneal metastases and were managed without further surgery. The remaining 10 patients underwent laparoscopic diversion followed by chemoradiation and subsequent resection. This small series illustrates the potential value of this strategy for patients with locally advanced tumors.

Laparoscopic colon resection, on the other hand, has received much attention in the literature. Concerns about port site recurrence and long operative times initially hindered its acceptance. A rapidly growing number of studies have suggested that laparoscopic resection is technically feasible, oncologically adequate, and associated with shorter hospitalization, quicker recovery, and less pain. A prospective, randomized trial is currently in progress to definitively prove these benefits.[63] A potential pitfall of laparoscopic resection is the loss of sensitivity for liver and nodal metastasis afforded by laparotomy. Laparoscopic ultrasound has been proposed as an adjunct to laparoscopic resection and was shown to have a sensitivity of 100% for liver and 94% for nodal metastases, compared to 75% and 6%, respectively, for laparoscopy alone.[64]

Perhaps the most obvious role for laparoscopic staging in the management of colorectal cancer is its role in the assessment of liver metastases. It is clear that the complete resection of colorectal metastases to liver confers a survival benefit and even long-term survival in a minority of patients.[65] The consensus on what is "resectable" has evolved from small, single-lobe lesions to essentially any technically feasible resection(s) that leave an adequate hepatic remnant. Nevertheless, as many as 40% selected for surgery are found unresectable at laparotomy. The goals of preoperative staging are, therefore, very similar to those for primary hepatic malignancies, and most studies of LUS for liver tumors have included both primary and metastatic lesions.[66–69] A key difference is that, for metastatic lesions, as many as two-thirds of patients are found to be unresectable because of extrahepatic disease such as local recurrence, nodal metastases, or peritoneal implants, whereas only one-third are due to underestimated intrahepatic extent.[70] Laparoscopy allows for identification of extrahepatic disease, while LUS examines the liver for evidence of technical unresectability, as discussed next for primary liver tumors. When specifically studied in 47 patients under evaluation for resection of colorectal metastases, laparoscopy alone identified 13% as unresectable, with half due to multifocality and half due to peritoneal metastasis; LUS identified another 25% as unresectable for reasons of multifocality, location precluding resection, and misdiagnosis.[71] Of the patients who subsequently underwent laparotomy, 79% underwent resection, whereas 75% of patients with unresectable disease were spared laparotomy. LUS may thus be as valuable for metastatic liver tumors as for primary tumors.

Hepatobiliary Cancer

As for pancreatic, gastric, and colon cancer, surgery is still the mainstay of therapy for primary malignancies of the liver and biliary tree. For hepatocellular carcinoma (HCC), the most common primary malignancy, only 20% are resectable at the time of diagnosis, and local recurrence develops in approximately one-half of patients after curative resection.[72] HCC is locally aggressive with frequent vascular invasion and formation of satellite lesions. Even if technically feasible, hepatectomy often leaves the cirrhotic patient with insufficient hepatic reserve. Intrahepatic cholangiocarcinoma, the second most common primary liver malignancy, is also characterized by extensive local disease and regional lymph node involvement at presentation. Gallbladder cancer is rarely diagnosed preoperatively but is usually an incidental finding at laparotomy or on pathological examination following cholecystectomy. The early onset of biliary obstruction associated with hilar and distal cholangiocarcinoma often allows more timely diagnosis and greater resectability. Distal cholangiocarcinoma is more similar to, although less aggressive than, pancreatic adenocarcinoma in its propensity for vascular and nodal involvement. Therefore, this discussion focuses on the staging of primary hepatic and proximal biliary malignancies, for which imaging of hepatic anatomy is crucial.

Unlike the other GI malignancies discussed, surgery is rarely necessary for palliation of liver tumors, either primary or metastatic. Nonresectional therapies, such as percutaneous ethanol injection (PEI) and transcatheter arterial chemoembolization (TACE) achieve satisfactory local recurrence rates, which, for small tumors, are not significantly different than those for resection.[73] Cryotherapy, frequently utilized for metastatic liver tumors, has been shown in at least one series to have benefit for HCC as well.[74] Effective and less invasive palliation is available for many patients with unresectable disease. Therefore, laparotomy to confirm unresectability often entails unnecessary expense and morbidity without additional benefit.

Despite the increasing quantity and quality of radiologic imaging modalities, many surgical explorations encouter unresectable tumors due to unsuspected spread or multifocality. CT and US remain the primary imaging modalities.[75] Intravenous contrast improves the sensitivity of CT, and numerous enhancement techniques exist, such as dual-phase imaging, delayed scanning, and arterial portography. Arterial portography (CTAP) has been shown to be more than 90% sensitive for the detection of metastatic liver lesions.[75] Spiral CT is less invasive and allows for dual-phase imaging but is less sensitive.[76] In addition to the limitations of resolution inherent to CT, the cirrhotic liver is prone to pseudolesions as a result of laminar flow perfusion defects and focal fatty deposits, resulting in a high false-positive rate.[77] US provides useful vascular information such as anatomy, flow, and patency but is highly operator dependent and generally less sensitive than CT. MRI may help in the differentiation of hemangiomata and in the detection of lesions less than 1 cm, but its role is not yet well defined.[78] None of these imaging studies is sensitive for the detection of nodal and small-volume peritoneal disease.

The exact number and size of lesions as well as their relationships to vascular and biliary structures are crucial for deciding whether and how much to resect. Although preoperative imaging may identify some patients as unresectable, laparotomy with intraoperative ultrasound (IOUS) has become the gold standard for the determination of resectability. Concomitant cirrhosis can be determined by inspection. Suspicious nodal and peritoneal lesions can be confirmed by biopsy. Direct contact with the liver surface allows visualization of lesions as small as 3 to 5 mm.[79] Doppler imaging can localize vascular structures and identify tumor thrombi. With sensitivity as high as 98%,[80] IOUS accurately delineates anatomy and yields information that results in a change in the operative procedure in almost 50% of patients.

Laparoscopy may obviate the need for laparotomy in some patients through more accurate diagnosis and staging. The preoperative diagnosis of liver tumors is not always certain preoperatively; laparoscopy may yield extrahepatic primary sites in as many as one-third of patients thought to have primary liver tumors.[67] Although the incidence of extrahepatic dissemination is lower for primary than for metastatic liver tumors, diagnostic laparoscopy can identify the small percentage of patients with unsuspected peritoneal metastases. Laparoscopy alone can also detect evidence of unresectability, such as unsuspected cirrhosis or bilobar disease, that precludes further examination or laparotomy, in almost 10% of patients.[81]

The introduction of ultrasound to diagnostic laparoscopy in the early 1980s was, therefore, an ideal combination for the staging of liver tumors. Studies early in the past decade validated the idea that LUS, when performed in patients with potentially resectable liver lesions by a variety of imaging modalities, may spare a significant number of patients laparotomy.[28,82] As already mentioned, most recent studies of LUS for liver tumors have included both primary and metastatic tumors; one of these series also included several benign lesions[67] (Table 63.3). In the only series specifically examining HCC,[81] laparotomy was avoided because of definite, evidence of unresectability in 16% of patients undergoing laparoscopic ultrasound (LUS); 88% of patients who underwent laparotomy following LUS were resected compared to 68% of a nonrandomized control group. LUS was less accurate for tumors greater than 10 cm and

TABLE 63.3. Results of laparoscopic ultresound (LUS) for liver tumors.

Author	No. of patients	Percent avoiding laparotomy	Percent resected at laparotomy
Babineau et al. (1994)[66]	19	48	73
John et al. (1994)[67]	50	72	93
Barbot et al. (1997)[68]	23	30	93
Lo et al. (1998)[81]	91	16	88
Jarnagin et al. (2000)[69]	104	16	75

was least sensitive, in general, for tumor thrombi and invasion of adjacent organs.

Although the sensitivity of LUS compared favorably to open contact US in an in vitro model of hepatic lesions,[83] laparotomy with IOUS remains the gold standard. Technical refinements in laparoscopic ultrasound transducers may gradually overcome the differences in sensitivity. Meanwhile, for patients with radiographically resectable tumors, the ability to avoid laparotomy in 15% to 20% of patients following LUS warrants consideration of this strategy.

Conclusion

Laparoscopy is a useful tool for both staging and treatment of many GI malignancies. It is cost-effective and widely available. As technical advances continue, laparoscopic procedures both for staging and treatment should take on an even greater role in the management of these malignancies.

References

1. Sugarbaker P, Wilson R. Using celioscopy to determine stages of intra-abdominal malignant neoplasms. Arch Surg 1976;111:41–44.
2. Bleiburg H, Rozencweig M, Mathieu M, et al. The use of peritoneoscopy in the detection of liver metastases. Cancer 1978;41:863–867.
3. Cuschieri A, Hall A, Clark J. The value of laparoscopy in the diagnosis and management of pancreatic carcinoma. Gut 1978;19:672–677.
4. Phillips E, Frankin M, Carroll B, et al. Laparoscopic colectomy. Ann Surg 1992;216:702–707.
5. Ballesta-Lopez C, Bastida-Vila X, Catarci M, et al. Laparoscopic Billroth II distal subtotal gastrectomy with gastric stump suspension for gastric malignancies. Am J Surg 1996; 171:289–292.
6. Ono Y, Katoh N, Kinukawa T, et al. Laparoscopic nephrectomy, and adrenalectomy: Nagoya experience. J Urol 1994; 152:1962–1966.
7. Sussman L, Christie R, Whittle D. Laparoscopic excision of distal pancreas including insulinoma. Aus N Z J Surg 1996; 66:414–416.
8. Sugarbaker P, Corlew S. Influence of surgical techniques on survival in patients with colon cancer: a review. Dis Colon Rectum 1982;25:545–557.
9. Jones D, Li-Wu G, Reinhard M, et al. Impact of pneumoperitoneum on trocar site implantation of colon cancer in hamster model. Dis Colon Rectum 1995;38:1182–1188.
10. Hoffman G, Baker J, Doxey J, et al. Minimally invasive surgery for colorectal cancer: initial follow-up. Ann Surg 1996;223:790–798.
11. Reilly W, Nelson H, Schroeder G, et al. Wound recurrence following conventional treatment of colorectal cancer. A rare but perhaps underestimated problem. Dis Colon Rectum 1996;39:200–207.
12. Allendorf J, Bessler M, Kayton M, et al. Increased tumour establishment and growth after laparotomy versus laparoscopy in a murine model. Surg Endosc 1995;9:49–52.
13. Sand J, Marnela K, Airo I, Nordback I. Staging of abdominal cancer by local anesthesia outpatient laparoscopy. Hepato-Gastroenterology 1996;43:1685–1688.
14. Sener S, Fremgen A, Menck H, Winchester D. Pancreatic cancer: a report of treatment and survival trends for 100,313 patients diagnosed from 1985–1995, using the National Cancer Database. J Am Coll Surg 1999;189:1–7.
15. Watanapa P, Williamson R. Surgical palliation for pancreatic cancer: developments during the past two decades. Br J Surg 1992;79:8–20.
16. DeRooij P, Rogatko A, Brennan M. Evaluation of palliative surgical procedures in unresectable pancreatic cancer. Br J Surg 1991;78:1053–1058.
17. Warshaw A, Gu Z, Wittenberg J, Waltman A. Preoperative staging and assessment of resectability of pancreatic cancer. Arch Surg 1990;125:230–233.
18. Gulliver D, Baker M, Cheng C, et al. Malignant biliary obstruction: efficacy of thin-section dynamic CT in determing resectability. AJR Am J Roentgenol 1992;159:503–507.
19. Freeny P, Traverso L, Ryan J. Diagnosis and staging of pancreatic adenocarcinoma with dynamic computed tomography. Am J Surg 1993;165:600–606.
20. Fuhrman G, Charnsangavej C, Abbruzzese J, et al. Thin-section contrast-enhanced computed tomography accurately predicts the resectability of malignant pancreatic neoplasms. Am J Surg 1994;167:104–113.
21. Conlon K, Dougherty E, Klimstra D, et al. The value of minimal access surgery in the staging of patients with potentially resectable peripancreatic malignancy. Ann Surg 1996; 223:134–140.
22. Dooley W, Cameron J, Pitt H, et al. Is preoperative angiography useful in patients with periampullary tumors? Ann Surg 1990;211:649–655.
23. Howard T, Chin A, Streib E, et al. Value of helical computed tomography, angiography, and endoscopic ultrasound in determining resectability of periampullary carcinoma. Am J Surg 1997;174:237–241.
24. Keogan M, Tyler D, Clark L, et al. Diagnosis of pancreatic carcinoma: role of FDG PET. AJR Am J Roentgenol 1998;171:1565–1570.
25. Fernandez-del Castillo C, Rattner D, Warshaw A. Further experience with laparoscopy and peritoneal cytology in the staging of pancreatic cancer. Br J Surg 1995;82:1127–1129.
26. John T, Greig J, Carter D, Garden O. Carcinoma of the pancreatic head and periampullary region. Tumor staging with laparoscopy and laparoscopic ultrasonography. Ann Surg 1995;221:156–164.
27. Holzman M, Reintgen K, Tyler D, Pappas T. The role of laparoscopy in the management of suspected pancreatic and periampullary malignancies. J Gastrointest Surg 1997;1: 236–244.
28. Cuesta M, Meijer S, Borgstein P, et al. Laparoscopic ultrasonography for hepatobiliary and pancreatic malignancy. Br J Surg 1993;80:1571–1574.
29. Murugiah M, Paterson-Brown S, Windsor J, et al. Early experience of laparoscopic ultrasonography in the man-

agement of pancreatic carcinoma. Surg Endosc 1993;7:177–181.

30. Bemelman W, De Wit L, Van Delden O, et al. Diagnostic laparoscopy combined with laparoscopic utrasonography in staging of cancer of the pancreatic head region. Br J Surg 1995;82:820–824.

31. Minnard E, Conlon K, Hoos A, et al. Laparoscopic ultrasound enhaces standard laparoscopy in the staging of pancreatic cancer. Ann Surg 1998;228:182–187.

32. John T, Wright A, Allan P, et al. Laparoscopy with laparoscopic ultrasonography in the TNM staging of pancreatic carcinoma. World J Surg 1999;23:870–881.

33. Fernandez-del Castillo C, Warshaw A. Laparoscopic staging and peritoneal cytology. Surg Oncol Clin N Am 1998;7:135–142.

34. Lillemoe K, Cameron J, Yeo C, et al. Pancreaticoduodenectomy: does it have a role in the palliation of pancreatic cancer? Ann Surg 1996;223:718–728.

35. Willet C, Lewandrowski K, Warshaw A, et al. Resection margins in carcinoma of the head of the pancreas: implications for radiation therapy. Ann Surg 1993;217:144–148.

36. Group GTS. Further evidence of effective adjuvant combined radiation and chemotherapy following curative resection. Cancer 1980;59:2006–2010.

37. Spitz F, Abruzzese J, Lee J, et al. Preoperative and postoperative chemoradiation strategies in patients treated with pancreaticoduodenectomy for adenocarcinoma of the pancreas. J Clin Oncol 1997;15:928–937.

38. Yeung R, Weese J, Hoffman J, et al. Neoadjuvant chemoradiation in pancreatic and duodenal carcinoma: a phase II study. Cancer 1993;72:2124–2133.

39. White R, Lee C, Anscher M, et al. Preoperative chemoradiation for patients with locally advanced adenocarcinoma of the pancreas. Ann Surg Oncol 1998;6:38–45.

40. Moertel C, Frytak S, Hahn R, et al. Therapy of locally unresectable pancreatic carcinoma: a randomized comparison of high dose (6000 rads) radiation alone, moderate dose radiation (4000 rads) + 5-fluorouracil, and high-dose radiaion + 5-fluorouracil. The Gastrointestinal Tumor Study Group. Cancer 1981;48:1705–1710.

41. Sarr M, Cameron J. Surgical palliation of unresectable carcinoma of the pancreas. World J Surg 1984;8:906–918.

42. Bornman P, Harries-Jones E, Tobias R, et al. Prospective controlled trial of transhepatic biliary endoprosthesis versus biliary bypass surgery for incurable carcinoma of the head of the pancreas. Lancet 1986;1:69–71.

43. Shepherd H, Royle G, Ross A, et al. Endoscopic biliary endoprosthesis in the palliation of malignant obstruction of the distal common bile duct: A randomized trial. Br J Surg 1988;75:1166–1168.

44. Andersen J, Sorneson S, Kruse A, et al. Randomized trial of endoscopic endoprosthesis versus operative bypass in malignant obstructive jaundice. Gut 1989;30:1132–1135.

45. Smith A, Dowsett J, Russell R, et al. Randomised trial of endoscopic stenting versus surgical bypass in malignant low bileduct obstruction. Lancet 1994;344:1655–1660.

46. Adam A, Cherry N, Roddie M, et al. Self-expandable stainless steel endoprostheses: for treatment of malignant bile duct obstruction. AJR Am J Roentgenol 1991;156:321–325.

47. Keymling M, Wagner J, Vakil N, Knyrim K. Relief of malignant duodenal obstruction by percutaneous insertion of a metal stent. Am J Gastroenterol 1993;39:439–441.

48. Espat N, Brennan M, Conlon K. Patients with laparoscopically staged unresectable pancreatic adenocarcinoma do not require subsequent surgical biliary or gastric bypass. J Am Coll Surg 1999;188:649–657.

49. Wanebo H, Kennedy B, Chmiel J, et al. Cancer of the stomach: a patient case study by the American College of Surgeons. Ann Surg 1993;218:583–592.

50. Botet J, Lightdale C, Zauber A, et al. Preoperative staging of gastric cancer: comparison of endoscopic US and dynamic CT. Radiology 1991;181:419–425.

51. Smith J, Brennan M, Botet J, et al. Preoperative endoscopic ultrasound can predict the risk of recurrence after operation for gastric carcinoma. J Clin Oncol 1993;11:2380–2385.

52. Stell D, Carter C, Stewart I, Anderson J. Prospective comparison of laparoscopy, ultrasonography and computed tomography in the staging of gastric cancer. Br J Surg 1996;83:1260–1262.

53. Asencio F, Aguilo J, Salvador J, et al. Video-laparoscopic staging of gastric cancer. A prospective multicenter comparison with noninvasive techniques. Surg Endosc 1997;11(12):1153–1158.

54. Bartlett D, Conlon K, Gerdes H, Karpeh M. Laparoscopic ultrasonography: the best pretreatment staging modality in gastric adenocarcinoma? Case report. Surgery 1995;118:562–566.

55. Conlon K, Karpeh M. Laparoscopy and laparoscopic ultrasound in the staging of gastric cancer. Semin Oncol 1996;23:347–351.

56. Smith A, John T, Garden O, Brown S. Role of laparoscopic ultrasonography in the management of patients with oesophagogastric cancer. Br J Surg 1999;86(8):1083–1087.

57. Burke E, Karpeh M, Conlon K, Brennan M. Laparoscopy in the management of gastric adenocarcinoma. Ann Surg 1997;225(3):262–267.

58. Goh P, So J. Role of laparoscopy in the management of stomach cancer. Semin Surg Oncol 1999;16(4):321–326.

59. Wilke H, Preusser P, Fink U, et al. Preoperative chemotherapy in locally advanced and nonresectable gastric cancer: a phase II study with etoposide, doxorubicin, and cisplatin. J Clin Oncol 1989;7:1318–1326.

60. Romijn M, van Overhagen H, Spillenaar Bilgen E, et al. Laparoscopy and laparoscopic ultrasonography in staging of oesophageal and cardial carcinoma. Br J Surg 1998;85(7):1010–1012.

61. Bonavina L, Incarbone R, Lattuada E, et al. Preoperative laparoscopy in management of patients with carcinoma of the esophagus and of the esophagogastric junction. J Surg Oncol 1997;65:171–174.

62. Koea J, Guillem J, Conlon K, et al. Role of laparoscopy in the initial multimodality management of patients with near-obstructing rectal cancer. J Gastrointest Surg 2000;4:105–108.

63. Stocchi L, Nelson H. Laparoscopic colectomy for colon cancer: trial update. J Surg Oncol 1998;68:255–267.

64. Goletti O, Celona G, Galatioto C, et al. Is laparoscopic sonography a reliable and sensitive procedure for staging

colorectal cancer? A comparative study. Surg Endosc 1998; 12:1236–1241.

65. Scheele J, Stangl R, Altendorf-Hofmann A. Hepatic metasteses from colorectal carcinoma: impact of surgical resection on the natural history. Br J Surg 1990;77:1241–1246.

66. Babineau T, Lewis D, Jenkins R, et al. Role of staging laparoscopy in the treatment of hepatic malignancy. Am J Surg 1994;167:151–155.

67. John T, Greig J, Crosbie J, et al. Superior staging of liver tumors with laparoscopy and laparoscopic ultrasound. Ann Surg 1994;220:711–719.

68. Barbot D, Marks J, Feld F, et al. Improved staging of liver tumors using laparoscopic intraoperative ultrasound. J Surg Oncol 1997;64:63–67.

69. Jarnagin W, Bodniewicz J, Dougherty E, et al. A prospective analysis of staging laparoscopy in patients with primary and secondary hepatobiliary malignancies. J Gastrointest Surg 2000;4:34–43.

70. Sugarbaker P. Surgical decision making for large bowel cancer metastatic to the liver. Radiology 1990;174:621–626.

71. Rahusen F, Cuesta M, Borgstein P, et al. Selection of patients for resection of colorectal metastases to the liver using diagnostic laparoscopy and laparoscopic ultrasonography. Ann Surg 1999;230:31–37.

72. Fuster J, Garcia-Valdecasas J, Grande L, et al. Hepatocellular carcinoma and cirrhosis: results of surgical treatment in a European series. Ann Surg 1996;223:297–302.

73. Liu C, Fan S. Nonresectional therapies for hepatocellular carcinoma. Am J Surg 1997;173:358–365.

74. Zhou X, Yu Y, Tang Z, et al. An 18-year study of cryosurgery in the treatment of primary liver cancer. Asian J Surg 1992; 15:43–47.

75. Karl R, Morse S, Halpert R, Clark R. Preoperative evaluation of patients for liver resection: appropriate CT imaging. Ann Surg 1993;217:226–232.

76. Irie T, Takeshita K, Wada Y, et al. CT evaluation of hepatic tumors: comparison of CT with arterial portography, CT with infusion hepatic arteriography and simultaneous use of both techniques. AJR Am J Roentgenol 1995;164:1407–1412.

77. Moran B, O'Rourke N, Plant G, Rees M. Computed tomographic portography in preoperative imaging of hepatic neoplasms. Br J Surg 1995;82:669–671.

78. Kruskal J, Kane R. Imaging of primary and metastatic liver tumors. Surg Oncol Clin N Am 1996;5:231–260.

79. Bismuth H, Castaing D, Garden O. The use of operative ultrasound in surgery of primary liver tumors. World J Surg 1987;11:610–614.

80. Paul M, Sibingamulder L, Cuesta M, et al. Impact of intraoperative ultrasonography on treatment strategy for colorectal cancer. Br J Surg 1994;81:1660–1663.

81. Lo C, Lai E, Liu C, et al. Laparoscopy and laparoscopic ultrasonosgraphy avoid exploratory laparotomy in patients with hepaticellular carcinoma. Ann Surg 1998;227:527–532.

82. Miles W, Paterson-Brown S, Garden O. Laparoscopic contact hepatic ultrasonography. Br J Surg 1992;79:419–420.

83. Cozzi P, McCall J, Jorgensen J, Morris D. Laparoscopic vs. open ultrasound of the liver: an in vitro study. Hepatobiliary Pancreat Surg 1996;10:87–89.

Index